Vitamin D

Vitamin D

D. E. M. LAWSON
University of Cambridge and Medical Research Council MRC Nutrition Unit, Cambridge

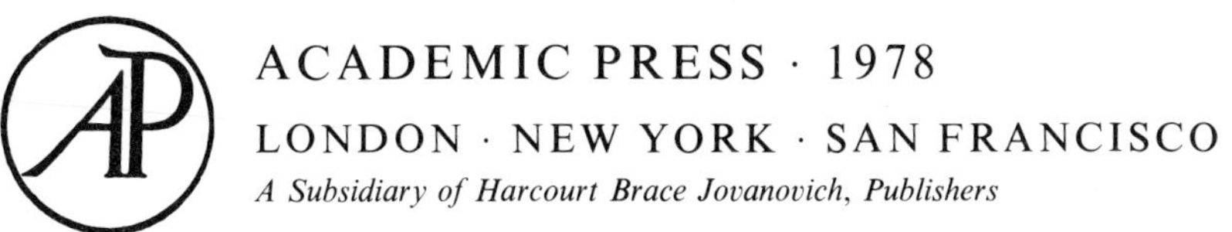

ACADEMIC PRESS · 1978
LONDON · NEW YORK · SAN FRANCISCO
A Subsidiary of Harcourt Brace Jovanovich, Publishers

ACADEMIC PRESS INC. (LONDON) LTD
24/28 Oval Road
London NW1

United States Edition published by
ACADEMIC PRESS INC.
111 Fifth Avenue
New York, New York 10003

Library of Congress Catalog Number: 77–77145
ISBN: 0–12–439850–2

Printed in Great Britain by William Clowes & Sons Limited
London, Beccles and Colchester

Preface

In the sixty years since the discovery of vitamin D our understanding of its biochemistry and physiology has occurred in phases. The first phase followed on the work of Mellanby in 1919 on the development of an animal model of rickets. From his demonstration of the curative power of certain foods the idea developed that rickets is a deficiency disease due to the lack of vitamin D. During this phase the vitamin was eventually isolated, its chemical structure established and the importance of ultraviolet light in its formation appreciated. In the thirty year period from 1935 progress in vitamin D research was intermittent, mainly involving delineation of the physiological actions of the vitamin.

The second phase of vitamin D research began in the late 1960s and has resulted in a complete change in attitude to the problems posed by this substance. It is now recognised that vitamin D is simply the precursor of a new steroid hormone, 1,25-dihydroxyvitamin D and that it is this substance which controls the translocation of calcium through the cells of intestine, bone and kidney. Vitamin D itself is only an essential metabolite with the unique property of being formed by ultraviolet light rather than by an enzyme. The trophic hormone for 1,25-dihydroxyvitamin D is parathyroid hormone and each of these two agents is now known to regulate the secretion of the other. Attention has now turned to the influence of other hormones on 1,25-dihydroxyvitamin D synthesis.

This book reviews the information which has been accumulated so rapidly during this period. One chapter covers the chemistry of vitamin D and its metabolites and this is followed by a discussion of the metabolism of the vitamin in animals. A recurrent theme in several chapters is the control of the various hydroxylation reactions which the vitamin undergoes. Other chapters deal with the function of vitamin D metabolites in intestine and bone. The realisation of the existence of this complex endocrinological system for the control of calcium homeostasis has had implications for clinicians in the understanding of the aetiology, and in the treatment of the diverse medical conditions which arise in man and in which calcium metabolism is uncontrolled. These aspects are also reviewed. In all cases the authors of the chapters are some of those who have been most closely involved with this research. It should be appreciated that valuable though these discoveries may be in themselves, they also reveal that much is still to be learned about the mechanisms by which calcium homeostasis is maintained, the control of this process, and the role of the vitamin D metabolites in bone growth. It is hoped that by reviewing and collecting together the newer information, it will act as a source book for other investigators and encourage them to contribute to the solution of these stimulating physiological problems with their important clinical implications.

April 1978 *D. E. M. Lawson*

List of Contributors

Dr. J. E. Aaron, Medical Research Council Mineral Metabolism Unit, The General Infirmary, Great George Street, Leeds LS1 3EX, England

Dr P. A. Bell, Tenovus Institute for Cancer Research, The Welsh National School of Medicine, The Heath, Cardiff CF4 4XX, Wales

Dr M. J. Barnes, Medical Research Council Connective Tissue Team, Department of Pathology, University of Cambridge, Tennis Court Road, Cambridge CB2 1QP, England

Professor H. F. DeLuca. Department of Biochemistry, College of Agricultural and Life Sciences, University of Wisconsin-Madison, Madison, Wisconsin 53706, USA

Dr C. S. Fullmer, Department of Physical Biology, New York State College of Veterinary Medicine, Cornell University, Ithaca, New York 14853, USA

Dr M. F. Holick, Department of Biochemistry, College of Agricultural and Life Sciences, University of Wisconsin-Madison, Madison, Wisconsin 53706, USA

Dr D. E. M. Lawson, University of Cambridge and Medical Research Council, Dunn Nutritional Laboratory, Milton Road, Cambridge CB4 1XJ, England

Dr E. B. Mawer, Department of Medicine, University of Manchester, Manchester M13 9WL, England

Professor, A. W. Norman, Department of Biochemistry, University of California, Riverside, California 92502, USA

Dr J. A. Parsons, National Institute for Medical Research, Mill Hill, London NW7 1AA, England

Professor S. W. Stanbury, Department of Medicine, University of Manchester, Manchester M13 9WL, England

Dr A. N. Taylor, Department of Physical Biology, New York State College of Veterinary Medicine, Cornell University, Ithaca, New York 14853, USA

Professor R. H. Wasserman, Department of Physical Biology, New York State College of Veterinary Medicine, Cornell University, Ithaca, New York 14853, USA

Contents

1 The Chemistry of the Vitamins D

PHILIP A. BELL

1 Introduction

The term 'vitamin D' refers to a group of seco-steroids with antirachitic properties, possessing in common a conjugated triene system of double bonds, of which cholecalciferol (vitamin D_3) (1, Fig. 1) and ergocalciferol (vitamin D_2) (2, Fig. 1) are the best-known examples.

Cholecalciferol, the naturally occurring antirachitic factor in fish liver oils, does not meet the classical definition of a vitamin, for it can be synthesised in mammals by the action of sunlight on its precursor, 7-dehydrocholesterol (3, Fig. 1), present in skin. Only when skin irradiation is insufficient must the balance of the requirement be met from dietary sources. The recent demonstration of the existence in mammals of a physiological control mechanism affecting the metabolism of cholecalciferol, as well as studies of its mechanism of action, reinforce the view that cholecalciferol is a vitamin imposed on man by civilisation.

Ergocalciferol occupies an anomalous position. Commercially more important than cholecalciferol as a food additive for man and livestock because of the ready availability from yeast of ergosterol (4, Fig. 1), its precursor, it is really a synthetic analogue of the naturally occurring antirachitic factor, cholecalciferol. Its pre-eminent position arises not only from the availability of its precursor, but also from a historical accident. It was observed that antirachitic activity could be generated in many foodstuffs and vegetable oils by irradiation with ultraviolet light (Steenbock and Black, 1924; Hess and Weinstock, 1924), and that a component of the sterol fraction was involved (Hess *et al.*, 1925; Steenbock and Black, 1925; Rosenheim and Webster, 1925). Consequently investigations centred on cholesterol and led to the conclusion that ergosterol, present as an impurity, was the true precursor of the antirachitic factor (Pohl, 1927; Rosenheim and Webster, 1927; Windaus *et al.*, 1927). Although this conclusion was subsequently shown to be erroneous, since 7-dehydrocholesterol was also present, ergocalciferol has continued to be the starting material in many chemical investigations. Fortunately much of the information obtained is equally applicable to cholecalciferol, and of course its metabolites, provided that due allowance is made for the differing properties of the side chains.

A NOMENCLATURE

The nomenclature used in this chapter follows the IUPAC rules for steroid nomenclature (IUPAC, 1969), although for simplicity trivial names are utilised as much as possible. The accepted trivial names, cholecalciferol and ergocalciferol, are used in place of vitamin D_2 and vitamin D_3; isomers and derivatives of these compounds are distinguished by subscript numerals following the trivial name to indicate their relationship to vitamin D_2 or vitamin D_3, e.g. tachysterol$_2$, lumisterol$_3$. In discussions of properties of the seco-steroid nucleus which are unaffected by the nature of the side chain, the prefix or subscript numeral indicating the nature of the side chain is omitted, e.g. calciferol, tachysterol.

In numbering the carbon atoms of these seco-steroids the numbering (and configurational designation) of the atoms and substituents in the parent steroid is retained, but when the structures are drawn the use of solid or broken lines to denote bonds to substituents which lie above or beneath the plane of the molecule denotes actual geometric configuration. Thus cholecalciferol (1, Fig. 1), by relation to cholesterol, is known as 9,10-seco-5,7,10(19)cholestatrien-3β-ol, but the 3-hydroxyl group is represented in its true geometrical position, beneath the plane of the molecule.

Configurations at asymmetric centres are specified according to the *R,S* notation by application of the sequence-rule procedure of Cahn *et al.* (1966).

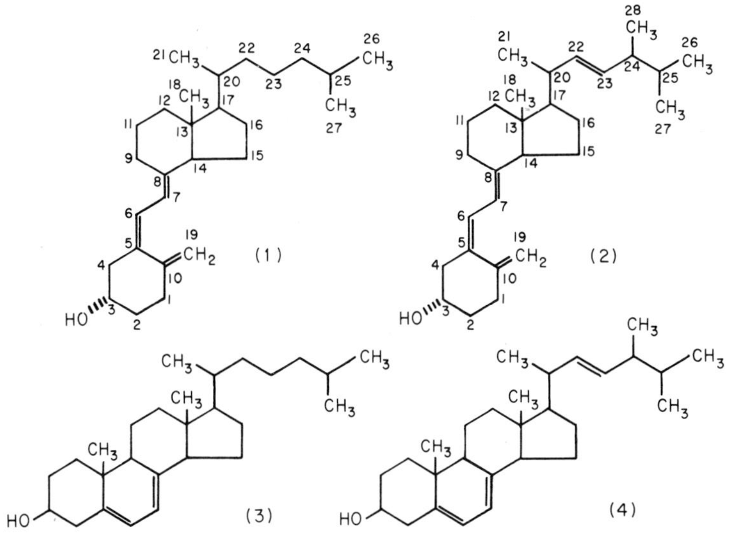

Fig. 1. Cholecalciferol, ergocalciferol and their precursors

Configurations about double bonds are specified by the *E,Z* notation (Blackwood *et al.*, 1968). To apply this latter notation, the priority of the groups attached to each of the carbon atoms of the double bond is assessed by application of sequence-rule procedures. If the two groups of higher priority are on the same side of the double bond then the configuration is *Z*; if they are on opposite sides the configuration is *E*. The *Z* and *E* notation corresponds to *cis* and *trans* respectively, but is applicable in cases where the *cis/trans* notation leads to ambiguities. Thus the full notation of cholecalciferol (1, Fig. 1) is 9,10-seco-(5*Z*,7*E*)-5,7,10(19)-cholestatrien-3β-ol.

II The Classical Vitamins D: Ergocalciferol and Cholecalciferol

A ERGOCALCIFEROL

The isolation of a pure, crystalline, active compound from irradiated ergosterol was accomplished in 1932 by two groups of workers, one led by Windaus in Germany (Windaus *et al.*, 1932a), the other by Bourdillon in England (Askew *et al.*, 1932). The name 'vitamin D_2' was adopted for the active compound by Windaus, whereas the British workers gave their product the name 'ergocalciferol'. (Vitamin D_1 was an earlier preparation consisting of a 1:1 complex of the active compound with lumisterol, an inactive isomer (Windaus *et al.*, 1931).)

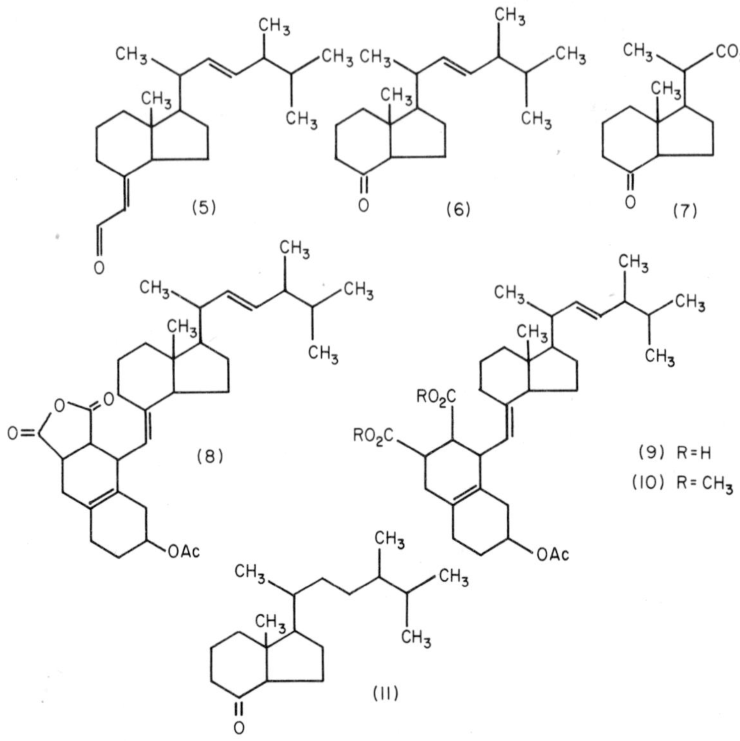

Fig. 2. Degradation products of ergocalciferol

Once the structure of ergosterol (4, Fig. 1) had been established (Windaus *et al.*, 1934), the structure of ergocalciferol (2, Fig. 1) was determined by orthodox degradative procedures. Initial characterisation had shown ergocalciferol to be a secondary alcohol reducible with sodium in ethanol to a dihydro-derivative (Windaus *et al.*, 1932a). Catalytic hydrogenation resulted in the consumption of four moles of hydrogen (Kuhn and Moller, 1934), and titration of the dihydro-derivative with perbenzoic acid confirmed this measurement (Von Reichel and Deppe, 1936). Diels' hydrocarbon was not produced from ergocalciferol on selenium dehydrogenation, and therefore it did not contain the steroid nucleus intact (Lettré, 1934); since elemental analysis of ergocalciferol showed no change in elemental composition compared with ergosterol, it was concluded that the additional centre of unsaturation was introduced by ring cleavage.

Oxidation of ergocalciferol with permanganate or chromic acid gave the $\alpha\beta$-unsaturated C_{21}-aldehyde (5, Fig. 2) and the ketone (6, Fig. 2); ozonolysis gave formaldehyde and the acid (7, Fig. 2) (Heilbron and Spring, 1935;

Heilbron *et al.*, 1935, 1936; Windaus and Grundmann, 1936). These reactions showed unsaturation in the 5,6- and 7,8-positions of the nucleus and the 22,23-position of the side chain and constituted strong evidence that the C_{10}-methyl group of ergosterol was converted to a methylene group in ergocalciferol. These conclusions were confirmed (Windaus and Thiele, 1936) by conversion of ergocalciferyl acetate to the maleic anhydride adduct (8, Fig. 2), which was in turn converted to the dicarboxylic acid (9, Fig. 2) and its dimethyl ester (10, Fig. 2). Platinum dehydrogenation of the diacid (9, Fig. 2) gave naphthalene and naphthalene-2-carboxylic acid. Selenium dehydrogenation of the dimethyl ester (10, Fig. 2) gave 2,3-dimethylnaphthalene, and partial hydrogenation of the ester followed by ozonolysis gave the saturated ketone (11, Fig. 2). The only arrangement of the double bonds in a triene system which would account for these degradation products is the 9,10-seco-5,7,10(19)-ergostatriene nucleus.

The stereochemistry of ergocalciferol was elucidated by x-ray crystallography of the 4-iodo-5-nitrobenzoate ester (Crowfoot and Dunitz, 1948; Hodgkin *et al.*, 1963); the molecule was shown to possess the 5*Z*,7*E*-configuration (2, Fig. 1), with the C_{19}-methylene out of the plane of the 5,7-diene to reduce steric strain. This configuration gives rise to ultraviolet absorption with a maximum at 265 nm ($\varepsilon = 18\,300$), similar to that of model hexatrienes of the same conformation. In the proton magnetic resonance spectrum the value of the coupling constant for the C_6-C_7 protons provides a further indication that the molecule possesses a similar conformation in solution (Delaroff *et al.*, 1963).

B CHOLECALCIFEROL

In a series of bioassays of irradiated ergosterol and irradiated cholesterol Waddell (1934) observed that irradiated ergosterol was much less effective in the chick than an amount of irradiated cholesterol giving the same response as irradiated ergosterol in rats. He concluded that the provitamin present as a trace contaminant in cholesterol is not ergosterol. Callow (1934) had predicted that an antirachitic compound derived from the cholestane rather than the ergostane series might exist in nature, and this compound was synthesised by Windaus *et al.* (1935). Cholesteryl acetate (12, Fig. 3) was oxidised with chromic acid to 7-oxocholesteryl acetate (13, Fig. 3), which was reduced in a Meerwein–Ponndorf reaction to a mixture of diols. The main component of this mixture was 7β-hydroxycholesterol (14, Fig. 3), the dibenzoate of which gave 7-dehydrocholesteryl benzoate (15, Fig. 3) on pyrolysis. On irradiation with ultraviolet light the free sterol (3, Fig. 1) gave an oil, from which the active product was isolated as the crystalline 3,5-dinitrobenzoate (Windaus *et al.*, 1936). The free compound (1, Fig. 1), later

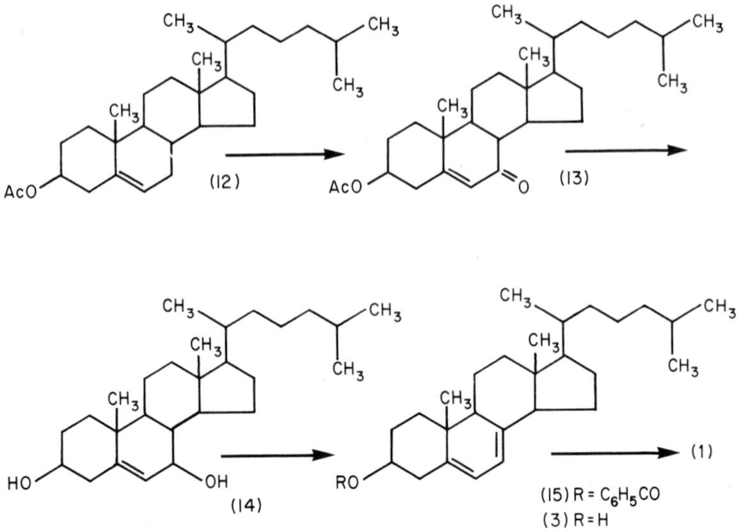

Fig. 3. Synthesis of cholecalciferol (Windaus)

obtained in a crystalline form (Schenck, 1937), is known as vitamin D_3, or cholecalciferol.

The antirachitic factor from tuna liver oil has been isolated using the techniques of solvent partition and chromatography on alumina (Brockmann, 1936). A 3,5-dinitrobenzoate and, subsequently, the free compound were obtained and shown to be identical with synthetic cholecalciferol and its ester (Brockmann and Busse, 1938). Thus the naturally occurring vitamin in tuna liver oil is cholecalciferol, and the naturally occurring provitamin in foodstuffs is 7-dehydrocholesterol. Confirmation that 7-dehydrocholesterol is the true provitamin from animal sources came with its isolation from pig skin (Windaus and Bock, 1937).

III The Irradiation Pathway

A PHOTOCHEMICAL AND THERMAL ISOMERISATIONS

From irradiated solutions of ergosterol Windaus and his collaborators isolated two compounds isomeric with ergocalciferol: lumisterol$_2$ (16, Fig. 4), the 9β,19α-stereoisomer of ergosterol (Windaus *et al.*, 1932b), and tachysterol$_2$ (17, Fig. 4), the 5(10),6,8-triene isomeric with ergocalciferol

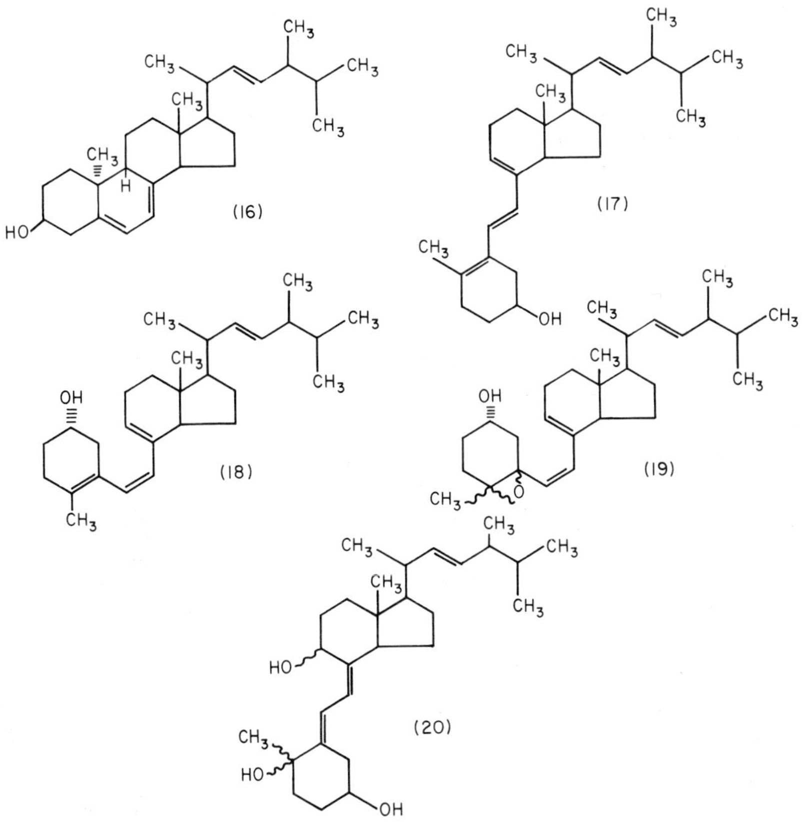

Fig. 4. Isomers of ergocalciferol and their derivatives

(Windaus *et al.*, 1932c). The analogous compounds in the cholecalciferol series were subsequently isolated (Windaus *et al.*, 1938, 1939).

These compounds were initially assumed to be intermediates in the photochemical reaction pathway from ergosterol to ergocalciferol, i.e.

$$\text{Ergosterol} \rightarrow \text{lumisterol}_2 \rightarrow \text{tachysterol}_2 \rightarrow \text{ergocalciferol}$$

However, in 1948 Velluz reported that irradiations performed below 20°C, in contrast to the irradiations performed at 50°C by Windaus, gave little ergocalciferol. When these irradiated solutions were warmed in the dark, major amounts of ergocalciferol were generated (Velluz *et al.*, 1948, 1949a). The ultimate step in the formation of ergocalciferol is therefore a thermal rather than a photochemical process. The labile precursor, pre-ergocalciferol (18, Fig. 4) was isolated in 1949 (Velluz and Amiard, 1949); in warm neutral solvents it is converted reversibly into ergocalciferol which represents approximately 75–80% of the resulting equilibrium mixture (Velluz *et al.*, 1949b; Verloop *et al.*, 1957).

Pre-ergocalciferol was shown to contain four double bonds, but it did not yield the aldehyde (5, Fig. 2) or the ketone (6, Fig. 2) on oxidation, nor did it show the infrared absorption characteristic of an exocyclic methylene group. The most remarkable property of this isomer was its ultraviolet absorption, which showed a maximum (262 nm) similar to that of ergocalciferol, but with a much reduced intensity (Velluz and Amiard, 1955). Pre-ergocalciferol was shown to be the 6*Z*-(*cis*)isomer of tachysterol$_2$ (Koevoet *et al.*, 1955), which had already been identified as a 6*E*-(*trans*) substance, since the pre-ergocalciferol was readily transformed into tachysterol$_2$ by iodine, a standard catalyst for *Z*/*E*(*cis*/*trans*) interconversion (Koevoet *et al.*, 1955). The energetically unfavourable *trans*/*cis* isomerisation can be effected by ultraviolet light (Velluz *et al.*, 1955a, b). Further evidence for the structure (18, Fig. 4) was derived from a study of the mono-epoxide (19, Fig. 4) of pre-ergocalciferol (Velluz *et al.*, 1955a, c). The dienoid light absorption of the epoxide confirmed that pre-ergocalciferol is a conjugated triene, and when the epoxide ring is opened with acid an anionotropic shift occurs, giving the triol (20, Fig. 4), which, as shown by light-absorption data, contains an intercyclic diene system.

B PHOTOCHEMICAL REACTIONS AT LOW TEMPERATURES

When first isolated, pre-ergocalciferol was assumed to fit into the Windaus irradiation sequence after tachysterol, i.e.

$$\text{Ergosterol} \rightarrow \text{lumisterol}_2 \rightarrow \text{tachysterol}_2 \rightarrow \text{pre-ergocalciferol}$$

However, the evidence of its 6*Z*- configuration ruled out this possibility, since pre-ergocalciferol rather than tachysterol$_2$ should be formed on ring opening of lumisterol$_2$. Another difficulty had been hinted at previously by Hodgkin and Sayre (1952) with regard to the ergosterol → lumisterol$_2$ sequence: they thought it unlikely that the steric position of the C_{19}-methyl group could change (epimerise) without the C_9-C_{10} or the C_5-C_{10} bond being broken. This discrepancy was resolved by the finding that tachysterol$_2$, ergosterol and lumisterol$_2$ were formed on irradiating pre-ergocalciferol, demonstrating not only that pre-ergocalciferol should occupy a central place in any irradiation scheme, but also that the reactions are reversible (Velluz *et al.*, 1955b, d).

Confirmation of these findings has come from the comprehensive studies of Havinga and his collaborators. Tracer experiments with radioactive ergosterol were followed by a series of kinetic studies in which each of the four

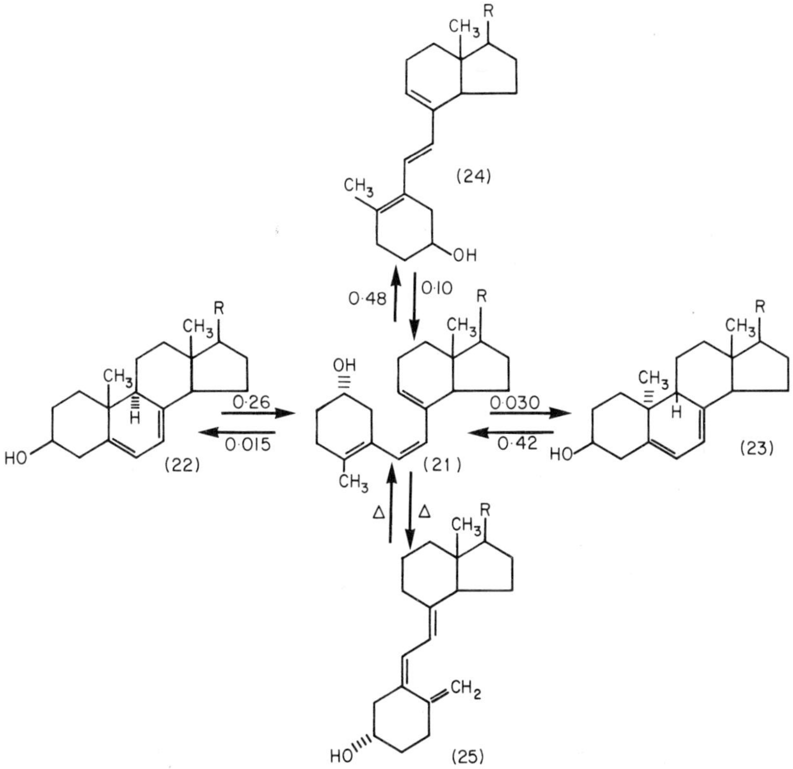

Fig. 5. Thermal and photochemical isomerisations of precalciferol (with quantum yields)

isomers, ergosterol, lumisterol$_2$, tachysterol$_2$, and pre-ergocalciferol, were irradiated separately in dilute solution at around 0°C, and the composition of the reaction mixture was determined as a function of the degree of photochemical conversion (Havinga *et al.*, 1955). Extrapolation of the percentage composition of each reaction mixture to zero time indicated both quantitatively and qualitatively the primary products formed from each of the compounds by photochemical conversion. Thus, ergosterol was converted to the extent of 85% into pre-ergocalciferol and 15% into other products, probably over-irradiation products (Rappoldt and Havinga, 1960). Similarly, lumisterol$_2$ yielded 100% of pre-ergocalciferol (Rappoldt, 1960a), pre-ergocalciferol gave over 90% of tachysterol$_2$ and 5% of ergosterol, and tachysterol$_2$ gave 70% of pre-ergocalciferol, the balance probably consisting of lumisterol$_2$ (Rappoldt, 1960b; Havinga *et al.*, 1960). The uncertainties concerning the formation of lumisterol were eventually clarified by the demonstration that irradiation of tritiated precholecalciferol, but not of tritiated tachysterol$_3$, gave lumisterol$_3$ (Sanders and Havinga, 1964).

These observations have led to the currently accepted irradiation scheme (Fig. 5). Precalciferol (21, Fig. 5) can cyclise to the provitamin (22, Fig. 5) and also to the $9\beta,19\alpha$-stereoisomer lumisterol (23, Fig. 5); alternatively it can undergo the reversible *Z/E* (*cis/trans*) photoisomerisation to the 6*E*-isomer tachysterol (24, Fig. 5). The cyclisation reactions are remarkably stereospecific, yielding exclusively the 9,10-*anti*-isomers. The quantum yields shown were determined for solutions in ether at 5°C using light of wavelength 253.7 nm (Havinga, 1973). Utilising these quantum yields and the extinction coefficients of the various isomers, the composition of the steady state can be calculated; these theoretical values are in good agreement (Table 1) with the measured composition of the quasi-stationary state obtained on continued irradiation (Havinga, 1973; Boomsma *et al.*, 1975). A true stationary state is never obtained because of the formation of 'over-irradiation' products.

Table 1. Composition of the photostationary state

Compound	Percentage of total	
	Calculated	Experimental
Tachysterol$_3$	76	75
Precholecalciferol	19.5	20
Lumisterol$_3$	2.5	2.5
7-Dehydrocholesterol	2	1.5

The nature of the photochemical intermediates has been studied; investigations of fluorescence spectra at 80°K led to the conclusion that the photoisomerisations occur via the excited singlet state (Havinga *et al.*, 1960; Havinga and Schlatmann, 1961), conclusions confirmed by the observation that the presence of a triplet sensitiser has an effect only on the *Z/E* (*cis/trans*) isomerisation, which then occurs with very different values for the quantum yields (Snoeren *et al.*, 1970). Advantage has recently been taken of this observation to increase the yield of precalciferol obtained after irradiation. Photolysis of ergosterol followed by a second irradiation in the presence of the triplet sensitiser fluorenone resulted in an increase in the yield of ergocalciferol from 11% to 35% (Eyley and Williams, 1975). The mechanisms of the photochemical interconversions have been further explored using model hexatrienes. The pattern of photoproducts is dependent on the conformational equilibrium in the ground state, interconversion between singlet

Table 2. Effect of size and configuration of the D ring on the calciferol/precalciferol equilibrum

Structure of calciferol analogue	Percentage in calciferol form
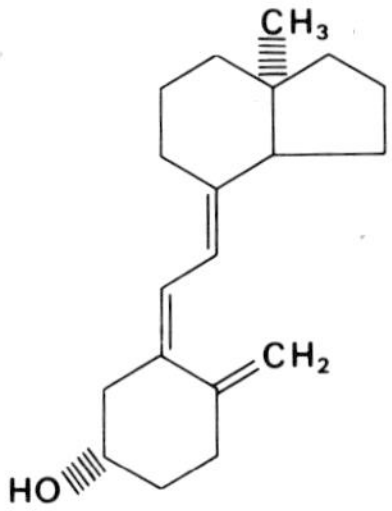 CH_3 CH_2 HO	5%
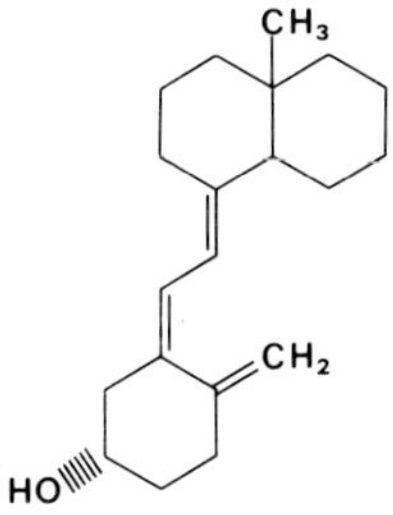 CH_3 CH_2 HO	35%
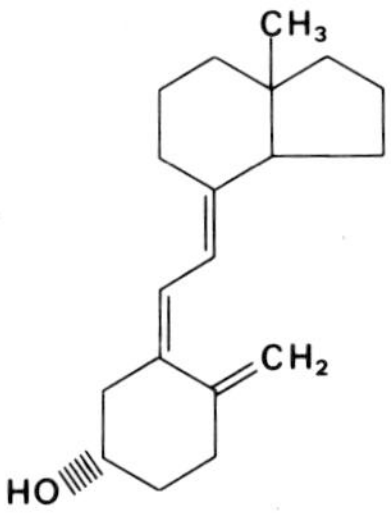 CH_3 CH_2 HO	80%
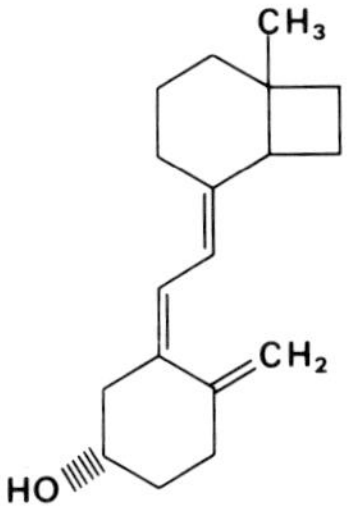 CH_3 CH_2 HO	100%

excited states being prevented by high rotational barriers which exist about bonds having considerable double bond character. Thus, for (3*Z*)-hexa-1,3,5-triene, which exists predominantly in the *tZt* conformation ($\varepsilon = 41\,000$), the photoisomerisation is simply *Z*/*E* isomerisation. When the *cZc* form predominates in the ground state, as in 2,5-dimethyl-(3*Z*)-hexa-1,3,5-triene ($\varepsilon = 12\,300$), cyclised products can be obtained in addition to the *E*-isomer (Vroegop *et al.*, 1973). This situation clearly reflects that occurring with precalciferol.

C THERMAL ISOMERISATIONS: THE PRECALCIFEROL CALCIFEROL EQUILIBRIUM

The thermal equilibrium between precalciferol (21, Fig. 5) and calciferol (25, Fig. 5) favours the calciferol form; the percentage of cholecalciferol in equilibrium with precholecalciferol ranges from 98 % at −20°C to 78 % at 80°C (Hanewald *et al.*, 1961). The rate constants for the reactions have been determined and have been shown to be independent of the nature of the solvent, of acidic or basic catalysis, and of factors known to affect free radical processes (Verloop *et al.*, 1957; Velluz *et al.*, 1957a). This evidence, together with the kinetic parameters (ΔH = 19 Kcal/mole; ΔS = −12 e.u.), led to the postulate that the reaction is intramolecular and occurs via a rigid cyclic transition state (Verloop *et al.*, 1957; Legrand and Mathieu, 1957). Confirmation of this pathway has come from studies with [19-^{3}H]pre-cholecalciferol (Akhtar and Gibbons, 1965). Thermal isomerisation of the tritiated compound occurred without loss of radioactivity and, from the distribution of radioactivity in the isolated cholecalciferol, it was concluded that the transition state is non-stereospecific, the 9α- and 9β-hydrogen atoms being equivalent. The transition state, originally proposed on steric considerations, is also favourable on orbital symmetry relationships (Woodward and Hoffmann, 1965).

The effect of molecular structure on the position of the precalciferol/calciferol equilibrium has been investigated. It has been suggested that in pre-ergocalciferol or precholecalciferol, the presence of a *trans*-attached D ring and a C_8—C_9 double bond gives rise to a strained molecule, and that the isomerisation to an exocyclic double bond would reduce the strain (Schlatmann *et al.*, 1964). Support for this view has come from a study of the position of equilibrium in model compounds having *trans*-attached D rings of different sizes, or having a *cis*-attached D ring, or no D ring at all. As predicted, the more strained the D ring, the more the equilibrium shifts in favour of the calciferol form (Table 2).

IV Isomerisation Reactions of the Calciferols

A THERMAL ISOMERISATIONS: PYRO- AND ISOPYRO-CALCIFEROLS

Above 100°C the calciferol system can ring-close, almost certainly via pre-calciferol, to produce irreversibly the 9,10 *syn*-isomers of ergosterol (or 7-dehydrocholesterol). In contrast the photochemical ring closure produces the *anti*-isomers, ergosterol and lumisterol$_2$, by a reversible process. The *syn*-isomer having the 9α,19α-configuration is known as pyrocalciferol (26, Fig. 6),

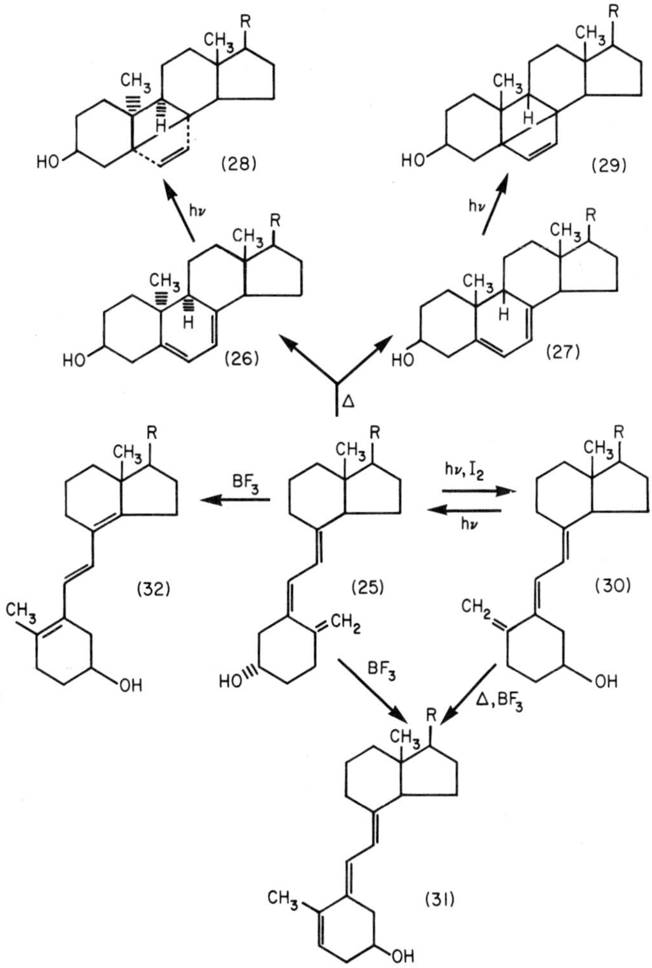

Fig. 6. Isomerisation reactions of the calciferols

and that having the 9β,19β-configuration is isopyrocalciferol (27, Fig. 6). On photoisomerisation these compounds isomerise to the corresponding bicyclohexene derivatives (28, 29, Fig. 6), but no ring opening occurs due to steric hindrance (Dauben and Fonken, 1959). These photoisomerisations can be reversed thermally, probably driven by the release of strain energy from the bicyclic compounds (Bloothoofd-Kruisbeek and Lugtenburg, 1972).

B *CIS-TRANS* ISOMERISATIONS

The calciferols, that is, the isomers having the 5*Z*,7*E*-configuration, will undergo *Z*/*E* (*cis*/*trans*) isomerisation. Verloop *et al.* (1955, 1959) found that treatment of ergocalciferol or cholecalciferol with small amounts of iodine in non-polar solvents under exposure to diffuse daylight affords the 5*E*-isomers, commonly known as the 5,6-*trans*-calciferols (30, Fig. 6). The reverse transformation has been accomplished photochemically (Inhoffen *et al.*, 1957a).

Further isomerisation of the 5,6-*trans*-calciferols occurs on heating at 180°C (Kobayashi, 1967a); for obvious steric reasons ring closure does not occur, but instead isomerisation takes place to yield isocalciferol (31, Fig. 6). The latter compound is also a product of the acid-catalysed isomerisation of calciferol or 5,6-*trans*-calciferol (Inhoffen *et al.*, 1956), as is another isomer, isotachysterol (32, Fig. 6) (Inhoffen *et al.*, 1954). In reactions catalysed by mineral or Lewis acids it appears that 5,6-*trans*-calciferol, isocalciferol, and isotachysterol are produced sequentially (Inhoffen *et al.*, 1956; Kobayashi, 1967b), the exocyclic 1(10),5,7-triene (31, Fig. 6) presumably being less stable than the 5(10),6,8(14)-isomer (32, Fig. 6). This reaction is the basis of the antimony trichloride colour test for vitamin D (Nield *et al.*, 1940; Wilkie *et al.*, 1958). The photoisomerisation of isotachysterol produces a 6*Z*-isomer, *cis*-isotachysterol, which can be converted back to the *trans* form (32, Fig. 6) with iodine and light (Verloop *et al.*, 1960).

Table 3. Stereochemistry and ultraviolet absorption of calciferol isomers

Compound	Configuration of conjugated triene	Preferred conformation	λ_{max}(nm)	ε_{max}
Calciferol	5*Z*,7*E*,10(19)-	*cZt*	265	18 300
5,6-*Trans*-calciferol	5*E*,7*E*,10(19)-	*cEt*	273	24 300
Isocalciferol	1(10),5*E*,7*E*-	*tEt*	286.5	44 100
Precalciferol	5(10),6*Z*,8-	*cZt*	263	9 120
Cis-isotachysterol	5(10),6*Z*,8(14)-	*tZt*	253	14 270
Tachysterol	5(10),6*E*,8-	*cEt*	281	24 600
Isotachysterol	5(10),6*E*,8(14)-	*tEt*	288.5	45 300

The isomers of calciferol display characteristic ultraviolet spectral properties, which are listed in Table 3. Clear regularities can be observed, both in the wavelengths of maximum absorption and also in extinction coefficients, which are in agreement with the assigned conformations and with the spectral characteristics of model hexatrienes of similar conformation. From this table it is apparent that *cis*-isocalciferol, the 5*Z*-isomer of isocalciferol, remains to be discovered. The *E*-(*trans*)stereoisomers, with the exception of 5,6-*trans*-calciferol, display some degree of fine structure in their ultraviolet absorption spectra, apparent as shoulders in the spectrum of tachysterol and as well-defined subsidiary peaks in the spectra of isocalciferol and isotachysterol.

C APPLICATIONS: GAS–LIQUID CHROMATOGRAPHY

The gas–liquid chromatography (glc) of steroids and seco-steroids is of necessity performed at high temperatures; since these are the conditions under which many isomerisation reactions of the calciferol nucleus can occur, the study of the glc behaviour of these compounds is of considerable interest.

Ziffer *et al.* (1960) showed that glc of the calciferols at temperatures in the range 200–250°C gives rise to two elution peaks resulting from formation of pyro- and isopyrocalciferols (26 and 27, Fig. 6). Isotachysterol and isocalciferol do not undergo cyclisation and are eluted unchanged, but 5,6-*trans*-calciferol, while not cyclising, is subject to thermal isomerisation to give isocalciferol (Kobayashi, 1967a), presumably because of the greater stability of the 1(10)-double bond. Tachysterol is, however, not isomerised to isotachysterol on glc.

Most studies of the glc behaviour of the calciferols and their isomers have utilised non-polar silicone oil stationary phases. With such phases distinct regularities in retention times can be observed dependent on the nature of both the nucleus and the side chain. Some typical data using OV-1 as the stationary phase are given in Table 4 to illustrate these regularities. It can be seen that for the four isomeric 5,7-dienes the order of elution is pyrocalciferol $<$ lumisterol $<$ isopyrocalciferol $<$ procalciferol, both for the free sterols and their trimethylsilyl ethers. Trimethylsilylation leads to an increase in retention time for the provitamins (retention factor $=1.22$) and for the isopyrocalciferols (retention factor $=1.17$), but to a decrease in retention times for the lumisterols and pyrocalciferols (retention factors $=0.94$ and 0.93, respectively). The order of elution for the non-cyclised seco-steroids is isocalciferol $<$ tachysterol $<$ isotachysterol; trimethylsilylation has little effect on the behaviour of these compounds (retention factors $=0.96$, 1.03, 0.99, respectively).

The structure of the side chain has a pronounced effect on retention times; while modifications of the number or oxidation state of the carbon atoms alter

Table 4. Glc data for some calciferol isomers and precursors

The data were obtained using a Pye 104 gas chromatograph with flame ionisation detection, with a 5ft column of 3% OV-1 on Gas-Chrom Q at 240°C. Retention times are expressed relative to 5α-cholestane (1.00, 6 min) (Bell, P. A. and Branch, W., unpublished results)

Side chain =	Relative retention time			
	H_3C–CH(R)–CH₂CH₂CH₂–CH(CH_3)–CH_3 (a)	H_3C–CH(R)–CH=CH–CH(CH_3)–CH(CH_3)–CH_3 (b)	H_3C–CH(R)–CH₂CH₂CH₂–C(OH)(CH_3)–CH_3 (c)	H_3C–CH(R)–CH₂CH₂CH₂–C(OTMS)(CH_3)–CH_3 (d)
R =				
Δ^5-Sterol	1.85	2.06	2.98	—
,TMS ether	2.22	2.50	3.61	4.74
Pyrocalciferol	2.02	2.26		
,TMS ether	2.48	2.75		
Lumisterol	1.69	1.87		
,TMS ether	1.59	1.76		
Pyrocalciferol	1.64	1.78	2.63	—
,TMS ether	1.50	1.59	2.41	3.14
Isopyrocalciferol	1.81	2.01	2.93	—
,TMS ether	2.12	2.32	3.48	4.51
Tachysterol	2.44	2.69		
,TMS ether	2.51	2.77		
5,6-*Trans*-calciferol	2.27	2.55	3.68	—
,TMS ether	2.23	2.37	3.52	4.64
Isocalciferol	2.27	2.55	3.68	—
,TMS ether	2.23	2.37	3.52	4.64
Isotachysterol	2.55	2.90	4.08	—
,TMS ether	2.56	2.82	4.02	5.06

Mean retention factors for side chain substitution

(a) ⟶ (b): 1.10

(a) ⟶ (c): 1.61

(a) ⟶ (d): 2.08

the retention times relatively little, introduction of a 25-hydroxyl group more than doubles them. The effect of trimethylsilylating the 25-hydroxyl group is greater than the effect of silylating the 3-hydroxyl group.

V Oxidation and Reduction Reactions of the Calciferol Nucleus

Partial reduction of calciferol, precalciferol, or tachysterol affords mixtures of dihydro-derivatives which have hypercalcemic properties. These reduction products therefore have been quite extensively studied, but the majority of such investigations were conducted before the advent of modern physical techniques for structural analysis, and so in many cases doubts still exist as to correct configurations or conformations. The confusion in this area is such that systematic reinvestigation would be of great value.

A variety of methods for partial reduction have been utilised, of which those of most value appear to be electron reduction with lithium in liquid ammonia or partial catalytic hydrogenation with Raney nickel catalyst. The products of reduction appear to be similar, regardless of whether the starting material is tachysterol, calciferol or precalciferol, and include compounds designated as dihydrotachysterol and dihydrocalciferols I–VI.

Dihydrotachysterol (33, Fig. 7), physiologically the most active of these derivatives, was first prepared by reduction of tachysterol$_2$ with sodium and propanol (Von Werder, 1939), but lithium and liquid ammonia are now the reducing agent of choice (Westerhof and Keverling Buisman, 1956; Van de Vliervoet *et al.*, 1956). The structure of dihydrotachysterol was established by chemical and infrared spectroscopic evidence (Westerhof and Keverling Buisman, 1957, 1959), and has been confirmed very recently by high resolution proton magnetic resonance spectroscopy (Wing *et al.*, 1974). Also physiologically active is dihydrocalciferol II (34, Fig. 7), obtained by partial hydrogenation of ergo- or cholecalciferol with Raney nickel catalyst (Schubert, 1954). Dihydrocalciferol II has an ultraviolet absorption spectrum virtually identical to that of dihydrotachysterol, and therefore clearly has the same 7*E*-configuration. Westerhof and Keverling Buisman (1959) suggested that dihydrocalciferol II is the 5*Z*-isomer of dihydrotachysterol and showed that Oppenauer oxidation of dihydrocalciferol II gave an $\alpha\beta$-unsaturated ketone (35, Fig. 7) which in turn gave an enol acetate reducible with borohydride to a mixture of dihydrocalciferol II and dihydrotachysterol. Subsequently Irmscher (1960) confirmed this hypothesis by demonstrating the iodine-catalysed isomerisation of dihydrocalciferol II to dihydrotachysterol. Dihydrocalciferol II exists preferentially as the conformer in which the 3-hydroxyl group and the C_{19}-methyl are both in the axial orientation (Schubert, 1956); this energetically unfavourable conformation is adopted as a result of steric hindrance in the alternative conformation with an equatorial C_{19}-methyl group.

Also obtained by Raney nickel hydrogenation is a third isomer, designated dihydrocalciferol IV (Westerhof and Keverling Buisman, 1957). This compound has the same ultraviolet spectrum as dihydrotachysterol and dihydrocalciferol II and possesses an equatorial hydroxyl group, but gives a different ketone on Oppenauer oxidation from that given by those isomers. Believing that the possibility of *cis-trans* isomerisation during the reduction was remote, Westerhof and Keverling Buisman (1957) therefore postulated structure 36 (Fig. 7) for dihydrocalciferol IV. An alternative stereochemical assignment (37, Fig. 7), first suggested by Von Werder (1957), has been confirmed recently (Okamura *et al.*, 1974a) by proton magnetic resonance spectroscopy.

A reduction product having no conjugated diene system, dihydrocalciferol I (38, Fig. 7) is obtained as one component of reduction mixtures from

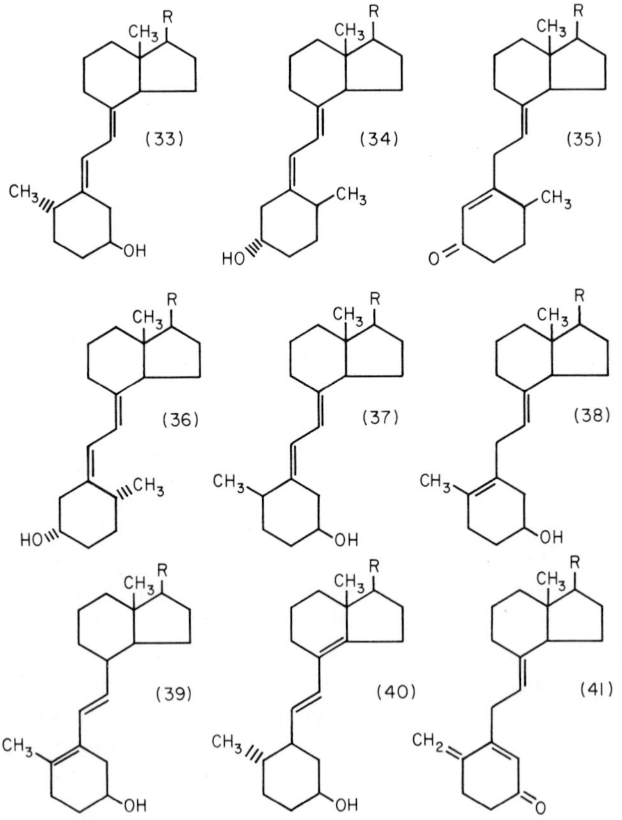

Fig. 7. Oxidation and reduction products of the calciferols

calciferol or tachysterol. This substance was first obtained by Windaus *et al.* (1932a), and its structure established by Von Werder (1939). Dihydrocalciferol I gives the ketone (35) on Oppenauer oxidation (Westerhof and Keverling Buisman, 1959).

Two other dihydro-derivatives of calciferol are dihydrocalciferols V and VI (Westerhof and Keverling Buisman, 1957). Structures 39 (Fig. 7) and 40 (Fig. 7) respectively are proposed for these isomers; evidence has been produced suggesting that they may be formed via isotachysterol produced by isomerisation of calciferol prior to reduction (Furst, 1965).

The partial oxidation of calciferol has not been studied as extensively as the partial reduction; Oppenauer oxidation gives the conjugated ketone (41, Fig. 7) which cannot be converted back to calciferol by enol acetylation and borohydride reduction (Trippett, 1955). Attack on the conjugated triene system can be achieved with lead tetra-acetate to give a 5,6-dihydroxy-derivative (Windaus and Riemann, 1942), or with neutral or weakly alkaline permanganate to give a 7,8-dihydroxy-derivative (Yu *et al.*, 1958), but the configurations of these derivatives have not been established.

VI Synthesis of Ergocalciferol, Cholecalciferol and Isomers

Although ergocalciferol and cholecalciferol may readily be synthesised by irradiation of their steroid 5,7-diene precursors, their preparation by partial or total synthesis utilising methods which emphasise their trienoid nature has been actively studied, particularly by the groups led by Inhoffen and by Lythgoe.

Early investigations of the partial synthesis of ergocalciferol utilised the aldehyde (5, Fig. 8) obtained by oxidation of ergocalciferol. Inhoffen *et al.* (1954) found that this compound could readily be condensed with 4-hydroxycyclohexanone (42, Fig. 8) to give a mixture of epimers of the trienolone (43 and 44, Fig. 8). As was already known from studies with model compounds, the terminal methylene group could not be introduced into the 3β-epimer (43, Fig. 8) by means of elimination reactions; thus thermal dehydration of the diol (45, Fig. 8) formed from the ketone and methyllithium gave not 5,6-*trans*-ergocalciferol (46, Fig. 8) but iso-ergocalciferol (47, Fig. 8) (Inhoffen *et al.*, 1954), presumably because of the difficulty of introducing such a relatively high energy bond as the exocyclic double bond by reactions subject to Saytzeff-type control (Brown *et al.*, 1954). However, the publication by Wittig and Schollkopf (1954) of a method of synthesis of olefins from carbonyl compounds and alkylidenetriphenylphosphoranes provided the key to the synthesis of the calciferols.

In the procedure followed by Inhoffen *et al.* (1955, 1957b, 1958a) the 3β-epimer of the ketone (43, Fig. 8) was separated from the 3α-epimer by

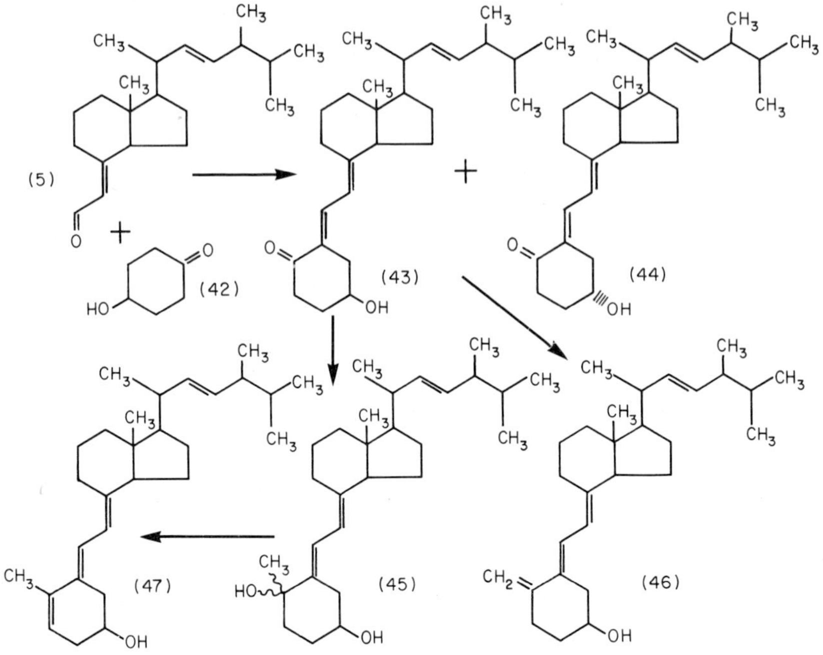

Fig. 8. Synthetic routes to ergocalciferol

chromatography on alumina and, on treatment with methylenetriphenylphosphorane, gave the corresponding C_{19}-methylene derivative, 5,6-*trans*-ergocalciferol (46, Fig. 8). The 5*E*,7*E*-(*cis*/*cis*)-configuration was deduced from the evidence of ultraviolet absorption spectra and of Oppenauer oxidation. In the final step of the synthesis the 5,6-*trans*-isomer was photoisomerised to the 5,6-*cis*-isomer using glass filters which transmitted the radiation necessary for isomerisation but prevented further photochemical decomposition of the product (Inhoffen *et al.*, 1957a).

The same series of reactions was utilised by Lythgoe and his group although the photoisomerisation and epimer separation were performed at different stages (Harrison and Lythgoe, 1957, 1958). The epimeric mixture (43 and 44, Fig. 8) was photoisomerised, the methylene group introduced, and the epimers then separated by chromatography as their 3,5-dinitrobenzoates.

The analogous partial synthesis of cholecalciferol from the corresponding aldehyde in the cholecalciferol series was accomplished in a similar manner (Inhoffen, 1958; Inhoffen *et al.*, 1959a) and was subsequently expanded into a total synthesis by synthesis of the aldehyde (Inhoffen *et al.*, 1958b, 1959b, c; Inhoffen, 1960).

These syntheses afford very low overall yields and are dependent on photochemical transformations and so studies have continued in an attempt to find a purely chemical route to the calciferols. This has been achieved (Dixon *et al.*, 1970; Dawson *et al.*, 1971b) by a synthesis in which the central double bond is formed via an acetylenic intermediate. (*S*)-3-Hydroxymethyl-4-methylcyclohex-3-en-1-ol (48, Fig. 9) was prepared from 5-methoxy-2-methylbenzoic acid in 14% yield (Dixon *et al.*, 1971), and was then converted into the enyne, (*S*)-3-ethynyl-4-methylcyclohex-3-en-1-ol (49, Fig. 9) in 30% yield (Dawson *et al.*, 1971a). This enyne was converted to its trimethylsilyl ether and, as its lithium derivative, was reacted with the chloroketone (51, Fig. 9), prepared (Littlewood *et al.*, 1971) from the diol (50, Fig. 9) which was itself

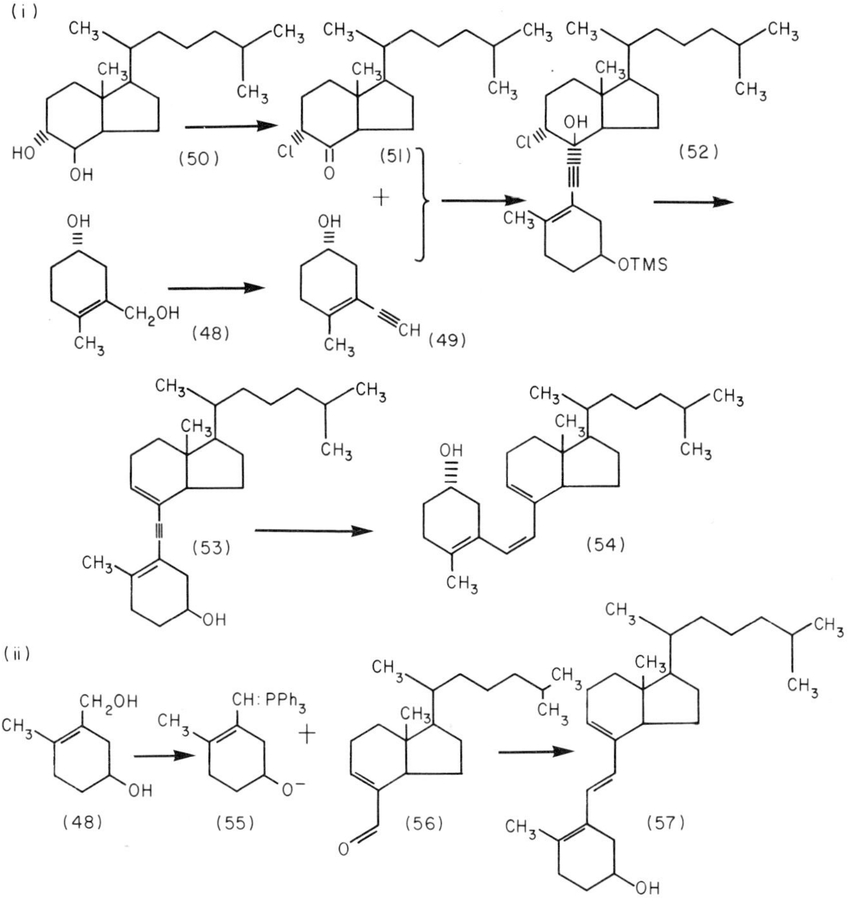

Fig. 9. Synthetic routes (i) to precholecalciferol, and (ii) to tachysterol$_3$

obtained by total synthesis (Bolton *et al.*, 1971), to give the chlorohydrin (52, Fig. 9). Removal of the protecting group followed by treatment with bis(ethylenediamine)chromium (II) afforded the dienyne (53, Fig. 9) which was semihydrogenated with Lindlar's catalyst to give precholecalciferol (54, Fig. 9), and hence cholecalciferol by thermal isomerisation. The overall yield in this synthesis is much higher than previous ones; the yield of precholecalciferol is 21 % from the chloroketone (51, Fig. 9).

One other total synthesis which should be mentioned is that of tachysterol$_3$ (Davidson *et al.*, 1963, 1967). The optically active diol (48, Fig. 9) was converted into the phosphorane (55. Fig. 9) which reacted with the aldehyde (56, Fig. 9), obtained by chemical degradation of cholesterol (Davidson *et al.*, 1964) and subsequently by total synthesis (Littlewood *et al.*, 1971), to give tachysterol$_3$ (57, Fig. 9).

VII Metabolites of Cholecalciferol

A 25-HYDROXYCHOLECALCIFEROL

25-Hydroxycholecalciferol (58, Fig. 10) was first isolated in 1968 and the structure established by high resolution mass spectrometry and by proton magnetic resonance spectroscopy (Blunt *et al.*, 1968a, b). The tertiary hydroxyl group at C_{25} is relatively unreactive and so does not interfere with the usual synthetic route to precalciferol by irradiation of a steroid 5,7-diene; the problem is simply one of introducing the 25-hydroxyl group into the 5,7-diene or its precursors.

The simplest synthetic route starts from 25-oxo-26-norcholesteryl acetate (59, Fig. 10). Introduction of the Δ^7-double bond is achieved by allylic bromination and dehydrobromination for which the favoured reagents are 1,3-dibromo-5,5-dimethylhydantoin (DDH) as brominating agent and trimethyl phosphite or *s*-collidine as dehydrobrominating agent. The 25-hydroxyl group and the C_{27}-methyl group are formed in a Grignard reaction with methylmagnesium iodide (Blunt and DeLuca, 1969; Halkes and Van Vliet, 1969). The sequence of these reactions is not critical, and all variations on the sequence have been followed as shown in Fig. 10.

Several other routes to the 25-hydroxylated sterols (60 or 62, Fig. 10) have been reported. Campbell *et al.* (1969) started from 3β-hydroxycholenic acid (64, Fig. 10), which was converted to the 25-homoester (66, Fig. 10) by means of an Arndt-Eistert rearrangement of the diazoketone (65, Fig. 10). Allylic bromination and dehydrobromination gave the diene (67, Fig. 10), which gave the diol (62, Fig. 10) on treatment with methylmagnesium iodide. These syntheses utilise as starting materials by-products of the oxidation of cholesterol that are now difficult to obtain. Ikekawa and his collaborators (Morisaki *et al.*,

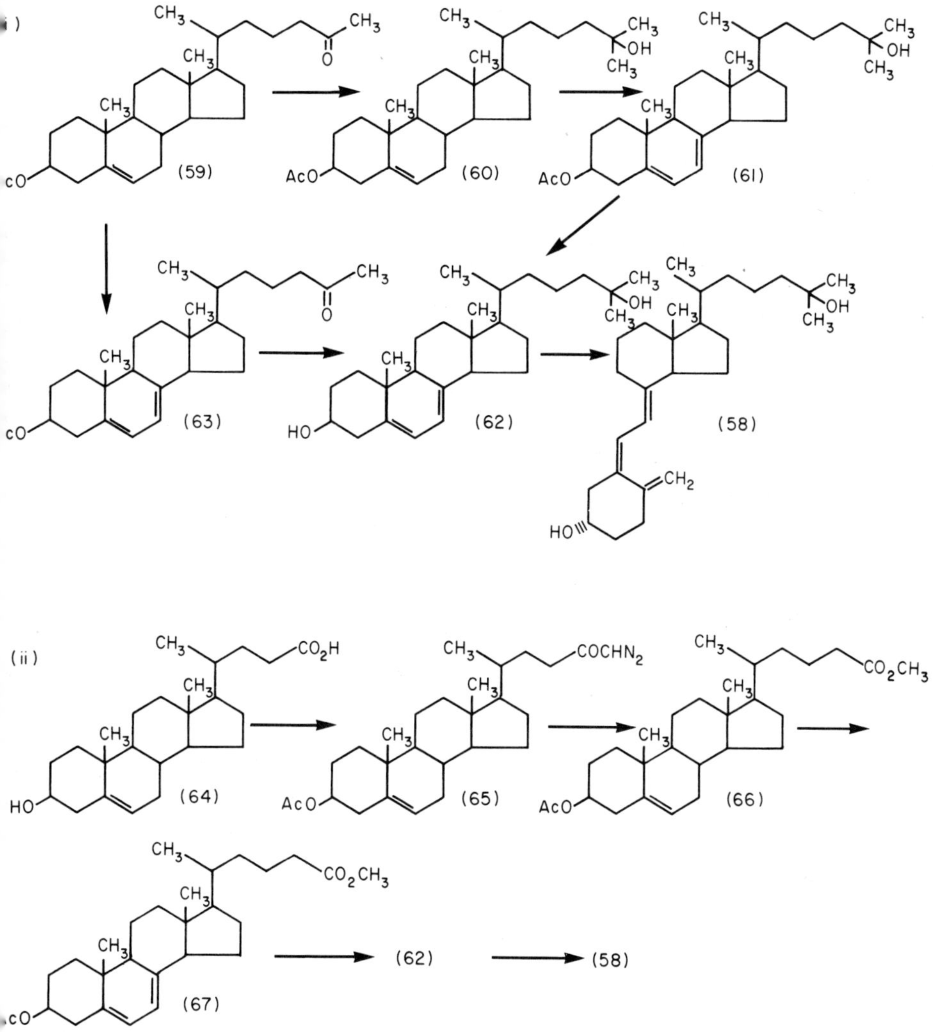

Fig. 10. Synthetic routes to 25-hydroxycholecalciferol from oxidation products of cholesterol

1973a) have explored alternative routes to 25-hydroxycholesterol starting from desmosterol acetate (69, Fig. 11), which is available by degradation of fucosterol (68, Fig. 11). These routes depend on the greater reactivity of the 24,25-bond as compared with the 5,6-double bond. The most convenient route is by oxymercuration of desmosteryl acetate with mercuric acetate in tetrahydrofuran, followed by demercuration with sodium borohydride. This

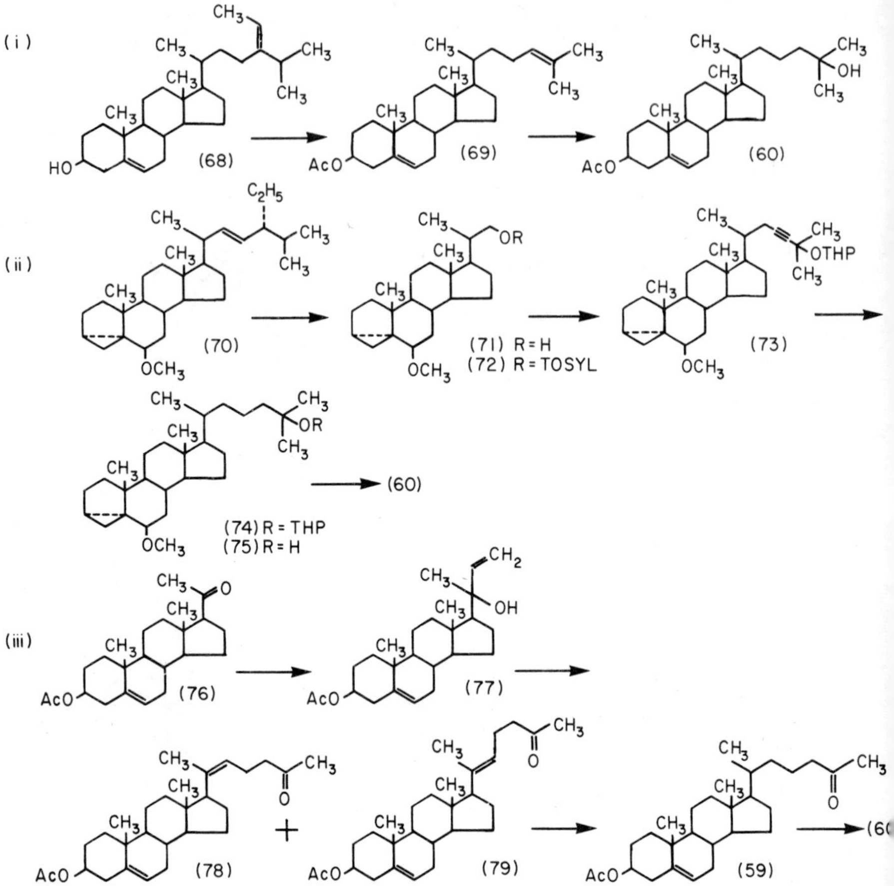

Fig. 11. Alternative routes to 25-hydroxycholesterol

method gives 25-hydroxycholesteryl acetate in 85% yield from desmosterol (Morisaki *et al.*, 1973a). Alternatively, selective epoxidation at C_{24}-C_{25} followed by lithium aluminium hydride reduction and reacetylation gives 60 (Fig. 10) in 50% yield.

Some alternative routes from readily available steroids have been explored by Uskokovic and his coworkers. Ozonolysis of the *i*-methyl ether (70, Fig. 11) derived from stigmasterol gave the alcohol (71, Fig. 11), which, as its tosylate (72, Fig. 11), gave the acetylene (73, Fig. 11) when reacted with the lithium derivative of 3-methyl-1-butyn-3-yl tetrahydropyranyl ether. Hydrogenation over platinum oxide or palladised charcoal gave the saturated side chain (74, Fig. 11) without hydrogenolysis at C_{25}. After removal of the tetrahydropyranyl group, treatment of the 25-hydroxy-derivative (75, Fig. 11) with glacial acetic acid at 70°C gave 25-hydroxycholesteryl 3β-acetate (60, Fig. 10) in 30% overall yield (Partridge *et al.*, 1974).

In another synthesis the same group used 3β-acetoxypregn-5-en-20-one (76, Fig. 11) as the starting material (Narwid *et al.*, 1974a). Treatment with vinylmagnesium chloride in dichloromethane at −78°C gave the 20*S*-allylic alcohol (77, Fig. 11). The Carroll rearrangement was performed on this alcohol using diketene or ethyl acetoacetate to give a mixture of *cis*- and *trans*-keto olefins (78 and 79, Fig. 11) in 60–70% yield. Hydrogenation with platinum oxide catalyst gave a mixture of 20*R*- and 20*S*-ketones, from which the required 20*R*-compound (59, Fig. 10) was separated by crystallisation. A Grignard reaction with methylmagnesium iodide then gave 25-hydroxycholesteryl acetate (60, Fig. 10).

From 25-hydroxycholecalciferol, other isomers and derivatives have been prepared by methods identical to those used for cholecalciferol itself. They include 5,6-*trans*-25-hydroxycholecalciferol (Holick *et al.*, 1972a; Lawson and Bell, 1974), 25-hydroxy-isotachysterol$_3$ (Holick *et al.*, 1973a), 25-hydroxy-isocholecalciferol and 25-hydroxydihydrotachysterol$_3$ (Suda *et al.*, 1970a; Lawson and Bell, 1974).

B 24,25-DIHYDROXYCHOLECALCIFEROL

A polar metabolite of cholecalciferol, first isolated from the plasma of pigs given large doses of cholecalciferol (Suda *et al.*, 1970b) and subsequently prepared *in vitro* (Holick *et al.*, 1972b) by incubation of chick kidney homogenates with 25-hydroxycholecalciferol, was identified as 24,25-dihydroxycholecalciferol (80, Fig. 12). The ultraviolet absorption spectrum, gas-liquid chromatographic behaviour, and typical mass spectral fragmentation pattern established that the compound was a derivative of cholecalciferol

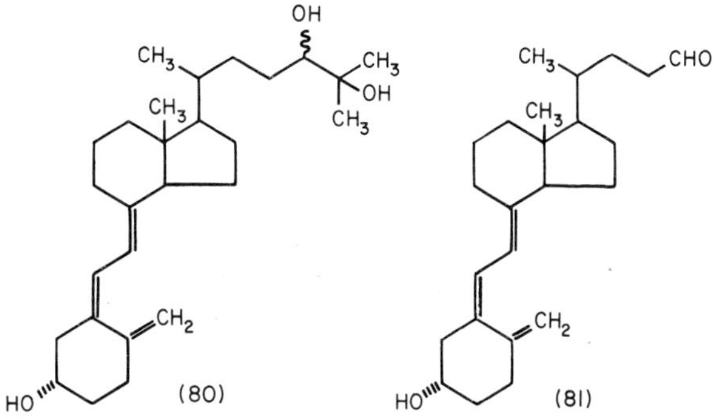

Fig. 12. 24,25-Dihydroxycholecalciferol and its periodate oxidation product

containing two additional hydroxyl groups in the side chain. Formation of a diacetate under mild conditions suggested the presence of two primary or secondary hydroxyl groups and one tertiary hydroxyl, which was shown to be located at C_{25} by the presence of fragments in the mass spectrum due to cleavage between C_{24} and C_{25}. Treatment of the compound with periodate gave rise to a product which, from its mass spectrum, could only be the aldehyde (81, Fig. 12), which could only have resulted by cleavage of a vicinal diol (Holick *et al.*, 1972b).

This metabolite has been synthesised, starting from 25-oxo-26-norcholesteryl acetate or from desmosteryl acetate. The ketone (59, Fig. 13) has been converted (Lam *et al.*, 1973) into a mixture of *cis*- and *trans*-enol acetates (82, Fig. 13), which were converted via the 24-bromo- and 24-iodo-derivatives into the 24-acetoxy-25-ketone (83, Fig. 13). A Grignard reaction with methylmagnesium iodide gave a mixture of 24,25-dihydroxycholesterols (84, Fig. 13), epimeric at C_{24}, which were then subjected to the usual sequence of reactions to give 24,25-dihydroxycholecalciferol (80, Fig. 13), obtained in 3% overall yield. One point worthy of note is that the 5,7-diene was purified by formation of the triazoline adduct of its triacetate; this adduct is readily separable from the 4,6-diene and from the starting material by chromatography and can be cleaved with metal hydrides. The separation of Δ^5- and $\Delta^{5,7}$-compounds is otherwise a difficult procedure. The 24*R*- and 24*S*-epimers present in the synthetic material have subsequently been separated by high-pressure liquid chromatography on silica gel as their tri-trimethylsilyl derivatives (Tanaka *et al.*, 1975a); the stereochemistry was determined for the separated 24*R*- and 24*S*-epimers of 24,25-dihydroxycholesterol (Seki *et al.*,

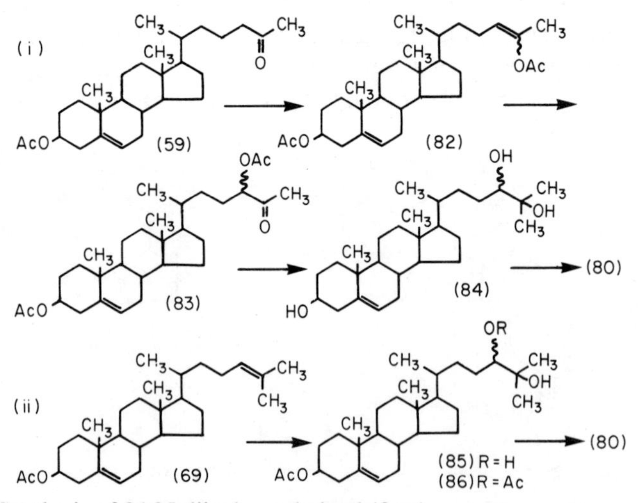

Fig. 13. Synthesis of 24,25-dihydroxycholecalciferol

1975). The natural material appears to be the 24*R*-epimer in that this epimer shows all the actions of cholecalciferol whereas the 24*S*-epimer is effective only in stimulating intestinal calcium transport (Tanaka *et al.*, 1975b).

In an alternative synthesis starting from desmosteryl acetate (69, Fig. 13), Redel and Bell have prepared the epimers of 24,25-dihydroxycholesteryl 3β-acetate (85, Fig. 13) by selective osmylation at Δ^{24} (Redel *et al.*, 1974a, 1975). The empimeric composition of the diacetate (86, Fig. 13) was determined by the addition of the chiral europium complex, tris-3-(trifluoromethylhydroxymethylene)-*d*-camphorato-europium, to a solution of the diacetate in carbon tetrachloride. This addition resulted in the proton magnetic resonance signal due to the acetate group at carbon-24 being resolved into two peaks of equal intensity, which indicated that approximately equal proportions of the 24*R*- and 24*S*-diastereoisomers were present. Introduction of the Δ^7-double bond and irradiation were performed by standard methods; it seems unlikely that the relative proportions of the diastereoisomers were changed in the course of these reactions. The diol (85, Fig. 13) has also been prepared by cleavage of the 24,25-epoxide of desmosteryl acetate with sulphuric acid (Seki *et al.*, 1973).

C 25,26-DIHYDROXYCHOLECALCIFEROL

From the plasma of chickens and pigs given tritiated cholecalciferol yet another hydroxylated metabolite has been isolated (Suda *et al.*, 1970c). The ultraviolet spectrum and mass spectra of this metabolite showed that the calciferol nucleus was intact and that two additional hydroxyl functions had been inserted into the side chain. Derivative formation established that one of these hydroxyl groups was tertiary, and mass spectral evidence indicated that the compound was a 25,26-dihydroxy-derivative (87, Fig. 14). This assignment was confirmed by periodate cleavage to the ketone (88, Fig. 14). The configuration at carbon-25 remains unknown.

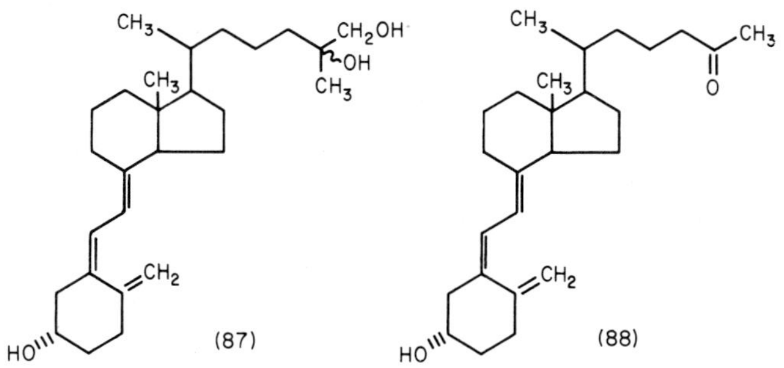

Fig. 14. 25,26-Dihydroxycholecalciferol and its periodate oxidation product

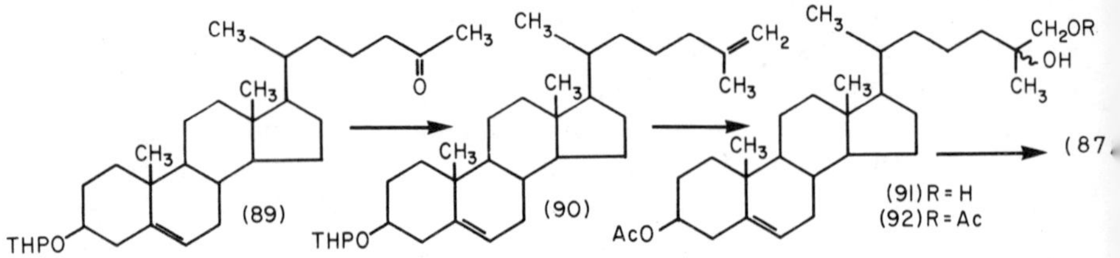

Fig. 15. Synthesis of 25,26-dihydroxycholecalciferol

This metabolite has been synthesised by Redel *et al.* (1973, 1974b) from the tetrahydropyranyl ether of 25-oxo-26-norcholesterol (89, Fig. 15), which was converted in a Wittig reaction to the 5,25-diene (90, Fig. 15). Hydrolysis and acetylation of the product were followed by selective osmylation of the Δ^{25}-double bond to give 25,26-dihydroxycholesteryl 3β-acetate (91, Fig. 15). The epimeric composition of the 3,26-diacetate (92, Fig. 15) was determined by proton magnetic resonance using a chiral europium complex, as for the 24,25-diol, and was shown to be an approximately equal mixture of 25*R*- and 25*S*-epimers. Subsequent steps in the synthesis were performed using standard methods, and the structure (87, Fig. 14) for the product was established by degradative and physicochemical methods. A similar route to the diol (91, Fig. 15) has been followed by other workers (Seki *et al.*, 1973).

D 1,25-DIHYDROXYCHOLECALCIFEROL AND 1-HYDROXYCHOLECALCIFEROL

The studies leading up to the isolation and identification of 1,25-dihydroxycholecalciferol will be described fully in subsequent chapters. The structure was established simultaneously by two laboratories (Lawson *et al.*, 1971a; Holick *et al.*, 1971a, b) and rests on a combination of mass spectral and degradative evidence, and on the distribution of tritium in labelled precursors. The mass spectrum of the compound showed a molecular ion at m/e 416 (632 for the tri-trimethylsilyl ether) indicating that two additional hydroxyl functions had been inserted into the molecule. Cleavage of the side chain gave a fragment with m/e 287, indicating that only one hydroxyl group was present in the side chain, and additional peaks due to cleavage between C_{24} and C_{25} located this hydroxyl at C_{25}. The remaining hydroxyl groups were located in the A ring by the detection of a specific fragment in the mass spectrum due to the A ring and carbons 6, 7 and 19. In cholecalciferol, cleavage of the C_7-C_8 bonds leads to a fragment with m/e 136 and a fragment at m/e 118 (136-H_2O). In the dihydroxy-compound, these peaks were replaced by peaks at 152 and 134, together with a peak at 116 (152-2H_2O).

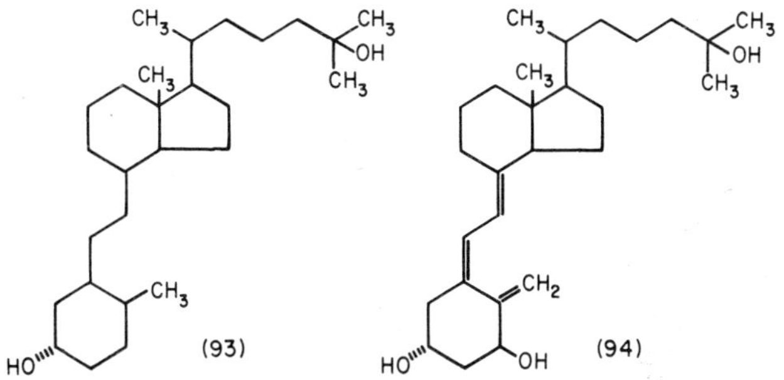

Fig. 16. 1α,25-Dihydroxycholecalciferol and its hydrogenation product

The Cambridge workers prepared the metabolite by incubation of 25-hydroxy[26-^{14}C, 1-^{3}H]cholecalciferol with a chick kidney homogenate and demonstrated that the product had lost at least 80% of the tritium originally present in the 25-hydroxycholecalciferol (Lawson *et al.*, 1971a). 25-Hydroxy-[1-^{3}H]cholecalciferol was prepared biosynthetically from [1-^{3}H]cholecalciferol, in which the tritium had been established to be located exclusively at the 1-position, with 85% in the 1α- and 15% in the 1β-position (Bell and Kodicek, 1970). This evidence, subsequently corroborated (Norman *et al.*, 1971), suggested that the remaining hydroxyl group is located at carbon-1, probably in the α-position. DeLuca and his collaborators investigated the location of the hydroxyl group by chemical methods. Catalytic reduction of the compound gave a hexahydro-diol, chromatographically identical with 93 (Fig. 16); hydrogenolysis of a hydroxyl group must therefore have occurred, and the hydroxyl must have been located in a position allylic to the triene system, on carbon-1 or carbon-4. The metabolite failed to react with periodate, however, which eliminated carbon 4 (and also carbon-2); thus, the metabolite must be 1,25-dihydroxycholecalciferol (94, Fig. 16). Confirmation of this proposed structure has come from synthesis; the medical and biological importance of this derivative has prompted several synthetic studies, and synthetic 1α,25-dihydroxycholecalciferol has been shown to be identical in chemical and biological properties with the metabolite (Semmler *et al.*, 1972).

The major problem in the synthesis of 1α,25-dihydroxycholecalciferol is that of introducing the 1α-hydroxyl function into the cholestane ring system while retaining the ability to generate the Δ^{5}-double bond subsequently. This problem has been successfully solved in syntheses which make use of established reactions, but most spectacularly by Barton and collaborators using an elegant and novel reaction sequence.

In the conventional synthetic routes, the 25-hydroxyl group was introduced at an early stage. DeLuca's group started from *i*-homocholanic acid methyl

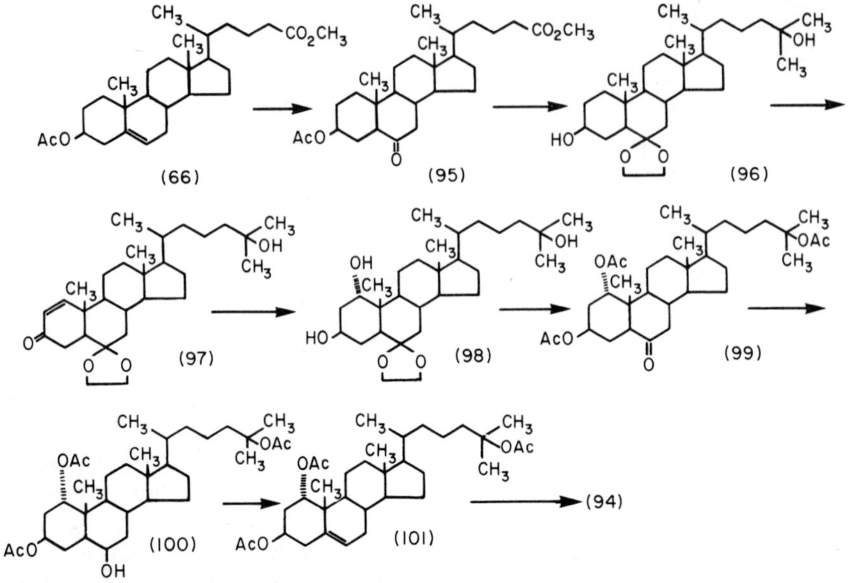

Fig. 17. Synthesis of 1α,25-dihydroxycholecalciferol (DeLuca)

ether, which was readily converted to the cholenic acid derivative (66, Fig. 17) in high yield (Semmler *et al.*, 1972). Nitration, reduction, and acid hydrolysis led to the ketone (95, Fig. 17), the key intermediate for subsequent functionalisation of ring B. After protection of the ketone as the ketal, a Grignard reaction led to the 25-hydroxy-derivative (96, Fig. 17). Oxidation of this compound with chromium trioxide in pyridine gave the 3-ketone, and bromination and dehydrobromination gave the Δ^1-3-ketone (97, Fig. 17). Epoxidation of this unsaturated ketone gave a 1α,2α-epoxide which was reduced with lithium aluminium hydride. Chromatography of the reduction product gave only the 1α,3α,25-triol, although the 1α,3β,25-triol might have been expected to be the major product. Semmler *et al.* (1972) have suggested that the 1α,3β,25-triol was lost on chromatography because of its high polarity. To obtain the desired 3β-isomer, the 1α,3α,25-triol was selectively oxidised with *N*-bromosuccinimide in pyridine and *t*-butanol, to give the 3-ketone. Reduction of this ketone with sodium borohydride then afforded the desired 1α,3β,25-triol (98, Fig. 17). Acetylation and mild acid hydrolysis gave the tri-acetoxy-ketone (99, Fig. 17) which on reduction with sodium borohydride gave the 6β-alcohol (100, Fig. 17). Dehydration of this alcohol with phosphorus oxychloride in pyridine then gave the Δ^5-compound (101,

Fig. 17), which was readily converted by the standard procedures of allylic bromination and dehydrobromination to the 5,7-diene. Irradiation of the 5,7-diene as its triacetate, followed by thermal isomerisation and hydrolysis, finally afforded the desired 1α,25-dihydroxycholecalciferol (94, Fig. 16), identical in chemical and biological properties with the natural metabolite.

In a related synthesis, only taken as far as 1α,25-dihydroxycholesterol, Japanese workers retained functionality at carbon-6 as the 6β-acetate (Rubio-Lightbourn *et al.*, 1973). Hydroboration of the dipyranyl ether (102, Fig. 18) of 25-hydroxycholesterol (Morisaki *et al.*, 1973a) gave a mixture of 5α,6α- and 5β,6β-isomers in which the 6α-hydroxy isomer (103, Fig. 18) predominated. Oxidation of the mixture of isomers, followed by borohydride reduction, led to the desired 5α,6β-isomer (104, Fig. 18). Protection of the 6β-hydroxyl function as its acetate and removal of the tetrahydropyranyl groups gave the 3β,25-diol-6β-acetate (105, Fig. 18). Oxidation of the 3β-hydroxyl

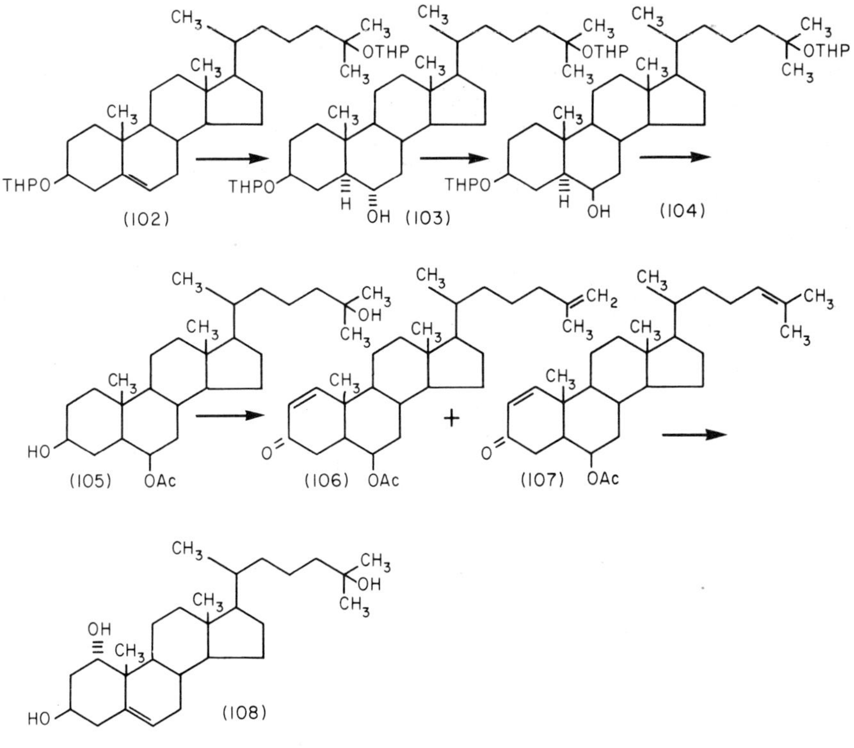

Fig. 18. Alternative synthesis of 1α,25-dihydroxycholesterol

group was followed by introduction of the Δ^1-double bond by α-bromination and dehydrobromination, but unfortunately under the conditions used by these workers dehydration at C_{25} also occurred, to give a mixture of dienes (106 and 107, Fig. 18).

These workers nevertheless proceeded with their synthesis using this mixture of dienes; formation of the 1α,2α-epoxide was followed by borohydride reduction of the 3-ketone to give predominantly the 3β-isomer. Protection of this group as the tetrahydropyranyl ether, saponification of the 6β-acetate, and dehydration with phosphorus oxychloride then afforded the Δ^5-compounds. Reduction of the epoxide with lithium aluminium hydride and removal of the protecting groups then gave the 1α,3β-diol. Reintroduction of the 25-hydroxyl group was then achieved by oxymercuration and demercuration, to give 1α,25-dihydroxycholesterol (108, Fig. 18).

A similar synthesis has recently been reported, also starting from 25-hydroxycholesterol and using a 6β-hydroxy-intermediate which was subsequently protected as its mesyl derivative; dehydration at C_{25} did not occur to the extent found by the Japanese workers (Narwid *et al.*, 1974b).

Even without the problems encountered, these syntheses are long, involved, and require separation of isomers at several stages. From a consideration of the well-known deconjugation reactions of Δ^4-3-ketosteroids, Barton *et al.* (1973) were led to speculate that, if a 4,6-dien-3-one such as 109 (Fig. 19) were reduced with lithium and ammonia in the presence of an effective proton source, an alternating sequence of reductions and protonations (Fig. 19) might lead to the desired 1α,3β-dihydroxy-Δ^5-compound (110, Fig. 19). This scheme was first shown to work for 1α,2α-epoxycholesta-1,4-dien-3-one and was subsequently applied to the synthesis of 1α,25-dihydroxycholesterol and 1α,25-dihydroxycholecalciferol (Barton *et al.*, 1974; Morisaki *et al.*, 1973b). Dehydrogenation of 25-hydroxycholesterol with dichlorodicyanobenzoquinone gave 25-hydroxycholesta-1,4,6-trien-3-one which, on treatment with

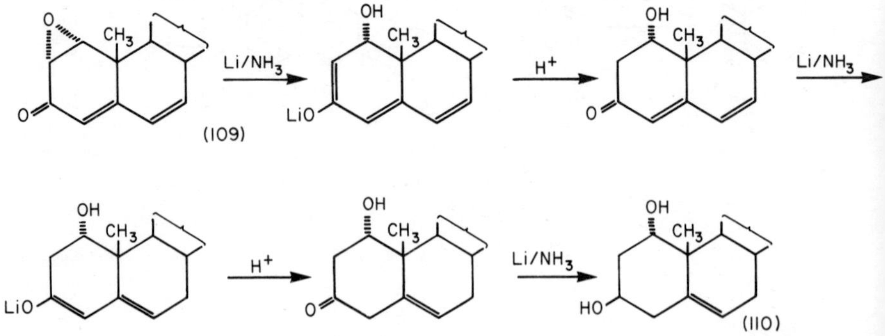

Fig. 19. Effect of a sequence of reductions and protonations on an unsaturated epoxide

alkaline hydrogen peroxide, gave the 1α,2α-epoxide. Treatment of this epoxide with large excesses each of lithium metal and ammonium chloride in a refluxing mixture of ammonia and tetrahydrofuran then gave, by the reaction sequence outlined in Fig. 19, 1α,25-dihydroxycholesterol in good yield. After conversion to the 1α,3β-diacetate, allylic bromination and dehydrobromination by the usual procedures led to the 5,7-diene. Irradiation, thermal isomerisation and saponification then gave the desired 1α,25-dihydroxycholecalciferol, obtained crystalline for the first time.

The related compound, 1α-hydroxycholecalciferol, has also been synthesised. Interest in this particular compound stems largely from the view that it may be biologically active after *in vivo* conversion to the 1α,25-dihydroxy-compound (a conversion which occurs in the liver) even when kidney function is impaired. From a commercial viewpoint the starting material, cholesterol, is readily available. Thus 1α-hydroxycholecalciferol has been synthesised by Barton *et al.* (1973) and by application of DeLuca's route to 1α,25-dihydroxycholecalciferol, utilising cholesterol as starting material (Holick *et al.*, 1973b). In addition, syntheses of 1α-hydroxycholesterol utilising conventional procedures have been reported (Pelc and Kodicek, 1970; Morisaki *et al.*, 1973c; Furst *et al.*, 1973).

The deconjugation reactions of unsaturated steroid ketones have been used to advantage in two recent syntheses (Kaneko *et al.*, 1974a, b). Cholesta-1,4-dien-3-one was deconjugated with potassium *t*-butoxide in dimethylsulphoxide followed by protonation, to give the unstable $\Delta^{1,5}$-3-ketone. Reduction with calcium borohydride in ethanol at −10°C gave the corresponding 3β-alcohol, which on hydroboration and oxidation with alkaline peroxide gave 1α-hydroxycholesterol and 2α-hydroxycholesterol, each in 15–20% yield (Kaneko *et al.*, 1973). Formation of the diacetate was followed by allylic bromination, dehydrobromination, and hydrolysis, to give 1α,3β-dihydroxycholesta-5,7-diene in 20% yield, and hence 1α-hydroxycholecalciferol. The authors suggested that the relatively low yield of the 5,7-diene was due to elimination of acetic acid at carbon-1 during the dehydrobromination procedure, and have subsequently published a synthesis of the 5,7-diene which elegantly overcomes this problem by using cholesta-1,4,6-trien-3-one (111, Fig. 20) as starting material. Deconjugation and reduction afford 3β-hydroxycholesta-1,5,7-triene (112, Fig. 20), which is converted to the triazoline adduct (113, Fig. 20) to protect the conjugated diene. Reaction of this adduct with 2 moles of *m*-chlorperbenzoic acid in chloroform gives the 1α,2α-epoxide (114, Fig. 20), which on refluxing with lithium aluminium hydride in tetrahydrofuran gives 1α,3β-dihydroxycholesta-5,7-diene (115, Fig. 20) in 5% overall yield (Kaneko *et al.*, 1974b).

Most interesting of these syntheses of 1α-hydroxycholecalciferol is the total

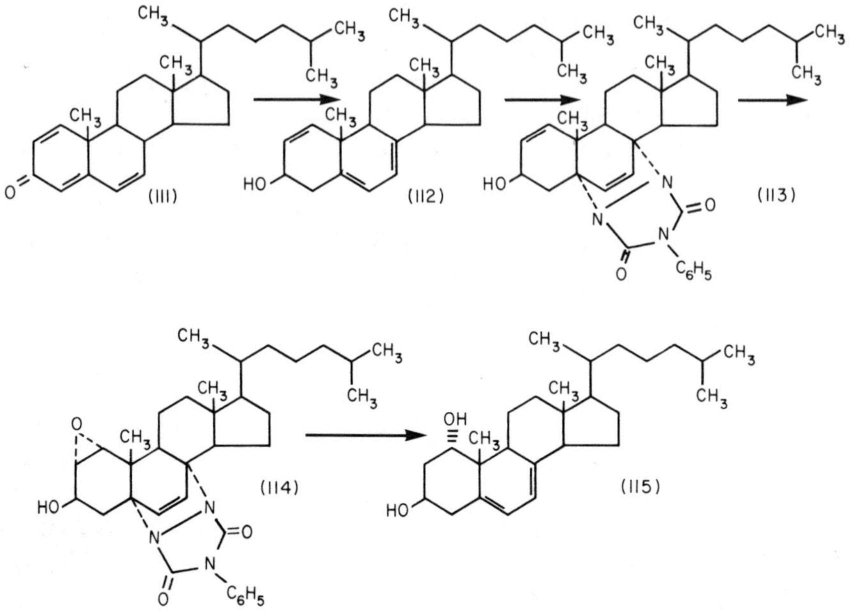

Fig. 20. Preparation of 1α,3β-dihydroxycholesta-5,7-diene via deconjugation reactions

synthesis reported recently by Harrison *et al.* (1973, 1974). These workers have converted the optically active lactone (116, Fig. 21) into the dihydroxy-acid (117, Fig. 21), and thence into the chloro-diene (118, Fig. 21), and the protected enyne (119, Fig. 21). The lithium derivative of this latter compound was reacted with 9α-chloro-des-*AB*-cholestan-8-one (51, Fig. 21) to give 120 (Fig. 21), which was converted, by methods already discussed for the total synthesis of cholecalciferol, into 1α-hydroxycholecalciferol (121, Fig. 21).

Yet another route to 1α-hydroxycholecalciferol has been devised in which cholecalciferol was treated with selenium dioxide and hydrogen peroxide in dioxane (B. Pelc, private communication). Four isomeric 1-hydroxycholecalciferols (1α-hydroxy-,1β-hydroxy-, 5*Z*- or 5*E*-) were obtained in low yield and were chromatographically separated and purified.

E 1,24,25-TRIHYDROXYCHOLECALCIFEROL

This metabolite has been produced *in vivo* in rats given 25-hydroxycholecalciferol and *in vitro* by incubation of 24,25-dihydroxycholecalciferol with chick

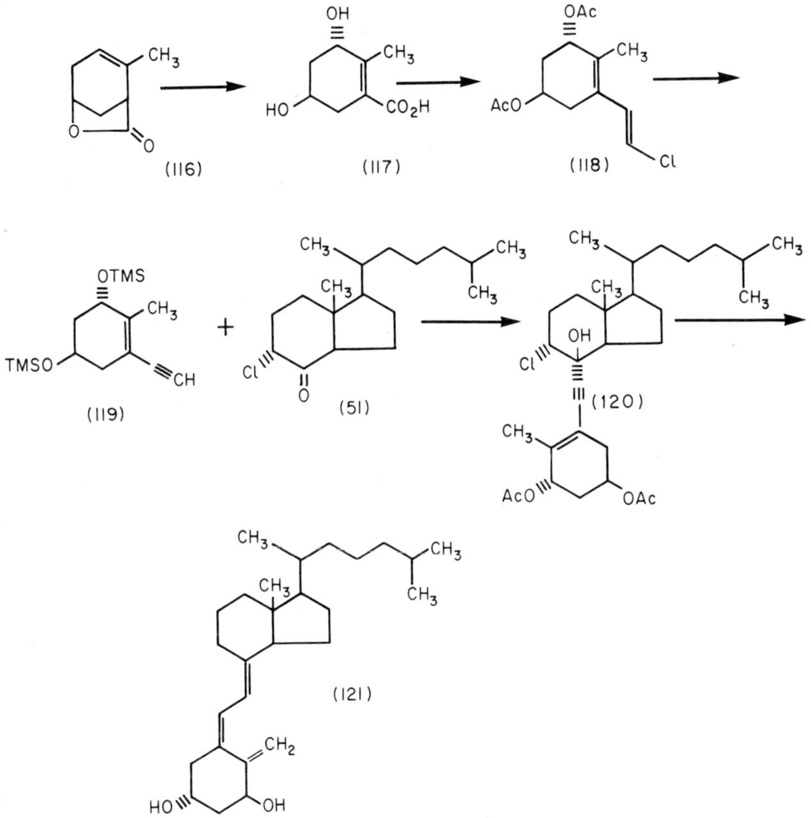

Fig. 21. Total synthesis of 1α-hydroxycholecalciferol

kidney homogenates (Holick *et al.*, 1973c). It has been identified by means of ultraviolet absorption spectrophotometry, mass spectrometry, and by its reaction with periodate. The 24*R*- and 24*S*-epimers have recently been synthesised (Ikekawa *et al.*, 1975a). 24,25-Dihydroxycholesterol was converted, through the 4,6-trien-3-one and its 1α,2-epoxide, into 1α,24ξ,25-trihydroxycholesterol. The C-24 epimers were separated and converted into (24R)-and (24S)-1α, 24,25,-trihydroxycholecalciferol in the usual way.

The synthesis of 1α,24-dihydroxycholecalciferol from 24-oxocholesterol has also been described (Morisaki *et al.*, 1975). The hydroxyl group at C-1 was inserted by Barton's procedure, and the monohydroxy-3,24-dibenzoate formed from resolution of the two C-24 epimers by silica gel column chromatography. The 1α,24-dihydroxycholecalciferol epimers were then formed in the usual manner.

VIII Calciferol Analogues

The preparation of analogues of the calciferols has received limited attention until recently, probably because most modifications have resulted in decreased biological activity. In addition, in many cases the products of irradiation have not been separated and purified, but have been subjected to biological assay as crude irradiation mixtures, with the presence of a calciferol analogue often being demonstrated spectroscopically.

Such modifications as have been prepared have mostly been those affecting the structure of the side chain or the group at the 3-position and have therefore involved little original chemistry. Modifications at the 3-position include the 3α-hydroxy-epimer and the 3β-thiol analogue and are listed in Table 5. Many modifications of the side chain have been reported, and these too are listed in Table 5. The identification of metabolites of cholecalciferol hydroxylated in the side chain has acted as a spur for further studies but, of the hydroxylated analogues produced to date, only 25-hydroxy-24-norcholecalciferol and 24-hydroxycholecalciferol have demonstrated significant biological activity; the only other side chain analogue with significant activity is 22,23-dihydro-ergocalciferol (vitamin D_4).

Relatively few modifications of the calciferol nucleus have been reported. Pelc (1974) has prepared 4α-hydroxycholecalciferol, and also the isomers of 1-hydroxycholecalciferol discussed in a previous section. 2α-Hydroxycholecalciferol has recently been prepared by hydroboration of cholesta-1,5-dien-3β-ol with 9-borabicyclo-(3.3.1)nonane followed by oxidation with alkaline hydrogen peroxide. Following acetylation of the product, the usual sequence of bromination, dehydrobromination, and irradiation led to the vitamin analogue (Kaneko *et al.*, 1975). Velluz and Amiard (1961) have prepared 11α-hydroxycholecalciferol. From considerations of structure-activity relationships, it has become apparent that the analogue possessing the 1α-hydroxyl group but lacking the hydroxyl group at the 3-position would be of interest, and this compound, 3-deoxy-1α-hydroxycholecalciferol, has recently been synthesised (Lam *et al.*, 1974; Okamura *et al.*, 1974b). In what is probably the most efficient route to this compound, 1α,2α-epoxycholesta-4,6-dien-3-one, the key intermediate in the synthesis of 1α-hydroxycholecalciferol by Barton's procedure, is reduced with lithium aluminium hydride to cholesta-4,6-dien-1α,3β-diol (Mitra *et al.*, 1974). Reduction of the diol with lithium in liquid ammonia then gives 1α-hydroxycholest-5-ene in 37% yield. The usual sequence of allylic bromination and dehydrobromination, irradiation, and thermal isomerisation gives 3-deoxy-1α-hydroxycholecalciferol, which has biological activity similar to that of 1α-hydroxycholecalciferol itself.

Table 5. Some analogues of the calciferols

(*a*) Modifications at the 3-position

Substituent	References
3α-OH, 3β-H	Windaus & Buchholz, 1939; Windaus & Naggatz, 1939; Aberhart *et al.*, 1976
3β-SH, 3α-H	Bernstein & Sax, 1951; Strating & Backer, 1950
3β-OH, 3α-CH_3	Strating, 1952; Strating & Backer, 1951
3β-CH_2OH, 3α-H	Strating, 1952; Strating & Backer, 1951
3β-CO_2CH_3, 3α-H	Strating, 1952; Strating & Backer, 1951

(*b*) Modifications of the side chain

Substituent at 17β-	References
H	Velluz *et al.*, 1957b
OH	Velluz *et al.*, 1957b; Butenandt *et al.*, 1938; Dimroth & Paland, 1939
$CH\cdot(CH_3)\cdot CH_2\cdot CH_2CO_2H$	Haslewood, 1939
$CH\cdot(CH_3)\cdot CH_2\cdot CH_2\cdot CH(C_2H_5)\cdot CH(CH_3)_2$	Haslewood, 1939
$CH\cdot(CH_3)\cdot CH_2\cdot(CH_2)_2\cdot CH_2\cdot CH_3$	Alberti *et al.*, 1949, 1950
$CH\cdot(CH_3)\cdot CH_2\cdot CH_2\cdot CH(CH_3)\cdot CH(CH_3)_2$	Windaus & Trautmann, 1937
$CH\cdot(CH_3)\cdot CH_2\cdot(CH_2)_2\cdot CH_2\cdot CH_2\cdot CH(CH_3)_2$	Louw *et al.*, 1955
$CH\cdot(CH_3)\cdot CH_2\cdot(CH_2)_3\cdot CH_2\cdot CH(CH_3)_2$	Louw *et al.*, 1955
$CH\cdot(CH_3)\cdot CO\cdot N(CH_3)_2$	Louw *et al.*, 1955
$CH\cdot(CH_3)\cdot CH_2\cdot N(CH_3)_2$	Louw *et al.*, 1955
$C\cdot(CH_3)\cdot OH\cdot CH_2\cdot CH_2\cdot CH_2\cdot C(CH_3)_2OH$	Bontekoe *et al.*, 1970
$C\cdot(CH_3)\cdot OH\cdot CH_2\cdot CH_2\cdot CH_2\cdot CH(CH_3)OH$	Bontekoe *et al.*, 1970
$CH\cdot(CH_3)\cdot CH_2\cdot CH_2\cdot CH_2\cdot OH$	Bontekoe *et al.*, 1970
$CH\cdot(CH_3)\cdot CH_2\cdot(CH_2)_2\cdot CH_2\cdot OH$	Bontekoe *et al.*, 1970; Holick *et al.*, 1975
$CH\cdot(CH_3)\cdot CH_2\cdot CH_2\cdot CH_2\cdot CH(CH_3)OH$	Bontekoe *et al.*, 1970; Holick *et al.*, 1975
$CH\cdot(CH_3)\cdot CHOH\cdot CH_2\cdot CH(CH_3)\cdot CH(CH_3)_2$	Crump *et al.*, 1973
$CH\cdot(CH_3)\cdot CH_2\cdot CH_2\cdot C(CH_3)_2OH$	Holick *et al.*, 1972a
$CH\cdot(CH_3)\cdot CH_2\cdot CH_2\cdot CHOH\cdot CH(CH_3)$ [24*R*- and 24*S*-]	Ikekawa *et al.*, 1975b; Tanaka *et al.*, 1975b.

IX Synthesis of Radioactive Calciferols

The synthesis of radioactively labelled compounds for use in metabolic studies or in competitive binding assays requires a somewhat different experimental approach from that required for normal chemical syntheses. Conflicting requirements for high stability, specificity of labelling, high specific activity, and overall cost-effectiveness have in some way to be reconciled; the development of syntheses of radioactively labelled calciferols illustrates several aspects of this specialised area of synthetic organic chemistry.

Optimum stability and specificity of labelling can best be attained using carbon-14, but this in many cases means incorporating the isotope at an early stage of the synthesis. Thus Havinga and Bots (1954) prepared [3-^{14}C]cholecalciferol from [3-^{14}C]cholestenone; similarly the commercially available [4-^{14}C]cholecalciferol originates from the synthesis of [4-^{14}C]cholestenone (Fujimoto, 1951; Heard and Ziegler, 1951). [4-^{14}C]Ergocalciferol has similarly been prepared (Pelc and Kodicek, 1972b). Although high specificity can be attained by these methods the specific activity is low, as is the efficiency of the synthesis in terms of incorporation of radioactivity into the final product. Biosynthetic procedures have also been used for the preparation of [^{14}C]ergocalciferol but result in more general labelling (Kodicek, 1959; Schaltegger, 1960; Imrie *et al.*, 1967).

High specific activities can best be obtained using tritium. The introduction of tritium can be accomplished by one of several general methods: exchange with hydrogens already present, replacement of other substituents, or direct addition to unsaturated linkages. Isotype exchange by the Wilzbach technique (Wilzbach, 1957) or by platinum-catalysed exchange with tritiated acetic acid (Peng, 1963; Parekh and Wasserman, 1965; Thompson *et al.*, 1966) has the advantage that it can be performed on cholecalciferol itself, but the distribution of the label is unknown, as is its stability.

Substitution reactions have been widely used, though they can suffer from considerable disadvantages. Thus treatment of 3β-benzoyloxy-6-bromo-5-cholesten-7-one (122, Fig. 22) with zinc and [^{3}H]acetic acid gave the 6-tritiated intermediate (123, Fig. 22), while reduction of this intermediate (non-tritiated) with sodium [^{3}H]borohydride gave the 7-tritiated intermediate (124, Fig. 22), both of which were readily converted into the corresponding tritiated 7-dehydrocholesterols, and subsequently into [6-^{3}H]- or [7-^{3}H]cholecalciferol (Callow *et al.*, 1966). The disadvantages of these procedures are that the zinc-acetic acid procedure requires a large excess of the tritium donor and that, in borohydride reductions, a maximum of 25% of the activity is incorporated. Metal hydride reductions may also be subject to adverse isotope effects (Chauduri *et al.*, 1962). Nevertheless such reactions can sometimes be employed with success as the recent studies on the metabolism of the clinically useful analogue, 1-hydroxycholecalciferol, have shown. Treatment of 1α,3β-diacetoxy-5α-cholestan-6-one with sodium [^{3}H]boro-hydride for three days gave the [6-^{3}H]intermediate which was converted into the 7-dehydrocholesterol derivative by treatment with phosphorus oxychloride followed by bromination and dehydrobromination. Irradiation of this provitamin derivative and saponification gave 1α-hydroxy-[6-^{3}H]-cholecalciferol of high specific activity (Holick *et al.*, 1976).

Catalytic reduction of a double bond with tritium gas is inherently more efficient than other techniques and can give very high specific activities. The most efficient syntheses of tritiated calciferols have utilised this procedure, in most cases inserting tritium into the 1- and 2-positions (Callow *et al.*, 1966; Neville and DeLuca, 1966). [1,2-$^3H_2$]Cholecalciferol has been prepared from [1,2-$^3H_2$]cholesterol, which was in turn prepared via partial heterogeneous catalytic tritiation of cholesta-1,4-dien-3-one to the 4-en-3-one, but this reaction gives poor yields of the partially reduced product. Higher yields in the

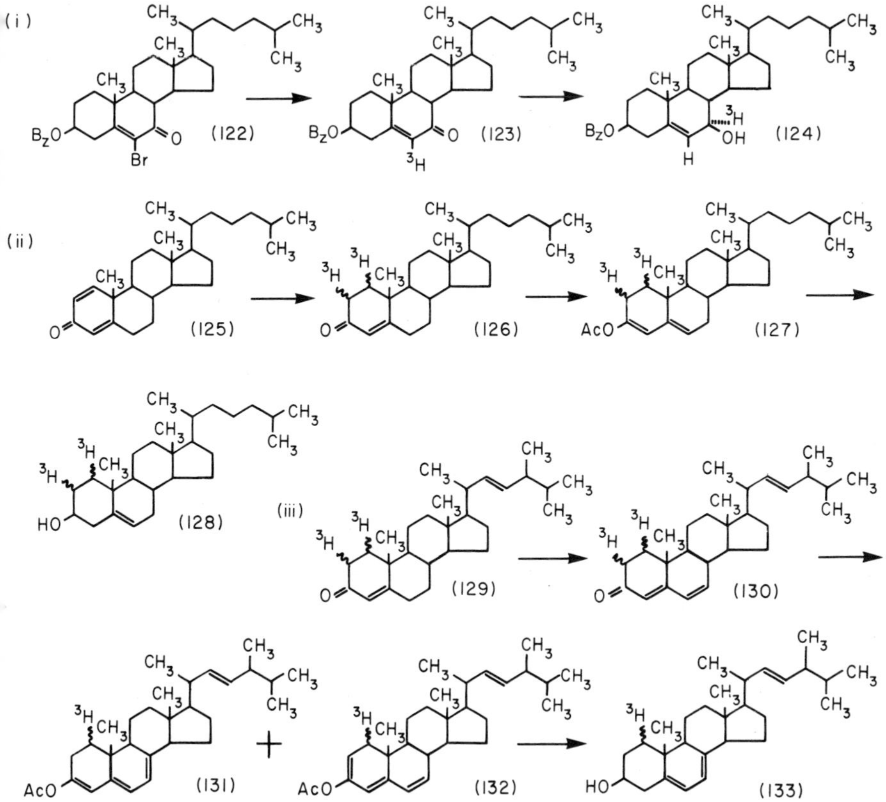

(i) (122) → (123) → (124)

(ii) (125) → (126) → (127) → (128)

(iii) (129) → (130) → (131) + (132) → (133)

Fig. 22. Intermediates in the synthesis of tritiated calciferols

tritiation procedure may be obtained by reduction of 5α-cholest-1-en-3-one to 5α-cholestan-3-one; [1-^{3}H]cholecalciferol was prepared (Callow *et al.*, 1966) by this procedure via [1,2-$^{3}H_2$]cholestan-3-one, from which tritium in the 2-position was removed by alkali equilibration. This gain in yield at one stage is, however, offset by the decrease in overall yield caused by the additional steps necessary for conversion into cholest-4-en-3-one.

Improvements in this synthesis were brought about by the introduction of the homogeneous hydrogenation catalyst, tristriphenylphosphinerhodium chloride, which enables the partial reduction of steroid 1,4-dien-3-ones to be performed with high yields. Thus partial reduction of cholesta-1,4-dien-3-one (125, Fig. 22) with tritium gas afforded the 1,2-tritiated compound (126, Fig. 22) which was converted by standard methods into the enol acetate (127, Fig. 22), cholesterol (128, Fig. 22), 7-dehydrocholesterol, and finally [1,2-$^{3}H_2$]cholecalciferol (Lawson *et al.*, 1971b). In an interesting variation of this procedure, Pelc and Kodicek (1971) prepared [1,2-$^{3}H_2$]ergost-4-en-3-one (129, Fig. 22) by essentially the same procedure, but then converted this compound into isoergosterone (130, Fig. 22). Enol acetylation gave a mixture of the enol acetates (131 and 132, Fig. 22), which on reduction with sodium borohydride gave ergosterol (133, Fig. 22) in 50% yield from (130, Fig. 22). Subsequent irradiation gave [1-^{3}H]ergocalciferol, tritium having been lost from the 2-position in the course of the enol acetylation.

Tritium insertion in the 1- and 2-positions also lends itself to determination of the tritium localisation by using the variety of known stereospecific transformations of the A and B rings of steroids. These techniques have been applied to the [1-^{3}H]- and [1,2-$^{3}H_2$]cholesterol used as precursors for the corresponding tritiated cholecalciferols (Bell and Kodicek, 1970), and Pelc and Kodicek (1972a) subsequently applied similar procedures to [1-^{3}H]ergosterol. [1-^{3}H]Cholesterol and [1-^{3}H]ergosterol showed an almost identical distribution of tritium, with about 85% being in the 1α-position and 15% in the 1β-position. Less than 2% of the total radioactivity was located elsewhere. [1,2-$^{3}H_2$]Cholesterol showed an uneven distribution of tritium between the 1- and 2-positions, with approximately 60% at position 1 (45% 1α- and 15% 1β-). It was assumed that changes in the distribution of radioactivity would be unlikely to occur during the course of subsequent reactions, so that this distribution would apply to the calciferols produced. These assumptions have been validated (E. A. Evans, private communication) using triton nuclear magnetic resonance spectometry, whereby it has been shown that the distribution of tritium in a sample of [1,2-$^{3}H_2$]cholecalciferol is 53.4% 1α- 9.1% 1β-, and 37.5% (2(α+β)-, in good agreement with the data obtained by degradative procedures. [22,23-$^{3}H_2$]-22,23-Dihydroergocalciferol has also been prepared by similar methods, by tritiation of the maleic anhydride adduct of ergosterol (DeLuca *et al.*, 1968).

25-Hydroxycholecalciferol is especially suitable for radiochemical syntheses as tritium or carbon-14 can obviously be inserted using radioactive Grignard reagents. Thus [^{3}H]methylmagnesium iodide can be caused to react with 25-oxo-26-norcholesteryl acetate or the corresponding 5,7-diene (Suda *et al.*, 1971); as the subsequent irradiation step proceeds in low yield, it is clearly advantageous to delay insertion of the radioactive component until a stage after the photochemical reaction. Bell and Scott (1973) used this principle in a synthesis in which 25-oxo-26-norcholecalciferyl acetate was reacted with [^{3}H]methylmagnesium iodide to give, after saponification, 25-hydroxy-[26,27-^{3}H]cholecalciferol of specific activity 10.6 Ci/m-mole. This synthesis has produced labelled material with the highest activity of any calciferol analogue yet achieved. 25-Hydroxy-[26,27-^{14}C]cholecalciferol has been prepared by similar methods (Bell and Scott, unpublished).

Other compounds related to the calciferols have been obtained in a radioactive form either by isomerisation of the appropriately labelled calciferol, e.g. 5,6-*trans*-[4-^{14}C]- and 5,6-*trans*-[1,2-$^{3}H_2$]cholecalciferol, and 25-hydroxy-5,6-*trans*-[26,27-^{14}C]cholecalciferol, or by conversion of a labelled isomer obtained on irradiation, e.g. [1,2-$^{3}H_2$]dihydrotachysterol$_3$ (Lawson and Bell, 1974).

X Conformation and Structure-Activity Relationships

Geometric and configurational isomerism among the calciferols has been discussed in the earlier sections but a further aspect of the isomerism of these molecules comes from conformational isomerism, resulting from rotation about single bonds. The preferred conformations of these substances in a given physical state have been established in recent years, using high-resolution proton magnetic resonance spectrometry and chemical shift techniques. This information on the preferred conformations of these seco-steroids may give some insight into structure-activity relationships.

Precalciferol and tachysterol may obviously adopt different conformations by rotation around the 5,6- or 7,8-single bonds respectively; application of the Nuclear Overhauser Effect has shown that the conformations shown in Fig. 5 are the preferred ones in solution (Lugtenburg and Havinga, 1969; Sanders *et al.*, 1969). Conformational equilibria can not only occur as a result of rotation around one single bond, but can also occur in ring systems. The cyclohexane ring system is the classic example, where dynamic equilibria are possible between different 'chair' or 'boat' conformations. In the case of the calciferols the implications of these considerations have only recently been appreciated. The structure of ergocalciferol was first studied by physical methods by Hodgkin and co-workers, who analysed the structure of the 4′-iodo-5′-nitrobenzoate ester by x-ray crystallography (Crowfoot and Dunitz, 1948;

Hodgkin *et al.*, 1963). Their analysis established that, in the crystal, the structure was as shown in (a), Fig. 23, with the ester group in an equatorial position, and the terminal methylene below the plane of the co-planar 5,7-diene. What was perhaps not widely appreciated about this structure was that this conformation is the result of the presence of the bulky ester substituent, which adopts the energetically favourable equatorial position. That this is so has been recently demonstrated by the x-ray crystallographic analysis of an analogue of calciferol, 3,20-*bis*(ethylenedioxy)-9,10-secopregna-5,7,10(19)-triene (Knobler *et al.*, 1972). In this compound no directive influence affects the 3-position and in the crystal it adopts the conformation having the terminal methylene group above the plane of the 5,7-diene. In solution a rapid equilibrium would be expected between these two forms (Havinga, 1973), that having the methylene above the plane (axial hydroxyl) (b, Fig. 23) and that having the methylene below the plane (equatorial hydroxyl) (a, Fig. 23), and this has now been confirmed by high resolution proton magnetic resonance studies (Wing *et al.*, 1974). Utilising 300 MHz p.m.r. spectroscopy, these authors analysed the coupling between the 3α- and 4β-hydrogens of cholecalciferol in solution. In the form of the A-ring with the hydroxyl group in the equatorial position, the 3α- and 4β-hydrogens are *trans*-diaxial, whereas with the hydroxyl group in the axial position these protons are *trans*-diequatorial. From model compounds it is known that *trans*-diaxial protons give couplings of $\sim$11 Hz, whereas *trans*-diequatorial protons give couplings of $\sim$4 Hz. In cholecalciferol the coupling was observed to be 7.4 Hz, which implies that about half of the molecules are in each of the two possible conformations. In dihydrotachysterol$_3$, however, the coupling is 10.0 Hz, which implies that the form with the equatorial hydroxyl group is favoured, a result predictable on the basis of conformational theory since the alternative conformation requires both the 3β-hydroxyl and 19-methyl groups to be in the energetically unfavourable axial conformation. An analysis of the compounds known to possess biological activity in anephric animals (in which 1-hydroxylation is considered not to occur) indicates that all such compounds possess a hydroxyl group located equatorially in a position geometrically corresponding to the 1-hydroxyl group of 1α,25-dihydroxycholecalciferol, but do not require a hydroxyl nor a C_{19}-methylene in positions geometrically corresponding to the 3β-hydroxyl or C_{19}-methylene groups of 1α,25-dihydroxycholecalciferol. The importance of the *pseudo*-1-hydroxyl group being equatorially located has been emphasised by Okamura *et al.* (1974a); they point out that dihydrocalciferol IV will preferentially adopt a conformation in which the hydroxyl group occupies an axial position because of the stronger preference of the C_{19}-methyl group for an equatorial orientation, and that this correlates with the known lesser activity of this compound relative to dihydrotachysterol. They have extended this argument for the

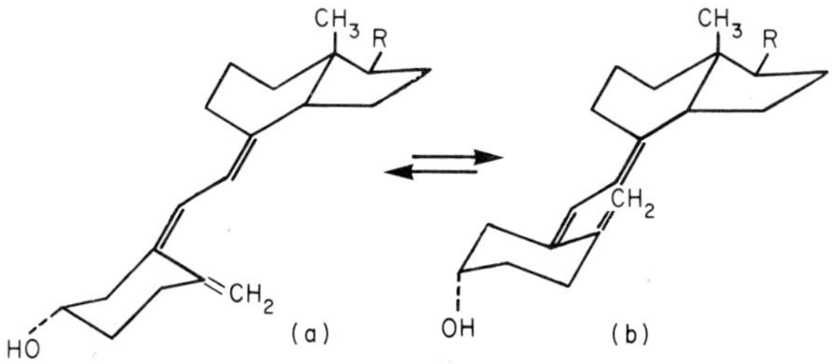

Fig. 23 Conformational equilibrium between forms of calciferol with (a) equatorial 3β-hydroxyl, and (b) axial 3β-hydroxyl

importance of an equatorial 1-hydroxyl or *pseudo*-1-hydroxyl group in affording biological activity by pointing out that in the case of 1α,25-dihydroxycholecalciferol the two possible conformations of the A-ring can only have an equatorial-axial or axial-equatorial combination of the 1α- and 3β-hydroxyl groups and, since the steric environments of the two hydroxyls are similar, then the two conformations should be essentially similar and present in equal proportions. In more recent studies using p.m.r. spectroscopy (Wing *et al.*, 1975), this group have now shown that the conformational equilibrium in 1α-hydroxycholecalciferol is shifted slightly to favour the axial 3β-hydroxyl, with approximately 56% having this conformation. 1α-Hydroxyepicholecalciferol has also been prepared and studied by similar techniques; due to hydrogen bonding the 1α-, 3β-diaxial form is favoured in this case (Okamura and Pirio, 1975; Sheves *et al.*, 1975). The 3-deoxy analogue however should be biased in favour of the form with the 1α-hydroxyl group in the equatorial conformation (Okamura *et al.*, 1974a).

These studies are of considerable interest, but much further work is required to delineate the precise structural requirements for biological activity. If one compares the requirements for activity in the calciferol series with those for another group of hormones, for example the glucocorticoids, it is of interest to note that studies with corticosteroids have led to the conclusion that while only one hydroxyl group (the 11β-hydroxyl) is obligatory for biological activity to be expressed, other hydroxyl groups function to increase the affinity of the hormone for the tissue receptor (Munck *et al.*, 1972) and thus lower the concentration needed for maximum response. Similarly, it may well be that the 25-hydroxyl and 3β-hydroxyl groups of 1α,25-dihydroxycholecalciferol increase the affinity of the compound for its tissue receptor. In support of these ideas are the studies of Brumbaugh and Haussler (1973) on the interaction of calciferols with tissue receptors. In their assay, 1α-hydroxycholecalciferol is only 1/450 as effective as 1α,25-dihydroxycholecalciferol in displacing radioactive 1α,25-dihydroxycholecalciferol from the receptor.

If the receptor discriminates between equatorial and axial conformations at position 1, it seems unlikely that the effect of varying the conformational equilibrium will be to affect the intrinsic activity; rather it will alter the apparent affinity of the compound for the receptor, since two equilibria have to be considered:

$$[\text{axial form}] \rightleftarrows [\text{equatorial form}]$$

and

$$[\text{equatorial form}] \rightleftarrows [\text{receptor-bound equatorial form}]$$

Amplification of these ideas requires studies with isolated receptors as well as intact animals, but that their application is not only of interest to biologists has already been demonstrated by the fact that the lack of biological activity of isocholecalciferol in anephric animals has caused its assigned structure to be questioned (Holick *et al.*, 1973a).

References

Aberhart, D. J., Chu, J. Y. R. and Hsu, A. C. T. (1976). *J. Org. Chem.* **41**, 1067.

Akhtar, M. and Gibbons, C. J. (1965). *J. Chem. Soc.* 5964.

Alberti, C. G., Camerino, B. and Mamoli, L. (1949). *Helv. Chim. Acta* **32**, 2038.

Alberti, C. G., Camerino, B. and Mamoli, L. (1950). *Helv. Chim. Acta* **33**, 229.

Askew, F. A., Bourdillon, R. B., Bruce, H. M., Callow, R. K., Philpot, J. St. L. and Webster, T. A. (1932). *Proc. Roy. Soc. Ser. B.* **109**, 488.

Barton, D. H. R., Hesse, R. H., Pechet, M. M. and Rizzardo, E. (1973). *J. Amer. Chem. Soc.* **95**, 2748.

Barton, D. H. R., Hesse, R. H., Pechet, M. M. and Rizzardo, E. (1974). *J. Chem. Soc. Chem. Commun.* 203.

Bell, P. A. and Kodicek, E. (1970). *Biochem. J.* **116**, 755.

Bell, P. A. and Scott, W. P. (1973). *J. Labelled Cpds.* **9**, 339.

Bernstein, S. and Sax, K. J. (1951). *J. Org. Chem.* **16**, 685.

Blackwood, J. E., Gladys, C. L., Loening, K. L., Petrarca, A. E. and Rush, J. E. (1968). *J. Amer. Chem. Soc.* **90**, 509.

Bloothoofd-Kruisbeek, A. M. and Lugtenburg, J. (1972). *Rec. Trav. Chim. Pays-Bas* **91**, 1364.

Blunt, J. W. and DeLuca, H. F. (1969). *Biochemistry* **8**, 671.

Blunt, J. W., DeLuca, H. F. and Schnoes, H. K. (1968a). *Chem. Commun.* 801.

Blunt, J. W., DeLuca, H. F. and Schnoes, H. K. (1968b). *Biochemistry* **7**, 3317.

Bolton, I. J., Harrison, R. G. and Lythgoe, B. (1971). *J. Chem. Soc.* **C**, 2950.

Bontekoe, J. S., Wignall, A., Rappoldt, M. P. and Roborgh, J. R. (1970). *Int. J. Vitam. Res.* **40**, 589.

Boomsma, F., Jacobs, H. J. C., Havinga, E. and Van der Gen, A. (1975). *Tetrahedron Lett.* 427.

Brockmann, H. (1936). *Hoppe-Seyler's Z. Physiol. Chem.* **241**, 104.

Brockmann, H. and Busse, A. (1938). *Naturwissenschaften* **26**, 122.

Brown, H. C., Brewster, J. H. and Schechter, H. (1954). *J. Amer. Chem. Soc.* **76**, 467.

Brumbaugh, P. F. and Haussler, M. R. (1973). *Life Sci.* **13**, 1737.

Butenandt, A., Hausmann, E. and Paland, J. (1938). *Ber. Deut. Chem. Ges.* **71**, 1316.
Cahn, R. S., Ingold, C. and Prelog, V. (1966). *Angew. Chem. Internat. Ed. Engl.* **5**, 385.
Callow, R. K. (1934). *Scient. J. Roy Coll. Sci.* **4**, 41.
Callow, R. K., Kodicek, E. and Thompson, G. A. (1966). *Proc. Roy Soc. Ser. B.* **164**, 1.
Campbell, J. A., Squires, D. M. and Babcock, J. C. (1969). *Steroids* **13**, 567.
Chauduri, A. C., Harada, Y., Shimiza, K., Gut, M. and Dorfman, R. I. (1962). *J. Biol. Chem.* **237**, 703.
Crowfoot, D. and Dunitz, J. D. (1948). *Nature* (London) **162**, 608.
Crump, D. R., Williams, D. H. and Pelc, B. (1973). *J. Chem. Soc. Perkin I* 2731.
Dauben, W. G. and Fonken, G. J. (1959). *J. Amer. Chem. Soc.* **81**, 4060.
Davidson, R. S., Littlewood, P. S., Medcalfe, T., Waddington-Feather, S. M., Williams, D. H. and Lythgoe, B. (1963). *Tetrahedron Lett.* 1413.
Davidson, R. S., Gunther, W. H. H., Waddington-Feather, S. M. and Lythgoe, B. (1964). *J. Chem. Soc.* 4907.
Davidson, R. S., Waddington-Feather, S. M., Williams, D. H. and Lythgoe, B. (1967). *J. Chem. Soc.* **C**, 2534.
Dawson, T. M., Dixon, J., Littlewood, P. S. and Lythgoe, B. (1971a). *J. Chem. Soc.* **C**, 2352.
Dawson, T. M., Dixon, J., Littlewood, P. S., Lythgoe, B. and Saksena, A. K. (1971b). *J. Chem. Soc.* **C**, 2960.
Delaroff, V. P., Rathle, P. and Legrand, M. (1963). *Bull Soc. Chim. Fr.* 1739.
DeLuca, H. F., Weller, M., Blunt, J. W. and Neville, P. F. (1968). *Arch. Biochem. Biophys.* **124**, 122.
Dimroth, K. and Paland, J. (1939). *Ber. Deut. Chem. Ges.* **72**, 187.
Dixon, J., Littlewood, P. S., Lythgoe, B. and Saksena, A. K. (1970). *Chem. Commun.* 993.
Dixon, J., Lythgoe, B., Siddiqui, I. A. and Tideswell, J. (1971). *J. Chem. Soc.* **C**,1301.
Eyley, S. C. and Williams, D. H. (1975). *J. Chem. Soc. Chem. Commun.* 858.
Fujimoto, G. I. (1951). *J. Amer. Chem. Soc.* **73**, 1856.
Furst, A., Labler, L., Meier, W. and Pfoertner, K.-H. (1973). *Helv. Chim. Acta* **56**, 1708.
Furst, W. (1965). *Pharm. Zentralhalle* **104**, 381.
Halkes, S. J. and Van Vliet, N. P. (1969). *Rec. Trav. Chim. Pays-Bas* **88**, 1080.
Hanewald, K. H., Rappoldt, M. P. and Roborgh, J. R. (1961). *Rec. Trav. Chim. Pays-Bas* **80**, 1003.
Harrison, I. T. and Lythgoe, B. (1957). *Proc. Chem. Soc.* 261.
Harrison, I. T. and Lythgoe, B. (1958). *J. Chem. Soc.* 837.
Harrison, R. G., Lythgoe, B. and Wright, P. W. (1973). *Tetrahedron Lett.* 3649.
Harrison, R. G., Lythgoe, B. and Wright, P. W. (1974). *J. Chem. Soc. Perkin I* 2654.
Haslewood, G. A. D. (1939). *Biochem. J.* **33**, 454.
Havinga, E. (1973). *Experientia* **29**, 1181.
Havinga, E. and Bots, J. P. L. (1954). *Rec. Trav. Chim. Pays-Bas* **73**, 393
Havinga, E. and Schlatmann, J. L. M. A. (1961). *Tetrahedron* **16**, 146.
Havinga, E., Koevoet, A. L. and Verloop, A. (1955). *Rec. Trav. Chim. Pays-Bas* **74**, 1230.
Havinga, E., De Kock, R. J. and Rappoldt, M. P. (1960). *Tetrahedron* **11**, 276.
Heard, R. D. H. and Ziegler, P. (1951). *J. Amer. Chem. Soc.* **73**, 4036.
Heilbron, I. M. and Spring, F. S. (1935). *Chem. Ind.* (London) **54**, 795.

Heilbron, I. M., Jones, R. N., Samant, K. M. and Spring, F. S. (1936). *J. Chem. Soc.* 905.
Heilbron, I. M., Samant, K. M. and Spring, F. S. (1935). *Nature* (London) **135**, 1072.
Hess, A. F. and Weinstock, M. (1924). *J. Biol. Chem.* **62**, 301.
Hess, A. F., Weinstock, M. and Helman, F. D. (1925). *J. Biol. Chem.* **63**, 305.
Hodgkin, D. C. and Sayre, D. (1952). *J. Chem. Soc.* 4561.
Hodgkin, D. C., Rimmer, B. M., Dunitz, J. D. and Trueblood, K. N. (1963). *J. Chem. Soc.* 4945.
Holick, M. F., Schnoes, H. K. and DeLuca, H. F. (1971a). *Proc. Nat. Acad. Sci. U.S.* **68**, 803.
Holick, M. F., Schnoes, H. K., DeLuca, H. F., Suda, T. and Cousins, R. J. (1971b). *Biochemistry* **10**, 2799.
Holick, M. F., Garabedian, M. and DeLuca, H. F. (1972a). *Biochemistry* **11**, 2715.
Holick, M. F., Schnoes, H. K., DeLuca, H. F., Gray, R. W., Boyle, I. T. and Suda, T. (1972b). *Biochemistry* **11**, 4251.
Holick, M. F., DeLuca, H. F., Kasten, P. M. and Korycka, M. B. (1973a). *Science* **180**, 964.
Holick, M. F., Semmler, E. J., Schnoes, H. K. and DeLuca, H. F. (1973b). *Science* **180**, 190.
Holick, M. F., Kleiner-Bossaller, A., Schnoes, H. K., Kasten, P. M., Boyle, I. T. and DeLuca, H. F. (1973c). *J. Biol. Chem.* **248**, 6691.
Holick, M. F., Garabedian, M., Schnoes, H. K. and DeLuca, H. F. (1975). *J. Biol. Chem.* **250**, 226.
Holick, M. F., Tavela, T. E., Holick, S. A., Schnoes, H. K., DeLuca, H. F. and Gallagher, B. M. (1976). *J. Biol. Chem.* **251**, 1020.
Ikekawa, N., Morisaki, M., Koizumi, N., Kato, Y. and Takeshita, T. (1975a). *Chem. Pharm. Bull.* (Japan) **23**, 695.
Ikekawa, N., Morisaki, M., Koizumi, N., Sawamura, M., Tanaka, Y. and DeLuca, H. F. (1975b). *Biochem. Biophys. Res. Commun.* **62**, 485.
Imrie, M. H., Neville, P. F., Snellgrove, A. W. and DeLuca, H. F. (1967). *Arch. Biochem. Biophys.* **120**, 525.
Inhoffen, H. H. (1958). *Angew. Chem.* **70**, 576.
Inhoffen, H. H. (1960). *Angew. Chem.* **72**, 875.
Inhoffen, H. H., Bruckner, K. and Grundel, R. (1954). *Chem. Ber.* **87**, 1.
Inhoffen, H. H., Kath, J. F. and Bruckner, K. (1955). *Angew. Chem.* **67**, 276.
Inhoffen, H. H., Quinkert, G., Hess, H.-J. and Erdmann, H. M. (1956). *Chem. Ber.* **89**, 2273.
Inhoffen, H. H., Quinkert, G., Hess, H.-J. and Hirschfeld, H. (1957a). *Chem. Ber.* **90**, 2544.
Inhoffen, H. H., Kath, J. F., Sticherling, W. and Bruckner, K. (1957b). *Justus Liebigs Ann. Chem.* **603**, 25.
Inhoffen, H. H., Irmscher, K., Hirschfeld, H., Stache, U. and Kreutzer, A. (1958a). *Chem. Ber.* **91**, 2309.
Inhoffen, H. H., Schutz, S., Rossberg, P., Berges, O., Nordsiek, K.-H., Plenio, H. and Horoldt, E. (1958b). *Chem. Ber.* **91**, 2626.
Inhoffen, H. H., Irmscher, K., Stache, U. and Kreutzer, A. (1959a). *J. Chem. Soc.* 385.
Inhoffen, H. H., Burkhardt, H. and Quinkert, G. (1959b). *Chem. Ber.* **92**, 1564.
Inhoffen, H. H., Irmscher, K., Friedrich, G., Kampe, D. and Berges, O. (1959c). *Chem. Ber.* **92**, 1772.

Irmscher, K. (1960). *Naturwissenschaften* **47**, 425.

IUPAC (1969). *Biochem. J.* **113**, 5.

Kaneko, C., Yamada, S., Sugimoto, A., Ishikawa, M., Sasaki, S. and Suda, T. (1973). *Tetrahedron Lett.* 2339.

Kaneko, C., Yamada, S., Sugimoto, A., Eguchi, Y., Ishikawa, M., Suda, T., Suzuki, M., Kakuta, S. and Sasaki, S. (1974a). *Steroids* **23**, 75.

Kaneko, C., Sugimoto, A., Eguchi, Y., Yamada, S., Ishikawa, M., Sasaki, S. and Suda, T. (1974b). *Tetrahedron* **30**, 2701.

Kaneko, C., Yamada, S., Sugimoto, A., Ishikawa, M., Suda, T., Suzuki, M. and Sasaki, S. (1975). *J. Chem. Soc. Perkin I* 1104.

Knobler, C., Romers, C., Braun, P. B. and Hornstra, J. (1972). *Acta Cryst. Ser. B.* **28**, 2097.

Kobayashi, T. (1967a). *J. Vitaminol.* (Japan) **13**, 255.

Kobayashi, T. (1967b). *J. Vitaminol.* (Japan) **13**, 268.

Kodicek, E. (1959). *In* 'Ciba Found. Symp. on Biosynthesis of Terpenes and Sterols' (Ed. Wolstenholme, G. E. W. and O'Connor, M.) p. 173, J. & A. Churchill Ltd., London.

Koevoet, A. L., Verloop, A. and Havinga, E. (1955). *Rec. Trav. Chim. Pays-Bas* **74**, 788.

Kuhn, R. and Moller, E. F. (1934). *Angew. Chem.* **47**, 145.

Lam, H. Y., Schnoes, H. K., DeLuca, H. F. and Chen, T. C. (1973). *Biochemistry* **12**, 4851.

Lam, H. Y., Onisko, B. L., Schnoes, H. K. and DeLuca, H. F. (1974). *Biochem. Biophys. Res. Commun.* **59**, 845.

Lawson, D. E. M. and Bell, P. A. (1974). *Biochem. J.* **142**, 37.

Lawson, D. E. M., Fraser, D. R., Kodicek, E., Morris, H. R. and Williams, D. H. (1971a). *Nature* (London) **230**, 228.

Lawson, D. E. M., Pelc, B., Bell, P. A., Wilson, P. W. and Kodicek, E. (1971b). *Biochem. J.* **121**, 673.

Legrand, M. and Mathieu, J. (1957). *C.R. Acad. Sci.* **245**, 2502.

Lettré, H. (1934). *Justus Liebigs Ann. Chem.* **511**, 280.

Littlewood, P. S., Lythgoe, B. and Saksena, A. K. (1971). *J. Chem. Soc.* **C**, 2955.

Louw, D. F., Strating, J. and Backer, H. J. (1955). *Rec. Trav. Chim. Pays-Bas* **74**, 1540.

Lugtenburg, J. and Havinga, E. (1969). *Tetrahedron Lett.* 2391.

Mitra, M. N., Norman, A. W. and Okamura, W. H. (1974). *J. Org. Chem.* **39**, 2931.

Morisaki, M., Rubio-Lightbourn, J. and Ikekawa, N. (1973a). *Chem. Pharm. Bull.* (Japan) **21**, 457.

Morisaki, M., Rubio-Lightbourn, J., Ikekawa, N. and Takeshita, T. (1973b). *Chem. Pharm. Bull* (Japan) **21**, 2568.

Morisaki, M., Bannai, K. and Ikekawa, N. (1973c). *Chem. Pharm. Bull.* (Japan) **21**, 1853.

Morisaki, M., Koizumi, N., Ikekawa, N., Takeshita, T. and Ishimoto, S. (1975). *J. Chem. Soc. Perkin I* 1421.

Munck, A., Wira, C., Young, D. A., Mosher, K. M., Hallahan, C. and Bell, P. A. (1972). *J. Steroid Biochem.* **3**, 567.

Narwid, T. A., Cooney, K. E. and Uskokovic, M. R. (1974a). *Helv. Chim. Acta* **57**, 771.

Narwid, T. A., Blount, J. F., Iacobelli, J. A. and Uskokovic, M. R. (1974b). *Helv. Chim. Acta* **57**, 781.

Neville, P. F. and DeLuca, H. F. (1966). *Biochemistry* **5**, 2201.

Nield, C. H., Russell, W. C. and Zimmerli, A. (1940). *J. Biol. Chem.* **136**, 73.

Norman, A. W., Myrtle, J. F., Midgett, R. J., Nowicki, H. G., Williams, V. and Popjak, G. (1971). *Science* **173**, 51.
Okamura, W. H. and Pirio, M. R. (1975). *Tetrahedron Lett.* 4317.
Okamura, W. H., Norman, A. W. and Wing, R. M. (1974a). *Proc. Nat. Acad. Sci. U.S.* **71**, 4194.
Okamura, W. H., Mitra, M. N., Wing, R. M. and Norman, A. W. (1974b). *Biochem. Biophys. Res. Commun.* **60**, 179.
Parekh, C. K. and Wasserman, R. H. (1965). *J. Chromatogr.* **20**, 407.
Partridge, J. J., Faber, S. and Uskokovic, M. R. (1974). *Helv. Chim. Acta* **57**, 764.
Pelc, B. (1974). *J. Chem. Soc. Perkin I* 1436.
Pelc, B. and Kodicek, E. (1970). *J. Chem. Soc.* **C**, 1624.
Pelc, B. and Kodicek, E. (1971). *J. Chem. Soc.* **C**, 3415.
Pelc, B. and Kodicek, E. (1972a). *J. Chem. Soc. Perkin I* 244.
Pelc, B. and Kodicek, E. (1972b). *J. Chem. Soc. Perkin I* 2980.
Peng, C. T. (1963). *J. Pharm. Sci.* **52**, 861.
Pohl, R. (1927). *Naturwissenschaften* **15**, 433.
Rappoldt, M. P. (1960a). *Rec. Trav. Chim. Pays-Bas* **79**, 392.
Rappoldt, M. P. (1960b). *Rec. Trav. Chim. Pays-Bas* **79**, 1012.
Rappoldt, M. P. and Havinga, E. (1960). *Rec. Trav. Chim. Pays-Bas* **79**, 369.
Redel, J., Bell, P., Delbarre, F. and Kodicek, E. (1973). *C.R. Acad. Sci. Ser. D.* **276**, 2907.
Redel, J., Bell, P., Delbarre, F. and Kodicek, E. (1974a). *C.R. Acad. Sci. Ser. D.* **278**, 529.
Redel, J., Bell, P. A., Bazely, N., Calando, Y., Delbarre, F. and Kodicek, E. (1974b). *Steroids* **24**, 463.
Redel, J., Bazeley, N., Calando, Y., Delbarre, F., Bell, P. A. and Kodicek, E. (1975). *J. Steroid Biochem.* **6**, 117.
Rosenheim, O. and Webster, T. A. (1925). *Lancet* 1025.
Rosenheim, O. and Webster, T. A. (1927). *Biochem. J.* **21**, 389.
Rubio-Lightbourn, J., Morisaki, M. and Ikekawa, N. (1973). *Chem. Pharm. Bull.* (Japan) **21**, 1854.
Sanders, G. M. and Havinga, E. (1964). *Rec. Trav. Chim. Pays-Bas* **83**, 665.
Sanders, G. M., Pot, J. and Havinga, E. (1969). *Fortschr. Chem. Org. Naturstoffe* **27**, 131.
Schaltegger, H. (1960). *Helv. Chim. Acta* **43**, 1448.
Schenck, F. (1937). *Naturwissenschaften* **25**, 159.
Schlatmann, J. L. M., Pot, J. and Havinga, E. (1964). *Rec. Trav. Chim. Pays-Bas* **83**, 1173.
Schubert, K. (1954). *Naturwissenschaften* **41**, 231.
Schubert, K. (1956). *Biochem. Z.* **327**, 507.
Seki, M., Rubio-Lightbourn, J., Morisaki, M. and Ikekawa, N. (1973). *Chem. Pharm. Bull.* (Japan) **21**, 2783.
Seki, M., Koizumi, N., Morisaki, M. and Ikekawa, N. (1975). *Tetrahedron Lett.* 15.
Semmler, E. J., Holick, M. F., Schnoes, H. K. and DeLuca, H. F. (1972). *Tetrahedron Lett.* 4147.
Sheves, M., Berman, E., Freeman, D. and Mazur, Y. (1975). *J. Chem. Soc. Chem. Commun.* 643.
Snoeren, A. E. C., Daha, M. R., Lugtenburg, J. and Havinga, E. (1970). *Rec. Trav. Chim. Pays-Bas* **89**, 261.
Steenbock, H. and Black, A. (1924). *J. Biol. Chem.* **61**, 405.

Steenbock, H. and Black, A. (1925). *J. Biol. Chem.* **64**, 263.
Strating, J. (1952). *Rec. Trav. Chim. Pays-Bas* **71**, 822.
Strating, J. and Backer, H. J. (1950). *Rec. Trav. Chim. Pays-Bas* **69**, 909.
Strating, J. and Backer, H. J. (1951). *Rec. Trav. Chim. Pays-Bas* **70**, 389.
Suda, T., Hallick, R. B., DeLuca, H. F. and Schnoes, H. K. (1970a). *Biochemistry* **9**, 1651.
Suda, T., DeLuca, H. F., Schnoes, H. K., Ponchon, G., Tanaka, Y. and Holick, M. F. (1970b). *Biochemistry* **9**, 2917.
Suda, T., DeLuca, H. F., Schnoes, H. K., Tanaka, Y. and Holick, M. F. (1970c). *Biochemistry* **9**, 4776.
Suda, T., DeLuca, H. F. and Hallick, R. B. (1971). *Anal. Biochem.* **43**, 139.
Tanaka, Y., DeLuca, H. F., Ikekawa, N., Morisaki, M. and Koizumi, N. (1975a). *Arch. Biochem. Biophys.* **170**, 620.
Tanaka, Y., Frank, H., DeLuca, H. F., Koizumi, N. and Ikekawa, N. (1975b). *Biochemistry* **14**, 3293.
Thompson, G. R., Lewis, B. and Booth, C. C. (1966). *J. Clin. Invest.* **45**, 94.
Trippett, S. (1955). *J. Chem. Soc.* 370.
Van de Vliervoet, J. L. J., Westerhof, P., Keverling Buisman, J. A. and Havinga, E. (1956). *Rec. Trav. Chim. Pays-Bas* **75**, 1179.
Velluz, L. and Amiard, G. (1949). *C.R. Acad. Sci.* **228**, 692.
Velluz, L. and Amiard, G. (1955). *Bull. Soc. Chim. Fr.* 205.
Velluz, L. and Amiard, G. (1961). *C.R. Acad. Sci.* **253**, 603.
Velluz, L., Petit, A. and Amiard, G. (1948). *Bull. Soc. Chim. Fr.* 1115.
Velluz, L., Amiard, G. and Petit, A. (1949a). *Bull. Soc. Chim. Fr.* 362.
Velluz, L., Amiard, G. and Petit, A. (1949b). *Bull. Soc. Chim. Fr.* 501.
Velluz, L., Amiard, G. and Goffinet, B. (1955a). *Bull. Soc. Chim. Fr.* 1341.
Velluz, L., Amiard, G. and Goffinet, B. (1955b). *C.R. Acad. Sci.* **240**, 2156.
Velluz, L., Amiard, G. and Goffinet, B. (1955c). *C.R. Acad. Sci.* **240**, 2076.
Velluz, L., Amiard, G. and Goffinet, B. (1955d). *C.R. Acad. Sci.* **240**, 2326.
Velluz, L., Amiard, G. and Goffinet, B. (1957a). *Bull. Soc. Chim. Fr.* 882.
Velluz, L., Amiard, G. and Goffinet, B. (1957b). *C.R. Acad. Sci.* **244**, 1794.
Verloop, A., Koevoet, A. L. and Havinga, E. (1955). *Rec. Trav. Chim. Pays-Bas* **74**, 1125.
Verloop, A., Koevoet, A. L. and Havinga, E. (1957). *Rec. Trav. Chim. Pays-Bas* **76**, 689.
Verloop, A., Koevoet, A. L., Van Moorselaar, R. and Havinga, E. (1959). *Rec. Trav. Chim. Pays-Bas* **78**, 1004.
Verloop, A., Corts, G. J. B. and Havinga, E. (1960). *Rec. Trav. Chim. Pays-Bas* **79**, 164.
Von Reichel, S. and Deppe, M. (1936). *Hoppe-Seyler's Z. Physiol. Chem.* **239**, 143.
Von Werder, F. (1939). *Hoppe-Seyler's Z. Physiol. Chem.* **260**, 119.
Von Werder, F. (1957). *Justus Liebigs Ann. Chem.* **603**, 15.
Vroegop, P. J., Lugtenburg, J. and Havinga, E. (1973). *Tetrahedron* **29**, 1393.
Waddell, J. (1934). *J. Biol. Chem.* **105**, 711.
Westerhof, P. and Keverling Buisman, J. A. (1956). *Rec. Trav. Chim. Pays-Bas* **75**, 453.
Westerhof, P. and Keverling Buisman, J. A. (1957). *Rec. Trav. Chim. Pays-Bas* **76**, 679.
Westerhof, P. and Keverling Buisman, J. A. (1959). *Rec. Trav. Chim. Pays-Bas* **78**, 659.
Wilkie, J. B., Jones, S. W. and Kline, O. L. (1958). *J. Amer. Pharm. Assoc. Sci. Ed.* **47**, 385.
Wilzbach, K. E. (1957). *J. Amer. Chem. Soc.* **79**, 1013.
Windaus, A. and Bock, F. (1937). *Hoppe-Seyler's Z. Physiol. Chem.* **245**, 168.

Windaus, A. and Buchholz, K. (1939). *Ber. Deut. Chem. Ges.* **72**, 597.
Windaus, A. and Grundmann, W. (1936). *Justus Liebigs Ann. Chem.* **524**, 295.
Windaus, A. and Naggatz, J. (1939). *Justus Liebigs Ann. Chem.* **542**, 204.
Windaus, A. and Riemann, U. (1942). *Hoppe-Seyler's Z. Physiol. Chem.* **274**, 206.
Windaus, A. and Thiele, W. (1936). *Justus Liebigs Ann. Chem.* **521**, 160.
Windaus, A. and Trautmann, G. (1937). *Hoppe-Seyler's Z. Physiol. Chem.* **247**, 185.
Windaus, A., Hess, A., Rosenheim, O., Pohl, R. and Webster, T. A. (1927). *Chemiker-Ztg.* **51**, 113.
Windaus, A., Luttringhaus, A. and Deppe, M. (1931). *Justus Liebigs Ann. Chem.* **489**, 252.
Windaus, A., Linsert, O., Luttringhaus, A. and Weidlich, G. (1932a). *Justus Liebigs Ann. Chem.* **492**, 226.
Windaus, A., Dithmar, K. and Fernholz, E. (1932b). *Justus Liebigs Ann. Chem.* **493**, 259.
Windaus, A., Von Werder, F. and Luttinghaus, A. (1932c). *Justus Liebigs Ann. Chem.* **499**, 188.
Windaus, A., Inhoffen, H. H. and Von Reichel, S. (1934). *Justus Liebigs Ann. Chem.* **510**, 248.
Windaus, A., Lettré, H. and Schenck, F. (1935). *Justus Liebigs Ann. Chem.* **520**, 98.
Windaus, A., Schenck, F. and Von Werder, F. (1936). *Hoppe-Seyler's Z. Physiol. Chem.* **241**, 100.
Windaus, A., Deppe, M. and Wunderlich, W. (1938). *Justus Liebigs Ann. Chem.* **533**, 118.
Windaus, A., Deppe, M. and Roosen-Runge, C. (1939). *Justus Liebigs Ann. Chem.* **537**, 1.
Wing, R. M., Okamura, W. H., Pirio, M. R., Sine, S. M. and Norman, A. W. (1974). *Science* **186**, 939.
Wing, R. M., Okamura, W. H., Rego, A., Pirio, M. R. and Norman, A. W. (1975). *J. Amer. Chem. Soc.* **97**, 4980.
Wittig, G. and Schollkopf, U. (1954). *Chem. Ber.* **87**, 1318.
Woodward, R. B. and Hoffmann, R. (1965). *J. Amer. Chem. Soc.* **87**, 2511.
Yu, W., Hung-Shiun, T., Jing-Jain, H., Yung-Chi, C. and Yao-Tseng, H. (1958). *Acta Chim. Sinica* **24**, 134.
Ziffer, H., VandenHeuvel, W. J. A., Haahti, E. O. A. and Horning, E. C. (1960). *J. Amer. Chem. Soc.* **82**, 6411.

2 Metabolism of Vitamin D

MICHAEL F. HOLICK AND HECTOR F. DELUCA

I Metabolites

A 25-HYDROXYCHOLECALCIFEROL

In the early 1590s Kodicek and coworkers (Kodicek, 1955; Kodicek and Ashby, 1954, 1960a, b; Kodicek *et al.*, 1960, 1961) reasoned that, in order to understand the mode and sites of action of vitamin D, investigations into storage, distribution and metabolism were required. They approached this problem by synthesising [G-^{14}C]ergocalciferol with a specific activity of 0.46 mCi/mmole, and after administration of pharmacological doses to rats, the fate of the label was investigated by the determination of the radioactivity in the tissues and excreta and by autoradiography of sections of tissue. Analogous work was also reported by Schaltegger (1960) and in monkeys by Blumberg *et al.* (1960). Kodicek and coworkers also attempted, by reversed phase chromatography, detection of biologically active metabolites of ergocalciferol. From these studies, it was concluded that calciferol was probably biologically active in itself and that further metabolism was for the purpose of degradation.

Norman and DeLuca (1963) prepared randomly labelled tritiated cholecalciferol and ergocalciferol having specific activities of 7.3 and 3.25 mCi/mmole respectively. These materials allowed the detection of at least three metabolites possessing some antirachitic activity (Norman *et al.*, 1964). Two years later Neville and DeLuca (1966) reported the synthesis of high specific activity [1,2-^{3}H]cholecalciferol. Using physiological amounts of this labelled compound (0.25 μg/rat), Lund and DeLuca demonstrated in serum, liver and bone the existence of a polar metabolite of calciferol (metabolite IV) which possessed biological activity at least equal to that of cholecalciferol (Lund and DeLuca, 1966; Morii *et al.*, 1967). They also demonstrated that the relative amount of the metabolite IV material is markedly increased as the dosage of the vitamin is decreased. However, the absolute amount of this material could be increased in blood by increasing the dosage of cholecalciferol. Utilising this fact, Blunt *et al.* (1968) gave four hogs 6.25 mg of cholecalciferol daily for a period of 26 days and then collected their blood. The blood was treated with sodium oxalate and the cells removed by centrifugation. Sufficient ammonium

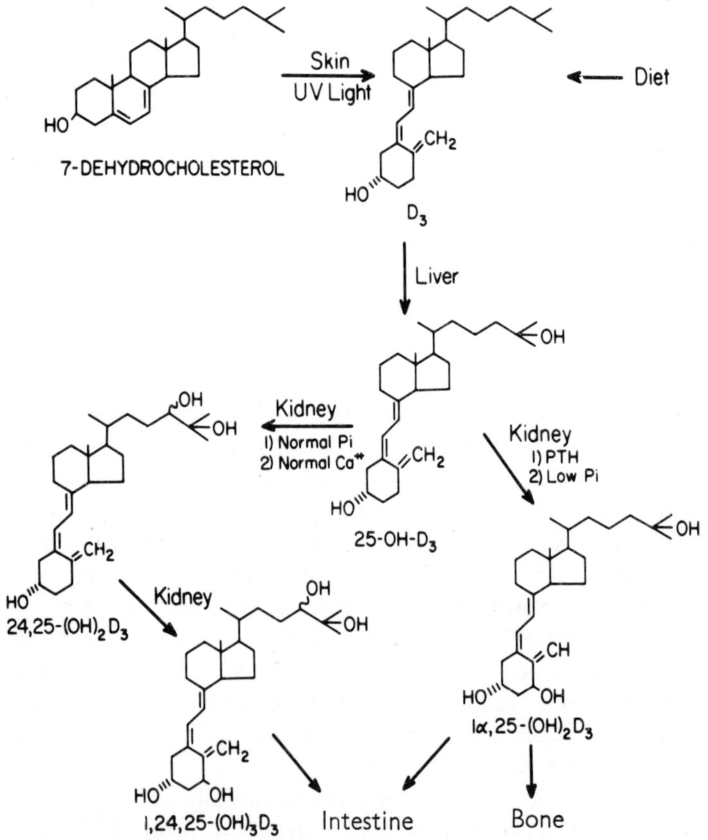

Fig. 1. Schematic summary of the origin of cholecalciferol and its various biologically active metabolites

sulfate was added to the plasma to achieve a 65–70% saturation. The precipitate was collected and extracted with methanol-chloroform. A radioactive extract was prepared in the same fashion from a hog that had received [1,2-^{3}H]cholecalciferol. The extracts were combined and chromatographed first on silicic acid columns and then on liquid-liquid Celite partition chromatographic columns. The metabolite (1.2 mg) was isolated in pure form and identified as the 25-hydroxy derivative (25-hydroxycholecalciferol) by means of mass spectrometry, nuclear magnetic resonance spectrometry and ultraviolet absorption spectrophotometry (Fig. 1). That was followed by the successful isolation and identification of 25-hydroxyergocalciferol using similar procedures (Suda *et al.*, 1969). The major site for the 25-hydroxylation was subsequently shown to take place in the liver (Ponchon *et al.*, 1969; Horsting and DeLuca, 1969).

B 1,25-DIHYDROXYCHOLECALCIFEROL

1 *Formation.* At first it was believed that 25-hydroxycholecalciferol was the metabolically active form of vitamin D. However, it was soon evident that it is metabolised rapidly to more polar products. Thus Haussler *et al.* (1968) reported a cholecalciferol metabolite more polar than the 25-hydroxymetabolite in the intestinal nuclear fraction of chicks given [^{3}H] cholecalciferol, and other evidence for the existence of this metabolite was subsequently reported by Lawson *et al.* (1969) and by Ponchon *et al.* (1970). With [1-^{3}H]cholecalciferol, Lawson *et al.* (1969) learned that during formation of the intestinal metabolite, the 1α-^{3}H was lost which led them to suggest that this metabolite had either a ketone or hydroxyl group on C-1.

The synthesis of labelled 25-hydroxycholecalciferol had been accomplished both biologically in the whole animal (Lawson *et al.*, 1969) and chemically (Suda *et al.*, 1971) and these preparations have been used in a number of studies to follow the metabolism of 25-hydroxycholecalciferol and to show that after a dose of this latter compound the main polar metabolite appeared in intestine and bone within 30 min (Lawson *et al.*, 1969; Cousins *et al.*, 1970a, b). The biological activity of the polar metabolite was established before its identity was fully known (Kodicek *et al.*, 1970; Myrtle *et al.*, 1970) so that it soon became clear that not only did the polar metabolite have all the actions of calciferol but that it acted more quickly than the vitamin in stimulating intestinal calcium transport (Haussler *et al.*, 1971; Omdahl *et al.*, 1971; Myrtle and Norman, 1971).

At first it was believed that the concentration of this metabolite could be increased by dosing pigs with large amounts of cholecalciferol and isolating the polar metabolite. Using this approach the isolation and identification of 21,25-dihydroxycholecalciferol and 25,26-dihydroxycholecalciferol from porcine plasma was reported (Suda *et al.*, 1970a, b). Although large doses of

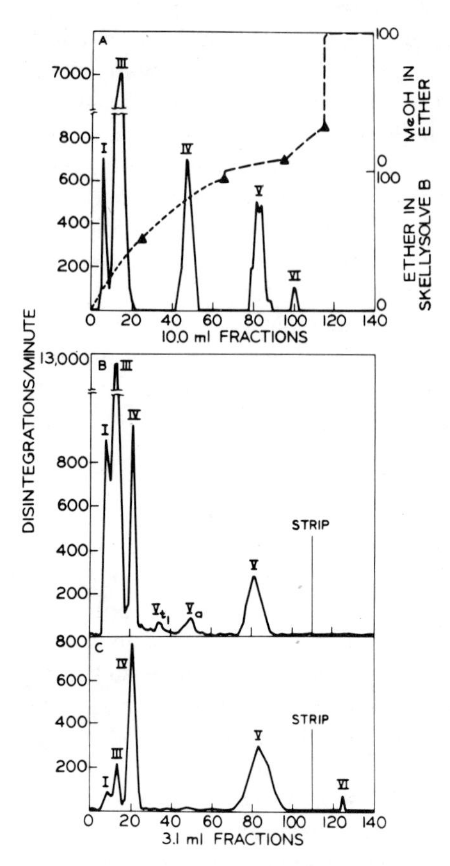

Fig. 2. Comparison of the chromatography of intestinal lipid extracts from groups of 3 chickens that received [1,2-^{3}H]cholecalciferol. A, Silicic acid chromatography of an intestinal lipid extract from chickens that received 2.5 μg of [1,2-^{3}H]cholecalciferol. B, Sephadex LH-20 ($CHCl_3$: Skellysolve B, 65:35) chromatography of intestinal lipid extract from chickens that received 2.5 μg of [1,2-^{3}H]cholecalciferol. C, Sephadex LH-20 chromatography of intestinal lipid extract from chickens that received 0.25 μg of [1,2-^{3}H]cholecalciferol. (Reproduced with permission from Holick and DeLuca, 1971)

21,25-dihydroxycholecalciferol appeared to have preferential activity in mobilising calcium from the bone while 25,26-dihydroxycholecalciferol appeared to have its greatest effect in stimulating intestinal calcium transport, it was clear that neither of these metabolites was the polar metabolite found in intestine. In fact, Lawson *et al.* (1971) reported that the '1α-tritium-deficient' metabolite could not be increased above 1 ng/g of intestinal tissue with increasing doses of cholecalciferol and that the other tissues, including blood, had much less of this metabolite.

In 1971 a new chromatographic system for calciferol metabolites using Sephadex LH-20 slurried and developed in 65:35 chloroform-Skellysolve B was developed (Holick and DeLuca, 1971). With this technique it was possible to demonstrate (Holick and DeLuca, 1971; Omdahl *et al.*, 1971) that the polar metabolite in the intestine as determined by silicic acid chromatography was composed of three metabolites when large doses of the vitamin were given but was homogeneous when a physiological dose (0.25 μg) was given (Fig. 2). It became obvious from these experiments that large doses of cholecalciferol would not result in increased amounts of the polar metabolite, denying investigators this approach to increasing the concentration of the metabolite. Instead it was necessary to dose large numbers of animals with a physiological amount of [1,2-^{3}H]cholecalciferol and attempt isolation of the metabolite from one of the target tissues, namely the intestine. Realising the difficulty in such an isolation, Fraser and Kodicek (1970) used an *in vitro* approach utilising the loss of ^{3}H from [4-^{14}C, 1α-^{3}H 25-hydroxycholecalciferol during formation of the metabolite to aid them in their search for the correct tissue. This approach was taken in the author's laboratory as well but failed because the rat was used as the source of tissue. In retrospect rat tissues possess a potent inhibitor of this system (Section IIB1) which unknowingly thwarted our *in vitro* attempts (Botham *et al.*, 1974). Fraser and Kodicek utilised chick tissue and were successful.

Even though it was reported by Cousins *et al.* (1970a) that metabolite V appeared in the intestine as early as 0.5 h after an intravenous dose of [26,26-^{3}H]-25-hydroxycholecalciferol, each of the laboratories was unable to generate the metabolite *in vitro* with this tissue. Homogenates from several tissues of chickens including liver, adrenal, parathyroid, ultimobronchial bodies and bones were tested by Fraser and Kodicek (1970) but they were unable to demonstrate a conversion of 25-hydroxycholecalciferol to the 'tritium deficient' metabolite by these tissues. Instead they found that the conversion of 25-hydroxycholecalciferol to this polar metabolite was carried out by homogenates of chicken kidneys. They injected [4-^{14}C, 1α-^{3}H]25-hydroxycholecalciferol to nephrectomised rats and clearly demonstrated that the 'tritium-deficient' metabolite was made solely by kidney tissue. These results were quickly confirmed in 1971 by Gray *et al.* (1971).

2 *Isolation and Identification*. In 1971, two years after it was first observed that the polar intestinal metabolite was biologically active, two laboratories simultaneously reported its structural identification. Starting with 1500 chickens dosed at 2.5 μg of [1,2-^{3}H]cholecalciferol, Holick *et al.* (1971a, b) collected the small intestines and extracted them with MeOH–$CHCl_3$ obtaining 10 μg of the metabolite in 22 g of lipid. After approximately ten

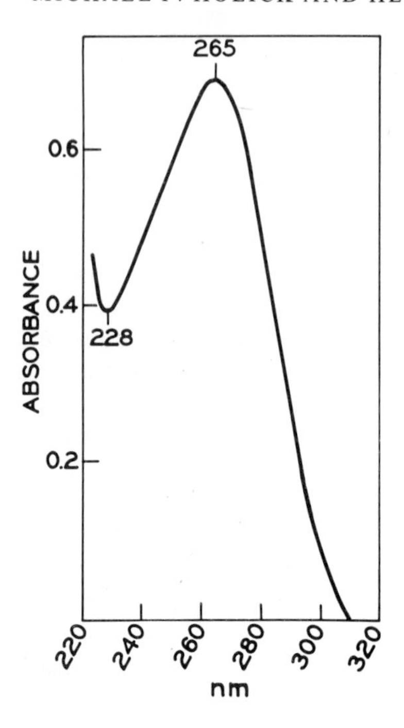

Fig. 3. Ultraviolet absorption spectrum of the 5,6-*cis*-triene system for cholecalciferol and its metabolites

purification procedures using liquid-gel partition chromatography and gel permeation chromatography with Sephadex LH-20 and Biobeads S-X8, the metabolite (8 μg) was isolated. However, complete purification was not achieved until the chromatographic properties of the metabolite were changed by making the C-25 trimethylsilyl ether derivative. This derivative chromatographed sufficiently differently from contaminants for final purification. The monosilyl ether derivative was hydrolysed to yield 2 μg of pure metabolite. The ultraviolet spectrum of the isolated metabolite showed λ_{max}265 nm and λ_{min}228 nm (Fig. 3), leaving little doubt that the 5,6-*cis* triene system was still intact (Blunt *et al.*, 1968; Holick and DeLuca, 1974). The mass spectrum of the metabolite and its tri-trimethylsilyl ether derivative (Fig. 4) showed molecular ion peaks at m/e 416 and 632 respectively, demonstrating the presence of three hydroxyl functions in the molecule. The intense fragment at m/e 131 in the mass spectrum of the trimethylsilyl ether derivative established one of the hydroxyls on C-25. It was further assumed that the 3β-hydroxyl of cholecalciferol was still intact, thus leaving one hydroxyl unaccounted for. Fragments at m/e 287, 269 (287-H_2O) and 251 (287-2H_2O) in the mass

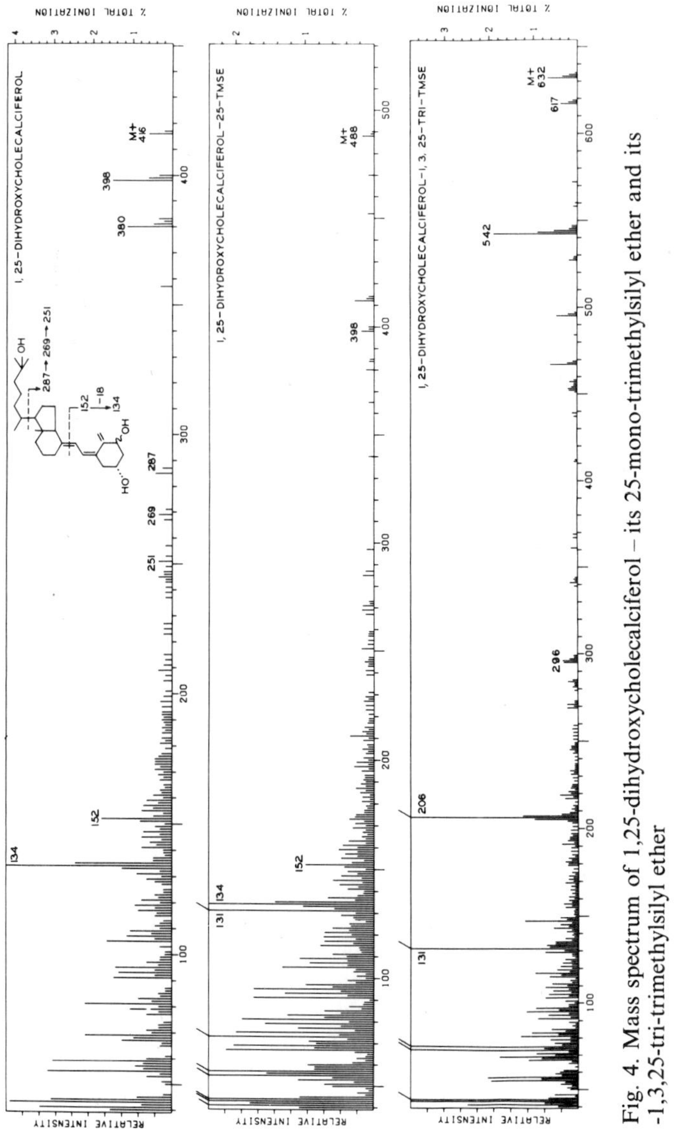

Fig. 4. Mass spectrum of 1,25-dihydroxycholecalciferol – its 25-mono-trimethylsilyl ether and its -1,3,25-tri-trimethylsilyl ether

spectrum of the metabolite corresponded to the loss of the entire side chain, that is, bond cleavage between C-17 and C-20. These fragments demonstrated that the additional hydroxyl was not in the side chain. The mass spectrum also showed prominent fragments at m/e 152 and 134 (152-H_2O) (due to ring A +C-6,C-7), which could only result from the addition of an oxygen function on ring A. The ultraviolet absorption spectrum ruled out C-6,C-7 and C-19 as possible positions. Therefore, the additional hydroxyl function had to be on C-1,2 or 4. Since positions on C-1 and C-4 were allylic to the 5,6-*cis*-triene system, it was possible to demonstrate by catalytic reduction with H_2 over PtO_2 that the extra hydroxyl in the A ring was on either C-1 or C-4 since the extra hydroxyl group in the A ring was eliminated by the reduction to yield hexahydro-25-hydroxycholecalciferol.

Treatment of the metabolite with sodium metaperiodate for 24 h at room temperature showed no reaction, while many vicinal hydroxy steroids showed the expected cleavage within 4 h thus eliminating both C-2 and C-4 as positions for the new hydroxyl. These data made it clear that the additional oxygen function had to be on C-1. Therefore, the physical data including the UV absorption spectra and mass spectrum and its chemical properties unequivocally demonstrated that the structure of the intestinal metabolite was the 1-hydroxy derivative of 25-hydroxycholecalciferol (Fig. 1).

Simultaneously Lawson *et al.* (1971) isolated 60 μg of the metabolite in approximately 30% purity from chicken kidney homogenates and reported that the metabolite has a λ_{max} of 269 nm and a λ_{min} at 232 nm. The mass spectrum of their metabolite showed molecular ion at m/e 416 and fragment peaks at m/e 287, 269, 251, 152 and 134. On the basis of the loss of 1α-^{3}H from the substrate, [1α-^{3}H, 4-^{14}C]25-hydroxycholecalciferol, they reasoned that the additional hydroxyl must be on C-1. These results led them to conclude that their tritium-deficient metabolite was 1,25-dihydroxycholecalciferol. A report appeared some time later confirming the mass spectral data on the metabolite (Norman *et al.*, 1971a). Evidence that the 1-hydroxyl of 1,25-dihydroxycholecalciferol is in the α position was provided by chemical synthesis. The chemically synthesised metabolite had physical properties and biological activity identical to the biosynthesised metabolite (Semmler *et al.*, 1972) confirming the structure as 1α,25-dihydroxycholecalciferol. However, until 1β-25-dihydroxycholecalciferol is prepared, certainty of the 1-hydroxyl configuration of the natural product is not absolute.

3 *Metabolism.* Although 1,25-dihydroxycholecalciferol can stimulate intestinal calcium transport and bone calcium mobilisation in anephric rats (Holick *et al.*, 1972b; Boyle *et al.*, 1972a), it was still possible that 1,25-dihydroxycholecalciferol might require further metabolic alteration before it can act at the target tissue level. Consequently Frolik and DeLuca (1971, 1972) prepared tritiated 1,25-dihydroxycholecalciferol from [26,27-^{3}H]-and

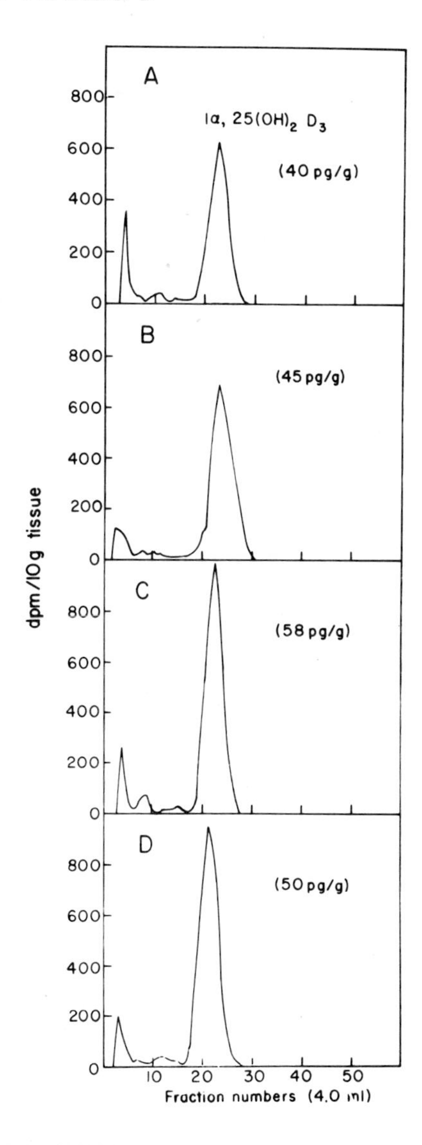

Fig. 5. Sephadex LH-20 ($CHCl_3$-Skellysolve B, 75:25) chromatographic profiles of intestinal lipid extracts from rats on diets with different calcium and phosphorus contents. Weanling rats were maintained on the various diets for 3 weeks and then received a pulse dose of 62.5 pmoles of [26,27-^{3}H]25-hydroxycholecalciferol. 96 h later the animals were sacrificed and the intestines were extracted for chromatography. Rats were maintained on a vitamin D-deficient diet with the following calcium and phosphorus content: A, 0.02% Ca, 0.30% P; B, 0.3% Ca, 0.3%P; C, 3% Ca, 0.3% P; D, 1,2% Ca, 0.1% P

[1,2-^{3}H] labelled 25-hydroxycholecalciferol, and dosed a physiological amount (62.5 pmoles) of each to vitamin D-deficient chickens and rats. At 6 h and 12 h later the blood, intestines and bones were collected, extracted and the extracts chromatographed on Sephadex LH-20. The results demonstrated that at a time the intestine was maximally transporting calcium in response to this metabolite, greater than 80% of the radioactivity in the intestine was 1,25-dihydroxycholecalciferol. No other metabolites were detected in significant quantity (Frolik and Deluca, 1971, 1972). It was also noted that at 6 h and 12h after dosing, when bone calcium mobilisation was maximally stimulated, only unaltered 1,25-dihydroxycholecalciferol was detected in that tissue. In a similar fashion Tsai *et al.* (1972) reported that after a dose of 312.5 pmoles of tritiated 1,25-dihydroxycholecalciferol the maximal accumulation in the intestine occurred 4 h later and that only one compound, 1,25-dihydroxy-cholecalciferol, was found between 4 h and 48 h after dosing.

Surprisingly rat intestinal calcium transport remains high for at least 7 days after a single 62.5 pmole dose of 1,25-dihydroxycholecalciferol (Holick *et al.*, 1973a). [26,27-^{3}H]1,25-Dihydroxycholecalciferol is found in the intestine even 4 days after a 62.5 pmole dose with greater than 80% of the lipid soluble radioactivity remaining as the hormone. Furthermore the amount of this compound remaining in the intestine at 4 days is unaffected by the calcium content of the diet (Fig. 5). At 96 h when the bone calcium mobilisation response had decreased considerably, 1,25-dihydroxycholecalciferol is also the prominent metabolite in that tissue independent of dietary calcium (Holick, Kasten-Schraufrogel, Tavela and DeLuca, unpublished results). These data suggest that once the active hormone, 1,25-dihydroxycholecalci-ferol, is provided, dietary and serum calcium does not influence further metabolism.

It is of some interest, therefore, that chronic oral administration of 1,25-dihydroxycholecalciferol in oily solutions to rats results in lack of bone responsiveness to the hormone in contrast to chronic intraperitoneal administration (Tanaka *et al.*, 1973). This is surprising since the bone of vitamin D-deficient rats responds equally well to either a single oral or an intravenous dose of 1,25-dihydroxycholecalciferol. Tritiated 1,25-dihydroxy-cholecalciferol given orally in oil to rats given previous chronic doses of the hormone appears in low concentrations in blood, bone and other organs in contrast to the same dose given to a vitamin D-deficient rat (Frolick and DeLuca, 1973). These results suggest that the hormone may induce a condition in intestine where it is rapidly metabolised or where it is poorly absorbed. Oddly enough chicks do not exhibit this phenomenon.

Recently Carre *et al.* (1974) have shown that cortisone induces rat intestine to convert 1,25-dihydroxycholecalciferol to a more polar metabolite which is biologically inactive. They suggest that cortisone may cause calciferol resistance by such a mechanism. These results, however, conflict with those of Kimberg *et al.* (1971) who did not detect this metabolite.

The availability of 25-hydroxy- and 1,25-dihydroxycholecalciferol labelled with ^{14}C at C-26,27 has been of value in demonstrating one of the metabolic pathways followed by the hormone (Kumar and DeLuca, 1976; Kumar *et al.*, 1976). ^{14}C labelled CO_2 was found in the expired air of both rats and chicks dosed with these labelled compounds. This pathway is peculiar to the hormone since $^{14}CO_2$ was not detected in anephric rats dosed with [26-^{14}C]25-hydroxycholecalciferol, The rate of formation of $^{14}CO_2$ is maximal in the first 4–8 h after the administration of [26-^{14}C]1,25-dihydroxycholecalciferol suggesting that this pathway may be of importance to the function of the hormone. Obviously much remains to be learned concerning the metabolism of 1,25-dihydroxycholecalciferol since no metabolites or excretary products have yet been identified.

C 24,25-DIHYDROXYCHOLECALCIFEROL

Utilising liquid gel partition chromatography which separates '21,25-dihydroxycholecalciferol' from the 1,25-dihydroxy-metabolite it was shown that the production of these two metabolites depended either directly or indirectly on the serum calcium concentration (Boyle *et al.*, 1971). In hypocalcaemic rats the major polar metabolite of 25-hydroxycholecalciferol found in the intestine, bone and blood is the 1,25-dihydroxy-metabolite. However, in rats which were either normocalcaemic or hypercalcaemic, 25-hydroxycholecalciferol was metabolised to a new metabolite which was thought to be 21,25-dihydroxycholecalciferol and designated as metabolite Va. In a similar fashion chicks maintained on a high calcium diet or on a diet in which strontium replaced calcium, metabolised 25-hydroxycholecalciferol to metabolite Va rather than 1,25-dihydroxycholecalciferol (Omdahl and DeLuca, 1971, 1972). Because nephrectomy markedly reduced metabolite Va production in rats maintained on either a high calcium or a normal calcium diet with cholecalciferol supplementation, the kidney appeared as the site of its biosynthesis (Boyle *et al.*, 1973). This point was established by the demonstration that kidney homogenates from chicks maintained on a high calcium, vitamin D-supplemented diet produce metabolite Va (Boyle *et al.*, 1973; Omdahl *et al.*, 1972).

1 *Isolation and Identification.* These observations provided the impetus to prepare enough of this metabolite for isolation and identification. Eleven micrograms of the metabolite was obtained from chicken kidney homogenates incubated with [26,27-^{3}H]25-hydroxycholecalciferol. The product was isolated and purified in a fashion similar to that used for the purification of 1,25-dihydroxycholecalciferol (Holick *et al.*, 1972a). The ultraviolet

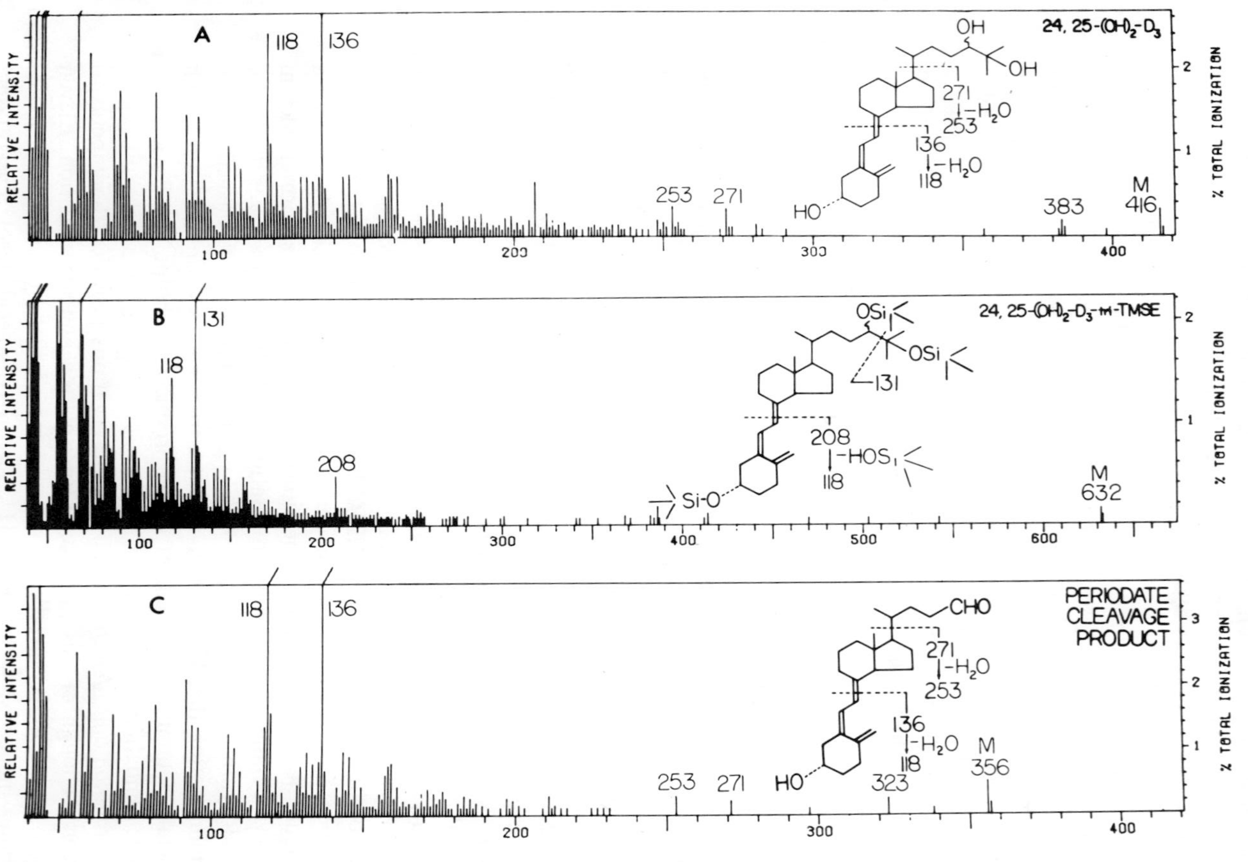

Fig. 6. Mass spectrum of A, 24,25-dihydroxycholecalciferol; B, its 3,24,25-tri-trimethylsilyl ether and C, 25,26,27-tris-nor-cholecalcifer-24-01

absorption for the metabolite showed a λ_{max}265 and λ_{min}228 nm (Fig. 3), demonstrating that the 5,6-*cis* triene system had not been altered. The mass spectrum of the metabolite (Fig. 6) showed a molecular ion m/e 416 suggesting the incorporation of an additional oxygen function into 25-hydroxycholecalciferol. Furthermore, the fragments at m/e 271 and 253 (271-H_2O) and m/e 136 and 118 (136-H_2O) are identical to those for cholecalciferol and its 25-hydroxy derivative (Blunt *et al.*, 1968), thus requiring that the additional oxygen function be on the side chain. Proof that the additional oxygen function on the side chain is a hydroxyl was provided by the mass spectrum of the trimethylsilyl ether derivative of the metabolite (Fig. 5), which showed a molecular ion m/e 632, demonstrating that there were three trimethylsilyl ether substituents on the molecule. The intense fragment m/e 131 firmly established that the C-25 hydroxyl remained. Upon treatment of the metabolite with periodate, 95% of the tritium on C-26 and C-27 was lost. The mass spectrum of the product from the periodate reaction (Fig. 5) showed a molecular ion at m/e 356 which could only result from the oxidative cleavage of the C-24, C-25 bond to yield a C-24 aldehyde. Therefore, it was concluded that the Va metabolite is the 24-hydroxy derivative of 25-hydroxycholecalciferol (Fig. 1).

The Va metabolite produced *in vivo* from hogs had been identified as 21,25-dihydroxycholecalciferol, which raised the question of two metabolites or misidentification of one. The Va metabolite isolated from hog blood showed an ultraviolet absorption spectrum and mass spectrum identical to those obtained for 24,25-dihydroxycholecalciferol. Furthermore, the porcine metabolite Va was also sensitive to periodate treatment and the mass spectrum of the resulting product was identical to that obtained for the *in vitro* generated 24,25-dihydroxycholecalciferol (Holick *et al.*, 1972a). These data demonstrated that this metabolite is also 24,25-dihydroxycholecalciferol and not the 21-hydroxy derivative of 25-hydroxycholecalciferol as originally believed (Suda *et al.*, 1970a). Final confirmation for this structural assignment was obtained when Seki *et al.* (1975) and Lam *et al.* (1973) synthesised 24,25-dihydroxycholecalciferol. The ultraviolet absorption spectrum, mass spectrum and the biological activity (Lam *et al.*, 1973) appeared identical to the biosynthesised material. Recently evidence has been obtained that the biosynthetic 24,25-dihydroxycholecalciferol has its 24-hydroxyl in the R sterioconfiguration (Tanaka *et al.*, 1975).

2 *Metabolism and Biological Activity.* The observation that 24,25-dihydroxycholecalciferol is the major circulating metabolite of cholecalciferol in normal and hypercalcaemic animals led Boyle *et al.* (1973) to examine the question as to whether 24,25-dihydroxycholecalciferol is capable of supporting growth, elevating serum calcium and calcifying bones of rats on a normal phosphorus diet. In this capacity 24,25-dihydroxycholecalciferol substitutes

well for the vitamin as it is capable of inducing intestinal calcium transport at dose levels similar to 25-hydroxycholecalciferol, but has little ability to mobilise calcium from bone. Furthermore, it appeared that 24,25-dihydroxycholecalciferol was metabolised to a more polar metabolite by the kidney before it elicited these biological responses and 1,24,25-trihydroxycholecalciferol (Fig. 1) was suggested as the structure for this new metabolite.

3 *Discrimination against* 24,25-*Dihydroxycholecalciferol by the Chicken.* (24R)-24,25-Dihydroxycholecalciferol produces only a minimal intestinal calcium transport response in chicks at doses up to 0.5 μg and at time intervals from 9–48 h. Furthermore, 1,24,25-trihydroxycholecalciferol although showing some stimulation of calcium transport was effective only 9 h after a dose (Holick *et al.*, 1967a). Because the 24-hydroxyl is on the same carbon as the C-28 methyl group of ergocalciferol, it is possible that such a substitution may trigger the discriminatory system and the 24-hydroxylated calciferols may be handled similarly to ergocalciferol in the fowl. Such a possibility is supported by the more rapid disappearance of [26,27-^{3}H]24,25-dihydroxycholecalciferol from the blood when compared to 25-hydroxycholecalciferol but whether the 24,25-dihydroxycholecalciferol is metabolised in the chick as an analogue of 25-hydroxyergocalciferol, however, must await further examination.

D 1,24,25-TRIHYDROXYCHOLECALCIFEROL

1 *Isolation and Identification.* Fifty micrograms of [26,27-^{3}H]24,25-dihydroxycholecalciferol isolated from the blood of pigs given large amounts of cholecalciferol (Suda *et al.*, 1971) was incubated with kidney homogenates obtained from chickens maintained on a rachitogenic diet. After several chromatographic steps, the metabolite was isolated in pure form and identified as 1,24,25-dihydroxycholecalciferol (Holick *et al.*, 1973a). The ultraviolet absorption spectrum of the metabolite, λ_{max}265 nm, was similar to those previously described for the 5,6-*cis*-triene system of cholecalciferol and its metabolites. The mass spectrum of the metabolite and its trimethylsilyl ether derivative (Fig. 7) showed molecular ion peaks at m/e 432 and 720 respectively, demonstrating that an additional hydroxyl function had been incorporated into the 24,25-dihydroxycholecalciferol. Furthermore, peaks at m/e 287, 269 (287-H_2O) and 251 (287-$2H_2O$) occurring from C-17, C-20 side chain cleavage in the mass spectrum of the metabolite confirmed the lack of an additional hydroxyl function on the side chain. The fragments of m/e 152 and 134 (152-H_20) (due to ring A plus C-6, C-7) in the mass spectrum of the metabolite and the corresponding fragments of m/e 296 and 206 (296-TMS-OH) in the mass spectrum of the tetra-trimethylsilyl ether derivative were

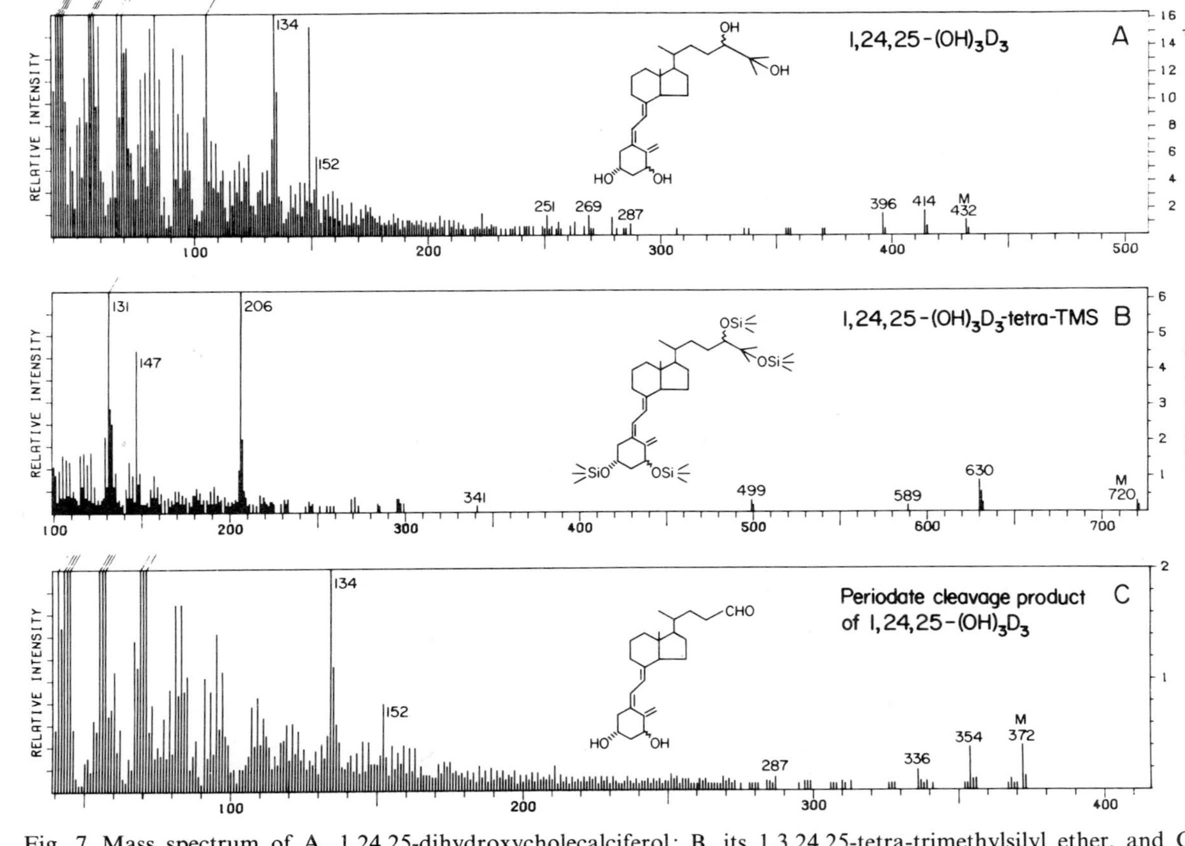

Fig. 7. Mass spectrum of A, 1,24,25-dihydroxycholecalciferol; B, its 1,3,24,25-tetra-trimethylsilyl ether, and C, periodate cleavage product of 1,24,25-dihydroxycholecalciferol

identical to fragments observed in the mass spectrum of 1,25-dihydroxy-cholecalciferol and its trimethylsilyl ether derivative, thus establishing an additional oxygen function in ring A. Periodate treatment of the metabolite yielded a product with a molecular ion peak at 272, corresponding to a C-24 aldehyde which results from the C-24, C-25 periodate cleavage. This demonstrated that the 24,25-hydroxyls were still present in the metabolite. Furthermore, peaks at m/e 152 and 134 firmly established that the additional hydroxyl function in ring A must be on C-1 since an additional hydroxyl function on either C-4 or C-2 would be vicinal to the hydroxyl on C-3 and thus be sensitive to periodate oxidation.

2 *Biological Activity*. To better understand the importance of this metabolite in calcium homeostasis, Holick *et al.* (1973a) examined the long-term

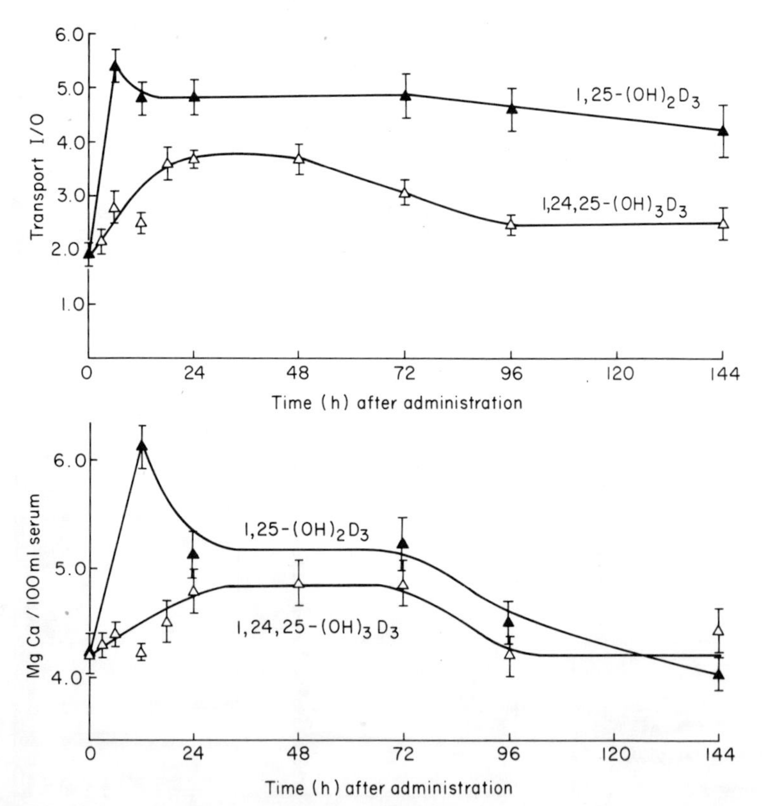

Fig. 8. A, Intestinal calcium transport and B, bone calcium mobilisation response of vitamin D-deficient rats to either 62.5 pmoles of 1,25-dihydroxy-(▲) or 1,24,25-trihydroxycholecalciferol (△). The vertical bars represent the standard error of the mean for 6 animals

biological activity of 1,24,25-dihydroxycholecalciferol in comparison to the 1,25-dihydroxy-metabolite in intestinal calcium transport, bone calcium mobilisation and calcification of bone. It can be seen in Fig. 8 that 62.5 pmoles of 1,24,25-dihydroxycholecalciferol first stimulates intestinal calcium transport 6 h after administration and that a maximum response is observed after 18 h, while 62.5 pmoles of 1,25-dihydroxycholecalciferol produces a maximum response at 6 h. Furthermore, 62.5 pmoles of 1,24,25-dihydroxycholecalciferol is 33% less active than the hormone in this system. The intestinal calcium transport level for the trihydroxy-metabolite began to decline at 72 h and by 96 h was down to control levels. The effectiveness of the hormone in the intestine is, therefore, much more prolonged than that of 1,24,25-dihydroxycholecalciferol.

The isolated trihydroxy-metabolite has minimal ability to mobilise calcium from bone. The response being maximal 24 h after dosing decreasing to control values by 72 h. In comparison, 1,25-dihydroxycholecalciferol produces a rapid response with a marked rise in serum calcium at 6 h with a sustained 1 mg% increase for 72 h after which time the serum calcium falls to control values (Fig. 8). The biopotency of this polar metabolite in comparison to the hormone can be observed in their ability to support calcification of rachitic rats. The antirachitic activity of 1,25-dihydroxycholecalciferol is 400 units/μg whereas for the trihydroxy-metabolite it is approximately 24 units/μg or about 20 times less active than the hormone in its ability to heal rachitic lesions. It is likely that 24,25-dihydroxycholecalciferol is recognised by the kidney 25-hydroxycholecalciferol-1α-hydroxylase and is a suitable substrate for the enzyme resulting in an analogue of 1,25-dihydroxycholecalciferol which retains the capacity to stimulate intestinal calcium transport but which has lost much of its bone calcium mobilising activity. Whether it has physiological significance or not remains unknown, but at the present time evidence of its physiological importance is at best disappointing.

E TISSUE DISTRIBUTION OF VITAMIN D AND ITS METABOLITES

Although much work has been carried out in this area with radioactive calciferol, conclusions are limited by the fact that the vitamin is rapidly metabolised to other metabolites. As a result, the distribution of radioactivity among the various organs becomes a very complex consideration. However, in spite of all of the negative features there are some general conclusions which can be drawn. It is clear that calciferol is absorbed in the intestinal tract primarily through the lacteal system (Avioli *et al.*, 1967). It is not clear which site in the intestine is responsible for the maximal rate of calciferol absorption since this appears to depend entirely upon the vehicle in which the vitamin is administered. Thus Schachter and coworkers (1964) concluded that calciferol must be absorbed primarily in the upper intestinal tract, whereas Kodicek and colleagues (1960) and Norman and DeLuca (1963) found that vitamin D was absorbed in the distal small intestine. The major difference was that Schachter *et al.* (1964) administered the [^{3}H]cholecalciferol in ethanol solutions whereas the other two groups administered the compound in vegetable oil.

Once absorbed, calciferol is probably carried in chylomicrons and on β-lipoproteins to the liver. The liver takes up as much as 60–80% of a dose of cholecalciferol given either orally or intravenously (Kodicek, 1960; Norman and DeLuca, 1963; Neville and DeLuca, 1966). Exactly which cells in the liver contain calciferol is not known. Some autoradiography has been carried out with large amounts of cholecalciferol (Kodicek, 1960), but more definitive experiments with physiological doses are needed before clear conclusions can be made.

In the liver and other tissues a small portion of the calciferol content at all time intervals is as long chain fatty acid esters of calciferol (Lund *et al.*, 1967; Fraser and Kodicek, 1968a, b). Evidence has been presented that the cholesterol esterifying enzymes of pancreatic juice and of plasma form these substances (Fraser and Kodicek, 1968c). About 1–1.5 h after the calciferol reaches the liver, it and its major metabolite, 25-hydroxycholecalciferol are released into the blood stream (Ponchon and DeLuca, 1969) primarily bound to specific transport protein (see chapter 5).

25-Hydroxycholecalciferol is further metabolised in the kidney to either 1,25-dihydroxy- or to 24,25-dihydroxycholecalciferol. In general the labelled metabolites and the vitamin are distributed in a similar manner among the tissues and organs. A major difference is that only cholecalciferol is taken up by the liver initially in large amounts. The hydroxylated compounds apparently do not enter the liver in a preferential manner with less than 4% of a dose appearing in that organ (Ponchon and DeLuca, 1969).

Of some interest is the fact that the intestine does not accumulate large amounts of either calciferol or any of its metabolites. The percent accumulation is below 10% and is often in the neighbourhood of 3–5%. This is also true for 1,25-dihydroxycholecalciferol, a recognised active form in that organ. A concentrating ability of the intestine and bone for the hormone relative to plasma levels might be expected. This is difficult to establish except that the intestine appears to accumulate 1,25-dihydroxycholecalciferol in contrast to 24,25-dihydroxycholecalciferol when given at equal levels (Boyle *et al.*, 1973). In any case, no more than 3–5% of the dose ever accumulates in that particular target tissue. The muscle and bone account for approximately 60% or more of the accumulation of a single dose of calciferol and its metabolites (Kodicek, 1955; Norman and DeLuca, 1963; Neville and DeLuca, 1966; Frolick and DeLuca, 1972).

There has been a great deal of discussion regarding the site of storage of calciferol. It has long been known that calciferol is one of the vitamins which is stored for long periods of time. Following a single dose of cholecalciferol, biological activity was detected in the livers of animals as long as six months later (Heymann, 1937). Primarily on the basis of these results and on the basis that the liver accumulates the initial dose of radioactive cholecalciferol, the idea that the liver is the major storage site for the vitamin has emerged. However, this has been questioned by Quarterman (1964) in his experiments with pigs. More recently work by Rosenstreich *et al.* (1971) has shown that upon chronic administration of radioactive cholecalciferol to rats the primary site of storage is the adipose tissue. This, therefore, makes even more understandable the persistence of calciferol in animals for long periods of time.

Little of the vitamin or its metabolites is excreted in the urine. Less than 5% of the total dose of cholecalciferol can be recovered in the urine (Neville and DeLuca, 1966; Avioli *et al.*, 1967; Kodicek, 1963). An interesting metabolite of cholecalciferol found in the urine is the sulphate conjugate. This is also found in relatively large quantities in the aqueous portion of milk (Sahashi *et al.*, 1969) and is reportedly synthesised primarily in liver (Higaki *et al.*, 1965).

The primary route of excretion of cholecalciferol appears to be through the bile and hence faeces (Blumberg *et al.*, 1960; Norman and DeLuca, 1963). The limited analysis so far carried out on the biliary metabolites indicates that a significant portion is present as a glucuronide (Bell and Kodicek, 1969) but not cholecalciferol glucuronide as originally proposed by Avioli *et al.* (1967).

F ERGOCALCIFEROL METABOLITES IN CHICKEN AND RAT

Steenbock and his colleagues (Steenbock *et al.*, 1932) were the first to recognise that vitamin D activity derived from ergosterol is not as effective as that in fish liver oils in the prevention of rickets in chicks. Waddell (1934) demonstrated that irradiated ergosterol is not as effective as irradiated impure cholesterol in preventing vitamin D-deficiency in chickens while both preparations were equally effective in the rat. He concluded that the provitamin in the cholesterol is not identical to ergosterol and that the chick discriminates between the two irradiation products. Although the ratio of the activity of cholecalciferol to that of ergocalciferol in the chick has been reported to range between 100:1 and 10:1, Chen and Bosmann (1964) established that cholecalciferol is about 10 times as active as ergocalciferol in curing rickets in chicks. This discrimination has also been observed in turkeys and in new-world monkeys (Hunt *et al.*, 1967). In contrast, rat, man and most other mammals respond equally as well to the two forms of the vitamin.

Following the administration of [U-^{14}C]ergocalciferol and of [1,2-

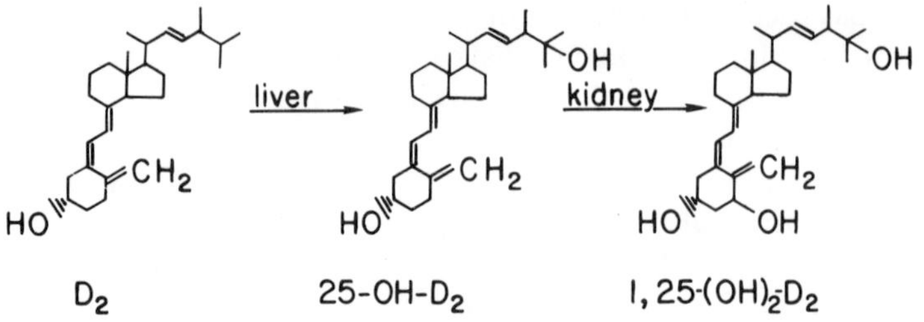

Fig. 9. Metabolism of ergocalciferol by the liver to its 25-hydroxymetabolite with subsequent conversion in the kidney to 1,25-dihydroxyergocalciferol

^{3}H]cholecalciferol to rachitic chicks the ^{14}C radioactivity disappears from the blood and tissues much more rapidly than the tritium radioactivity. The [^{14}C] appears in the bile and faecal excretory products which led to the suggestion that ergocalciferol or an active metabolite thereof is turned over more quickly than cholecalciferol thus explaining its decreased biological activity (Imrie *et al.*, 1967). It was later shown that chicks are capable of hydroxylating both ergo- and cholecalciferol on C-25 (Fig. 9), and that rachitic chicks also discriminate against 25-hydroxyergocalciferol in terms of biological activity (Drescher *et al.*, 1969).

In agreement with the conclusions of Drescher *et al.* (1969), Jones *et al.* (1975) have shown that chicken liver homogenates carry out the 25-hydroxylation of ergocalciferol at a rate equal to that found with cholecalciferol. Furthermore the chick kidney 25-hydroxycholecalciferol-1α-hydroxylase does not discriminate against 25-hydroxyergocalciferol.

Another possible site of discrimination against ergocalciferol and its metabolites is the binding capability of the plasma transport proteins (Belsey *et al.*, 1974). Although the carrier protein for 25-hydroxycholecalciferol binds ergo- and cholecalciferol equally well in rats, the affinity of the chick protein for 25-hydroxycholecalciferol is ten times greater than for 25-hydroxyergocalciferol. It is possible that poor binding of this latter metabolite results in its rapid metabolism to execretory products.

[3α-^{3}H]Ergocalciferol of high specific activity has been synthesised and converted *in vivo* into [3-^{3}H]25-hydroxyergocalciferol which together with the unlabelled metabolite obtained from porcine plasma has been incubated with kidney homogenates from rachitic chickens (Jones *et al.*, 1975). From such incubation mixtures, a polar metabolite was isolated in pure form and identified as 1,25-dihydroxyergocalciferol (Fig. 9). This metabolite was found to be as active as 1,25-dihydroxycholecalciferol in all systems known to be responsive to cholecalciferol in the rat and to have been between 10 and 20% of the activity of 1,25-dihydroxycholecalciferol in the chick (Jones *et al.*, 1976a). Thus discrimination by the chick against the ergocalciferol side chain persists in the metabolically active form of the vitamin. Two sources of this discrimination have been suggested. The target organ may respond poorly to 1,25-dihydroxyergocalciferol, alternatively the chick may possess a mechanism for rapidly metabolising C-24 substituted sterols resulting in a lower total tissue level of the 25-hydroxy- and 1,25-dihydroxy-metabolites of ergocalciferol (Jones *et al.*, 1976b).

II Regulation of Vitamin D Metabolism

A VITAMIN D-25-HYDROXYLASE

It is well-known that calciferol or some antirachitic substance is synthesised in the skin following ultraviolet activation of a precursor (DeLuca *et al.*, 1971). Since 7-dehydrocholesterol exists in abundant supply in the skin, it seems likely that its irradiation product is cholecalciferol, although it has never been isolated from this source and identified in a rigorous fashion. It is so far unknown whether the synthesis of cholecalciferol or antirachitic substances in the skin is under feed-back regulation.

The initial site of calciferol metabolism has been shown to be the liver where 25-hydroxylation occurs. A report from Tucker *et al.* (1973) has suggested that the vitamin is hydroxylated on C-25 in many tissues, especially intestine and kidney. The basis for their results was the incubation of intestinal or kidney homogenates from chicks with radioactive cholecalciferol and the recovery of a compound which comigrates with 25-hydroxycholecalciferol in standard chromatographic systems. These results were obtained at high substrate concentrations and have been confirmed in our laboratory (Bhattacharyya and DeLuca, 1973). However, hepatectomy of rats essentially eliminates the production of 25-hydroxycholecalciferol in this species (Olson, Knutson, Bhattacharyya and DeLuca, unpublished results; Ponchon *et al.*, 1969). Furthermore, hepatic homogenates have clear ability to catalyse the conversion of cholecalciferol to its 25-hydroxy-metabolite and the liver initially takes up most of the radioactive cholecalciferol and returns the 25-hydroxy-substance to the blood stream. Recent experiments using cellophane constriction of the portal vein followed by ligation of the hepatic artery have allowed the survival of rats for up to 12 h following removal of the liver. In such a model very little 25-hydroxycholecalciferol appears even though large concentrations of cholecalciferol are found in the plasma because of the absence of liver accumulation (Olson, Knutson, Bhattacharyya and DeLuca, unpublished results). It seems very likely, therefore, at least in the rat which is perhaps more representative of mammalian species, that the major site of 25-hydroxylation *in vivo* is the liver.

There has been some controversy regarding the idea that the 25-hydroxylase is feed-back regulated. In early work from Kodicek's laboratory as a result of using large amounts of cholecalciferol the 25-hydroxy-metabolite was not detected because its amount was small relative to the vitamin itself (Kodicek, 1960). In the work which led to the isolation and identification of 25-hydroxycholecalciferol, it was necessary to raise the dosage of cholecalciferol from 2.5 μg/day to 6 mg/day in order to raise the circulating level of 25-hydroxycholecalciferol from 1 unit of antirachitic activity per ml to 12 units per ml (Blunt *et al.*, 1968). Certainly these experiments illustrate that there is not a linear relationship between dosage of cholecalciferol and the amount of 25-hydroxycholecalciferol circulating in the plasma. In a series of experiments designed to test the idea that the 25-hydroxylase is regulated, Horsting and DeLuca (1969) and Bhattacharyya and DeLuca (1973) showed that the preadministration of radioactive cholecalciferol to rachitic or vitamin D-deficient rats markedly reduced the ability of hepatic homogenates to convert cholecalciferol to the 25-hydroxy-metabolite even though the substrate was of the same specific activity as the dose of radioactive cholecalciferol given to inhibit the 25-hydroxylation. These experiments illustrate clearly that regulation of some sort is taking place at the hepatic 25-hydroxylation stage. The nature of the inhibition of the 25-hydroxylase is not known although 25-hydroxycholecalciferol can serve as a product inhibitor (Horsting and DeLuca, 1969). However, the concentration of 25-hydroxycholecalciferol in the liver which inhibits the 25-hydroxylase is considerably smaller than that needed to exert product inhibition *in vitro*. It seems that inhibiting the 25-hydroxylase is related to the liver level of 25-hydroxycholecalciferol which must in some way feed-back regulate the cholecalciferol 25-hydroxylase. As the liver level of 25-hydroxycholecalciferol is depleted, the 25-hydroxylase is permitted to resume original activity. These results have been questioned on the basis of results obtained with chicks as Tucker *et al.* (1973) have shown that in this species the administration of 0.25 μg of cholecalciferol did not result in a diminution of the hepatic level of the 25-hydroxylase. Bhattacharyya and DeLuca (1974) have confirmed this observation and have shown in addition that the administration of more than 0.50 μg of cholecalciferol to deficient chickens will shut down the 25-hydroxylase in a manner very similar to that seen in the rat. There is, therefore, little doubt that regulation of the 25-hydroxylase can be demonstrated in the chick as well as the rat. Support of this has also been obtained by Haddad and his collaborators who have shown that the circulating level of 25-hydroxycholecalciferol is not related linearly to the dosage of cholecalciferol given (Haddad and Stamp, 1974). One must, therefore, consider that the initial entry of cholecalciferol into its metabolic sequence has a regulated step controlling the flow of the vitamin into its active metabolites.

B 25-HYDROXYCHOLECALCIFEROL-1α-HYDROXYLASE

1 *Characterisation of the 25-Hydroxycholecalciferol-1α-Hydroxylase.* Perhaps the most significant site for regulation of cholecalciferol metabolism is the 25-hydroxycholecalciferol-1α-hydroxylase in the kidney. Before discussing the regulation of this metabolic conversion, it is perhaps of importance to review the enzymology of the conversion. There is little doubt that this hydroxylation takes place exclusively in the kidney (Fraser and Kodicek, 1970; Gray *et al.*, 1971; Norman *et al.*, 1971b). Nephrectomy completely prevents the production of the hormone from 25-hydroxycholecalciferol. Furthermore, the only *in vitro* tissue preparation which will carry out the hydroxylation is the kidney (Fraser and Kodicek, 1970). The specific cell within the kidney at which hydroxylation occurs remains unknown; however, it has been conclusively shown that the mitochondria is the intracellular site of the 1α-hydroxylation reaction (Fraser and Kodicek, 1970; Gray *et al.*, 1972). This reaction is supported by internally generated NADPH which is probably generated by energy linked transhydrogenation from NADH (Ghazarian and DeLuca, 1974). Thus mitochondria with an intact respiratory and oxidative phosphorylation system are required for the 25-hydroxycholecalciferol-1α-hydroxylation. The specific requirement for NADPH has been clearly demonstrated in calcium swollen mitochondria which permits the entry of reduced pyridine nucleotides from external sources into the mitochondria. NADH will not support the hydroxylation in this system whereas NADPH is virtually as effective as hydroxylation in intact mitochondria with succinate or malate as the substrate. The 25-hydroxycholecalciferol-1α-hydroxylase has been conclusively demonstrated by the work of Ghazarian *et al.* (1974) to be dependent upon a cytochrome P-450. The first evidence for a cytochrome-P-450 component was obtained by Fraser and Kodicek (1970) who demonstrated that this system is carbon monoxide sensitive. Ghazarian and DeLuca (1974) extended the observation and demonstrated that the carbon monoxide inhibition is light reversible, an observation which has recently been confirmed (Henry and Norman, 1974). In addition, Ghazarian *et al.* (1974) have shown that amino glutethimide and metyrapone, inhibitors of cytochrome P-450 reactions, inhibit the 1α-hydroxylation of 25-hydroxycholecalciferol *in vitro*. Convincing spectral evidence was also presented that chick kidney mitochondria contain a cytochrome P-450. The 1α-hydroxylase enzyme has been solubilised and the isolated cytochrome P-450 fraction combined with beef adrenadoxin and beef flavoprotein together with a source of NADPH. This reconstituted system carries out *in vitro* 1α-hydroxylation of 25-hydroxycholecalciferol conclusively demonstrating the dependence of the 1α-hydroxylase on cytochrome P-450. In addition, classical $^{18}O_2$ experiments have been carried out (Ghazarian *et al.*, 1973), which demonstrate that the

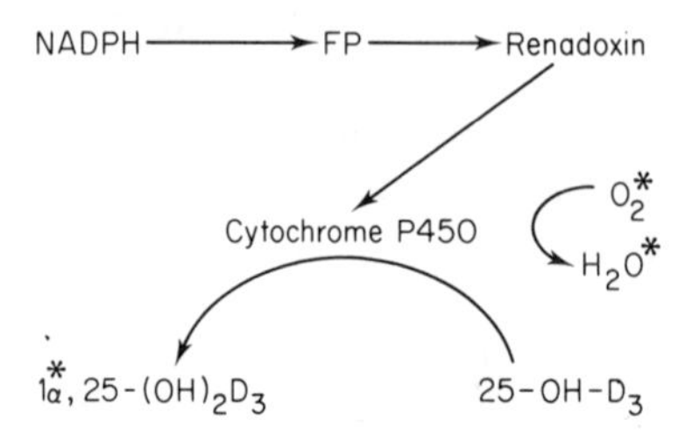

Fig. 10. Proposed biochemical mechanism of 1-hydroxylation of 25-hydroxycholecalciferol

1α-hydroxylase is a mixed-function oxidase with the oxygen appearing in the 1,25-dihydroxycholecalciferol coming from molecular oxygen. It seems clear that the 25-hydroxycholecalciferol-1α-hydroxylase has at least three components, namely a flavoprotein, an iron sulfur protein, renal ferredoxin, and a cytochrome P-450 (Fig. 10).

Although experiments with nephrectomised animals have shown that the kidney is the site of 1,25-dihydroxycholecalciferol formation in the rat *in vivo* (Gray *et al.*, 1971) it has not yet been possible to demonstrate this reaction with rat kidney tissue *in vitro*. The presence of inhibitory factor in rat tissues particularly serum and intestine has been reported (Botham *et al.*, 1974) and a similar factor but with much less activity is present in chick tissues. This factor is a protein and has been isolated from rat serum by the usual purification procedures for proteins (Botham *et al.*, 1976). Various mechanisms have been considered by which this inhibition can occur and all but some have been eliminated. It appears that the inhibitor is also the plasma 25-hydroxycholecalciferol binding protein and it may therefore act by binding the substrate more strongly than the 1-hydroxylase enzyme. Certainly the reduction in the velocity of the 1-hydroxylase-enzyme in the presence of the inhibitor can be explained by substrate binding. The physiological significance of this inhibition is not clear.

2 *Regulation of 25-Hydroxycholecalciferol-1α-Hydroxylase Activity*. (*a*) Role of Dietary Calcium and the Nicolaysen Endogenous Factor. It has long been known that animals and man placed on a low calcium diet develop high rates of intestinal calcium absorption whereas those on a high calcium diet develop low rates of absorption (Nicolaysen *et al.*, 1953). Furthermore, the needs for calcium by the skeleton somehow are interpreted by the intestine by showing high rates of intestinal calcium absorption. This led Nicolaysen

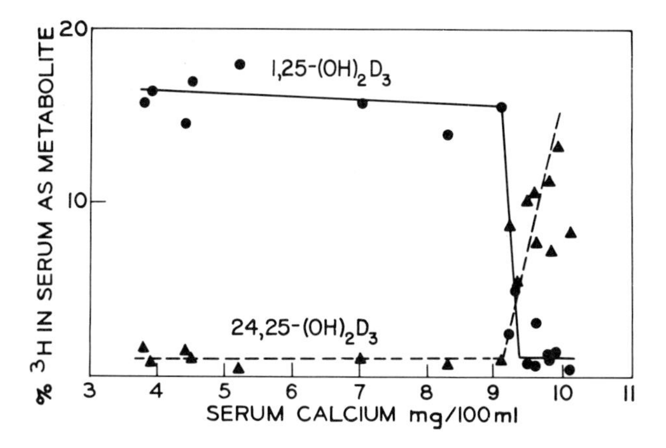

Fig. 11. The relationship of serum calcium concentration to the ability of rats to produce 1,25-dihydroxycholecalciferol from 25-hydroxycholecalciferol. Animals were fed diets containing various amounts of calcium and phosphorus with and without cholecalciferol for three weeks. At that time all animals received an intravenous injection of [26,27-^{3}H]25-hydroxycholecalciferol. 12 h later blood was taken from each animal, extracted and chromatographed to reveal the metabolites formed. All animals regardless of treatment were used in this plot. Note the sharp switch-over point at 9.5 mg% calcium. Under hypocalcaemic conditions the major metabolite of 25-hydroxycholecalciferol is the hormonal metabolite while norma- and hypercalcaemic conditions promote the production of 24,25-dihydroxycholecalciferol

and collaborators to postulate the existence of a hormone, termed the 'endogenous factor', which is secreted by the skeleton and which instructs the intestine of the skeletal needs for calcium. This factor was shown to be found only in animals given vitamin D (Nicolaysen, 1953). This led to an examination of the possibility that the endogenous factor might be 1,25-dihydroxycholecalciferol. Animals fed low dietary calcium produce large amounts of 1,25-dihydroxycholecalciferol, whereas those on a high calcium diet produce only small amount of the hormone (Boyle *et al.*, 1971). In addition, when the 1,25-dihydroxycholecalciferol synthesis was prevented by dietary calcium, another metabolite appeared which was identified as 24,25-dihydroxycholecalciferol (Holick *et al.*, 1972a). In agreement with the idea that 1,25-dihydroxycholecalciferol represents Nicolaysen's 'endogenous factor', Omdahl and DeLuca (1973) and Ribovich and DeLuca (unpublished results) demonstrated in chicks and rats that the ability to adapt to dietary calcium is eliminated by the administration of an exogenous source of 1,25-dihydroxycholecalciferol. Thus the 1,25-dihydroxycholecalciferol is the messenger that the intestine receives in response to the need for calcium.

The synthesis of 1,25-dihydroxycholecalciferol in intact animals is, therefore, related to serum calcium concentration (Fig. 11) and rats having a normal serum calcium level make both the 1,25- and 24,25-dihydroxy-metabolites (Boyle *et al.*, 1972b). However, in rats that are even slightly hypocalcaemic the synthesis of 1,25-dihydroxycholecalciferol is stimulated whereas the synthesis of the 24,25-dihydroxy-metabolite is inhibited. On the other hand, as the rats become hypercalcaemic, the synthesis of the 1,25-dihydroxycholecalciferol is shut off and the synthesis of the 24,25-dihydroxy-cholecalciferol is stimulated. This plot shows the true feed-back nature of serum calcium concentration on the synthesis of the hormone.

(*b*) Role of Parathyroid Hormone and Calcitonin. The hypocalcaemic stimulus of 1,25-dihydroxycholecalciferol synthesis is mediated by the parathyroid glands (Garabedian *et al.*, 1972; Fraser and Kodicek, 1973; Rusmussen *et al.*, 1972). It now seems clear that in response to hypocalcaemia,

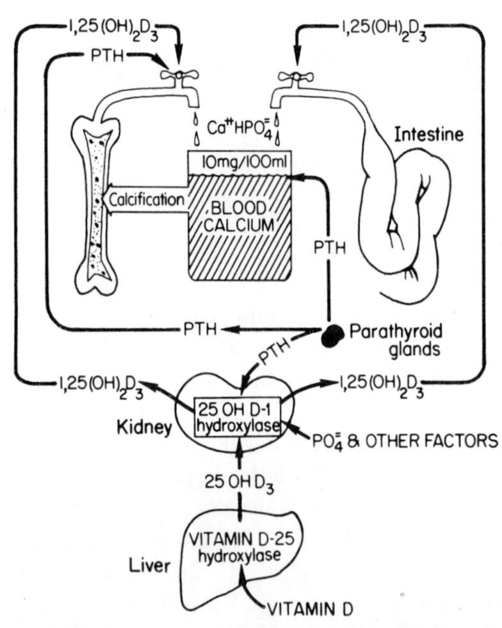

Fig. 12. Schematic representation of the hormonal control loop for calciferol metabolism and function. A reduction in the serum calcium from 10 mg/100 ml serum prompts a proportional secretion of parathyroid hormone that acts to stimulate the synthesis of 1,25-dihydroxycholecalciferol in kidney. This metabolite is taken up by the intestine to aid the absorption of calcium. Parathyroid hormone plus the hormone acts on the bone to effect bone calcium mobilisation. As the serum calcium increases towards normal (10 mg/100 ml serum) parathyroid secretion is diminished and so too is the synthesis of 1,25-dihydroxycholecalciferol

the parathyroid glands secrete parathyroid hormone which by some unknown mechanism triggers the synthesis of 1,25-dihydroxycholecalciferol. This steroid hormone then stimulates calcium absorption and bone calcium mobilisation restoring serum calcium to normal (Fig. 12). The mobilisation of calcium from bone requires the presence of both 1,25-dihydroxycholecalciferol and parathyroid hormone while the intestinal calcium transport system reponds to 1,25-dihydroxycholecalciferol without parathyroid hormone (Garabedian *et al.*, 1974a). In fact, parathyroid hormone has no direct effect on intestinal calcium transport. Thus its effect on calcium absorption is entirely mediated by the stimulation of 1,25-dihydroxycholecalciferol synthesis.

MacIntyre and his colleagues (Galante *et al.*, 1972a) have attempted to

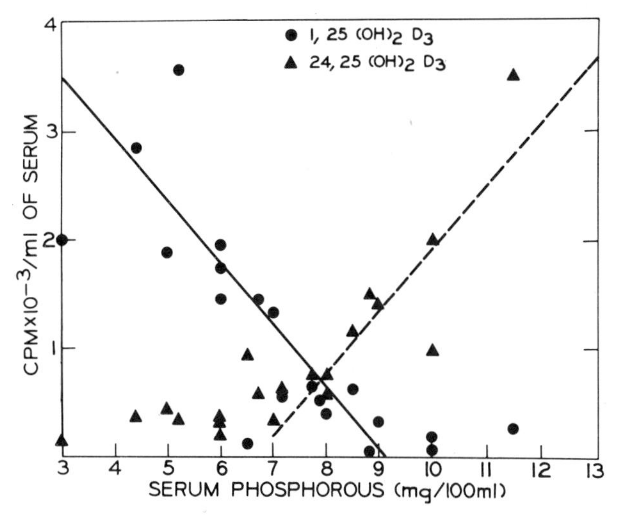

Fig. 13. The relationship of serum phosphorus concentration to the ability of rats to produce 1,25-dihydroxycholecalciferol from the 25-hydroxy precursor. For this plot thyroparathyroidectomised rats were prepared in the following diverse manners. (1) They were fed a high calcium, low phosphorus diet for 2 weeks and then given 325 pmoles 25-hydroxycholecalciferol orally 24 h prior to thyroparathyroidectomy. (2) They were fed a high calcium, adequate phosphorus diet for 2 weeks and were given 325 pmoles 25-hydroxycholecalciferol orally every day for 5 days prior to thyroparathyroidectomy. The rats from these two groups were shifted to various diets. All rats were injected with 325 pmoles [26,27-^{3}H]25-hydroxycholecalciferol and 12 h later their serum was taken for serum calcium, serum phosphorus and chromatographic analysis of ^{3}H labelled 25-hydroxycholecalciferol metabolites. The serum phosphorus is plotted versus production of 24,25-dihydroxy or 1,25-dihydroxycholecalciferol for all rats regardless of treatment. No correlation is found between metabolite levels and serum calcium concentration. (Reproduced with permission from Tanaka and DeLuca, 1973)

show that excessive amounts of parathyroid hormone actually inhibit the synthesis of 1,25-dihydroxycholecalciferol. This observation is difficult to place in physiological perspective and furthermore has not been substantiated by work in other laboratories. It may, however, play some role in pathological states in which large amounts of circulating parathyroid hormone are found such as in hyperparathyroidism.

So far two groups have reported regulation of calciferol metabolism by calcitonin. Galante *et al.* (1972b) with large amounts of calcitonin, have demonstrated that there is a stimulation of 1,25-dihydroxycholecalciferol synthesis whereas Rasmussen *et al.* (1972), using isolated renal tubules, have demonstrated a depression in the synthesis of the hormone, by the *in vitro* addition of the hormone. However, *in vivo* experiments which are critically addressed to the question of whether calcitonin plays a regulatory role in cholecalciferol metabolism are lacking.

(*c*) Dietary Phosphate. It is known that phosphate depletion stimulates intestinal calcium absorption (Morrissey and Wasserman, 1971). At least a partial basis for this has been put forth by Tanaka and DeLuca (1973) who demonstrated that in addition to parathyroid hormone, hypophosphataemia can also stimulate the synthesis of 1,25-dihydroxycholecalciferol. In thyroparathyroidectomised rats, reduction of serum inorganic phosphate by dietary deprivation or other means to levels of less than 8 mg/100 ml stimulates the synthesis of 1,25-dihydroxycholecalciferol (Fig. 13). The mechanism of this stimulation remains unknown, but nevertheless phosphate deprivation can stimulate the synthesis of 1,25-dihydroxycholecalciferol and inhibit the synthesis of 24,25-dihydroxycholecalciferol (Baxter and DeLuca, 1976). This development is of particular importance in view of the fact that 1,25-dihydroxycholecalciferol can be shown to function in the stimulation of intestinal phosphate transport (Chen *et al.*, 1974) and in the elevation of serum inorganic phosphate (Tanaka and DeLuca, 1974). Thus one can visualise that the 1,25-dihydroxycholecalciferol may be a hormone involved in phosphate metabolism as well as in calcium metabolism (DeLuca, 1974a).

The idea that phosphate deprivation on one hand and parathyroid hormone, which blocks renal tubular reabsorption of phosphate, both stimulate synthesis of 1,25-dihydroxycholecalciferol has led to the suggestion that both might function in a similar way by decreasing the renal cellular level of inorganic phosphate (Tanaka and DeLuca, 1973). A reduced renal cell level of inorganic phosphate would stimulate the synthesis of the 1,25-dihydroxycholecalciferol. Measurements of renal cortex levels of inorganic phosphate have tended to support these suggestions, but additional information will be necessary before this hypothesis can be accepted.

Throughout the course of this discussion it is apparent that as the synthesis of 1,25-dihydroxycholecalciferol is depressed either by the absence of parathyroid hormone or by the presence of inorganic phosphate, the synthesis of 24,25-dihydroxycholecalciferol is increased in a compensatory manner. It must be emphasised as it was originally shown by Boyle *et al.* (1971), that regulation of the 25-hydroxycholecalciferol renal hydroxylase takes place only in animals maintained on a source of vitamin D. Such a regulation is not apparent in the vitamin D-deficient animal. The vitamin D-deficient kidneys contain little or no 25-hydroxycholecalciferol-24-hydroxylase. It is interesting to note that the kidney is not the sole site of synthesis of the 24,25-dihydroxycholecalciferol since recent work by Garabedian *et al.* (1974b) has shown that other tissues can make this metabolite. Additional work in our laboratory has also confirmed that 25-hydroxycholecalciferol-24-hydroxylase can be found in other tissues (Tanaka and DeLuca, unpublished results).

The fact that the 24-hydroxylase is absent in the vitamin D-deficient state has led to an examination of the idea that some form of vitamin D might well induce the formation of the 24-hydroxylase system. Conclusive proof of this has not yet been obtained although it can be readily demonstrated that the administration of 1,25-dihydroxycholecalciferol to vitamin D-deficient animals will within 6 h induce the ability to make 24,25-dihydroxycholecalciferol (Ghazarian *et al.*, 1975). Furthermore, 1,25-dihydroxycholecalciferol does increase RNA synthesis in kidney (Chen and DeLuca, 1973) and the stimulation of the 24-hydroxylase by 1,25-dihydroxycholecalciferol can be blocked with actinomycin D (Tanaka and DeLuca, unpublished results). The regulation, therefore of the renal 25-hydroxycholecalciferol hydroxylases is a complex system that is not understood at the molecular level. Attempts have been made to demonstrate that the regulation is a simple ionic inhibition or activation of the hydroxylases in the kidney (Horiuchi *et al.*, 1974; Norman, 1974; MacIntyre *et al.*, 1975). Although simple experiments which show that the addition of calcium or phosphate will either inhibit or stimulate the *in vitro* 1α-hydroxylation have been carried out, these experiments are inconclusive and carry with them many difficulties in interpretation of the results (Ghazarian *et al.*, 1975; Suda *et al.*, 1973; Galante, *et al.*, 1973; DeLuca, 1974b). The regulation *in vivo* requires many hours, which makes it unlikely that it is an ionic activation or inhibition mechanism. More likely the synthesis or degradation of the hydroxylases is the regulating phenomenon and that in the absence of vitamin D it is possible that the messenger RNA for the 25-hydroxycholecalciferol-24-hydroxylase is absent. In any case although we understand that the parathyroid hormone, serum levels of inorganic phosphate and 1,25-dihydroxycholecalciferol itself play an important role at the physiological level in regulating the renal 25-hydroxycholecalciferol hydroxylases, the molecular mechanism of this regulation or even the cellular mechanism of these regulations, remains largely unknown and will likely represent an important area of investigation in the next several years.

III Analogues of Cholecalciferol and Metabolites

A SIDE CHAIN ANALOGUES

Windaus and coworkers (1935, 1936) were the first to synthesise calciferol analogues differing in their side chain structures. They successfully synthesised an analogue of ergosterol which had a choleserol side chain and reported that one of its irradiation products possessed about the same antirachitic potency as ergocalciferol. However, when the side chain was replaced by a hydroxyl function (Dimroth and Paland, 1939) or by a bile acid side chain (Haslewood, 1939), the compounds were devoid of vitamin D activity. When the Δ^{22} of ergocalciferol was reduced, the resulting compound, vitamin D_4, had 75% of the biological activity of cholecalciferol in rats and about 10% in the case of chicks (Windaus and Trautman, 1937; DeLuca *et al.*, 1968). With the realisation that vitamin D_3 must be converted to 1,25-dihydroxycholecalciferol before it can function, came the possibility that the failure of such

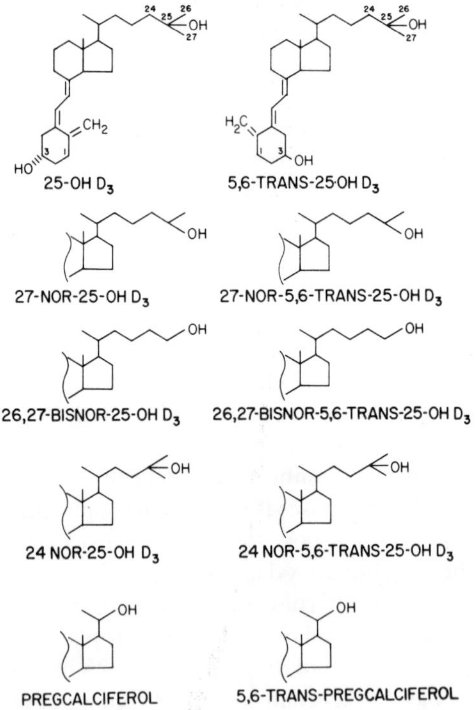

25-OH D_3 | 5,6-TRANS-25-OH D_3

27-NOR-25-OH D_3 | 27-NOR-5,6-TRANS-25-OH D_3

26,27-BISNOR-25-OH D_3 | 26,27-BISNOR-5,6-TRANS-25-OH D_3

24 NOR-25-OH D_3 | 24 NOR-5,6-TRANS-25-OH D_3

PREGCALCIFEROL | 5,6-TRANS-PREGCALCIFEROL

Fig. 14. The structures of the various side chain analogues of 25-hydroxycholecalciferol

analogues to function might be due to a failure of the side chain hydroxylation or 1α-hydroxylation.

By synthesising analogues with the 25-hydroxyl group, the failure of function which might be due to a failure of 25-hydroxylation could be eliminated. The 24-nor-,27-nor- and 26,27-bisnor-25-hydroxycholecalciferol were synthesised and shown to be capable of stimulating intestinal calcium transport and bone calcium mobilisation in rats but had only 1–10% of the activity of 25-hydroxycholecalciferol (Fig. 14). However, these analogues are biologically inactive at a 25 μg dose level in anephric rats, suggesting that they are hydroxylated by the kidney 25-hydroxycholecalciferol-1α-hydroxylase before they can function. Additional evidence that this hydroxylation occurs was suggested by the fact that rotation of the A ring of the 27-nor-and 26,27-bisnor-25-hydroxycholecalciferol by a *cis-trans* isomerisation, which places the 3β-hydroxyl in a pseudo-1α-hydroxy position, partially restores the intestinal calcium transport and bone calcium mobilisation activity in anephric rats. When the side chain is replaced by a hydroxyl (Fig. 14), no

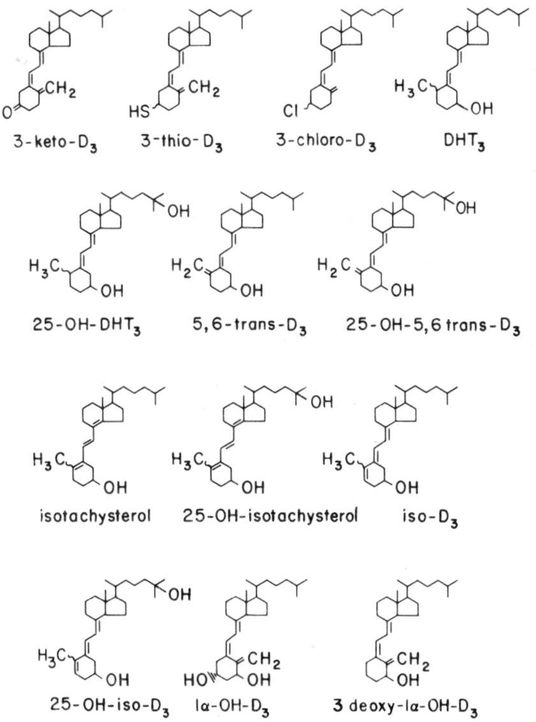

3-keto-D_3 3-thio-D_3 3-chloro-D_3 DHT_3

25-OH-DHT_3 5,6-trans-D_3 25-OH-5,6 trans-D_3

isotachysterol 25-OH-isotachysterol iso-D_3

25-OH-iso-D_3 Iα-OH-D_3 3 deoxy-Iα-OH-D_3

Fig. 15. The structures of the various A ring analogues and isomers of cholecalciferol and its 25-hydroxy-metabolite

biological activity in either the intestine or bone is found. In order to rule out that the lack of activity might be due to the inability of the kidney to hydroxylate this analogue in the 1α-position, the 5,6-*trans* isomer was made and found to be biologically inactive at dosages of 25 μg or less (Holick *et al.*, 1975a).

Crump *et al.* (1973) and Bontekoe *et al.* (1970) prepared 22-hydroxy-vitamin D_4, 27-nor- and 26,27-bisnor-25-hydroxycholecalciferol and noted that these analogues were biologically inactive based on tests for antirachitic activity. It is now clear that 27-nor- and 26,27-bisnor-cholecalciferol have biological activity suggesting that it is necessary to test analogues of calciferol not only for antirachitic activity, but also for intestinal calcium transport and bone calcium mobilisation before they can be considered biologically inactive.

The side chain analogue investigations demonstrate that optimal activity of 25-hydroxycholecalciferol requires an intact side chain. Some slight modification of side chain structure is tolerated, but most alterations markedly diminish biological activity. This reduction in activity is probably not due to failure of 1-hydroxylation since the 5,6-*trans* derivatives are not more active than the 5,6-*cis* forms. However, an unequivocal decision on this cannot be made until the 1α-hydroxy derivatives of each of these analogues are prepared. The recent demonstration that the 24-nor-1α,25-dihydroxycholecalciferol is essentially inactive at a 2.5 μg dose gives considerable support to the concept that an intact side chain is of great importance to 1,25-dihydroxycholecalciferol function (Reeve, Lam, Schnoes and DeLuca, in preparation).

B A-RING ANALOGUES OF CHOLECALCIFEROL AND 1,25-DIHYDROXYCHOLECALCIFEROL

1 *3β-Hydroxyl Group*. The β-hydroxyl group at C-3 has been replaced by a keto function (Windaus and Bucholz, 1938), a sulfhydryl (Bernstein and Sax, 1951) and a halogen (Bernstein *et al.*, 1949) and in each case these replacements eliminated vitamin D activity of the molecule (Fig. 15). Again the inactivity may be due to a failure of 25- and 1α-hydroxylations.

2 *Dihydrotachysterols*. One of the most important analogues of calciferol was discovered by von Werder (1939). He reduced tachysterol with sodium/propanol to yield dihydrotachysterol (Fig. 15) and other reduction products (chapter 1,V). Although this compound possessed only 0.2% of the antirachitic activity of cholecalciferol, it is more effective than large doses of the vitamin in the elevation of serum calcium of hypoparathyroid animals and man (Roborgh and DeMan, 1960; Harrison *et al.*, 1968). The 25-hydroxy derivative of dihydrotachysterol (Fig. 15) has been synthesised and is biologically more active than dihydrotachysterol$_3$ on a weight basis, which

suggests that the 25-hydroxy derivative may be the active form. Additionally since ring A is rotated 180° during reduction to dihydrotachysterol$_3$, the 3β-hydroxy is located somewhere near the spacial position occupied by the 1α-hydroxyl of 1,25-dihydroxycholecalciferol. It is, therefore, understandable that nephrectomised animals respond to either dihydrotachysterol$_3$ (Harrison and Harrison, 1972) or 25-hydroxydihydrotachysterol$_3$ (Hallick and DeLuca, 1972).

3 *Isomers of Cholecalciferol.* During the 1950s and early 1960s much effort was directed to the synthesis and characterisation of various isomers of cholecalciferol (chapter 1, IVB). In their attempts to devise a new method for the synthesis of ergocalciferol, Inhoffen *et al.* (1954) reported the synthesis of two triene isomers of ergocalciferol, isoergocalciferol and isotachysterol$_2$ (Fig. 15). A year later Verloop and coworkers (1955) reported the synthesis of the 5,6-*trans* isomer of cholecalciferol (Fig. 15) by iodine catalysis and showed that its biological activity in chickens was about 3% that of cholecalciferol (Verloop *et al.*, 1959). In 1972 Holick *et al.* (1972c, d) compared the structure of 5,6-*trans*-cholecalciferol to dihydrotachysterol$_3$ and 1,25-dihydroxycholecalciferol. Although ring A is substantially different from either the hormone or dihydrotachysterol$_3$, it does have a hydroxyl in the general position occupied by the 1-hydroxyl of 1,25-dihydroxycholecalciferol. Unlike cholecalciferol or its 25-hydroxy-metabolite, 5,6-*trans*-cholecalciferol can stimulate both intestinal calcium transport and bone calcium mobilisation in anephric rats, thus serving as a true analogue of 1,25-dihydroxycholecalciferol. In vitamin D-deficient animals, 2.5 μg of this analogue is capable of eliciting an intestinal calcium transport response as early as 3 h after its administration and shows a small but significant bone calcium mobilisation response after 3 h and a maximum response at 12 h. Since it has been demonstrated that the 25-hydroxy derivatives of dihydrotachysterol$_3$, ergo- and cholecalciferol are biologically more active on a weight basis than their non-hydroxylated analogues (Suda *et al.*, 1970c; Blunt *et al.*, 1968), it was of interest to see if this might also be the case with 5,6-*trans*-cholecalciferol. Although on a weight basis the 25-hydroxy derivative did not appear to be more active than its parent compound in stimulating intestinal calcium transport in anephric rats, this derivative had less activity in mobilising calcium from bones of anephric rats (Holick *et al.*, 1972d). Since isocholecalciferol and isotachysterol also have their A ring rotated 180° so that the 3β-hydroxyl function is in a *pseudo* 1α-hydroxy position, these isomers were synthesised and tested for their biological potency (Holick *et al.*, 1973b). Isotachysterol (Fig. 15) and its 25-hydroxy derivative are capable of stimulating intestinal calcium transport and bone calcium mobilisation in anephric rats similar to 5,6-*trans*-cholecalciferol and are 10–100 times less active than cholecalciferol on a weight basis. However, isocholecalciferol (Fig. 15) and its 25-hydroxy derivative are not

capable of stimulating either intestinal calcium transport or bone calcium mobilisation in anephric rats.

C 1-HYDROXY DERIVATIVES

1 1-*Hydroxycholecalciferol.* The most promising analogue of 1,25-dihydroxycholecalciferol is 1α-hydroxycholecalciferol (Fig. 15). This analogue is much less difficult to prepare chemically than 1,25-dihydroxycholecalciferol and is less expensive to make in large quantities (Holick *et al.*, 1973c: Barton *et al.*, 1973; Kaneko *et al.*, 1974; chapter 1,VIIB). Unlike the other 1α-hydroxy analogues 1α-hydroxycholecalciferol is about half as active on weight basis as 1,25-dihydroxycholecalciferol in promoting intestinal calcium transport, bone calcium mobilisation and in its ability to heal rachitic lesions in rats. In the chick and the rat the time course and biological activity in intestinal calcium transport and in the chick bone calcium mobilisation activity of 1-hydroxy- and 1,25-dihydroxycholecalciferol are equal (Haussler *et al.*, 1973; Holick *et al.*, 1973c). However, the bone calcium mobilisation response in the rat to 1-hydroxycholecalciferol is clearly much slower than the response to the hormone (Holick *et al.*, 1973c). A comparison has been made of the amount of 1α-hydroxy- and of cholecalciferol required to achieve a steady level of intestinal calcium transport, bone mineralisation and bone calcium mobilisation in the rat (Holick *et al.*, 1975b). The biological potency of 1α-hydroxycholecalciferol is between 2–5 times that of cholecalciferol in rats and thus is about half as active as 1,25-dihydroxycholecalciferol (Tanaka *et al.*, 1973).

There were a number of indications in the literature that 1-hydroxycholecalciferol is effective in the target tissues through conversion to the 1,25-dihydroxy-metabolite before [6-^{3}H]1-hydroxycholecalciferol became available to conclusively demonstrate this conversion (Holick *et al.*, 1976b, c). Studies in this laboratory have shown that 1-hydroxycholecalciferol is about equally as active as 25-hydroxycholecalciferol in mobilising calcium from foetal tibia in culture (Stern *et al.*, 1975), whereas the hormone is about 1000–5000 times more active than 25-hydroxycholecalciferol suggesting the importance of a 25-hydroxyl group for activity (Raisz *et al.*, 1972). In addition on the basis of a chromatin binding assay for the hormone, Zerwekh *et al.* (1974) have concluded that 25-hydroxylation is necessary for expression of the activity in 1-hydroxycholecalciferol.

The only finding suggesting that 1-hydroxycholecalciferol could act unchanged has been obtained with cultures of embryonic chick intestine (R. A. Corradino, personal communication) but this system responds to large amounts of several metabolites of cholecalciferol apparently without their undergoing further metabolism (Corradino, 1973). The experiments with [6-

^{3}H]1-hydroxycholecalciferol showed that the biological activity of this substance is largely, if not exclusively due to its conversion to [6-^{3}H]1,25-dihydroxycholecalciferol. The latter substance appears in the intestine and bone of both rats and chicks before the maximal response of the tissues to the steroid is observed. Over 80 % of the radioactivity in these tissues is found as the hormone. The utilisation of 1-hydroxycholecalciferol may not be as great after an oral dose as after an intravenous dose since less radioactivity is found in bone and blood in the former case. The intestine has similar levels of the hormone whichever route the 1-hydroxycholecalciferol is administered (Holick *et al.*, 1976b, c).

2 3-*Deoxy-*1α-*hydroxycholecalciferol.* The synthesis of 3-deoxy-1α-hydroxycholecalciferol (Fig. 15) has been described and it has been shown that this analogue is capable of stimulating intestinal calcium transport. (Lam *et al.*, 1974). Although the 3-deoxy-1α-hydroxycholecalciferol shows some bone calcium mobilising activity *in vivo* it is virtually inactive in bone culture experiments, at least in concentrations of 10^{-6} M or less, while 1α-hydroxycholecalciferol has activity at about 10^{-9} M (Stern, Tanaka, Schnoes and DeLuca, unpublished results). Furthermore, it has little or no activity in healing rickets or in elevating serum phosphorus concentration of rachitic rats (Reeve, Schnoes and DeLuca, unpublished results). Other workers have also synthesised this substance (Okamura *et al.*, 1974), but have found a stimulation of calcium absorption in the chick which was inexplicably greater than that found by Lam *et al.* (1974). They used this observation to suggest that the more active configuration of the 1α-OH group is equitorial. Since the 3-deoxy-1α-hydroxycholecalciferol has little activity in the mobilisation of calcium from bone and on the mineralisation of bone, this hypothesis at best must be restricted to intestinal calcium transport. Whether there is validity for such a hypothesis for this system as well must await more definitive work.

3 *Conclusion.* The recent interest in the synthesis of analogues of cholecalciferol and its metabolites has led to the following conclusion about structural activity relationships. 1. The 5,6-*cis*-triene is not absolutely required for maintenance of biological responsiveness but its modification markedly reduces its effectiveness. 2. Minor alterations in the side chain length are permissible but they also markedly reduce biological activity while removal of the entire side chain renders all vitamin D compounds inactive. 3. The 3β-hydroxy function is not needed for intestinal calcium transport once a 1α-hydroxy or a *pseudo* 1α-hydroxy is in the molecule. However, its absence markedly reduces activity in bone and in the elevation of serum phosphorus. Although it is clear that the systems responsive to vitamin D differ in their structural requirements it appears that the 1α- and 3β hydroxyls along with an intact side chain with a 25-hydroxy and a *cis*-triene structure are all required for maximum biological responsiveness on a weight basis. To date there is no

analogue of cholecalciferol that is more biologically potent on a weight basis than the natural hormone 1,25-dihydroxycholecalciferol.

D SUMMARY

In the past decade it has been shown that cholecalciferol must be converted to its 25-hydroxy-metabolite in the liver and then to 1,25-dihydroxycholecalciferol in the kidney before it can function in calcium and phosphate metabolism. Its further metabolism and function awaits elucidation and the function of other known metabolites of cholecalciferol remain to be learned. For calcium metabolism, however, it is clear that 1,25-dihydroxycholecalciferol is a calcium mobilising hormone whose synthesis is regulated by 1,25-dihydroxycholecalciferol itself, parathyroid hormone and serum phosphorus concentration. Analogue studies show that for optimal activity in all its functions, 3β and 1α-hydroxy groups are needed as well as a *cis*-triene and an intact side chain with a 25-hydroxyl group. Possibly the intestinal calcium transport system does not require a hydroxy group at C-3 and C-25, but more experiments are needed for such a conclusion.

References

Avioli, L. V., Lee, S. W., McDonald, J. E., Lund, J. and DeLuca, H. F. (1967). *J. Clin. Invest.* **46**, 983.

Barton, D. H. R., Hesse, R. H., Pechet, M. M. and Rizzardo, E. (1973). *J. Am. Chem. Soc.* **95**, 2748.

Baxter, L. A. and DeLuca, H. F. (1976). *J. Biol. Chem.* **251**, 3158.

Bell, P. A. and Kodicek, E. (1969). *Biochem. J.* **115**, 663.

Belsey, R. E., DeLuca, H. F. and Potts, J. T. (1974). *Nature* (London) **247**, 208.

Bernstein, S. and Sax, K. J. (1951). *J. Org. Chem.* **16**, 685.

Bernstein, S., Oleson, J. J., Ritter, H. B. and Sax, K. J. (1949). *J. Am. Chem. Soc.* **71**, 2576.

Bhattacharyya, M. H. and DeLuca, H. F. (1973). *J. Biol. Chem.* **248**, 2969.

Bhattacharyya, M. H. and DeLuca, H. F. (1974). *Biochem. Biophys. Res. Commun.* **59**, 734.

Blumberg, A., Aebi, H., Hurni, H. and Schönholzer, G. (1960). *Helv. Physiol. Acta* **18**, 56.

Blunt, J. W., DeLuca, H. F. and Schnoes, H. K. (1968). *Biochemistry* **7**, 3317.

Bontekoe, J. S., Wignall, A., Rappoldt, M. P. and Roborgh, J. R. (1970). *Int. J. Vitamin Res.* **40**, 589.

Botham, K. M., Ghazarian, J. G., Kream, B. E. and DeLuca, H. F. (1976). *Biochemistry* **15**, 2130.

Botham, K. M., Tanaka, Y. and DeLuca, H. F. (1974). *Biochemistry* **113**, 4961.

Boyle, I. T., Gray, R. W. and DeLuca, H. F. (1971). *Proc. Nat. Acad. Sci. USA* **68**, 2131.

Boyle, I. T., Miravet, L., Gray, R. W., Holick, M. F. and DeLuca, H. F. (1972a). *Endocrinol.* **90**, 605.

Boyle, I. T., Gray, R. W., Omdahl, J. L. and DeLuca, H. F. (1972b). *In* 'Endocrinology 1971' (Ed. S. Taylor) pp. 468–476. Wm. Heinemann Medical Books Ltd., London.
Boyle, I. T., Omdahl, J. L., Gray, R. W. and DeLuca, H. F. (1973). *J. Biol. Chem.* **248**, 4174.
Carre, M., Ayigbede, O., Miravet, L. and Rasmussen, H. (1974). *Proc. Nat. Acad. Sci. USA* **71**, 2996.
Chen, P. S., and Bosmann, H. B. (1964). *J. Nutr.* **83**, 133.
Chen, T. C. and DeLuca, H. F. (1973). *Arch. Biochem. Biophys.* **156**, 321.
Chen, T. C., Castillo, L., Korycka-Dahl, M. and DeLuca, H. F. (1974). *J. Nutr.* **104**, 1056.
Corradino, R. A. (1973). *Science* **179**, 402.
Cousins, R. J., DeLuca, H. F., Suda, T., Chen, T. and Tanaka, Y. (1970a). *Biochemistry* **9**, 1453.
Cousins, R. J., DeLuca, H. F. and Gray, R. W. (1970b). *Biochemistry* **9**, 3649.
Crump, D. R., Williams, D. H. and Pelc, B. (1973). *J. Chem. Soc Perkin Trans.* **I**, 2731.
DeLuca, H. F. (1974a). *Fed. Proc.* **33**, 2211.
DeLuca, H. F. (1974b). *Am. J. Med.* **57**, 1.
DeLuca, H. F., Weller, M., Blunt, J. W. and Neville, P. F. (1968). *Arch. Biochem. Biophys.* **124**, 122.
DeLuca, H. F., Blunt, J. W. and Rikkers, H. (1971). *In* 'The Vitamins' (Ed. W. H. Sebrell, Jr and R. S. Harris) pp. 213–230. Academic Press, New York.
Dimroth, K. and Paland, J. (1939). *Chem. Ber.* **72**, 187.
Drescher, D., DeLuca, H. F. and Imrie, M. H. (1969). *Arch. Biochem. Biophys.* **130**, 657.
Fraser, D. R. and Kodicek, E. (1968a). *Biochem. J.* **106**, 485.
Fraser, D. R. and Kodicek, E. (1968b). *Biochem. J.* **106**, 491.
Fraser, D. R. and Kodicek, E. (1968c). *Biochem. J.* **109**, 457.
Fraser, D. R. and Kodicek, E. (1970). *Nature* (London) **228**, 764.
Fraser, D. R. and Kodicek, E. (1973). *Nature New Biol.* (London) **241**, 163.
Frolik, C. A. and DeLuca, H. F. (1971). *Arch. Biochem. Biophys.* **147**, 143.
Frolik, C. A. and DeLuca, H. F. (1972). *J. Clin. Invest.* **51**, 2900.
Frolik, C. A. and DeLuca, H. F. (1973). *J. Clin. Invest.* **52**, 543.
Galante, L., MacAuley, S. J., Colston, K. W. and MacIntyre, I. (1972a). *Lancet* **i**, 985.
Galante, L., Colston, K. W., MacAuley, S. J. and MacIntyre, I. (1972b). *Nature* (London) **238**, 271.
Galante, L., Colston, K. W., Evans, I. M. A., Byfield, P. G. H., Matthews, E. W. and MacIntyre, I. (1973). *Nature* (London) **244**, 438.
Garabedian, M., Holick, M. F., DeLuca, H. F. and Boyle, I. T. (1972). *Proc. Nat. Acad. Sci USA* **69**, 1673.
Garabedian, M., Tanaka, Y., Holick, M. F. and DeLuca, H. F. (1974a). *Endocrinol.* **94**, 1022.
Garabedian, M., Pavlovitch, H., Fellot, C. and Balsan, S. (1974b). *Proc. Nat. Acad. Sci. USA* **71**, 554.
Ghazarian, J. G. and DeLuca, H. F. (1974). *Arch. Biochem. Biophys.* **160**, 63.
Ghazarian, J. G., Schnoes, H. K. and DeLuca, H. F. (1973). *Biochemistry* **12**, 2555.
Ghazarian, J. G., Jefcoate, C. R., Knutson, J. C., Orme-Johnson, W. H. and DeLuca, H. F. (1974). *J. Biol. Chem.* **249**, 3026.
Ghazarian, J. G., Tanaka, Y. and DeLuca, H. F. (1975). *In* 'Calcium Regulating Hormones' (Ed. R. V. Talmage, M. Owen and J. A. Parsons) pp. 381–390. Excerpta Medica, Amsterdam.

Gray, R., Boyle, I. and DeLuca, H. F. (1971). *Science* **172**, 1232.
Gray, R. W., Omdahl, J. L., Ghazarian, J. G. and DeLuca, H. F. (1972). *J. Biol. Chem.* **247**, 7528.
Haddad, J. G. and Stamp, T. C. B. (1974). *Am. J. Med.* **57**, 57.
Hallick, R. B. and DeLuca, H. F. (1972). *J. Biol. Chem.* **247**, 91.
Harrison, H. E. and Harrison, H. C. (1972). *J. Clin. Invest.* **51**, 1919.
Harrison, H. E., Harrison, H. C. and Lifshitz, F. (1968). *In* 'Parathyroid Hormone and Thyrocalcitonin (Calcitonin)' (Ed. R. V. Talmage and L. F. Belanger) pp. 455–460. Excerpta Medica, Amsterdam.
Haslewood, G. A. D. (1939). *Biochem. J.* **33**, 454.
Haussler, M. R., Myrtle, J. F. and Norman, A. W. (1968). *J. Biol. Chem.* **243**, 4055.
Haussler, M. R., Boyce, D. W., Littledike, E. T. and Rasmussen, H. (1971). *Proc. Nat. Acad. Sci. USA* **68**, 177.
Haussler, M. R., Zerwekh, J. E., Hesse, R. H., Rizzardo, E. and Pechet, M. M. (1973). *Proc. Nat. Acad. Sci. USA* **70**, 2248.
Henry, H. L. and Norman, A. W. (1974) *J. Biol. Chem.* **249**, 7529.
Heymann, W. (1937). *J. Biol. Chem.* **118**, 371.
Higaki, M., Takahashi, M., Suzuki, T. and Sahashi, Y. (1965). *J. Vitaminol* **II**, 266.
Holick, M. F. and DeLuca, H. F. (1971). *J. Lipid Res.* **12**, 460.
Holick, M. F. and DeLuca, H. F. (1974). *In* 'Advances in Steroid Biochemistry and Pharmacology' (Ed. M. H. Briggs and G. A. Christie) pp. 111–155. Academic Press, London and New York.
Holick, M. F., Schnoes, H. K. and DeLuca, H. F. (1971a). *Proc. Nat. Acad. Sci USA* **68**, 803.
Holick, M. F., Schnoes, H. K., DeLuca, H. F., Suda, T. and Cousins, R. J. (1971b). *Biochemistry* **10**, 2799.
Holick, M. F., Schnoes, H. K., DeLuca, H. F., Gray, R. W., Boyle, I. T. and Suda, T. (1972a). *Biochemistry* **11**, 4251.
Holick, M. F., Garabedian, M. and DeLuca, H. F. (1972b). *Science* **176**, 1146.
Holick, M. F., Garabedian, M. and DeLuca, H. F. (1972c). *Science* **176**, 1247.
Holick, M. F., Garabedian, M. and DeLuca, H. F. (1972d). *Biochemistry* **11**, 2715.
Holick, M. F., Kleiner-Bossaller, A., Schnoes, H. K., Kasten, P. M., Boyle, I. T. and DeLuca, H. F. (1973a). *J. Biol. Chem.* **248**, 6691.
Holick, M. F., DeLuca, H. F., Kasten, P. M. and Korycka, M. B. (1973b). *Science* **180**, 964.
Holick, M. F., Semmler, E. J., Schnoes, H. K. and DeLuca, H. F. (1973c). *Science* **180**, 190.
Holick, M. F., Garabedian, M., Schnoes, H. K. and DeLuca, H. F. (1975a). *J. Biol. Chem.* **250**, 226.
Holick, M. F., Kasten-Schraufrogel, P., Tavela, T. and DeLuca, H. F. (1975b). *Arch. Biochem. Biophys.* **166**, 63.
Holick, M. F., Baxter, L. A., Schraufragel, P. K., Tavela, T. E. and DeLuca, H. F. (1976a). *Biochemistry* **251**, 397.
Holick, M. F., Tavela, T. E., Holick, S. A., Schnoes, H. K., DeLuca, H. F. and Gallagher, B. M. (1976b). *J. Biol. Chem.* **251**, 1020.
Holick, S. A., Holick, M. F., Tavela, T. E., Schnoes, H. K. and DeLuca, H. F. (1976c). *J. Biol. Chem.* **251**, 1025.
Horiuchi, N., Suda, T., Sasaki, S., Ezawa, I., Sano, Y. and Ogata, E. (1974). *FEBS Lett.* **43**, 353.
Horsting, M. and DeLuca, H. F. (1969). *Biochem. Biophys. Res. Commun.* **36**, 251.

Hunt, R. D., Garcia, F. G. and Hegsted, D. M. (1967). *Lab. Animal Care* **17**, 222.
Imrie, M. H., Neville, P. F., Snellgrove, A. W. and DeLuca, H. F. (1967). *Arch, Biochem. Biophys.* **120**, 525.
Inhoffen, H. H., Bruckner, K. and Grundel, R. (1954). *Chem. Ber.* **87**, 1.
Jones, G., Schnoes, H. K. and DeLuca, H. F. (1975). *Biochemistry* **14**, 1250.
Jones, G., Baxter, L. A., DeLuca, H. F. and Schnoes, H. K. (1976a). *Biochemistry* **15**, 713.
Jones, G., Schnoes, H. K. and DeLuca, H. F. (1976b). *J. Biol. Chem.* **251**, 24.
Kaneko, C., Yamada, S., Sugimoto, A., Eguchi, Y., Ishikawa, M., Suda, T., Suzuki, M., Kakuta, S. and Sasaki, S. (1974). *Steroids* **23**, 75.
Kimberg, D. V., Baerg, R. D., Gershon, E. and Grandusius, R. T. (1971). *J. Clin. Invest.* **50**, 1309.
Kodicek, E. (1955). *Biochem. J.* **60**, XXV.
Kodicek, E. (1960). *In* 'Proceedings of the Fourth International Congress of Biochemistry' (Ed. E. W. Umbreit and H. Molitor) p. 198. Pergamon Press Ltd., London.
Kodicek, E. (1963). *In* 'The Transfer of Calcium and Strontium Across Biological Membranes' (Ed. R. H. Wasserman) p. 185. Academic Press, New York.
Kodicek, E. and Ashby, D. R. (1954). *Biochem. J.* **57**, xiii.
Kodicek, E. and Ashby, D. R. (1960a). *Biochem. J.* **75**, 17.
Kodicek, E. and Ashby, D. R. (1960b). *Biochem, J.* **76**, 14.
Kodicek, E., Cruickshank, E. M. and Ashby, D. R. (1960). *Biochem, J.* **76**, 15P.
Kodicek, E., Darmady, E. M. and Stranack, F. (1961). *Clin. Sci.* **20**, 185.
Kodicek, E., Lawson, D. E. M. and Wilson, P. W. (1970). *Nature* (London) **228**, 763.
Kumar, R. and DeLuca, H. F. (1976). *Biochem. Biophys. Res. Commun.* **69**, 197.
Kumar, R., Harnden, D. and DeLuca, H. F. (1976). *Biochemistry* **15**, 2420.
Lam, H. Y., Schnoes, H. K., DeLuca, H. F. & Chen, T. C. (1973). *Biochemistry* **12**, 4851.
Lam, H. Y., Onisko, B. L., Schnoes, H. K. and DeLuca, H. F. (1974). *Biochem. Biophys. Res. Commun.* **59**, 845.
Lawson, D. E. M., Wilson, P. W. and Kodicek, E. (1969). *Biochem. J.* **115**, 269.
Lawson, D. E. M., Fraser, D. R., Kodicek, E., Morris, H. R. and Williams, D. H. (1971). *Nature* (London) **230**, 228.
Lund, J. and DeLuca, H. F. (1966). *J. Lipid Res.* **7**, 739.
Lund, J., DeLuca, H. F. and Horsting, M. (1967). *Arch. Biochem. and Biophys.* **120**, 513.
MacIntyre, I., Galante, L. S., Colston, K. W., Evans, I. M. A., Larkins, R. G., MacAuley, S. J., Hillyard, C. J., Greenberg, P. B., Matthews, E. W. and Byfield, P. G. H. (1975). *In* 'Calcium Regulating Hormones' (Ed. R. V. Talmage, M. Owen and J. A. Parsons) p. 396. Excerpta Medica, Amsterdam.
Morii, H., Lund, J., Neville, P. F. and DeLuca, H. F. (1967). *Arch. Biochem. Biophys.* **120**, 508.
Morrissey, R. L. and Wasserman, R. H. (1971). *Am. J. Physiol.* **220**, 1509.
Myrtle, J. F. and Norman, A. W. (1971). *Science* **171**, 79.
Myrtle, J. F., Haussler, M. R. and Norman, A. W. (1970). *J. Biol. Chem.* **245**, 1190.
Neville, P. F. and DeLuca, H. F. (1966). *Biochemistry* **5**, 2201.
Nicolaysen, R., Eeg-Larsen, N. and Malm, O. J. (1953). *Physiol. Rev.* **33**, 424.
Norman, A. W. (1974). *Amer. J. Med.* **57**, 21.
Norman, A. W. and DeLuca, H. F. (1963). *Biochemistry* **2**, 1160.
Norman, A. W., Lund, J. and DeLuca, H. F. (1964). *Arch. Biochem. Biophys.* **108**, 12.

Norman, A. W., Myrtle, J. F., Midgett, R. J., Nowicki, H. G., Williams, V. and Popjak, G. (1971a). *Science* **173**, 51.
Norman, A. W., Midgett, R. J., Myrtle, J. F. and Nowicki, H. G. (1971b). *Biochem. Biophys. Res. Commun.* **42**, 1082.
Okamura, W. G., Mitra, M. N., Wing, R. M. and Norman, A. W. (1974). *Biochem. Biophys. Res. Commun.* **60**, 179.
Omdahl, J. L. and DeLuca, H. F. (1971). *Science* **174**, 949.
Omdahl, J. L. and DeLuca, H. F. (1972). *J. Biol. Chem.* **247**, 5520.
Omdahl, J. L. and DeLuca, H. F. (1973). *Physiol. Rev.* **53**, 327.
Omdahl, J. L., Holick, M., Suda, T., Tanaka, Y. and DeLuca, H. F. (1971). *Biochemistry* **10**, 2935.
Omdahl, J. L., Gray, R. W., Boyle, I. T., Knutson, J. and DeLuca, H. F. (1972). *Nature New Biol.* (London) **237**, 63.
Ponchon, G. and DeLuca, H. F. (1969). *J. Nutr.* **99**, 157.
Ponchon, G., Kennan, A. L. and DeLuca, H. F. (1969). *J. Clin. Invest.* **48**, 2032.
Ponchon, G., DeLuca, H. F. and Suda, T. (1970). *Arch. Biochem. Biophys* **141**, 397.
Quarterman, J. (1964). *Brit. J. Nutr.* **18**, 65.
Raisz, L. G., Trummel, C. L., Holick, M. F. and DeLuca, H. F. (1972). *Science* **175**, 768.
Rasmussen, H., Wong, M., Bikle, D. and Goodman, D. B. P. (1972). *J. Clin. Invest.* **51**, 2502.
Roborgh, J. R. and DeMan, T. J. (1960). *Biochem. Pharmacol.* **3**, 277.
Rosenstreich, S. J., Rich, C. and Volwiler, W. (1971). *J. Clin. Invest.* **50**, 679.
Schachter, D., Finkelstein, J. D. and Kowarski, S. (1964). *J. Clin. Invest.* **43**, 787.
Schaltegger, H. (1960). *Helv. Chim. Acta* **43**, 1448.
Seki, M., Koizumi, N., Morisaki, M. and Ikekawa, N. (1975). *Tetrahedron Lett.* **1**, 15.
Sahashi, Y., Suzuki, T., Higaki, M. and Asano, T. (1969). *J. Vitaminol.* **15**, 78.
Semmler, E. J., Holick, M. F., Schnoes, H. K. and DeLuca, H. F. (1972). *Tetrahedron Lett.* **40**, 4147.
Steenbock, H., Kletzien, S. W. F. and Halpin, J. G. (1932). *J. Biol. Chem.* **97**, 249.
Stern, P. H., Trummel, C. L., Schnoes, H. K. and DeLuca, H. F. (1975). *Endocrinol.* **97**, 1552.
Suda, T., DeLuca, H. F., Schnoes, H. K. and Blunt, J. W. (1969). *Biochemistry* **8**, 3515.
Suda, T., DeLuca, H. F., Schnoes, H. K., Ponchon, G., Tanaka, Y. and Holick, M. F. (1970a). *Biochemistry* **9**, 2917.
Suda, T., DeLuca, H. F., Schnoes, H. K., Tanaka, Y. and Holick, M. F. (1970b). *Biochemistry* **9**, 4776.
Suda, T., Hallick, R. B., DeLuca, H. F. and Schnoes, H. K. (1970c). *Biochemistry* **9**, 1651.
Suda, T., DeLuca, H. F. and Hallick, R. B. (1971). *Anal. Biochem.* **43**, 139.
Suda, T., Horiuchi, N., Sasaki, S., Ogata, E., Ezawa, I., Nagata, N. and Kimura, S. (1973). *Biochem. Biophys. Res. Commun.* **54**, 512.
Tanaka, Y. and DeLuca, H. F. (1973). *Arch. Biochem. Biophys.* **154**, 566.
Tanaka, Y. and DeLuca, H. F. (1974). *Proc. Nat. Acad. Sci. USA* **71**, 1040.
Tanaka, Y., DeLuca, H. F., Ikekawa, N., Morisaki, M. and Koizumi, N. (1975). *Arch. Biochem. Biophys.* **170**, 620.
Tanaka, Y., Frank, H. and DeLuca, H. F. (1973). *Endocrinol.* **92**, 417.
Tsai, H. C., Wong, R. G. and Norman, A. W. (1972). *J. Biol. Chem.* **247**, 5511.
Tucker, G., III, Gagnon, R. E. and Haussler, M. R. (1973). *Arch. Biochem. Biophys.* **155**, 47.

Verloop, A., Koevoet, A. L. and Havinga, E. (1955). *Recl. Trav. Chim. Pays-Bas* **74**, 1125.
Verloop, A., Koevoet, A. L., Van Moorsellar, R. and Havinga, E. (1959). *Recl. Trav. Chim. Pays-Bas* **78**, 1004.
von Werder, F. (1939). *Hoppe-Seyler's Z. Physiol Chem.* **260**, 119.
Waddell, J. (1934). *J. Biol. Chem.* **105**, 711.
Windaus, A. and Buchholz, K. (1938). *Hoppe-Seyler's Z. Physiol. Chem.* **256,** 273.
Windaus, A. and Trautman, G. (1937). *Hoppe-Seyler's Z. Physiol. Chem.* **247**, 185.
Windaus, A., Lettre, H. and Schenck, F. (1935). *Ann.* **520**, 98.
Windaus, A., Schenck, F. and von Werder, F. (1936). *Hoppe-Seyler's Z. Physiol. Chem.* **241**, 100.
Zerwekh, J. E., Brumbaugh, P. F., Haussler, D. H., Cork, D. J. and Haussler, M. R. (1974). *Biochemistry* **13**, 4097.

3 Calcium and Phosphorus Absorption

ANTHONY W. NORMAN

I General Considerations

A CALCIUM AND PHOSPHORUS HOMEOSTASIS

Calcium and phosphorus are the most abundant of the elements present in the body (Widdowson and Dickerson, 1964) and have accordingly been a topic of major concern for biologists, biochemists, physiologists and endocrinologists during the past three-quarters of a century. As can be seen by inspection of Table 1, these two elements play key roles in a wide spectrum of biological processes, and consequently a major problem for the living organism is to ensure an adequate supply of calcium and phosphorus to meet these bodily needs. It is essential to life that calcium and phosphorus be supplied on a continuing daily basis.

The primary means of acquiring phosphorus and calcium is via dietary intake and it is the main object of this chapter to review our current understanding of the mechanisms involved in the intestinal absorption of calcium and phosphorus. However, it would be naïve to simply focus on the intestine without appreciating that the problem of calcium and phosphorus absorption is of necessity interrelated to the larger problems of phosphorus and calcium homeostasis. Since these two elements are so important to the organism and since the problem of dietary excess in some ways may present as many potential problems as a dietary paucity, the organism has evolved a 'total body solution' to these problems over the length time of evolution, i.e.

Table 1. Biological calcium and phosphorus

I Utilisation

Calcium	*Phosphorus*
Body content (70 kg man has 1.2 kg of Ca^{2+})	Body content (70 kg man has 770 g of phosphorus)
Structural (Bone has 95 % of body Ca^{2+})	Structural (Bone has 90% of body inorganic phosphate (Pi))
Plasma (Ca^{2+}) = 2.5 mM	Plasma (Pi) = 2.3 mM
Muscle contraction	Intermediary metabolism (phosphorylated intermediates)
Nerve pulse transmission	Genetic information (DNA and RNA)
Blood clotting	Phospholipids
Membrane structure	Enzyme/protein components (phosphohistidine, phosphoserine)
Enzyme cofactors (amylase, trypsinogen, lipases, ATPases)	Membrane structure
Egg shell (birds)	

II Daily Requirements (70 kg man)

	Calcium[a] (mg)	Phosphorus[b] (mg)
Dietary intake	700	1200
Faecal excretion[c]	150	350–370
Urinary excretion[c]	550	

[a] Taken from Bronner (1964)
[b] Taken from Bartter (1964)
[c] Based on the listed intake level

the system of calcium and phosphorus homeostasis. The homeostasis mechanisms for these two elements involve the integrated action of the site of uptake – the intestine – with the site of major deposition – the bone – with the major site of excretion – the kidney. The coordinated operation of these three organs provides the minute-to-minute basis for regulating the tissue levels of calcium and phosphorus.

The subject of calcium and phosphorus homeostasis has been discussed in a multitude of reviews over the years; the following references giving other viewpoints and emphasis: Nicolaysen *et al.*, 1953; Nicolaysen and Eeg-Larson, 1953; Rasmussen and DeLuca, 1963; Bronner, 1964, 1972; Wasserman and Taylor, 1969, 1972; Wasserman, 1963.

It has been traditional in the past to consider the subjects of calcium and phosphorus separately; it is obvious that in terms of many of their physiological interactions that these ions are regulated in a coordinated manner. The consistency with which the blood in calcium is maintained by the organisms is remarkable (2.3–2.5 mM) and is achieved by interrelated endocrinological mechanisms at different sites in the body.

The acceptable phosphorus range in plasma is somewhat wider (0.8–2.2 mM) but this is perhaps not surprising as the phosphorus is in equilibrium not only with bone phosphate but with the phosphorus which is involved with the multitude of organic phosphorus containing compounds involved in intermediary metabolism. The traditional view has been that only parathyroid hormone acting at the renal level has an effect on phosphate homeostasis. However, as will become apparent, this view is currently under re-examination in a number of laboratories.

Three of the most important of the biological regulators of calcium and phosphorus metabolism are vitamin D (calciferol), parathyroid hormone and calcitonin. Significant developments and advances have been made in recent years concerning each of these controlling factors. It is likely that calciferol, which may be classified chemically as a steroid, acts in a manner similar to that of well-known steroid hormones such as oestrogen, aldosterone, and hydrocortisone (Norman, 1968). Also, there is considerable evidence to support the view that the active form of calciferol is a steroid hormone, 1,25-dihydroxycholecalciferol, which is produced by the kidney in response to various physiological signals (Norman, 1975 – see chapters 2 and 10). With this perspective in mind, it is possible to identify new relationships between vitamin D (in reality a hormone), its secretory organ (the kidney), the target tissues (the intestine and skeleton) and various disease states related to calcium homeostasis and vitamin D. Similarly with parathyroid hormone, there has been a continuing cascade of new information concerning the means of biosynthesis and secretion of this polypeptide hormone as well as to its metabolism at peripheral target tissues, the liver, the kidney, and bone (Reiss and Canterbury, 1974 – see chapter 10). Again with calcitonin, there is an increasing understanding of the importance it may play in both calcium and phosphorus metabolism (Segre and Potts, 1975 – see chapter 10). A new concept relates to the possible interaction between the intestinal gastrin hormone, and its effect on calcitonin release at times of dietary intake of calcium (Cooper *et al.*, 1972).

B DIETARY REQUIREMENTS FOR CALCIUM AND PHOSPHORUS

It is complicated to unequivocally determine the dietary requirements of calcium and phosphorus since the requirement for one ion is interdependent on the amounts of the other ion and indeed the other nutrients present in the diet. In many instances the requirements have been proven to vary markedly from species to species. The calcium intake of most humans varies between 200 and 1500 mg/day (Bronner, 1964). As will be discussed below, under the subject of adaptation, the fraction of this dietary calcium which is absorbed is under stringent regulation via physiological mechanisms which are influenced by 'the calcium demand' of the organism. Dietary phosphate intake in man also ranges from 600 to 2000 mg/day (Irving, 1964; Bartter, 1964). At present no specific evidence is available, suggesting that adaptation is a component of the intestinal absorption process for phosphorus. However, one complication relating to both calcium and phosphorus is their propensity for precipitation. That is to say, when calcium and phosphorus are present in relatively high quantities together, the various fractions of the other component may be dietarily unavailable due to precipitation and concomitant excretion.

C INTESTINAL MORPHOLOGY AND CYTOLOGY

1 *Microscopic Appearance.* Any studies that are designed to elucidate the biochemical parameters of intestinal calcium and phosphorus absorption must recognise the unique morphology of the intestinal columnar epithelial cells. These cells are highly differentiated to accomplish their special role in various absorptive processes. The lumen of the small intestine is composed of a multitude of finger-like projections which are termed villi. Typically these villi range from 0.5–1.5 nm in length and are composed principally of two types of cells, namely the columnar epithelial cell and the goblet or mucus-secreting cell. The latter is believed to be concerned with the secretion of mucopolysaccharide components present in the lumen of the intestine.

The apical surface of the columnar epithelial cells which is exposed towards the lumen is referred to as the brush border or microvillar membrane. These microvilli are approximately 1 μm long and 0.1 μm wide. As a consequence the surface area of the mucosa is increased 600-fold, as compared to the total area of a simple cylinder (Wilson, 1962). A variety of carbohydrate hydrolases and an alkaline phosphatase of the intestinal mucosal cell are known to be specifically associated with this brush border region (Miller and Crane, 1961; Norman *et al.*, 1970). This is believed to be the region of localisation of 'permeases' which are postulated as being involved in the absorption of materials into the cell. This outermost surface of the columnar epithelial cell is known to be covered with a filamentous mucopolysaccharide coat, termed the glycocalyx or 'fuzzy coat' (Ito, 1965). The specific function of the glycocalyx is not known at the present time, but some workers have reported that it is impregnated with knobs or spherical particles of 40 Å–60 Å in diameter, which can be stained by dyes specific for polysaccharides (Forstner, 1969, 1971). It has been suggested by Forstner (1971) that these surface knobs and filaments are identical with glycoproteins exhibiting disaccharidase, naphthalamadase, and alkaline phosphatase enzymatic activity.

Beneath the columnar epithelial cell lies the lymphatic and blood vascular systems. These systems project into each villus, and thus provide an efficient mechanism for the translocation of a substrate once it leaves the epithelial cells. Any efforts to describe the overall transport of phosphorus and calcium from the lumen of the intestine to the blood must then take account of this highly specialised and complicated cellular organisation.

It is possible to outline a path that phosphorus or calcium atoms may follow during their absorption process, and in so doing a number of factors have to be considered. These factors include the ionic state of the calcium, as it is transported, and the influence on this state of calcium chelating ions such as citrate and in addition that phosphate may form, or is capable of forming, covalent bonds with organic molecules. The next step would involve a possible interaction of these substances with the negatively charged mucopolysaccharide with its exposed sulfate groups. Subsequently the ions interact with and are transported across the microvillar membrane, but it is an unresolved question as to whether the mechanism involved is passive diffusion, carrier mediated transport or active transport. One factor which must be taken into account in any final description of this process is the negative electric potential on the inside of the cell with respect to the outside and this for calcium is an attractive force, while for phosphate, it would be a repulsive force. Similar considerations in a reverse manner would apply to the exit step at the basal side of the cell. Inside the cell a multitude of interactions may occur with obvious possibilities including mitochondrial and microsomal membranes. A most pertinent question is what role these intracellular organelles may have in the transcellular migration of phosphate and calcium. At the basal side of the cell, the movement of the substances through the membrane and the possible intervention of a sodium/potassium activated ATPase are problems that have been appreciated by a variety of investigators. Having left the cell, the ions must move through the interstitial space until finally encountering the endothelial cells of the blood capillaries. In terms of the three potential regulators or mediators of the intestinal absorption of calcium and phosphate, i.e. calciferol and its metabolites, parathyroid hormone and/or calcitonin, it is apparent that there are several possible sites in the process of translocation on which to exert specific actions.

2 *Cell Turn-over Time.* The cells on the villus are rapidly renewed. The musosal cells originate in a progenitor population in the crypt of Lieberkuhn and migrate towards the villi tips where they are extruded into the lumen. Only after epithelial cells enter the villus do they differentiate into fully functional absorptive cells. This differentiation process is characterised by a change of the RNA/protein ratio and a change in the activity of various enzymes as a function of the position of the epithelial cell on the villus. The undifferentiated cells in the crypt possess a high content of RNA (Webster and Harrison, 1969)

mainly in the form of free ribosomes. Their microvilli are sparse and blunted and contain a low activity of digestive enzymes, such as esterases, disaccharidases, and alkaline phosphatase (Palade, 1958; Dahlquist and Nordstrom, 1966; Nordstrom *et al.*, 1968). The enzymatic activities, esterase, leucine amino peptidase, invertase, and alkaline phosphatase, increase in a regular pattern with migration of epithelial cells towards the villus (Padykula, 1962; Lipkin and Bell, 1968). Intestinal epithelial cell turnover times of 30–48 h have been reported in mice, rats, chicks and humans. The rate of epithelial cell renewal increases when there is an increased demand for new cells, as in recovery from radiation injury, response to parasite infestation or adaptation to partial intestinal resection (Crane *et al.*, 1965). The rate of cell renewal is regulated by the cell proliferation in the crypt and cell loss at the extrusion zone. The molecular basis of this regulation is as yet poorly understood, but it is interesting to consider the possible intervention of cholecalciferol or its active metabolite, 1,25-dihydroxycholecalciferol in this process.

Administration of cholecalciferol to rachitic animals effects a 2.5–3.5 fold increase in intestinal calcium transport (Adams and Norman, 1970) with the increase occurring only after a time lag of 24–48 h (Norman, 1966). The present concept of the mechanism of action of calciferol involves at least two major time dependent processes which can partially account for this time lag (see chapter 5):

(*a*) Time required for the two-step metabolism of cholecalciferol to 1,25-dihydroxycholecalciferol.

(*b*) Time required for interaction of hormonal metabolite with its intestinal cytoplasmic and nuclear receptor (Norman and Henry, 1974) where it results in subsequent *de novo* synthesis or induction of proteins including calcium-binding protein (Wasserman *et al.*, 1968) alkaline phosphatase (Norman *et al.*, 1970) and an ATPase activated by calcium (Melancon and DeLuca, 1970; Holdsworth, 1970). The activity of all these proteins has been shown to increase in intestinal mucosal cells after administration of calciferol or 1,25-dihydroxycholecalciferol but it is possible that the appearance and loss of these proteins is dependent upon the rate of turnover of the mucosal cells themselves.

The following questions concerning the effect of calciferol on intestinal calcium transport have been considered:

(*i*) Does calciferol affect the physiology of the intestine?

(*ii*) Is such a change a prerequisite for the increase of intestinal calcium transport?

(*iii*) Is the turnover time of the intestinal epithelial cells a determining factor in the gradual increase or the decrease of calcium transport after a single dose of calciferol?

Attempts to answer these questions have been made on studies on the effect of calciferol treatment on intestinal mucosal cell turnover in the chick (Spielvogel *et al.*, 1972), and the rat (Birge and Alpers, 1973) respectively.

In the first study, three groups of chickens were prepared, namely a vitamin D-deficient group, a group vitamin D-replete for 100 h (i.e. first of all deficient and then given 12.5 μg of cholecalciferol every 48 h starting at 124 h before termination) and a third group that were normal chicks. The turnover time of ileal epithelial cells was found to be 90–98 h for the three groups. Treatment with the vitamin for more than 110 h resulted in an increase in villus length so that the villus of the normal chick was 30% longer than that of the vitamin D-deficient chicken. Since the total transit times were only slightly different in these three groups, the rates of migration were of necessity quite different, e.g. 7.0×10^{-3} cm/h for the normal as compared with 5.9×10^{-3} cm/h for vitamin D-replete and 4.3×10^{-3} cm/h in the vitamin D-deficient groups. Thus, there is clearly a trophic effect of cholecalciferol on the morphology of the villus of the ileum of the chick. A similar result was obtained by Birge and Alpers (1973) in their study in the rat where they reported an approximately 20% increase in villus length in cholecalciferol treated animals. The decrease in villus size in chicks or rats deficient in the vitamin is not surprising, since deficient animals are generally retarded in their rate of growth (Steenbock and Herting, 1955).

Another pertinent fact is that the stimulation of intestinal calcium transport and the rise of brush border enzyme activities are known to be maximal by 35–40 h after a single dose of cholecalciferol or in only 12–20 h when 1,25-dihydroxycholecalciferol is given. At this time, the villus size and rate of migration in the cholecalciferol or metabolite treated birds would not be significantly different from that of the deficient birds. Thus this result shows that the primary action of cholecalciferol increased calcium transport – is not dependent upon a change at the cellular level of the increase in cell size, number, or migration rate. Clearly, the vitamin and its metabolites have effects on the villus size and migration rate; however, comparison of the changes with time in the morphology with the changes in levels of the various proteins suggests that the effect of cholecalciferol on villus length and cell migration rate is not an absolute prerequisite for stimulation of intestinal calcium transport.

D TECHNIQUES FOR STUDYING CALCIUM AND PHOSPHORUS ABSORPTION

Over the years, a multitude of techniques have been devised which have permitted investigators to quantitate various facets of the intestinal absorption of phosphorus and calcium and these are summarised in Table 2. An excellent review on this subject has been produced (Berger, 1960). Basically two techniques have been developed, namely those in the intact animal, and those where a portion of the intestinal cells have been removed for study under more defined conditions *in vitro*. Before the 1960s, almost all techniques had to depend upon the use of stable isotopes and the use of conventional balance techniques where the input and output of calcium and phosphorus by the animal could be measured.

At the present time, two radioactive isotopes of calcium are available, namely calcium-45, a beta emitter (0.252 meV max) with a half-life of 152

Table 2. Methods for measuring intestinal calcium and phosphorus absorption

Method	*Reference*
I *in vivo*	
A Man	
1. Metabolic balance studies	(Liu and Chu, 1943; Stanbury and Lumb, 1962)
2. Faecal recovery of radiocalcium	(Blair *et al.*, 1954; Rich and Ivanovich, 1964)
3. Double isotope method (one given orally and the other i.v.)	
(*a*) Two separate doses of ^{47}Ca with external counting	(Curtis *et al.*, 1967; Litwak, 1969)
(*b*) ^{47}Ca and ^{45}Ca measured in plasma and/or urine	(DeGrazia and Rich, 1964; Szymendra *et al.*, 1972)
4. Plasma appearance after oral radio-calcium	(Heaney and Whedon, 1958)
B Experimental animals	
1. Isolated loops *in situ*	(Coates and Holdsworth, 1961; Scott, 1965; Hibberd and Norman, 1969)
2. Perfusion *in situ*	(Olson and DeLuca, 1969)
II *in vitro*	
A Transcellular transport	
1. Everted intestinal sacs	(Wilson and Wiseman, 1954; Schacter and Rosen, 1959)
2. Short circuit conditions	(Ussing, 1949; Adams and Norman, 1970)
3. Glass perfusion apparatus	(Adams and Norman, 1970)
B Cellular uptake studies	
(*a*) Unidirectional tissue uptake	(Martin and DeLuca, 1969a)

days, and a calcium-47 which is both a gamma emitter (1.31 meV, 0.81 meV, and 0.49 meV) and a beta emitter (1.98 meV, 0.67 meV) with a half-life of 4.53 days. There are also now available two radioactive isotopes of phosphorus. Phosphorus-32 is primarily used as a strong beta emitter (1.7 meV beta max) with a half-life of 14.3 days; while phosphorus-33 is a weak beta emitter (0.248 meV) with a half-life of 24.5 days (Lederer *et al.*, 1967).

In experimental animals, the primary technique *in vivo* has been the procedure of Coates and Holdsworth (1961) as modified by Hibberd and Norman (1969). In this technique, radioactive calcium or phosphorus is placed in an isolated loop in a selected region of the small intestine of an anaesthetised animal and at varying time periods later, the appearance of the isotope in the plasma is measured. Care must be exercised to obtain the plasma sample in a relatively short period of time after placing the isotope in the intestine, since it is well known that there is rapid exchange of both plasma calcium and phosphate with the readily exchangeable pools of these substances present in the bone. Thus, if the appearance of the isotope in the plasma is to be a measure of 'intestinal absorption', these measurements must be taken at an early enough time period before significant exchange and dilution of the isotope has occurred with nonradioactive ions present in the bone.

Conventional techniques utilised for studies *in vitro* on the intestinal absorption of calcium and phosphorus use either an everted intestinal sac as pioneered by Wilson and Wiseman (1954) or the short circuit conditions as originally defined by Ussing (1949). The sac technique involves evertion of the segment of the small intestine which presumably facilitates the oxygenisation of mucosal cells when they are incubated in a bath with solution available to both sides. Such sac preparations have been shown to maintain a number of physiological functions for at least an hour. The technique does, however, have certain disadvantages: for example, usually only one sample per sac is obtainable and the serosal volume is invariably quite small, ca. 0.5 ml, so that significant errors due to absorption and adsorption may occur. Further, the value obtained is not a rate, but a ratio of the equilibrium concentrations of the ions on the inside to those on the outside of the sac. Another problem associated with the small volume in the serosal compartment is that it may gain up to 0.2–0.3 ml of water in the course of the incubation period. This large volume change makes it difficult to ascertain whether one is studying the effect of water movement on phosphorus or calcium transport.

A significant improvement in technique is the apparatus originally described by Helbock *et al.* (1966) which was a modification of an earlier apparatus described by Ussing (1949). The numerous advantages of this technique over other *in vitro* techniques have been discussed (Adams and Norman, 1970), the principle ones being that the experiments can be run under short-circuit conditions and thus remove the extraneous effect of other electro-potentials. In addition, multiple samples can be taken as a function of time so that a rate of transport is quantitatively determined.

An alternative *in vitro* technique is that described by Martin and DeLuca (1969a), which also measures the rate of uptake of ions into the cell across the brush border membrane. The 'uptake apparatus' consists of two lucite sheets, one of which has a small orifice of approximately 0.5 cm diameter. An ileal segment of the tissue is placed serosal side down on the solid lucite sheet and the second sheet with the orifice is placed over the tissue with the hole centred over the tissue. The slides are held together with rubber and the edges pressed firmly together so that a silicone gasket present will form a seal round the edges. The sheets are then emersed in a beaker for incubation in a buffer solution containing the isotope. After incubation, the sheets are transferred to a second beaker containing an ice-cold wash buffer, dried and the exposed tissue is cut out with a $\frac{1}{4}$ inch cork borer. Thus, one can measure the presence of isotope in the excised piece of tissue which can only have been present by virtue of uptake across the exposed cellular membrane.

E CALCIUM AND PHOSPHORUS ABSORPTION: PROBLEM DEFINED

Before designing experiments to experimentally evaluate the complexities and realities of the intestinal absorption of calcium and phosphorus, it is possible to identify in a flow chart manner the various steps that one may anticipate

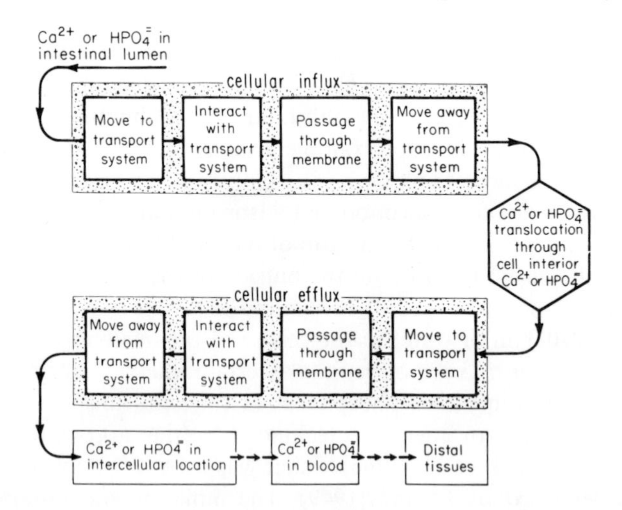

Fig. 1. Flow chart analysis of the process of transfer of calcium and phosphorus from the lumen of the intestine across the intestinal cell to the blood

that should or could be associated with this multi-stepped and multi-compartmental problem (Fig. 1). The problem reduces to the simple transfer of the ion in question from the lumen of the intestine across the intervening membranes to the plasma. Kinetically, one may follow this as disappearance of ion from the lumen or appearance of ion in the plasma. However, consideration of the various intervening membranes and compartments that one can postulate should be involved suggests that simple straightforward kinetic analysis may not expose the sophistication of the details of the overall process. There are basically three steps involved with the transport process – uptake across the extracellular membrane of the intestinal cell, then transport across the cell and efflux out of the cell across another cell membrane. However, each of the steps concerned with the membrane transfer may be divided into substeps, i.e. an interaction with the membrane, a passage through the membrane, and dissociation or release from the membrane. However, a further degree of complexity is that the two plasma membranes in question in the intestinal columnar epithelial cell are not identical. The composition and function of the brush border membrane is very different from that of the basal cell membrane. Also there are a multitude of potential interactions that may occur inside the cell as the ions are translocated through the cellular milleau. Any complete biochemical description then of calcium and phosphorus absorption must take account of these cellular 'facts of life'.

F EARLY FINDINGS ON CALCIUM AND PHOSPHORUS ABSORPTION (UP TO 1950)

Before the availability of radioactive calcium and phosphorus in the 1940s, it was difficult to establish unequivocally that one of the primary actions of calciferol was to promote or facilitate the intestinal absorption of calcium. One of the first papers to report studies concerned with defining the mechanism of intestinal absorption of calcium and phosphorus was that of Bergheim (1926). He pointed out that both phosphorus and calcium were secreted by the intestine and then subject to reabsorption at different intestinal locations. Other workers in this period made use primarily of balance studies in which the intake and the faecal and urinary levels of calcium and phosphorus were measured. These studies were carried out in children (Findlay *et al.*, 1920), in the rat (McClendon, 1922; Brown *et al.*, 1932), the chick (Bethke *et al.*, 1929), and in the dog (Jones, 1927). It was generally agreed that there was an increased loss of phosphorus and calcium in vitamin D-deficiency which resulted from primarily an increased output of these elements into the faeces.

It was not until the pioneering and most thorough studies of Nicolaysen, that the first direct causal relationship between calciferol and calcium absorption was unequivocally established. In a notable series of experiments he demonstrated the following:

(*a*) There was no alteration in the amount of calcium or phosphorus excreted into the faeces by vitamin D-deficient or normal rats in which a Thiery-Vella fistula was made of the entire colon (Innes and Nicolaysen, 1937).

(*b*) An intravenous injection of calcium was not followed by increased faecal calcium, but rather by a concomitant increased renal excretion of calcium in the urine. These results were independent of the vitamin D-status of the rats (Innes and Nicolaysen, 1937).

(*c*) Under conditions of dietary phosphorus deprivation, calciferol markedly stimulated intestinal calcium absorption in the rat, whereas following the withdrawal of dietary calcium, calciferol had no enhancing or inhibiting effect on phosphorus absorption (Nicolasen, 1937a,b). The latter result was obtained irrespective of whether the dietary phosphorus was inorganic or organic phosphate.

(*d*) In a pioneering experiment utilising isolated, ligated jejunal loops of rachitic and normal rats *in vivo*, Nicolaysen (1937a) found that the rate of absorption of calcium was markedly increased in normal rats as compared to vitamin D-deficient rats. Under similar conditions, the absorption of calcium from the abdominal cavity was identical in normal and deficient rats. This study clearly demonstrated for the first time the stimulatory effect of calciferol on intestinal calcium absorption.

Thus when radioactive calcium and phosphorus became available in the early 1940s, the ground work was laid for more sophisticated studies. One of the early tracer experiments utilising both orally and intraperitoneally administered $^{45}Ca^{2+}$ showed that the intestinal excretion of calcium was not affected by the vitamin D-status of the animal (Greenberg, 1945). Other studies by Migicovsky and Emslie (1947, 1949) in the chick, and by Carlsson (1951) and Lindquist (1952) in the rat utilising radioactive calcium, substantiated the earlier work of Nicolaysen that calciferol had a significant effect on intestinal calcium absorption in the rat.

Very little work was done in the period of time 1920–1950 that was specifically concerned with defining the mechanism of phosphate absorption. One of the first studies was conducted by Nicolaysen (1937a) utilising ligated intestinal loops *in situ*; he found that inorganic phosphate and sodium glycerol phosphate were absorbed equally well in normal and vitamin D-deficient rats. Later studies of Dols *et al.* (1938) in rachitic chick, Cohn and Greenberg (1939), or Manley and Morgareidy (1939) in the rat, and Shimotori and Morgan (1943) in dogs, utilising orally administered radioactive phosphorus noted no effect of calciferol on phosphorus absorption.

II Current Concepts of Calcium and Phosphorus Absorption

The physiological studies demonstrating the enhancing effect of calciferol on intestinal absorption of calcium and phosphorus have laid the groundwork for a rigorous biochemical examination of the detailed mechanism by which these two substances are moved across the small intestine. The problem is basically one of determining whether the transport of calcium and/or phosphorus is an active transport, i.e. occurs against an electrochemical gradient (Ussing, 1949), or passive transport, and what the detailed role of the hormones mentioned in Section III A, particularly calciferol, may be in these processes. Thus it may be that the vitamin or its hormonal metabolite acts as a direct effector and binds to some crucial membrane to change the conformation of protein components so that the membrane has an increased permeability to calcium, thus in essence facilitating a passive transfer. An alternative theory which is consistent in the hormone-like action of calciferol (see chapter 5) is that the vitamin or its metabolite may either induce the synthesis of the appropriate enzyme systems involved in an active transport system or induce the synthesis of a modified more permeable membrane (to calcium and/or phosphate). In this circumstance, as the vitamin or its metabolite are not directly involved in calcium transport, the question still remains as to how these cations and anions actually cross the cell membrane and interior of the cell. If calciferol induces the production of a transport system which may be either active or passive, it is pertinent also to know whether the parameters of the induced system are identical or different from the noninduced system (vitamin D-deficient animal). Calciferol may induce additional quantities of the same pre-existing system, alter components of an existing system, or initiate the production of a second calcium or phosphate transport system. There have been a multitude of papers and a variety of interpretations of the data on this subject.

Schacter's group began a series of investigations on intestinal calcium transport in 1959. These studies were a departure from the original whole animal experiments mentioned earlier which had been performed by Nicolaysen, Greenberg and others. Schacter used the everted sac technique to study calcium transport *in vitro*. The initial experiments on calcium transport were made in normal animals and it was only later that he attempted to evaluate the role of calciferol in this process. He found that calcium was transported against a concentration gradient in an everted sac prepared from the small intestine of rats (Schacter and Rosen, 1959). According to the criterion of Rosenberg and Wilbrandt (1957), this is indicative of active transport. Schacter's group later became interested in the calciferol aspect of the system when they found that deprivation of the vitamin decreased intestinal calcium transport. Using the everted sac method, it was found that the concentration ratio was 2.9 for the calciferol treated animals and only 1.1 for the deficient animals. The effect of various inhibitors on calcium transport in everted sacs from normal animals showed that cyanide, azide, dinitrophenol, iodoacetamide and malonate were effective in curtailing calcium transport. This suggested that metabolic energy was required for both the uptake and release steps (Schacter and Rosen, 1959). In other studies, efforts were made to define subcomponents of the overall transport process by separately measuring the uptake and release of calcium from intestinal slices. The mechanism was described as having a facilitated diffusion step at the musosal surface and an active pump located at the basal membrane of the columnar epithelial cells (Kimberg *et al.*, 1961).

Wasserman and colleagues studied *in vivo* flux rates in the normal rat, using the procedure of Curran and Soloman (1957) and provided evidence showing that the flux rate was greater than unity at all levels of calcium concentration. This indicated to these workers that calcium was actively transported in the intact animal (Wasserman *et al.*, 1961). Wasserman's laboratory also studied calcium flux *in vitro* in rachitic rats and chicks and found that cholecalciferol administration increased the plasma-to-lumen calcium flux in the chick ileum 2.7-fold, and in the rat duodenum 1.9-fold. As expected, the lumen-to-plasma flux was also increased, but it was only 1.3-fold for both the chick and the rat. These data suggested to Wasserman and co-workers that the major effect of cholecalciferol was not on a unidirectionally transport system, but that it operated only to increase diffusional permeability. It was suggested that this could be caused perhaps by some change in membrane structure or by synthesis of proteins specific for calcium (Wasserman *et al.*, 1966).

Harrison and Harrison (1960) found that the effect of cholecalciferol on calcium transfer *in vitro* in rats' intestine is not blocked by inhibitors of oxidative metabolism. This observation led to the conclusion that calciferol increases the rate of diffusion of calcium across the intestine. In other studies, Harrison and Harrison (1965) also found that calcium is actively transported in a rat duodenum as judged by the criterion of Rosenberg and Wilbrandt (1957). Later studies indicated that when calcium transfer was measured in tissue from which the mucosa had been removed (i.e. only the underlying serosa was present) there was no difference due to cholecalciferol administration. Consequently, the conclusion was drawn that the difference due to cholecalciferol treatment lay in the mucosal tissue as compared with the serosal tissue. In other related studies, the Harrisons found that active transport of calcium was observed when the everted intestinal loops were incubated in a buffer with a concentration of 26 mM Na^{+}, but not in the presence of 145 mM Na^{+}. Similar results were also reported from DeLuca's laboratory (Martin and DeLuca, 1969b; Martin *et al.*, 1969). The steroid was able to manifest the calciferol mediated stimulation of intestinal calcium transport even when the experiment was performed *in vitro* with *N*-ethylmaleimide present in the incubation solution (Hurwitz *et al.*, 1967). All of these results supported the original contention of Harrison and Harrison that the calciferol effect is not on a unidirectional pump for calcium, but rather that the membrane permeability of calcium is altered by calciferol treatment.

Calcium transport has been studied *in vitro* in cholecalciferol treated and deficient chicks. Using everted sacs, it was found that metabolic inhibitors and *N*-methylmaleimide (Sallis and Holdsworth, 1962) were able to inhibit calcium transport but that the cardiac glycoside ouabain when present in the mucosal solution was ineffective. Studies on the effect of temperature on calcium transport indicated that the cholecalciferol effect was not apparent at low temperatures. In everted sacs incubated at 38°C, cholecalciferol was found to increase the amount of calcium transferred to the serosal fluid and also to increase the amount of calcium found in the mucosal compartment. On the basis of this and other results, these workers concluded that calcium is pumped out of the epithelial cells by a process which is dependent on the energy of metabolism. A model was formulated in which calciferol was proposed to inhibit an active pump which returns calcium from the musosal cell to the lumen, thus bringing about a unidirectional transport of calcium (Holdsworth, 1965).

A summary of the major conclusions concerning calciferol mediated calcium transport obtained by laboratories other than that of the author is given in Table 3. As is apparent in this table, there are a variety of opinions on the mechanism of vitamin D mediated calcium transport.

There are also a variety of conflicting reports concerning the effect of calciferol on phosphorus absorption. A possible effect of the vitamin on this process was first noted by Carlson (1954) in studies carried out in rats. Under circumstances where the animals were fed a calcium-deficient diet, he concluded that the observed increase in phosphate absorption was due to a 'general improvement of the condition of the animal' and not due to a direct effect of the vitamin. Later, Harrison and Harrison (1961) reported that the absorption of phosphorus was activated by the presence of calcium and that phosphate absorption was less efficient in vitamin D-deficient animals as compared to the vitamin D-treated controls. On the other hand, using intestinal loops in rachitic chicks which were perfused *in vivo* (Sallis and Holdsworth, 1962), it was reported that the steroid had no effect on the intestinal absorption of radioactive phosphate.

The effects of calciferol on transport of inorganic phosphate into and across the intestinal mucosa of rats has been reported (Kowarsky and Schacter, 1969). Calciferol given to intact rats was found to selectively increase phosphate transport *in vitro* in the direction of mucosa to serosa. At

Table 3. Summary of studies on vitamin D mediated calcium transport

Investigator	Reference	Effect of vitamin D on calcium transport	Comments
Schacter	Schacter and Rosen, 1959; Schacter *et al.*, 1960; Kimberg *et al.*, 1961	Active transport	2-step mechanism with an uptake and a release with an effect on both processes
Wasserman	Wasserman *et al.*, 1961, 1966, 1968; Wasserman and Taylor, 1969	Increased diffusional permeability	Isolated CaBP implicated in calcium transport. CaBP is localised in the brush border region
Holdsworth	Sallis and Holdsworth, 1962; Holdsworth, 1970	Active transport	Vitamin D inhibits a metabolically operated pump that returns calcium from the mucosal cell to the lumen
Harrison and Harrison	1960, 1965	Altered permeability	The action of vitamin D may be a permeability change which potentiates an active calcium pump by the increased availability of calcium
Saltman	Helbock *et al.*, 1966	Not active (effect of vitamin D not investigated)	Calcium transport in mature rats was found to be nonactive according to the method of Ussing. Phosphate transport was active and could cause calcium to be actively transported
Walling and Rothman	1969	Active transport	Calcium transport, according to the method of Ussing gave flux ratios of 2.2 for +D and 1.4 for −D using rats as experimental animal
Krawitt and Schedl	1968	Active transport	Studied calcium transport in the small intestine *in vivo* perfusion. Transport against concentration gradient was seen in all segments.
DeLuca	Martin and DeLuca, 1969a; Martin *et al.*, [illegible]	Active transport	Found a Ca^{++}-stimulated ATPase in the intestinal brush borders which responds to vitamin D treatment

the time, it was claimed that the sterol acted directly in the intestine without prior activation; however, this seems untenable in view of the more recent information on the metabolism of calciferol. Further, they stated that phosphate transport was restricted to 'selective channels' in the mucosa; this conclusion was based on a complex interpretation of the relative specific activities of differing phosphate pools present in this tissue. Hence, the effect of calciferol on calcium transport had been reported by them to be maximal in the duodenum and independent of the presence of phosphate and since phosphate transport was found to be maximal in the jejumum, and independent of the presence of calcium, these workers concluded that the sterol has separate influences on these two intestinal transport mechanisms.

More recently, Wasserman and Taylor (1973) and Taylor (1974) studied the effects of cholecalciferol on the intestinal absorption of radioactive phosphate in the chick. They observed that phosphate was rapidly translocated across all segments of the small intestine and that cholecalciferol administration stimulated the process in each segment. It was claimed that the absorption of phosphate inhibited by the presence of arsenate, ethane diphosphonate (EHDP) and L-phenylalanine (an inhibitor of alkaline phosphatase). These workers stated that they could not detect the existence of a phosphate-binding protein comparable to the calcium-binding protein. The stimulation of phosphate uptake by calciferol in mucosal tissue was maximal at 16 hours, while stimulation of the complete transfer of phosphate from lumen to blood only became maximal at 48 hours.

Others have also interpreted their results as showing that cholecalciferol stimulates phosphate absorption independent of calcium absorption (Hurwitz and Barr, 1972). Their conclusion is based on results similar to that reported above by Kowarski and Schacter, i.e. the calciferol enhanced calcium absorption in the chick occurred mainly in the duodenum and that for phosphate mainly in the jejumum.

The most recent report on the relationship between calciferol and phosphate absorption is from the laboratory of DeLuca and co-workers (Chen *et al.*, 1974). These workers found that cholecalciferol and the metabolites 25-hydroxy- and 1,25-dihydroxycholecalciferol but not 24,25-dihydroxycholecalciferol stimulated phosphate transport independently of calcium transport in the rat. Phosphate transport was highest where there was also some stimulation by the presence of calcium – but in the jejunum phosphate transport was completely independent of the presence of calcium in the medium. Further, these workers concluded that since the 25-hydroxy-metabolite did not stimulate phosphate transport in an anephric animal, this supported the view that the active form of cholecalciferol which supported the phosphate transport was the renal metabolite 1,25-dihydroxycholecalciferol. As shown in panel D of Fig. 2, stimulation of intestinal phosphate transport

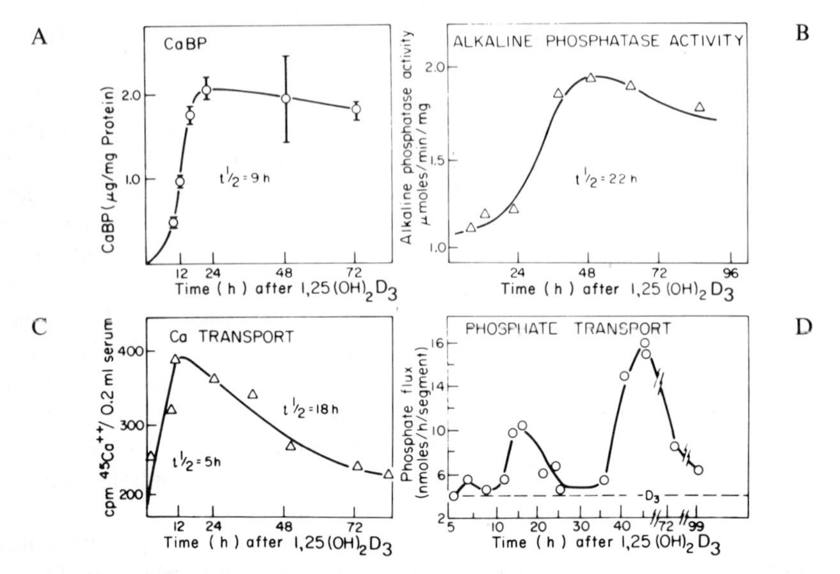

Fig. 2. Time course of several intestinal responses after treatment with 1,25-dihydroxycholecalciferol. In panels A, B, and C, chicks were treated orally with 325 pmoles (5U) of the hormone dissolved in 1,2-propanediol. A, Appearance of calcium binding protein (CaBP). CaBP was determined by immuno assay in the laboratory of Professor R. H. Wasserman, Cornell University. B, Increase in alkaline phosphatase activity of the intestinal brush border (Norman *et al.*, 1970). C, Increase in intestinal Ca^{2+} transport measured *in vivo* (Myrtle and Norman, 1971). D, Increase in stimulation of intestinal absorption of phosphate after administration of 1,25-dihydroxycholecalciferol (Mitsuyasu and Norman, unpublished observations)

directly in response to 1,25-dihydroxycholecalciferol has been observed (Mitsuyasu and Norman, unpublished observations). The kinetics of the response of phosphate transport to the administration of the hormone in which phosphate transport is increased more slowly that calcium transport is still unexplained.

In biochemical terms, the role of calcium in the regulation of calcium and phosphate absorption has been advanced by the metabolic studies described in the previous chapter. As discussed in detail in chapter 5, the effect of antibiotics such as actinomycin D on calciferol stimulated calcium absorption and the studies on the intracellular localisation are consistent with the hypothesis that the active form of calciferol regulates the expression of genetic information leading to the synthesis of enzymes for the alteration of the membrane structure necessary for calcium absorption (Norman, 1965; Zull *et al.*, 1965). The proof of such hypotheses depends upon establishing a correlation between the variations in protein levels and enzyme activities with the changes in calcium and phosphorus absorption in response to the vitamin or its active metabolite. Shown in Fig. 2 is the time course in the stimulation by 1,25-dihydroxycholecalciferol of intestinal calcium-binding protein (panel A), alkaline phosphatase (panel B), calcium absorption (panel C), and phosphate absorption (panel D). The dramatic difference in the time required for onset of action of these two latter processes suggests that they are dissociated from one another. However, it seems certain that these two changes are only part of a complex pattern of time dependent responses to 1,25-dihydroxycholecalciferol, which occurs in the intestinal mucosa, and that other changes will be discovered in the next few years.

III Factors Affecting Calcium and Phosphorus Absorption

A LOW CALCIUM DIET (ADAPTIVE RESPONSE)

The ability of the intestine to adapt to a low calcium diet by increasing the proportion of this element which is absorbed has been referred to already in Section IB and illustrated in Fig. 3, where three different examples of this phenomenon are shown. It has been found by Coburn *et al.* (1973), that this relationship can be observed in man (Fig. 3A) and it has been found in the chick by a number of investigators. The results reproduced in Fig. 3B show that at a high dietary level of calcium (1.8%) in a cholecalciferol repleted bird, there is a relatively low level of intestinal calcium absorption; whereas with a low dietary calcium level ($<0.05\%$), there is an approximate three-fold increase in the rate of calcium transport when cholecalciferol is administered. Thus the bird is able to adapt its rate of intestinal calcium transport to inversely reflect the amount of calcium in the diet. It is also apparent that the 'adaptation process' is dependent on the presence of the vitamin. In the presence of cholecalciferol (Fig. 3B) there is no marked change in the rate of transport of calcium as the dietary content of calcium is varied. The changes in the intestinal calcium transport which occur in chicks with increase in age and in rate of growth can be seen in Fig. 3C. For the first 30 days after hatching, at a time when the birds were actively growing and presumably had a high demand for calcium, there is a surprising fall in the rate of calcium transport when there is a ready dietary source of cholecalciferol. Thus the presence of the dietary vitamin ensures that the intestinal calcium transport systems may respond in an adaptive fashion to meet the demands placed on the calcium absorption system by the animal. Also shown in Fig. 3C is the response of a vitamin D-deficient chick given a single dose of cholecalciferol or 1,25-dihydroxycholecalciferol. Unfortunately, there are as yet no reports concerning attempts to assess a possible adaptation of the intestinal absorption of phosphorus.

The mechanism of this adaptive response can be understood on the basis of the control system regulating the production of 1,25-dihydroxycholecalciferol. The following findings are the source of this understanding:

1. The adaptive response is not shown by animals receiving either Sr^{2+} or actinomycin D and both these substances inhibit the formation of the hormone (Corradino and Wasserman, 1968; Corradino *et al.*, 1971; Omdahl and DeLuca, 1972).

2. A low calcium diet stimulates intestinal calcium flux and calcium-binding protein levels (Morrisey and Wasserman, 1971; Freund and Bronner, 1975).

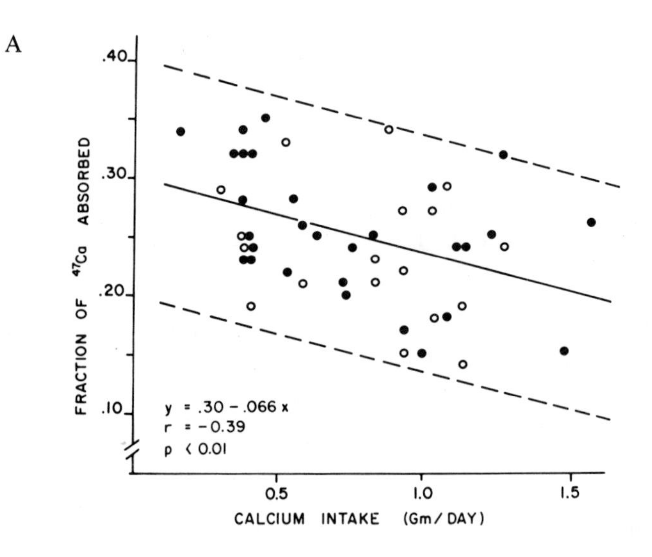

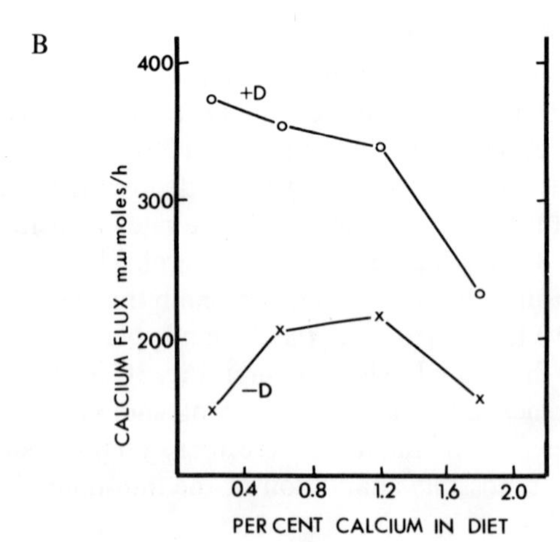

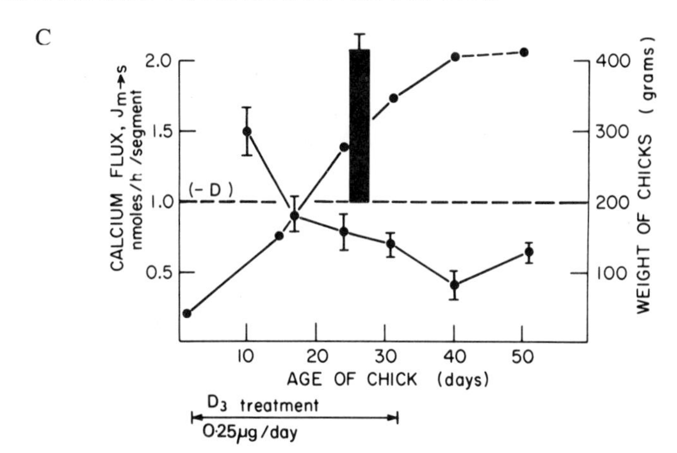

Fig. 3. A, The relationship between the fraction of ^{47}Ca absorbed and the previous habitual dietary intake of calcium in normal subjects. Each point represents a separate individual; males (●), females (○); the interrupted lines encompass the 95% confidence limits for individual values. Reproduced by the permission of the authors (Coburn *et al.*, 1973). B, Adaptation of calcium transport in chicks. Chicks were raised for 20 days on a standard rachitogenic diet, containing 0.6% Ca^{2+} (Norman and Wong, 1972), and then changed to diets containing 0, 0.6, 1.2, or 1.8% calcium, 0.4% phosphate. Half the birds received 0.37 μg of cholecalciferol (+D) daily, the other half received only 1,2-propanediol. After 5 days the rate of calcium flux was measured in ileal segments, *in vitro*, as described by Adams and Norman (1970). C, Changes in the activity of intestinal calcium transport with age or growth and vitamin D status. Groups of chicks were placed on a diet of 0.6% calcium, 0.4% phosphate and received 0.25 μg of cholecalciferol per day, from day 1 to day 32. The rate of intestinal calcium transport was measured, *in vitro*, in an apparatus similar to that of Ussing as described by Adams and Norman (1970). Other groups of chicks received no dietary calciferol for 21 days, at which time they exhibited the classical symptoms of rickets. At this point they received either 1.25 μg of cholecalciferol or 50 μg of 1,25-dihydroxycholecalciferol and their intestinal transport was measured either 24 h or 8 h later, respectively.

3. A tendency to a low plasma calcium level will result from a low calcium diet.

4. 1,25-Dihydroxycholecalciferol levels are raised in low plasma calcium situations (Hughes *et al.*, 1975) presumably through the action of parathyroid hormone.

In summary, therefore, a low dietary calcium level results in a tendency for plasma calcium levels to fall, thereby stimulating parathyroid hormone secretion and thus raising 1,25-dihydroxycholecalciferol levels in plasma. This latter hormone increases calcium flux by a stimulation of the absorption system, one component of which is calcium-binding protein (chapter 4).

B ANTIBIOTICS INCLUDING FILIPIN

Fundamental to our understanding of the mode of action of calciferol has been the results obtained with inhibitors of DNA directed RNA synthesis such as actinomycin D (Norman, 1965; Zull *et al.*, 1965; Norman *et al.*, 1969) and α-amanytin (Corradino, 1973) and it is hoped that a further insight into the action of calciferol on the mucosal membrane will result from studies with the polyene antibiotic filipin. Shown in Fig. 4 are more recent results obtained in the author's laboratory, demonstrating that actinomycin D is capable of blocking both cholecalciferol and 1,25-dihydroxycholecalciferol stimulated intestinal calcium transport. If actinomycin D is given intraperitoneally to rachitic chicks at the appropriate time prior to the intracardial administration of either cholecalciferol or its hormonal metabolite, there is inhibition of the characteristic stimulation of intestinal calcium transport which is observed within 24 h or 10 h respectively. As was reported in detail by Tsai *et al.*, 1973, this was not due to an inhibition by actinomycin D of the localisation of 1,25-dihydroxycholecalciferol in the intestine. It can be unequivocally demonstrated that there are normal quantities of this metabolite present in the intestine after administering actinomycin D to these birds.

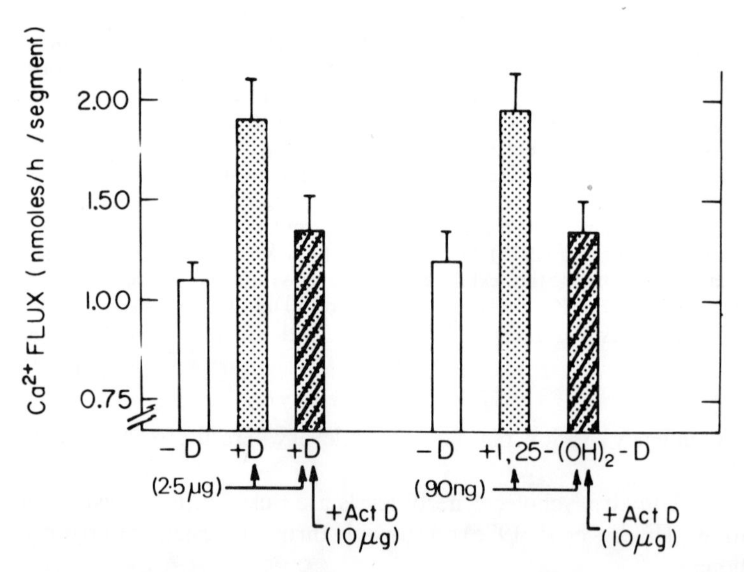

Fig. 4. Effect of actinomycin D on cholecalciferol or 1,25-dihydroxycholecalciferol stimulation of intestinal calcium transport. Indicated doses of the vitamin or of the hormone were given intracardially either 24 h or 10 h, respectively, before measurement of intestinal calcium transport, *in vitro*, according to the procedures of Adams and Norman (1970). Where indicated, a total of 10 μg of actinomycin D were administered intraperitoneally at intervals prior to the dose of the steroid.

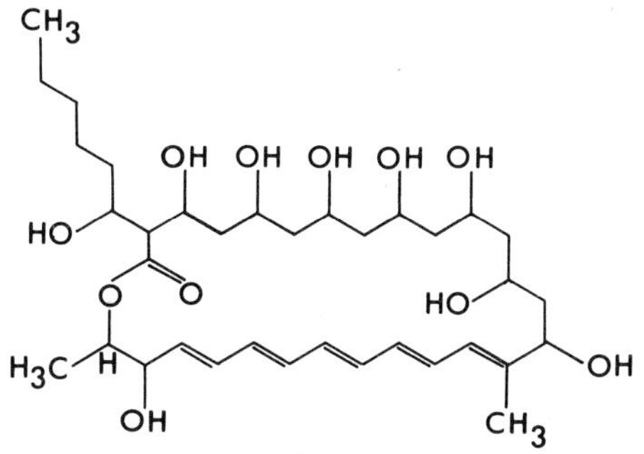

Fig. 5. Structure of the polyene antibiotic, filipin

As was the case with adaptation of intestinal absorption, there have been no reports to date concerning the ability of actinomycin D to block the intestinal absorption of phosphate.

Filipin was discovered during the course of investigations to find antibiotics which might either mimic the action of calciferol in the intestine or inhibit calcium absorption by a different mechanism than that of inhibiting protein synthesis. The consequences of filipin treatment *in vitro* have been found to be remarkably similar to the effect induced *in vivo* by cholecalciferol or 1,25-dihydroxycholecalciferol (Adams *et al.*, 1970).

There are some forty polyene antibiotics described in the literature (Norman *et al.*, 1976) and the structure of filipin is given in Fig. 5. Of all the antibiotics, amphotercin B, pimaricin, filipin, etruscomycin and nystatin have been most extensively studied (Van Zupthen *et al.*, 1971; Norman *et al.*, 1972a, b; Spielvogel and Norman, 1975). The structure of a polyene is characterised by the presence of a large lactone ring which has a number of conjugated double bonds on one side and multiple hydroxyl groups on the opposite side of the molecule. The biological effects of polyene antibiotics including filipin, have been shown conclusively by Kinsky *et al.* (1967); Demel *et al.* (1972) and Norman *et al.* (1972a, b; 1976) to result from their ability to increase the permeability of target membranes for selected small molecules. The molecular basis of this action of filipin is believed to be mediated by a selective interaction of the polyene antibiotic with membrane-bound sterols, specifically cholesterol. There results a stoichiometric 1:1 interaction between one molecule of the membrane bound cholesterol and one molecule of filipin to produce a molecular complex (Katzenstein *et al.*, 1974). It is known that this is a non-covalent interaction being primarily hydrophobic in nature. As a consequence of this polyene antibiotic-membrane bound sterol interaction, there results a selective change in the permeability properties of the

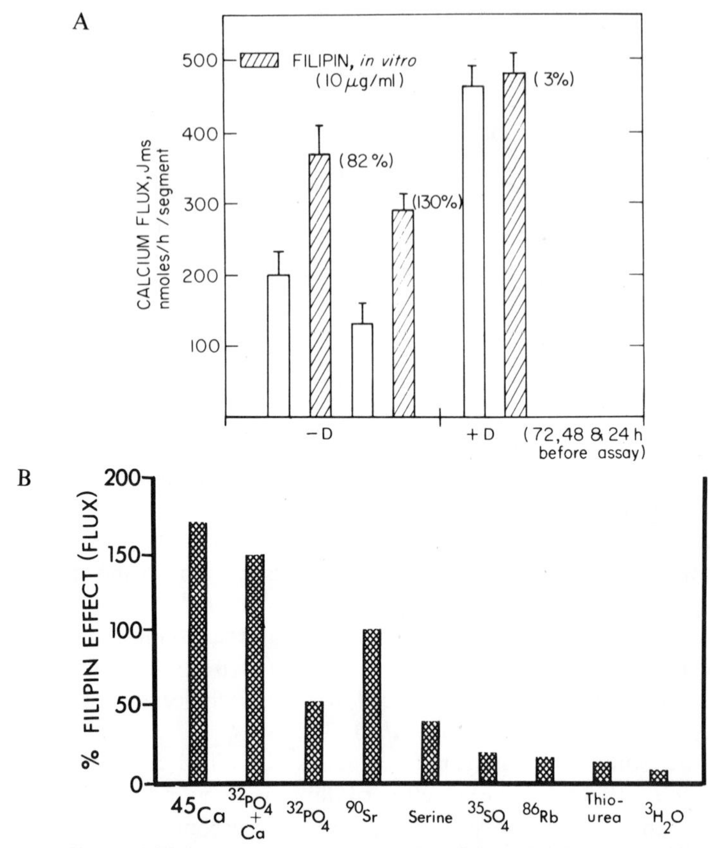

Fig. 6. Effects of filipin on transport properties of the chick ileum. A, Effect of filipin treatment *in vitro* on the intestinal transport of calcium. Segments of intestinal mucosa tissue were obtained from either vitamin D-deficient (−CC) or from chicks which had received 12.5 μg of cholecalciferol 72, 48, and 24 h before death (+CC). The intestinal segments were mounted in the transport chambers (see Adams and Norman, 1970), and filipin (▨, 10 μg/ml; ca. 10^{-5} M) was placed in the solution bathing only the mucosal surface of the tissue. 30 min later, the intestinal transport of calcium was measured, and calculated as calcium flux, $J_{m \to s}$ (nmoles per hour per segment). B, The effect of filipin *in vitro*, on the ileal flux of various ions and substances in the calciferol-deficient chick intestine. Experiments performed *in vitro* in the Ussing transport apparatus for all experiments except the strontium and rubidium flux experiments, which were performed in a glass transport apparatus (see Adams and Norman, 1970). The initial concentration of all ions and compounds tested was 0.10 mM except Rb^+ (0.2 mM) and water. The initial flux determination was made for each isotope for a 20 min period following the initial preincubation period. Filipin was added to the mucosal compartment to give a final concentration of 10 μg/ml. After a 20 min lag, the flux determination was made in the presence of filipin. The filipin effect was then measured as the percent increase of the flux rate due to filipin over the initial flux rate in the absence of filipin

membrane. A detailed discussion of the molecular basis for these changes has appeared (Spielvogel and Norman, 1975).

In Fig. 6 is shown some of the original data which suggested the value of using filipin *in vitro* as a tool to study calcium transport. As shown in Fig. 6A, filipin at concentrations of 10 μg/ml (ca. 1.7×10^{-5} M) stimulates the calcium flux, J_{ms}, of ileal tissue from vitamin D-deficient chicks by 150–200% but has little or no effect on J_{ms} of ileal tissue obtained from cholcalciferol-treated birds. As shown in Fig. 6B, the filipin treatment *in vitro* on ileal tissue obtained from vitamin D-deficient chicks is surprisingly specific for calcium as compared to water, thiourea, serine, phosphate, sulphate or rubidium. It should be emphasised that the data presented in Fig. 6B is the result of transport of the substance in question completely across the mucosal cells, i.e. its disappearance from the mucosal cells and its appearance on the serosal side. Filipin was shown to be the most effective of all the polyene antibiotics tested. No effect has ever been noted when filipin was placed in a solution bathing the serosal surface of the tissue; i.e. the effects of filipin occur only on the brush border or microvilli side of the intestinal columnar epithelial cell.

The consequences of incubating filipin *in vitro* with ileal tissue from vitamin D-deficient birds was found to mimic many aspects of cholecalciferol administration in terms of calcium transport (Table 4). Filipin, when placed in a solution bathing only the brush border side of the intestinal cell (*a*) induces an active translocation of calcium against an electrochemical gradient; (*b*)

Table 4. Comparison of the properties of the intestinal calcium transport system induced *in vivo* by vitamin D or by filipin applied *in vitro*[a]

	−D	−D+filipin *in vitro*[b]	+D
Active transport of calcium	No	Yes	Yes
Flux rate, J_{ms}/J_{ms}	0.96	1.8	2.2
Specificity for Ca^{2+} transport	—	Yes	Yes
Sensitivity to low temperature	—	Yes	Yes
N-Ethylmaleimide sensitivity	—	+	+
CaBP present	No	No	Yes
Alkaline phosphatase activity	Low	Unchanged	Increase
Effect sensitive to actinomycin D	No	No	Yes
Evidence that calciferol or filipin mediates an increased cellular uptake of Ca^{2+}	—	Yes	Yes
Calcium transport system is adaptive to dietary Ca^{2+} levels	No	No	Yes

[a] Taken from Adams and Norman (1970); Adams *et al.* (1970) and Wong *et al.* (1970)

[b] Filipin was added *in vitro*, to solution bathing ileal tissue from calciferol-deficient (−D) chicks

confers the property of cold sensitivity on the increased J_{ms} flux; (*c*) confers sensitivity to the sulfhydryl reagent *N*-ethylmaleimide on the increased J_{ms} flux and (*d*) interacts with the membrane bound carrier on the brush border side of the cell to effect an increased uptake of calcium into the cell (Adams and Norman, 1970; Adams *et al.*, 1970; Wong *et al.*, 1970).

Further, filipin was clearly shown not to be an ionophoretic compound for calcium, so that the enhanced calcium transport could not be ascribed to a direct interaction or chelation of calcium by filipin. It is also interesting to note the marked specificity of filipin for calcium in contrast to its lack of effect on phosphate.

Shown in Table 5 is a study of the effect of filipin treatment *in vitro* on the uptake of calcium into the mucosal cell itself. When ileal tissue was obtained from either vitamin D-deficient or vitamin D-treated chicks and then both tissues were separately treated with filipin under *in vitro* conditions, it was observed that there was a marked enhancement of the uptake of calcium into the cell in both tissue preparations. As with the transport process, the effect of filipin on the permeability of the membrane to calcium was specific to this ion as a variety of other anions, cations and organic molecules were not taken up by the mucosal cell. It should be noted, however, that the effect of filipin on calcium intake by intestinal mucosal cells can be observed irrespective of the vitamin status of the animal, in contrast to calcium flux across the whole cell which is affected by filipin only when the cells are obtained from vitamin D-deficient animals (Wong and Norman, 1975).

An attempt has been made to understand the mechanism by which the interaction of filipin with the intestinal brush border may result in such specific permeability changes. Aspects of the interaction to be taken into account include the time scale required to effect the filipin mediated permeability changes (<30 min for maximum response) and the finding that ileal segments

Table 5. Effect of filipin on calcium uptake by mucosal cells

Calciferol status	Rate of Calcium Uptake ±SE		Per cent increase
	−Filipin	+Filipin	
$-D_3$	4.82±0.34 (4)	9.25±1.10 (4)	92%
$+D_3$	9.84±0.67 (4)	16.3±0.92 (4)	60%

The experiments were performed, *in vitro*, in the uptake apparatus as described by Wong and Norman (1975) with an initial calcium concentration of 0.10 mM. Adjacent segments of a single ileum were preincubated for 30 min, with and without filipin (10 μg/ml). Rate of uptake was determined by placing the uptake apparatus in fresh medium containing 2.5 μCi of $^{45}Ca^{2+}$. Chicks termed $+D_3$ received 3 oral doses of 12.5 μg (32.5 moles) of cholecalciferol 72, 48 and 24 h before sacrifices.

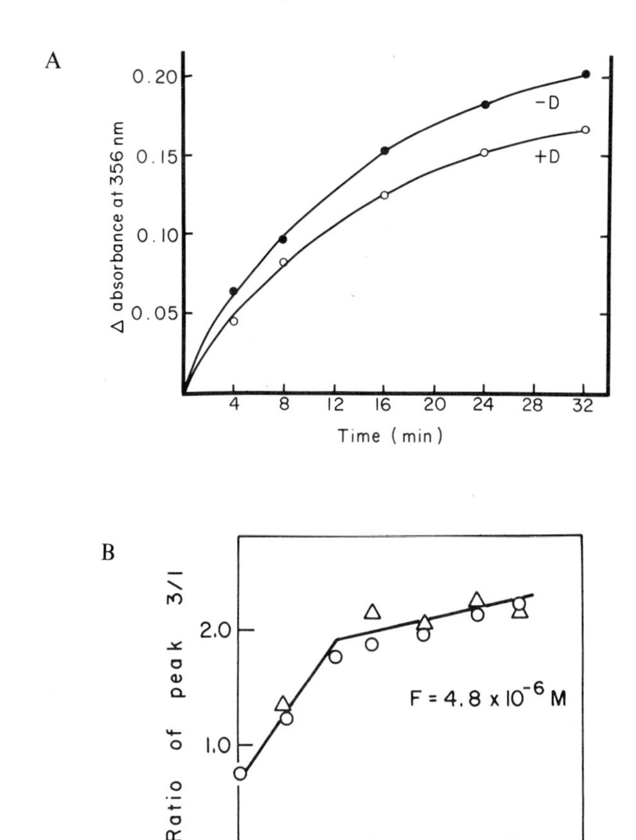

Fig. 7. A, Time course of binding of filipin, *in vitro*, to 8 cm everted intestinal ileal segments from vitamin D-treated and/or vitamin D-deficient chicks. Ileal segments + vitamin D were excised from vitamin D-treated chicks which had received a 12.5 μg oral dose of cholecalciferol 26 h before sacrifice. Filipin binding was monitored as described by Adams *et al.* (1970). B, Stoichiometry of interaction of filipin with brush border cholesterol. The filipin concentration was 4.8×10^{-6} M. The lower scale represents the cholesterol concentration as determined by Lieberman-Burchard analysis of the lipid extract of the same brush border preparations. Brush border preparations were obtained from groups of 15 vitamin D-deficient chicks (−D) or chicks repleted with 12.5 μg of cholecalciferol 72, 48, and 24 h before sacrifice (+D)

from cholecalciferol-treated and -deficient birds bind filipin equally well (Fig. 7A).

It has been shown (Norman *et al.*, 1972a, b) that the interaction of filipin with cholesterol results in a change in the ultraviolet spectrum of the filipin. This spectral change can be employed to determine both the stoichiometry of the interaction, or, if that is known, to determine the amount of cholesterol present in the tissue. Results of such an experiment are shown in Fig. 7B. It was of interest to ascertain if filipin reacting with cholesterol in brush border membranes obeys the same 1 : 1 stoichiometry. The question was examined by determining the total cholesterol concentration of bush border membranes after lipid extraction and observing the associated spectral change of filipin upon its reaction with aqueous samples of brush border containing cholesterol concentration 0.3–3 times that of the filipin concentration (Fig. 7B). When the spectral change of filipin is plotted against the brush border protein or cholesterol concentration a sharp break is evident at a cholesterol concentration of 4.6×10^{-6} M. Since filipin was applied at a final concentration of 4.8×10^{-6} M, a stoichiometry of 1:1 can be proposed for the complex of filipin and membrane cholesterol. Most importantly, it was found that brush border membranes obtained from the intestine of vitamin D-treated or vitamin D-deficient birds interacted *identically* with the polyene antibiotic.

In parallel studies, Spielvogel and Norman (1975) found that the application of filipin to liposome composed of phospholipids plus cholesterol resulted in a generalised increase in permeability for both anions (phosphate included) and cations (including calcium). This suggests that these model membranes which are devoid of protein do not show a specific filipin-mediated enhancement of calcium transport to the exclusion of phosphate transport. This strongly suggests that the protein component of the brush border membrane plays an important role in the determination of the selective calcium and phosphate permeability properties. Filipin is capable of selectively improving the permeability to calcium, as can calciferol or its metabolites but these metabolites have to act *in vivo*.

In Fig. 8 is given a schematic diagram showing the possible molecular basis of filipin's action in the brush border region of the mucosal cells of the intestine. The sum of the evidence summarised here and reported in detail elsewhere (Spielvogel, 1973; Wong *et al.*, 1970; Spielvogel and Norman, 1975) suggests that filipin is apparently able to effect a structural reorganisation of the brush border membrane of ileal tissue obtained from vitamin D-deficient chicks so that an increased uptake of calcium into the mucosal cell occurs. The consequences of the direct, filipin-mediated reorganisation of the brush border membrane are remarkably similar to the indirect, actinomycin D sensitive effect brought about by dietary calciferol or 1,25-dihydroxycholecal-

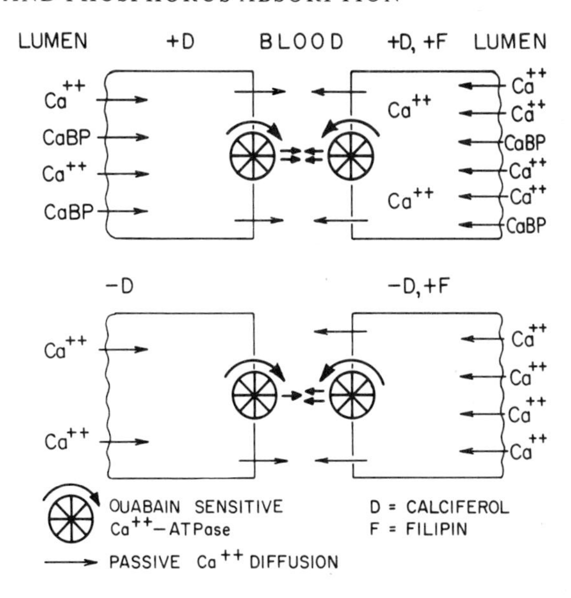

Fig. 8. Mechanism of action of polyene antibiotic filipin, *in vitro*, on intestinal epithelial cells. The top panels indicate schematically the effects of filipin in intestinal tissue from vitamin D-treated chicks; the bottom panels indicate the effects of filipin in the intestinal tissue from rachitic chicks

ciferol. A plausible hypothesis then for a part of the mechanism of action of 1,25-dihydroxycholecalciferol is that its administration to a vitamin D-deficient animal mediates by a process of induction the *de novo* synthesis of proteins, followed by a structural reorganisation of the brush border or microvillar membrane (chapter 5). These 'new' proteins could function in either a catalytic or structural role in the brush border membrane so as to result in a more efficient translocation of calcium and also possibly phosphate. It is also conceivable that the calciferol metabolites have independent selective effects to stimulate the absorption of phosphate. The finding that filipin, *in vitro*, can enhance the uptake of calcium in the ileum of cholecalciferol-treated chicks, but cannot change the overall rate of transport from the mucosal-to-serosal side, indicates that the rate-limiting step for the transport process is *not* at the brush border membrane. The rate limiting factor of the overall calcium transport could therefore be intracellular [the mitochondria are known to accumulate calcium rapidly (Rossi and Lehninger, 1963)] or at the basal membrane of the epithelial cells (Norman *et al.*, 1965). A ouabain-sensitive Na^+, K^+-activated ATPase located at the serosal side of the epithelial cell has been proposed as playing a role in the extrusion of calcium from the epithelial cells (Martin and DeLuca, 1969b; Wong, 1972; Birge *et al.*, 1972).

Filipin, upon interaction with a sterol in the brush border membrane, can cause a structural rearrangement of the membrane's components. Consequently, some negative binding sites at the mucosal side of the intestinal epithelial cell are perhaps uncovered. The increase of negative binding sites on the brush border membrane of vitamin D-treated and -deficient chicks enhances the concentration of calcium near this membrane. This is shown on the right-hand side of Fig. 8. More calcium enters the epithelial cells as a consequence of the filipin treatment. The calcium-binding protein present in the brush border region of vitamin D-treated chicks serves a similar purpose to that of filipin, in that it also increases the calcium concentration in the brush border membrane and in the intestinal epithelial cells. The ouabain-sensitive calcium pump located at the serosal side of intestinal epithelial cells actively transports the calcium into the blood stream. It is assumed that this process is rate limiting in the intestine of cholecalciferol or 1,25-dihydroxycholecalciferol treated chicks. Therefore, identical amounts of calcium will be translocated from the mucosal-to-serosal side in ileal segments obtained from cholecalciferol treated birds and intestines of cholecalciferol-treated or depleted chicks after incubation *in vitro* with filipin. However, less calcium will be transported by the intestinal epithelial cells obtained from rachitic chicks.

Shown in Fig. 9 is an integrated scheme which attempts to describe the overall process of calcium and phosphate absorption in the intestine. The

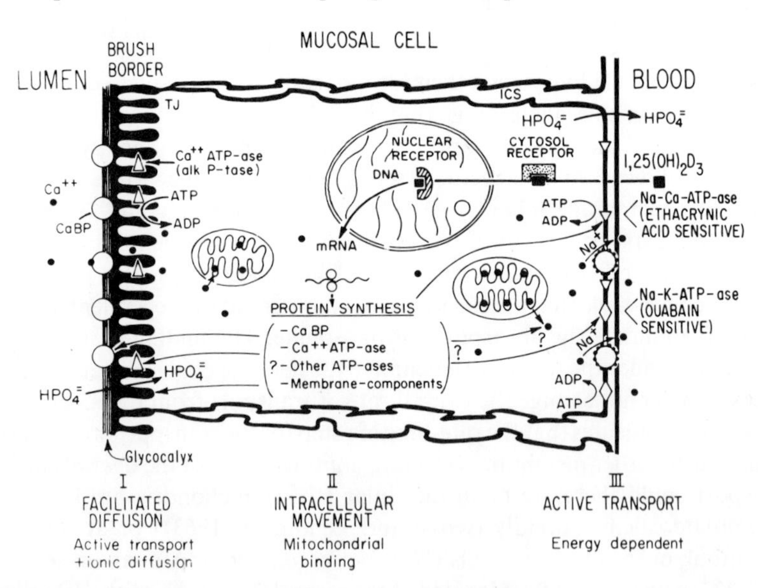

Fig. 9. Proposed mechanism of action of 1,25-dihydroxycholecalciferol in the intestine and its proposed effects on stimulation of intestinal calcium and phosphorus translocation

active transport system for calcium is dependent upon the intracellular availability of calcium, so that as the intracellular calcium concentration increases (either by filipin action *in vitro* or calciferol metabolite action *in vivo*), it is possible to envisage an increased efflux of calcium at the basal membrane side. It is known that the intracellular concentration of calcium is very low (10^{-6} to 10^{-7} M) and that most of the intracellular calcium is contained in the mitochondria (Thomas and Greenwalt, 1968). The increase in calcium in the intestinal epithelial cells is reflected by a more efficient supply of calcium to the $Na^{+}K^{+}$-activated ATPase which actively transports calcium into the underlying blood vessels. If this serosal pump operates unidirectionally, the ratio of flux of calcium from mucosa-to-serosa to the flux from serosa-to-mucosa would exceed 1.00 if the tissue was treated with filipin. It is also conceivable, however, that the K_m of this calcium pump limits the maximal amount of calcium which can be extruded at a given time interval. This will explain the finding that the filipin-mediated increase of calcium in the ileum of cholecalciferol-treated chicks was not reflected in an overall increase in calcium translocation. Since this active pump on the serosal side requires metabolic energy, this suggests that any interference with the translocation of substrates for cellular metabolism will inhibit both the calciferol and filipin-mediated active calcium transport in the intestine. This would explain the effects of *N*-ethylmaleimide and low temperature sensitivity of the calcium transport processes summarised in Table 4.

C MISCELLANEOUS FACTORS

An indication of the wide range of factors known to influence calcium absorption is given by the selection listed in Table 6. Some of these have been discussed in the previous two sections. In a review prepared by Wasserman and Taylor (1969), there is a detailed description of the effect on calcium absorption of lactose and related carbohydrates, amino acids and detergents including bile acids and cetrimide. As no developments have occurred since that review was prepared which causes our understanding of the effects of these substances on calcium absorption to be altered, they will not be considered further here.

Several plants have been recognised as being the cause of a general calcinosis in farm animals allowed to graze on them (Worker and Carrillo, 1967; Sansom *et al.*, 1971; Dirksen *et al.*, 1970; Wasserman, 1975). The condition is similar to calciferol intoxication. Subsequent studies showed that a wide range of animals are affected, including cow, horse, rabbit, rat and chick. The signs and symptoms vary somewhat from species to species but most show the following: hypercalcaemia, hyperphosphataemia, soft tissue calcification, muscle wasting and increased calcium absorption. The plants so

Table 6. Factors affecting the intestinal absorption of calcium or phosphorus

Lactose and other carbohydrates	Wasserman and Comar, 1959
Amino acids	Wasserman *et al.*, 1956
Solanum glaucophyllum (malacoxalon)	Humphreys, 1973
Ethane diphosphonate	Bonjour *et al.*, 1972, 1973; Krawitt *et al.*, 1974
Ethanol	Krawitt, 1973
Glucocorticoids	Krawitt, 1972
Peptide hormones	
Parathyroid hormone	Rasmussen, 1959; Shah and Drapper, 1966
Calcitonin	Olson *et al.*, 1972; tanzer and Navia, 1973
Metabolic inhibitors	
2,4-Dinotrophenol	Schacter and Rosen, 1959
Cyanide	
Iodoacetamide	Adams and Norman, 1970
Antibiotics	
Gene-active	Norman, 1965, 1966, Zull *et al.*, 1965
actinomycin D	
α-amanitin	Corradino, 1973
Membrane-active	Adams *et al.*, 1970; Wong and Norman, 1975
filipin	
Vitamin D	*loc. cit.*

far recognised as causing the disease are *Solanum glaucophyllum* (malacoxylon) (Worker and Carrilo, 1967), Cestrum diurnum (Wasserman, 1975) and *Tristeum flavescens* (Dirksen *et al.*, 1970). The most well-studied active principle is that from Glaucophyllum which can be extracted from the plant by water. A number of metabolic changes have been observed which show the active principle in the leaf to have 1,25-dihydroxycholecalciferol activity: raising plasma calcium and phosphorus levels (Mautalen, 1972; Uribe *et al.*, 1974); increasing calcium absorption (Sansom *et al.*, 1971; O'Donnell and Smith, 1973); raising calcium-binding protein levels (Lawson *et al.*, 1974); overcoming Sr^{2+} inhibition of vitamin D activity (Wasserman, 1974) and being active in anephric rats (Walling and Kimberg, 1975). Furthermore, Walling *et al.* (1975) have shown that the substance present in the aqueous extract of the plant can compete with 1,25-dihydroxycholecalciferol for the binding sites in the intestinal nuclei for the hormone. The recent report therefore that the aqueous extract of *S. glaucophyllum* contains 1,25-dihydroxycholecalciferol was not unexpected (Haussler *et al.*, 1976).

There have been numerous reports in the literature of the ability of diphosphonates to inhibit calciferol stimulated intestinal calcium transport

(Bonjour *et al.*, 1973). The administration of 10 mg of ethane diphosphonate (EHDP) to rats has been shown by Bonjour *et al.* (1972) to inhibit hypercalcaemia due to bone mobilisation and to dramatically decrease the absorption of calcium. The present basis of understanding the mode of action of EHDP is by virtue of its ability to inhibit the conversion of cholecalciferol to its active form, 1,25-dihydroxycholecalciferol. Thus the administration of the hormone but not of cholecalciferol to vitamin D-deficient animals treated with EHDP results in a marked stimulation of intestinal calcium transport. These results suggest that the basis of action of this drug is not at the intestinal level, but is principally at the renal level (Krawitt *et al.*, 1973) where the metabolic transformation of 25-hydroxycholecalciferol into 1,25-dihydroxycholecalciferol occurs.

The chronic administration of ethanol also effects an inhibition of the intestinal absorption of calcium in the duodenum (Krawitt, 1973). This inhibition was not reversed by cholecalciferol or the hormone metabolite, indicating that the effect of the ethanol is not concerned with the metabolism of the vitamin (Krawitt, 1975). It is suggested that the ethanol affects an intracellular site in the intestine which is involved in calcium absorption, a phcnomenon which is almost certainly not the explanation of the calcium malabsorption observed in chronic alcoholic patients where there is also massive liver damage.

It is also well established that an excess of glucocorticoids can reduce the intestinal absorption of calcium (Harrison and Harrison, 1960; Kimberg *et al.*, 1961) and it has been postulated by several workers that the glucocorticoids are 'antagonistic' to the action of calciferol. It has been shown that glucocorticoids will reduce the active transport of calcium by the duodenum of rats, will suppress brush border alkaline phosphotase activity but interestingly, calcium binding protein levels are unaffected (Kimberg *et al.*, 1971; Krawitt, 1972; Lukert *et al.*, 1973). Originally there was some discussion as to whether this antagonistic effect was a result of interference in the metabolism of calciferol to its active form, or whether it was the result of an independent 'end organ action' on the intestine. Recent studies indicate that the suppression of calcium transport is mediated independently of any direct interaction on the metabolism of cholecalciferol (Kimberg *et al.*, 1971; Favus *et al.*, 1973). This inhibitory action of cortisol on calcium transport is still unexplained.

Another aspect of intestinal calcium and phosphorus absorption which is the subject of many investigations concerns the effects of the peptide hormones, calcitonin and parathyroid hormone on this process.

The polypeptide hormone calcitonin is generally believed to act in preventing hypercalcaemia but the mechanisms by which it achieves this are not completely understood, although a possibility is an inhibition by calcitonin of bone resorption. In addition, an inhibitory effect of calcitonin on the calciferol induced increases in calcium absorption has been reported (Olson *et al.*, 1972). These authors showed that an acute infusion of a pharmacological dose of purified porcine calcitonin into rats produced an immediate drop in calcium absorption in animals given cholecalciferol but has no effect on calcium absorption in vitamin D-deficient animals. Also, Tanzer and Navia (1973) found that administration of calcitonin can inhibit the intestinal absorption of phosphate.

The possible role of parathyroid hormone in the overall process of intestinal calcium absorption is perhaps somewhat clearer. Several reports have appeared in the literature that support the view that the regulation of intestinal calcium absorption and the adaptation to dietary calcium by depravation is mediated in part by parathyroid hormone. Until recently, the site of action of the hormone on the transport process was believed to be unknown. However, it now appears likely that parathyroid hormone is a trophic hormone capable of stimulating the output by the kidney of 1,25-dihydroxycholecalciferol. This would result in an increased secretion of parathyroid hormone and concomitant increased renal production of 1,25-dihydroxycholecalciferol. The increased availability of the hormone to the intestine would have the potential of resulting in an increased biosynthesis of calcium-binding protein and other transport components and hence an increased absorption of calcium.

D DISEASE STATES OF MAN

It is only natural that in a process as complex as the one described above for calcium and phosphorus absorption that there should occur disease states which result from abberations of specific steps in the overall process (chapter 9). Table 7 lists the disease states known to occur in man, in which there is an alteration in the intestinal absorption of calcium and phosphorus.

Table 7. Disease states of man affecting calcium and phosphorus absorption

	Intestinal absorption	
	Increased	Decreased
Calcium	Sarcoidosis Idiopathic hypercalcaemia Hyperparathyroidism	Glucocorticoid antagonism Tropical sprue Chronic renal failure Hypoparathyroidism
Phosphorus	?	Rickets

Examination of this list will show that calcium absorption is far more prone to derangement than is phosphorus absorption. At present, there are no known diseases in man which can overtly be described to produce either an increase or a depression in the intestinal absorption of phosphorus.

The etiological basis of hyperparathyroidism and hypoparathyroidism have been discussed earlier in relation to their proposed effects on altering the metabolism of calciferol to its active hormonal form (chapter 2, IIB). Also, the possible basis of glucocorticoid antagonism has been mentioned. Chronic renal failure is always or usually characterised by an impaired intestinal absorption of calcium (Coburn *et al.*, 1973). This disease state too probably perturbs the metabolism of calciferol to its active forms. Thus, much, if not all, of the explanation for impaired intestinal calcium absorption in renal failure is due to a paucity of the active form of calciferol. Sarcoidosis is believed to result from a heightened intestinal sensitivity or responsiveness to small doses of calciferol. The primary clinical manifestation is a hypercalcaemia, and it has been postulated that this may result from an increased intestinal absorption of calcium. However, the precise biochemical explanation for the disease is not yet available. Tropical sprue is a disease characterised by an alteration in morphology of the brush border region of the intestinal mucosal cells and may be explicable in terms of a lack of absorptive cells. The functional basis for idiopathic hypercalcaemia is not presently known. However, individuals have documented elevated intestinal calcium absorption in this disease state.

E CONCLUDING REMARKS

It is clear that a detailed understanding at the molecular level of the intestinal absorption of calcium and phosphorus is a challenging problem to which there is not yet a completely definitive solution. It is apparent that the role of calciferol and its active metabolite, 1,25-dihydroxycholecalciferol, is firmly established in terms of its ability to stimulate or mediate an increased intestinal absorption of calcium. Further, there are a number of studies which strongly indicate the possibility that this steroid hormone also exerts an independent effect on intestinal absorption of phosphate. Many of the 'black box' complications of the multi-step process for transfer of these substances from the lumen of the intestine to the blood have at least been identified as existing. In some instances, notably the isolation of calcium-binding protein (chapters 4 and 5), a detailed study at the molecular level of a component of the transport system has in fact been accomplished. It remains to the future, however, to provide an equally detailed description of both the function and the composition of other components associated with or intimately involved with the intestinal absorption of phosphorus and calcium.

References

Adams, T. H. and Norman, A. W. (1970) *J. Biol. Chem.* **245**, 4421.
Adams, T. H., Wong, R. G. and Norman, A. W. (1970). *J. Biol. Chem.* **245**, 4432.
Bartter, F. C. (1964). *In* 'Mineral Metabolism' (Ed. C. L. Comer and F. Bronner) Vol. 2A, p. 315. Academic Press, New York and London.
Berger, E. Y. (1960). *In* 'Mineral Metabolism' (Ed. C. L. Comar and F. Bronner) Vol. 1, p. 249. Academic Press, New York and London.
Bergheim, O. (1926). *J. Biochem.* **70**, 51.
Bethke, R. M., Kennard, D. C., Kik, C. H. and Zinzalian, G. (1929). *Poult. Sci.* **8**, 257.
Birge, S. J. and Alpers, D. H. (1973). *Gastroenterology* **64**, 977.
Birge, S. J., Gilbert, A. and Avioli, L. V. (1972) *Science* **176**, 168.
Blair, M., Spencer, H., Swernov, J. and Laszlo, D. (1954). *Science* **120**, 1029.
Bonjour, J. P., Russell, R. G. C., Morgan, D. B. and Fleisch, H. A. (1972) *Amer. J. Physiol.* **224**, 1011.
Bonjour, J. P., DeLuca, H. F., Fleisch, H., Trechsel, U., Matejowec, L. A. and Omdahl, J. L. (1973). *Europ. J. Clin. Invest.* **3**, 44.
Bronner, F. (1964). *In* 'Mineral Metabolism' (Ed. C. L. Comar and F. Bronner) Vol. 2A, p. 341. Academic Press, New York and London.
Bronner, F. (1972). 'Engineering Principles in Physiology', Vol. 1, p. 227. Academic Press, New York and London.
Brown, H. B., Shohl, A. T., Chapman, E. E., Rose, C. S. and Saurwein, E. M. (1932). *J. Biol. Chem.* **98**, 207.
Carlsson, A. (1951). *Acta pharmac. tox.* **7** (suppl. 1), 1.
Carlsson, A. (1954). *Acta phys. Scandinav.* **31.**
Chen, T. C., Castillo, L., Korycka-Dahl, M. and DeLuca, H. F. (1974) *J. Nutr.* **98,** 1056.
Coates, M. E. and Holdsworth, E. S. (1961). *Brit. J. Nutr.* **15**, 131.
Coburn, J. W., Koppel, M. H., Brickman, A. S. and Massry, S. G. (1973) *Kidney Intl.* **3**, 264.
Cohn, W. E. and Greenberg, D. M. (1939). *J. Biol. Chem.* **130**, 625.
Cooper, C. W., Schwesinger, W. H., Mahgoub, A. M., Ontjes, D. A., Gray, T. K. and Munson, D. L. (1972). *In* 'Calcium, Parathyroid Hormone and the Calcitonins' (Ed. R. V. Talmage and P. L. Munson) p. 128. Excerpta Medica Amsterdam.
Corradino, R. A. (1973). *Nature* (London) **243**, 41.
Corradino, R. A., Ebel, J. G., Craig, P. H., Taylor, A. N. and Wasserman, R. H. (1971). *Calc. Tiss. Res.* **7**, 81.
Corradino, R. A. and Wasserman, R. H. (1968). *Arch. Biochem.* **126**, 957.
Crane, R. K., Forstner, G. and Eichholz, A. (1965). *Biochim. Biophys. Acta* **109**, 467.
Curran, P. F. and Solomon, A. K. (1957). *J. Gen. Physiol.* **41**, 143.
Curtis, F. K., Fellows, H. and Rich, C. (1967). *J. Lab. Clin Med.* **69**, 1036.
Dahlquist, A. and Nordstrom, C. (1966). *Biochim. Biophys. Acta.* **113**, 624.
DeGrazia, J. A. and Rich, C. (1964). *Metabolism* **13**, 650.
Demel, R. A., Bruckdorfer, K. R. and van Deenen, L. L. M. (1972). *Biochim. Biophys. Acta.* **255**, 311.
Dirksen, G., Plank, P., Spies, A., Hanichen, T. and Dammrich, K. (1970). *Deutsch Tierarztl Wschr.* **77**, 321.
Dols, M. J. L., Jansen, B. C. P., Sizoo, G. J. and DeVries, J. (1938). *Nature* (London) **139**, 1068.

Favus, M. J., Walling, M. W. and Kimberg, D. V. (1973). *J. Clin Invest.* **52**, 1680.
Findlay, L., Paton, D. N. and Sharpe, J. S. (1920). *Quart. J. Med.* **14**, 352.
Forstner, G. G. (1969). *Amer. J. Med. Sci.* **258**, 172.
Forstner, G. G. (1971). *Biochem. J.* **121**, 781.
Freund, T. and Bronner, F. (1975). *Amer. J. Physiol.* **228**, 861.
Greenberg, D. M. (1945). *J. Biol. Chem.* **157**, 99.
Harrison, H. E. and Harrison, H. C. (1960). *Amer. J. Physiol.* **199**, 265.
Harrison, H. E. and Harrison, H. C. (1961). *Amer. J. Physiol.* **201**, 1007.
Harrison, H. E. and Harrison, H. C. (1965). *Amer. J. Physiol.* **208**, 370.
Haussler, M. R., Wassermann, R. H., McCain, T. A., Perterlik, M., Bursac, K. M. and Hughes, M. R. (1976). *Life Sciences* **18**, 1049.
Heaney, R. P. and Whedon, G. D. (1958). *J. Clin. Endocrinol. Metab.* **18**, 1246.
Helbock, H. J., Forte, J. G. and Saltman, P. (1966). *Biochim. Biophys. Acta* **126**, 81.
Hibberd, K. A. and Norman, A. W. (1969). *Biochem. Pharmacol.* **18**, 2347.
Holdsworth, E. S. (1965). *Biochem. J.* **96**, 475.
Holdsworth, E. S. (1970). *J. Membr. Biol.* **3**, 43.
Hughes, M. R., Brumbaugh, P. F., Haussler, M. R., Wergedal, J. E. and Baylink, D. J. (1975). *Science* **190**, 578.
Humphreys, D. J. (1973). *Nature New Biology* (London) **246**, 156.
Hurwitz, S. and Barr, A. (1972). *Amer. J. Physiol.* **222**, 761.
Hurwitz, S., Harrison, H. C. and Harrison, H. E. (1967). *J. Nutr.* **91**, 319
Innes, J. R. M. and Nicolysen, R. (1937). *Biochem. J.* **31**, 101.
Irving, J. T. (1964). *In* 'Mineral Metabolism' (Ed. C. L. Comar and F. Bronner) Vol. 2A, p. 249. Academic Press, New York and London.
Ito, S. (1965). *J. Cell Biol.* **27**, 475.
Jones, M. R. (1927). *Amer. J. Physiol.* **79**, 694.
Katzenstein, I. P., Spielvogel, A. M. and Norman, A. W. (1974). *J. Antibiotics* **XXVII**, 943.
Kimberg, D. V., Schacter, D. and Scenker, H. (1961). *Amer. J. Physiol.* **200**, 1256.
Kimberg, D. V., Baerg, R. D., Gershon, E. and Graudusius, R. T. (1971). *J. Clin. Invest.* **50**, 1309.
Kinsky, S. C., Demel, R. A. and van Deenen, L. L. M. (1967). *Biochim. Biophys. Acta* **135**, 835.
Kowarski, S. and Schacter, D. (1969). *J. Biol. Chem.* **244**, 211.
Krawitt, E. L. (1972). *Biochim. Biophys. Acta* **274**, 179.
Krawitt, E. L. (1973). *Nature* (London) **243**, 88.
Krawitt, E. L. (1975). *Calc. Tiss. Res.* **18**, 119.
Krawitt, E. L. and Schedl, H. P. (1968). *Amer. J. Physiol.* **214**, 232.
Krawitt, E. L., Sampson, H. W., Kunin, A. S. and Matthews, J. L. (1974). *Calc. Tiss. Res.* **15**, 21.
Lawson, D. E. M., Wilson, P. W. and Smith, A. W. (1974). *Febs Letters* **45**, 122.
Lederer, C. M., Hollander, J. M. and Perlman, I. (1967). Table of Isotopes, sixth edition, John Wiley, New York.
Lindquist, E. (1952). *Acta Paediat., Stockh.* **41** (suppl. 86), 1.
Lipkin, M. and Bell, N. H. (1968). *In* 'Cell Proliferation' (Ed. C. F. Code) p. 2861. Washington, D.C.
Litwak, L. (1969). *Amer. J. Clin. Nutr.* **22**, 771.
Liu, S. H. and Chu, H. I. (1943). *Medicine* **22**, 103.
Lukert, B. P., Stanbury, S. W. and Mawer, E. B. (1973). *Endocrinol.* **93**, 718.
Manley, M. L. and Morgareidy, K. (1939). *J. Nutr.* **18**, 411.

Martin, D. L. and DeLuca, H. F. (1969a). *Arch. Biochem. Biophys.* **134**, 139.
Martin, D. L. and DeLuca, H. F. (1969b). *Amer. J. Physiol.* **216**, 1351.
Martin, D. L., Melancon, Jr., M. J. and DeLuca, H. F. (1969). *Biochem. Biophys. Res. Commun.* **35**, 819.
Mautalen, C. A. (1972). *Endocrinol.* **90**, 563.
McClendon, J. F. (1922). *Amer. J. Physiol.* **61**, 373.
Melancon, M. J. and DeLuca, H. F. (1970). *Biochemistry* **9**, 1658.
Migicovsky, B. B. and Emslie, A. R. G. (1947). *Arch. Biochem. Biophys.* **20**, 185.
Migicovsky, B. B. and Emslie, A. R. G. (1949). *Arch. Biochem. Biophys.* **13**, 325.
Miller, D. and Crane, R. K. (1961). *Anal. Biochem.* **2**, 284.
Morrisey, R. L. and Wasserman, R. H. (1971). *Amer. J. Physiol.* **220**, 1509.
Myrtle, J. F. and Norman, A. W. (1971). *Science* **171**, 79.
Nicolaysen, R. (1937a). *Biochem. J.* **31**, 107.
Nicolaysen, R. (1937b). *Biochem. J.* **31**, 122.
Nicolaysen, R. and Eeg-Larsen, N. (1953). *Vitam. and Horm.* **II**, 29.
Nicolaysen, R., Eeg-Larsen, N. and Malm, O. J. (1953). *Physiol. Rev.* **33**, 424.
Nordstrom, C., Dahlquist, A. and Josefsson, L. (1968). *J. Histochem. Cytochem.* **15**, 713.
Norman, A. W. (1965). *Science* **149**, 184.
Norman, A. W. (1966). *Amer. J. Physiol.* **211**, 829.
Norman, A. W. (1968). *Biol. Rev.* **43**, 97.
Norman, A. W. (1975). *Vitam. and Horm.* **32**, 325.
Norman, A. W. and Wong, R. G. (1972). *J. Nutr.* **102**, 1709.
Norman, A. W. and Henry, H. (1974). *Recent Progress in Horm. Res.* **30**, 431.
Norman, A. W., Bieber, L. L., Lindberg, D. and Boyer, P. D. (1965). *J. Biol. Chem.* **240**, 2855.
Norman, A. W., Haussler, M. R., Adams, T. H., Myrtle, J. F., Roberts, P. and Hibberd, K. A. (1969). *Amer. J. Clin. Nutr.* **22**, 396.
Norman, A. W., Mircheff, A. K., Adams, T. H. and Spielvogel, A. (1970). *Biochim. Biophys. Acta* **215**, 348.
Norman, A. W., Demel, R. A., DeKruyff, B., Geurts van Kessel, W. S. M. and van Deenen, L. L. M. (1972a). *Biochim. Biophys. Acta.* **290**, 1.
Norman, A. W., Demel, R. A., DeKruyff, B. and van Deenen, L. L. M. (1972b). *J. Biol. Chem.* **247**, 1918.
Norman, A. W., Spielvogel, A. M. and Wong, R. G. (1976). *In* 'Advances in Lipid Research' (Ed. D. Kritchevsky) Vol. 14, p. 127. Academic Press, New York and London.
O'Donnell, J. M. and Smith, M. W. (1973). *Nature* (London) **244**, 357.
Olson, E. B. and DeLuca, H. F. (1969). *Science* **165**, 405.
Olson, Jr. E. B., DeLuca, H. F. and Potts, Jr., J. T. (1972). *Endocrinol.* **90**, 151.
Omdahl, J. L. and DeLuca, H. F. (1972). *J. Biol. Chem.* **247**, 5520.
Padykula, H. A. (1962). *Fred. Proc.* **21**, 873.
Palade, G. E. (1958). *In* 'Frontiers in Cytology' (Ed. S. L. Palay) p. 283. Yale Univ. Press, New Haven, Conn.
Rasmussen, H. (1959). *Endocrinol.* **65**, 317.
Rasmussen, H. and DeLuca, H. F. (1963). *Ergebn. Physiol.* **53**, 108.
Reiss, E. and Canterbury, J. M. (1974). *Recent Prog. in Horm. Res.* **30**, 391.
Rich, C. and Ivanovich, P. (1964). *Northwest. Med.* **63**, 792.
Rosenberg, T. and Wilbrandt, W. (1957). *J. Gen. Physiol.* **41**, 289.
Rossi, C. S. and Lehninger, A. L. (1963). *Biochemische Zeit* **338**, 698.

Sallis, J. D. and Holdsworth, E. S. (1962). *Amer. J. Physiol.* **203**, 497.
Sansom, B. F, Jagg, M. J. and Dobereiner, J. (1971). *Res. Vet. Sci.* **12**, 604.
Schacter, D. and Rosen, S. M. (1959). *Amer. J. Physiol.* **196**, 357.
Schacter, D., Dowdle, E. B. and Schenker, H. (1960). *Amer. J. Physiol.* **198**, 263.
Scott, D. (1965). *Quart. J. Exp. Physiol.* **50**, 312.
Segre, V. and Potts, J. T. (1975). *In* 'Calcium Metabolism, Bone and Metabolic Bone Disease' (Ed. F. Kuhlencordt and H. P. Kruse) p. 285. Springer Verlag, Berlin and New York.
Shah, B. G. and Draper, H. H. (1966). *Amer. J. Physiol.* **211**, 963.
Shimotori, N. and Morgan, A. F. (1943). *J. Biol. Chem.* **147**, 201.
Spielvogel, A. M. (1973). Ph.D. Dissertation, University of California, Riverside.
Spielvogel, A. M. and Norman, A. W. (1975). *Arch. Biochem. Biophys.* **167**, 335.
Spielvogel, A. M., Farley, R. D. and Norman, A. W. (1972). *Exp. Cell Res.* **74**, 359.
Stanbury, S. W. and Lumb, G. A. (1962). *Medicine* **41**, 1.
Steenbock, H. and Herting, D. C. (1955). *J. Nutr.* **57**, 449.
Szymendra, J., Heaney, R. P. and Saville, P. (1972). *J. Lab. Clin. Med.* **79**, 570.
Tanzer, F. S. and Navia, J. M. (1973). *Nature New Biology* (London), **242**, 221.
Taylor, A. N. (1974). *J. Nutr.* **104**, 489.
Thomas, R. S. and Greenwalt, J. W. (1968). *J. Cell Biol.* **39**, 55.
Tsai, H. C., Midgett, R. J. and Norman, A. W. (1973). *Arch. Biochem. Biophys.* **157**, 339.
Uribe, A., Holick, M. F., Joregensen, N. A. and DeLuca, H. F. (1974). *Biochem. Biophys. Res. Comm.* **58**, 257.
Ussing, H. H. (1949). *Acta Physiol. Scand.* **19**, 43.
Van Zupthen, H., Demel, R. A., Norman, A. W. and van Deenen, L. L. M. (1971). *Biochim. Biophys. Acta.* **241**, 310.
Walling, M. W. and Kimberg, D. V. (1975). *Gastroenterol.* **69**, 200.
Walling, M. W. and Rothman, S. S. (1969) *Amer. J. Physiol.* **217**, 1144.
Walling, M. W., Kimberg, D. V., Lloyd, W., Wells, H., Procsal, D. A. and Norman, A. W. (1975). Proc. 2nd Vitamin D Workshop, p. 717. Walter de Gruyter.
Wasserman, R. H. (1963). *In* 'The Transfer of Calcium and Strontium Across Biological Membranes' (Ed. R. H. Wasserman) p. 211. Academic Press, New York and London.
Wasserman, R. H. (1974). *Science* **183**, 1092.
Wasserman, R. H. (1975). *Nutr. Revs.* **33**, 1.
Wasserman, R. H. and Comar, C. L. (1959). *Proc. Soc. Exp. Biol. Med.* **101**, 314.
Wasserman, R. H. and Taylor, A. (1969). *In* 'Mineral Metabolism' (Ed. C. L. Comar and F. Bronner) Vol. 3, p. 320. Academic Press, New York and London.
Wasserman, R. H. and Taylor, A. N. (1972). *Ann. Rev. Biochem.* **41**, 179.
Wasserman, R. H. and Taylor, A. N. (1973). *J. Nutr.* **103**, 586.
Wasserman, R. H., Comar, C. L. and Nold, M. M. (1956). *J. Nutr.* **59**, 371.
Wasserman, R. H., Kallfelz, F. A. and Comar, C. L. (1961). *Science* **133**, 883.
Wasserman, R. H., Taylor, A. N. and Kallfelz, F. A. (1966). *Amer. J. Physiol.* **211**, 419.
Wasserman, R. H., Corradino, R. A. and Taylor, A. (1968). *J. Biol. Chem.* **243**, 3978.
Webster, H. L. and Harrison, D. D. (1969). *Exptl. Cell Res.* **56**, 245.
Widdowson, E. M. and Dickerson, J. W. T. (1964). *In* 'Mineral Metabolism' (Ed. C. L. Comar and F. Bronner) Vol. 2A, p. 1. Academic Press, New York and London.
Wilson, T. H. (1962). 'Intestinal Absorption', Saunders, Philadelphia, Pa.
Wilson, T. H. and Wiseman, G. (1954). *J. Physiol.* **123**, 116.
Wong, R. G. (1972). Ph.D. Dissertation, University of California, Riverside.

Wong, R. G. and Norman, A. W. (1975). *J. Biol. Chem.* **250**, 2411.
Wong, R. G., Adams, T. H., Roberts, P. A. and Norman, A. W. (1970). *Biochim. Biophys. Acta* **219**, 61.
Worker, N. A. and Carrillo, B. J. (1967). *Nature* (London) **215**, 2411.
Zull, J. E., Czarnowska-Misztal, E. and DeLuca, H. F. (1965). *Science* **149**, 182.

4 The Vitamin D-Dependent Calcium-Binding Proteins

R. H. WASSERMAN, C. S. FULLMER
AND A. N. TAYLOR

I Introduction

Approximately 10 years ago, the first definitive evidence for the existence of a vitamin D-dependent calcium-binding protein appeared (Wasserman and Taylor, 1966). From equilibrium dialysis and competitive ion-exchange binding methods, it was shown that the administration of cholecalciferol to rachitic chicks caused an increase in the calcium-binding activity of crude extracts of intestinal mucosa. Further analysis clearly indicated that the calcium-binding activity was associated with a protein of molecular weight of about 28 000. Soon thereafter, a calcium-binding protein was shown to be present in the rat intestine that was responsive to cholecalciferol (Kallfelz *et al.*, 1967; Schachter, 1970), and this was followed by several investigations demonstrating the wide species distribution of the intestinal calcium-binding protein (CaBP).

Since its discovery, many experiments have been undertaken in order to determine if this unique protein plays a role in the calcium absorptive mechanism. Under several different nutritional and physiological conditions in which there was either a deficiency of calcium or an increased need for calcium, it was determined that the calcium-binding protein content of intestine varied in direct relation to the degree of calcium absorption (Wasserman and Corradino, 1973). This information suggested that the cholecalciferol-induced calcium-binding protein is significantly involved in the calcium-absorptive process. Simultaneously with the physiological investigations, several of these proteins have been isolated and partially characterised in terms of calcium-binding activity, amino acid composition and other properties, and the crystallisation of one such protein, the bovine CaBP, has been achieved. Also, in the interim, antisera was developed against a few of these proteins which provided a sensitive tool for their assay, a means of determining localisation, and for providing information on cross-reactivity of calcium-binding proteins from various species.

This review attempts to summarise present information on the intestinal calcium-binding protein and analogous proteins found in other tissues and organs. These proteins have, for the most part, a dependence on cholecalciferol for their synthesis. Previous reviews on this subject have appeared (Taylor and Wasserman, 1969; Wasserman and Corradino, 1973; Wasserman *et al.*, 1974a).

II Vitamin D-Dependency and Species Distribution of Calcium-Binding Protein

Considerable advances have been made towards uncovering the metabolism of vitamin D, and it is now established that the cholecalciferol molecule undergoes two significant hydroxylation reactions, the first is a liver-based 25-hydroxylation reaction and the second, a kidney-based 1α-hydroxylation reaction (Omdahl and DeLuca, 1973; Norman, 1974). The result of these transformations is the formation of the active or hormonal form of cholecalciferol, the 1α,25-dihydroxycholecalciferol. Other reactions are known to occur, such as the production of 24,25-dihydroxycholecalciferol and 25,26-dihydroxycholecalciferol, but the form most active in stimulating calcium transport is the 1,25-dihydroxycholecalciferol. Its formation is feed-back regulated (chapter 2 IIB).

Much attention has been given to the molecular action of calciferol and the available information for the chick indicates that cholecalciferol functions through the induction of the synthesis of a protein or proteins involved in calcium absorption. The evidence for *de novo* protein synthesis in the avian species has been previously reviewed (Wasserman and Corradino, 1973; Omdahl and DeLuca, 1973) and this evidence is summarised below: cytosol and nuclear receptors for 1,25-dihydroxycholecalciferol have been identified in chick intestinal cells (Brumbaugh and Haussler, 1973; Tsai and Norman, 1973; Lawson and Emtage, 1974); inhibitors of protein synthesis, such as actinomycin D and puromycin, inhibit the action of vitamin D (Norman, 1974; Lawson and Emtage, 1974); the studies of Emtage *et al.* (1974a, b) demonstrate that polysomes isolated from intestines of vitamin D-treated chicks are capable of synthesising calcium-binding protein whereas polysomes isolated from intestines of rachitic chicks did not have this capability; and the investigations of MacGregor *et al.* (1971) showing that the incorporation of C^{14}-labelled leucine into calcium-binding protein after cholecalciferol preceded an increase of calcium absorption. The organ culture studies from this laboratory demonstrated that, in embryonic chick intestine in organ culture, the addition of cholecalciferol or some of its metabolites to the culture

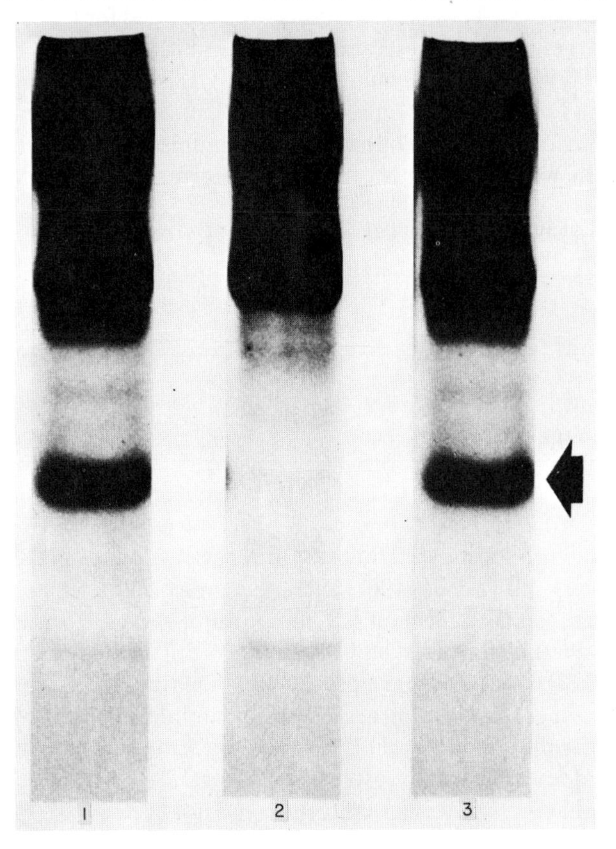

Fig. 1. Acrylamide discontinuous gel electrophoresis of calf intestinal mucosal supernatant solutions from: 1, normal calf; 2, rachitic calf; 3, rachitic calf administered cholecalciferol. Arrow denotes position of calcium-binding protein band. Electrophoresis toward the anode (bottom). See text for details

medium resulted in the synthesis of CaBP and enhanced ^{45}Ca uptake, processes that were sensitive to inhibitors of protein synthesis (Corradino and Wasserman, 1971a, b; Corradino, 1973a, b).

The calciferol-dependency of intestinal CaBPs in species other than the chick has been demonstrated by one method or another. Investigations with the calf indicated that, in this species, CaBP is either absent or present in very small amounts in vitamin D-deficient animals. In this study, calves were maintained on normal or rachitogenic diets (in the absence of sunlight) for about 4 months. Cholecalciferol (45 000 i.u.) was administered intramuscularly to one rachitic calf at 5 days and again at 4 days before killing. Duodena were removed from a normal, rachitic and cholecalciferol-dosed rachitic animal, scraped, homogenised, and the 30 000 × g supernatant solutions obtained. These supernatants were analysed for CaBP by analytical acrylamide gel electrophoresis and for calcium-binding activity by the Chelex-100 assay procedure (Wasserman *et al.*, 1968). It is evident from the results in Table 1 and Fig. 1 that very little, if any, CaBP remained in the rachitic animal under these conditions. Following the administration of cholecalciferol, CaBP levels were quickly restored to near normal levels.

Table 1. Calcium-binding activity of mucosal supernatant solutions from normal, rachitic and cholecalciferol-treated calves

	%S[a]	Total Protein (μg/ml)	CaPr/mg Protein[b]
Normal calf	63.5	10.27	0.16
Rachitic calf	21.9	10.01	0.02
Rachitic $+D_3$ calf	51.7	9.10	0.11

[a] %S is % ^{45}Ca retained in supernatant phase
[b] CaPr is ^{45}Ca bound to protein

The calciferol-dependency for the synthesis of a rat intestinal CaBP was first disclosed by Kallfelz *et al.* (1967) and later confirmed by others, including the extensive studies by Schachter (1970), Ooizumi *et al.* (1970), Harmeyer and DeLuca (1969), and Freund and Bronner (1975a). However, it was proposed that rat CaBP is derived from a pro-CaBP at the ribosomal or post-ribosomal level (Drescher and DeLuca, 1971a). The inhibition of the action of cholecalciferol by actinomycin D has been difficult to achieve consistently in the rat and an intestinal cytosol receptor for 1,25-dihydroxycholecalciferol similar to that present in chick epithelium has not been found (Reynolds *et al.*, 1975).

A species in which the calciferol-dependency of intestinal CaBP has not yet been demonstrated is the guinea pig (Chapman, 1974). Despite several months on a vitamin D-deficient diet (albeit adequate in calcium and phosphorus), intestinal CaBP was still evident in this species by the ion-exchange resin procedure and by examining acrylamide gel electrophoretic patterns. However, these guinea pigs also were *not* rachitic. The interpretation of these results is either: (*a*) residual stores of calciferol were adequate to prevent rickets and to maintain CaBP or (*b*) exogenous calciferol is not essential in this species to support adequate calcium absorption, bone formation and CaBP synthesis. Results of a recent study communicated to us by Dr Eric Lawson (Cambridge, England) also suggested the non-dependence of guinea pig CaBP on an exogenous source of vitamin D activity. In the Lawson experiment, serum 25-hydroxycholecalciferol levels were monitored and observed to fall to undetectable levels by a competitive binding assay. Yet, CaBP was still detectable. Studies of this apparent exception should prove significant in understanding the control of, and requirements for, the synthesis of CaBP.

A recent report attempts to emphasise the lack of correlation between CaBP and rickets in the pig (Harrison *et al.*, 1975). Duodenal CaBP (actually calcium-binding activity as determined by the ion-exchange resin method) was found to be somewhat lower but still detectable in pigs from vitamin D-deficient sows fed a vitamin D-deficient diet for 12 weeks. These animals, however, were normo-calcaemic and normo-phosphataemic, and showed no evidence of rickets. In another experiment, immature pigs were fed a vitamin D-deficient, calcium-deficient diet for 12 weeks. CaBP was somewhat higher than in the control group. Direct measurements of vitamin D content in liver indicated that the deficient group still had a residual vitamin D concentration of 1 μg/gm dry weight of tissue, which might be sufficient for CaBP formation. Rickets that did occur in these pigs was probably more related to the imposed deficiency of calcium and phosphorus than to a lack of vitamin D.

CaBP has been detected in species other than those mentioned above. Hurwitz *et al.* (1973) reported the presence of intestinal CaBP in turkeys; Wasserman and Taylor (1971), in the new-world monkey; Bar *et al.* (1976), in the Japanese quail; Fullmer and Wasserman (1975), in the horse and guinea pig; Hitchman and Harrison (1972), Alpers *et al.* (1972), Helmke *et al.* (1974), Menczel *et al.* (1971) and Morrissey *et al.* (1975) in man; and Taylor *et al.* (1968) in the dog.

With the availability of antisera specific to chick intestinal CaBP, it was a simple procedure to survey for the presence of immunologically reactive proteins, presumably CaBP, in other species. Intestinal extracts from some species known to contain CaBP by ion-exchange methodology did not cross react with anti-chick CaBP (rat, dog, cow, horse, pig, guinea pig, human). However, intestinal homogenates from a variety of species did react, indicating the presence of a protein(s) with determinant groups identical to chick CaBP. These included the duck, goose, Japanese quail, robin, frog, toad, turtle, bass and pike.

Thus, the absolute dependency of intestinal CaBP formation on calciferol or its metabolites has certainly been shown for several species, as documented above. However, an overall generalisation of the relationship of calciferol to CaBP formation is confounded by observations on the guinea pig and possibly the pig. These exceptions, after further detailed investigations, might either reveal an alternate non-calciferol-dependent mechanism of CaBP synthesis, or that some species can form cholecalciferol by non-photochemical means, or that sufficient calciferol was available to prevent rickets and support CaBP synthesis, despite the intake of an apparently vitamin D-deficient diet.

III Tissue Distribution of Calcium-Binding Protein

The intestine, considered to be the primary target organ of vitamin D, was the original tissue in which the vitamin D-induced CaBP was detected (Wasserman and Taylor, 1966). Subsequent studies documented its presence along the entire length of the small intestine (Taylor and Wasserman, 1970b).

The avian kidney also contains CaBP which increased in concentration after cholecalciferol administration to vitamin D-deficient chicks (Taylor and Wasserman, 1972), thus strengthening the contention that it too was a target organ of the vitamin, as had previously been proposed by others. Hermsdorf and Bronner (1975) have partially purified a calciferol-dependent calcium-binding protein from the kidney cortex of the rat. Its molecular weight was estimated to be 28 000, similar in molecular size to the chick intestinal protein but more than twice that in rat intestine. A kidney CaBP has also been reported in the dog (Sands and Kessler, 1971) and man (Piazolo *et al.*, 1971).

The shell gland (uterus) of the laying hen is an organ involved in the translocation of a considerable amount of calcium during egg-shell formation and was shown to contain a cholecalciferol-induced CaBP (Corradino *et al.*, 1968) providing the first direct evidence that this gland is responsive to the vitamin. Although some differences between the intestinal and uterine proteins of the chicken were previously claimed (Bar and Hurwitz, 1973), more recent investigations indicate that these are identical (Fullmer *et al.*, 1976).

When an immunohistochemical technique was applied to the pancreas by Morrissey *et al.* (1975), a positive reaction for CaBP in the cat, rat, mouse and chick was noted, the antisera employed were prepared against human kidney CaBP.

The mammary gland is another organ involved in the transfer of significant amounts of calcium. The presence of a calcium-binding protein in both rat and bovine mammary tissue has been reported (Bauman *et al.*, 1972). The concentration of the protein in mammary tissue was dependent on the lactational status of the animal, but no data was provided regarding its calciferol dependency.

The brain of the chick recently was shown to contain CaBP, which is apparently the same molecular species as that found in the intestine and kidney (Taylor, 1974a). The original report contained no evidence that the brain CaBP was dependent on cholecalciferol. However, more recent experiments have documented its responsiveness to the vitamin (Taylor, 1974b).

An extremely sensitive radioimmunoassay for pig CaBP has been developed by Murray *et al.* (1974) and used to obtain important information on the presence of CaBP in various tissues. With this assay, CaBP was readily detectable in duodenum and kidney but, in addition, there were significant concentrations in thyroid gland, liver, pancreas and blood (Murray *et al.*, 1975) (Table 2). The presence of CaBP in blood has important nutritional and physiological implications because changes in duodenal CaBP levels due to dietary manipulations were directly reflected by blood CaBP levels (Murray *et al.*, 1975). Specifically, it was shown that a low calcium diet fed to pigs increased intestinal CaBP by a factor of 2.0 and blood CaBP increased by a factor of 2.6. If this relationship holds in other situations and in other species,

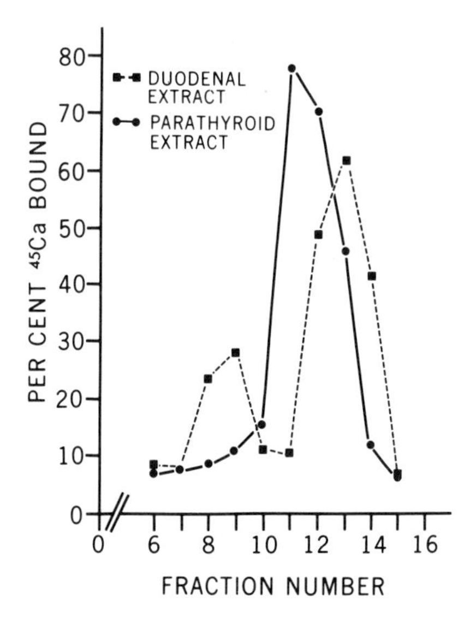

Fig. 2. Calcium-binding activity as measured by a competitive resin binding test, in fractions eluted from Sephadex G-50 chromatography of pig parathyroid and duodenal extracts. The calcium-binding activity of the parathyroid extract is eluted as a larger molecule than the major calcium-binding peak from a duodenal extract run later on the same column. (From Murray *et al.*, 1974)

a powerful tool will become available for readily assessing the vitamin D and calcium status of animals under various disease and nutritionally abnormal conditions.

The parathyroid gland of the pig also contains a calcium-binding protein, as first reported by Oldham *et al.* (1974). Studies by Murray *et al.* (1975) confirmed the presence of a calcium-binding entity in pig parathyroid glands but this was distinct from intestinal CaBP. As can be noted in Fig. 2, the molecular sizes of pig parathyroid CaBP and intestinal CaBP, as determined by gel filtration, were significantly different. Calcium-binding proteins have not been detected in chick or bovine parathyroid glands, using gel filtration procedures in conjunction with the ion exchange binding assay (Fullmer, Cohn and Wasserman, unpublished data).

Table 2. Radioimmunoassay of intestinal CaBP in various tissues and organs of the pig[a]

Tissue or organ	CaBP concentration (ng/g tissue, wet wt)
Duodenum	400 000–2 000 000
Kidney	2000–11 000
Thyroid	610–4300
Liver	400–1100
Pancreas	120–160
Plasma	30–80[b]

[a] From Murray *et al.*, 1975
[b] Plasma CaBP expressed as ng/ml

IV Cellular Localisation of Calcium-Binding Protein

Using the fluorescent antibody procedure, it was possible to localise CaBP at two distinct locations in chick intestine (Taylor and Wasserman, 1970a). The protein was present in the goblet cells and also associated with the absorptive surface of all of the intestinal epithelial cells. The exact site of CaBP location at the absorptive surface, i.e. the microvilli or the mucopolysaccharide surface coat material, could not be resolved because of the thickness of the histological sections and the resolution of the light microscope. Since the absorptive surface represents the first point of contact for the absorption of dietary calcium and a cellular site shown to be sensitive to vitamin D (Wasserman and Taylor, 1969), it was speculated that CaBP at this location represented the 'functional CaBP'. The significance of the goblet cell CaBP has not been established, but it is conceivable that the goblet cell represents a site of synthesis of the protein from which CaBP is subsequently extruded to become associated with the absorptive surface.

Immunohistochemical localisation of CaBP in human intestine has been studied by two groups (Helmke *et al.*, 1974; Morrissey *et al.*, 1975). Both studies utilised antisera prepared against CaBP isolated from human kidney. Fluorescence, claimed to be due specifically to CaBP, was observed at the absorptive surface and also in the basal region of epithelial cells in suction biopsy samples obtained from the duodenal region of persons 30–60 years of age (Helmke *et al.*, 1974). In addition, they noted that 25-hydroxycholecalciferol administration to rachitic children restored the normal pattern of fluorescence seen in healthy persons. A non-specific fluorescence was noted in the goblet cells. On the other hand, Morrissey *et al.* (1975), using perioxidase conjugated antisera, reported the presence of CaBP in the intercellular spaces of human jejunum. It appeared to be associated with the lateral and basal membranes with none or little at the absorptive surface.

The most recent studies have extended the number of species examined and provided the first ultrastructural localisation. CaBP was localised in pig intestine, employing anti-pig intestinal CaBP antiserum, in the cytoplasm of the absorptive cells and inconsistently at the absorptive surface, but not in goblet cells (Arnold *et al.*, 1976). A similar distribution pattern was observed in chick intestine in response to 1,25-dihydroxycholecalciferol (Morrissey *et al.*, 1978). They also noted CaBP in the cytoplasm of absorptive cells and in some nuclei, but not in globlet cells. The only published ultrastructural investigation supported the goblet cell site of CaBP (Taylor and McIntosh, 1977). Specific immuno-markers were seen in mucin granules in goblet cell theca and in underlying condensing vacuoles arising from the Golgi complex. No consistent localisation was observed at the microvillar border in the ultrastructural study.

It is obvious from this discussion that a unified concept does not exist for the immunological localisation of intestinal CaBP. Unfortunately, a complete understanding of CaBP's role in intestinal calcium transport depends, in part, on reliable knowledge of the true *in situ* site(s) of the protein.

Using the same immunohistological technique, Morrissey *et al.* (1975) reported the presence of CaBP in the kidney of the monkey, dog, cat, mouse, the chick and man, again using antisera prepared against CaBP isolated from human kidney. CaBP was associated with intracellular membranes or the cytosol of cells in both proximal and distal convoluted tubules, straight segments and in thin loops deep in the papilla, but not in cells of the glomerulus. In this laboratory, Lippiello (1974) observed CaBP to be predominantly associated with the distal tubular cells in bovine and chick kidney, using species-specific antisera.

CaBP has also been localised in the tubular gland cells of the shell gland (uterus) of the laying hen by the fluorescent antibody procedure, utilising antisera against chick intestinal CaBP (Lippiello and Wasserman, 1975). The gland cell localisation added support to the contention that they are the cells involved in calcium secretion during egg shell formation.

The pancreatic islets of cat, dog, rat, mouse and chick yielded a positive antibody reaction, indicating the presence of CaBP (Morrissey *et al.*, 1975). The distribution of the peroxidase reaction product suggested that CaBP was located intracellularly in the beta cells. The beta cell localisation is the same as that reported for the calcium ion by two different techniques and indicates that CaBP may be involved in the calcium fluxes in conjunction with insulin release.

V Quantitative Relationship between Calcium-Binding Protein and Cholecalciferol

The administration of varying amounts of cholecalciferol to the rachitic chick induced the formation of intestinal CaBP in direct correspondence to the amount of the vitamin given (Fig. 3). This has constituted the basis of a bioassay for cholecalciferol, using CaBP as the end point of that assay (Bar

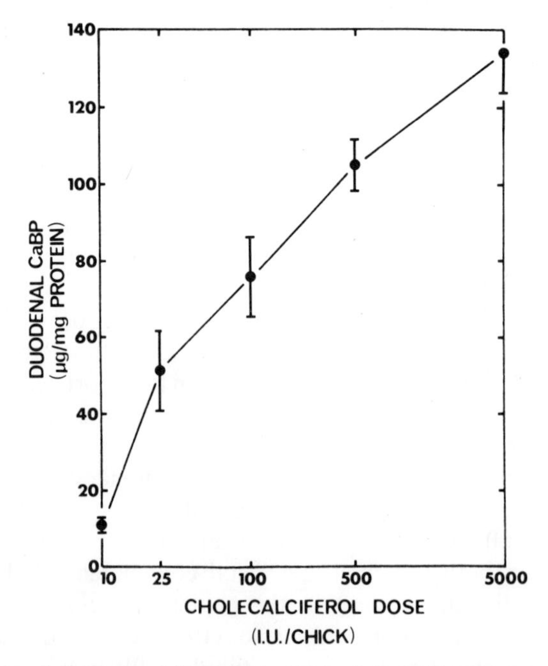

Fig. 3. Duodenal CaBP level in rachitic chicks injected intramuscularly with 10 to 5000 i.u. cholecalciferol/chick, 48 h prior to killing. Each value represents the mean ±SEM of six chicks

and Wasserman, 1974). The advantage of the CaBP-based assay is its sensitivity, specificity and reproducibility, and was used to determine the cholecalciferol content of commercial sources of the vitamin, such as cod-liver oil and a multiple vitamin preparation. The agreement between the stated concentration of vitamin D in these preparations by the manufacturer and that determined by the new vitamin D bio-assay was excellent. As an illustration (Table 3), cholecalciferol in cod liver oil was stated to contain 85 i.u. cholecalciferol per gm by the commercial distributor and the value from the bioassay was 84±9 i.u. cholecalciferol per gm. Subsequently, this assay has been employed to determine the cholecalciferol equivalency of two calcinogenic plants, *Solanum malacoxylon* (Wasserman *et al.*, 1974a) and *Cestrum diurnum* (Wasserman *et al.*, 1975).

Table 3. Bioassay of cholecalciferol equivalent in two commercial sources of the vitamin[a]

Source	Dose based on manufacturer's specifications	CaBP[b]	Estimated dose from CaBP-based assay
	i.u. cholecalciferol equivalent/chick	μg/mg protein	i.u. cholecalciferol-equivalent/chick
Cod-liver oil[c]	19.1	15.8±2.0	18.9
	38.2	20.1±2.3	32.0
Multiple vitamin drops[d]	40	22.6±0.8	42.9
	100	30.3±1.6	110.0

[a] Cholecalciferol equivalent source and standards given orally to 4-week-old vitamin D-depleted chicks 48 h before killing

[b] Mean±SEM of 5 chicks

[c] General Biochemicals, Chagrin Falls, Ohio; 85 i.u. cholecalciferol-equivalent per gram

[d] Pet Drops, Upjohn Co., Kalamazoo, Mich.; 1666 i.u. cholecalciferol-equivalent per gram

Bronner and Freund (1975) examined the relationship between intestinal CaBP synthesis and cholecalciferol administration to the vitamin D-deficient rat, and a similar direct correlation was also noted in this species. This has particular significance for the assay of different sources of calciferol, because the rat responds about equally to ergo- and cholecalciferol, whereas the chick has a relatively high specificity for the cholecalciferol form.

VI Calcium-Binding Protein during Embryonic Development

The appearance of CaBP in various tissues during embryonic development has been reported in the chick. The protein was detectable in the kidney tissue at day 10 and persisted therein through the hatching stage (Taylor and Wasserman, 1972). Initially most of the CaBP was associated with the intermediate kidney, the mesonephros, which regresses in size and function at about day 16. From day 10 to day 14, CaBP content of the definitive kidney, the metanephros, initially increased dramatically and then remained at nearly the same concentration through the hatching period. Despite the early appearance of kidney CaBP, intestinal calcium-binding protein in the chick embryo is not detectable until the day of hatch (day 21) at which time there is a rapid synthesis of the protein (Corradino *et al.*, 1969).

The reason for the inability of embryonic intestine to synthesise detectable quantities of CaBP is not known since the avian egg does contain choleciferol, and Moriuchi and DeLuca (1974) have indicated that conversion of the vitamin to 1,25-dihydroxycholecalciferol is apparent by day 18. Evidence was also given by Oku *et al.* (1975) that the 1,25-dihydroxycholecalciferol cytosol receptor can be detected in embryonic intestinal tissue by day 17. Further the direct injection of the hormone into the egg at 18 days of incubation can induce the synthesis of duodenal CaBP (Corradino and Wasserman, 1974). The above information suggests that the embryonic intestine contains the complete potential for synthesising CaBP but, for some reason, inadequate levels of the hormone are available to stimulate synthesis at this site. This contention is also borne out by the observation that, in organ culture, embryonic chick duodenum responded to 1,25-dihydroxycholecalciferol (also cholecalciferol and its 25-hydroxymetabolite) by an increase in ^{45}Ca uptake and the formation of CaBP by the tissue (Corradino, 1973a). The synthesis of CaBP in embryonic organ culture is inhibited by actinomycin D and α-amanitin (Corradino, 1973b) and, as detailed later, a relationship between the adenylate cyclase system, cholecalciferol, CaBP and calcium absorption was also proposed on the basis of observations made with this system (Corradino, 1974).

VII Purification Procedures for Calcium-Binding Proteins

The purification procedure originally developed for chick intestinal CaBP (Wasserman *et al.*, 1968) has, with modification, been successfully employed for the isolation of calcium-binding proteins from the cow, horse, guinea pig, pig (Fullmer and Wasserman, 1975), human intestine (Alpers *et al.*, 1972) and hen uterus (Fullmer *et al.*, 1976). The isolation procedure, in general, involves the preparation of an aqueous supernatant solution from a homogenate of mucosal tissue as the starting material. This is sequentially subjected to: (*a*) ammonium sulphate fractionation, (*b*) gel filtration column chromatography and (*c*) preparative discontinuous acrylamide gel electrophoresis. On occasion, due to the heat stability of calcium-binding proteins (Bredderman and Wasserman, 1974), heat treatment at 60°–70°C replaced the ammonium sulphate step in order to precipitate a significant amount of inactive protein.

Recently, a useful technique has been introduced by Hitchman and co-workers (1973), which takes advantage of an intrinsic charge difference in porcine CaBP with or without bound Ca^{2+}. Porcine mucosal supernatant solution, partially purified by heat treatment and gel filtration, is subjected to chromatography on DEAE-Sephadex at pH 7.0 in the presence of 1.0 mM Na_2EDTA and eluted with a linear NaCl gradient. Under these conditions, CaBP is eluted at a NaCl concentration slightly greater than 0.1 M. The CaBP-containing fractions are then concentrated, rinsed, and applied to a second DEAE-Sephadex column and eluted with buffer containing 1.0 mM $CaCl_2$ in place of the EDTA previously used. In this case, CaBP is not retained by the column matrix and appears in the void volume.

In this laboratory, we have been employing a technique similar to that of Hitchman *et al.* (*loc. cit.*) which provides quantities of highly purified mammalian CaBP with a minimum of time and sample manipulation. Bovine mucosal supernatant solutions are prepared in Tris buffer (pH 8.0) containing 50 mM NaCl and are subjected to continuous hollow fibre dialysis, using a

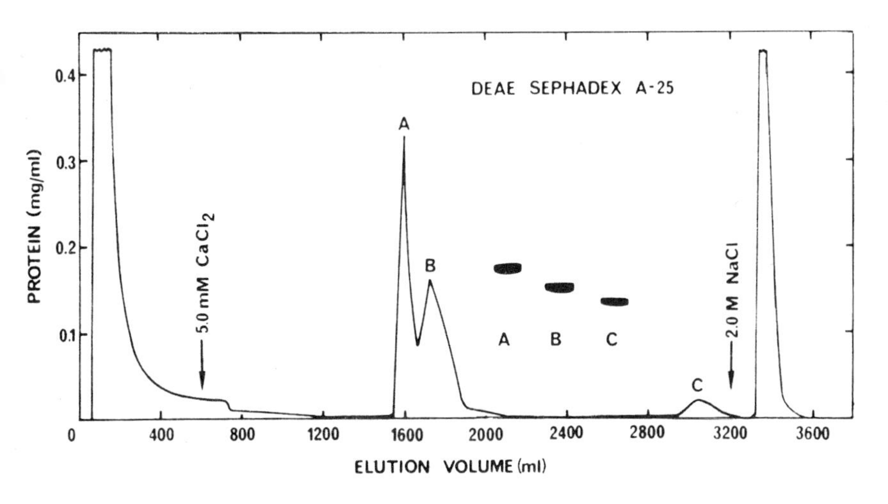

Fig. 4. The protein elution profile of bovine intestinal calcium-binding protein from DEAE Sephadex A-25 eluted with 5 mM $CaCl_2$. The protein peaks and acrylamide gels correspond to the three forms of bovine calcium-binding protein: A, Major form; B, Minor form, and C, Minor B form. Calcium-binding protein could not be detected immunologically in either the void volume peak or after stripping the column with 2 M NaCl. See text for details

HIDx-50 cartridge (Amicon Corp.). Bovine CaBP readily passes into the ultrafiltrate which is subsequently concentrated by ultrafiltration through a UM-2 membrane (Amicon Corp.). This concentrated preparation is applied to a 2.5 cm × 35 cm column of DEAE-Sephadex A-25 and eluted with aqueous buffer until protein is no longer detectable in the eluate. Elution is then begun with Tris buffer, containing 5.0 mM $CaCl_2$ and no NaCl. This buffer not only saturates the calcium-binding sites on the molecule and decreases the affinity of CaBP for the charged groups on the matrix, but precludes the further elution of slowly moving proteins by virtue of the reduced ionic strength. As shown in Fig. 4, CaBP is selectively released under these conditions. This method has been useful for the rapid and large scale purification of intestinal calcium-binding proteins from the cow, horse, pig and guinea pig.

VIII Characteristics of Calcium-Binding Protein from Various Species

The first vitamin D-dependent intestinal calcium-binding protein discovered and that most extensively studied has been that from the chick (Wasserman *et al.*, 1968). This CaBP has a molecular weight of about 28 000 Daltons, as estimated by gel filtration (Wasserman *et al.*, 1968; Fullmer and Wasserman, 1975), SDS acrylamide electrophoresis, and amino acid composition (Bredderman and Wasserman, 1974). Total amino acid analysis indicates a high content of dicarboxylic amino acids ($\sim 30\%$) as well as leucine and lysine (Bredderman and Wasserman, 1974; Fullmer and Wasserman, 1975) (Table 4). As expected from its high degree of water solubility, chick CaBP also shows a high content of polar residues. On the basis of amino acid composition, the protein has a calculated partial specific volume of 0.734 g/cm^3 and average charge per residue of 0.384. The isoelectric point has been calculated to be 4.2 and 1.0%, 1 cm extinction coefficient at 280 nm is 9.03 (Bredderman and Wasserman, 1974).

Detailed binding analyses of chick CaBP by equilibrium dialysis procedures and Scatchard plot methodology (Bredderman and Wasserman, 1974) have revealed the presence of 4 high-affinity calcium-binding sites with average affinity constants (K_a) for calcium of about 2×10^6 M^{-1}. As expected on the basis of the numerous side-chain carboxyl groups, about 32 low-affinity binding sites ($k_a \sim 10^2$ M^{-1}) were found. The pH-dependency of the binding reaction shows a slightly bi-phasic pH optimum for calcium-binding (at pH ~ 6.3, ~ 9.2) and the experimentally determined isoelectric point is pH 4.2–4.3 (Ingersoll and Wasserman, 1971), the latter agreeing with that calculated from the amino acid composition.

Table 4. Amino acid compositions of some calcium-binding proteins

Amino acid	Bovine	Equine	Porcine	Guinea pig	Chick	Hen uterus
Lysine	13	14	10–11	11–12	22–23	23
Histidine	0	0	0	0	4	4
Arginine	0	0	1	0	5–6	6
Aspartic acid	7	8–9	7–8	8	31–32	29
Threonine	2	0	1	2	9	9
Serine	8	7	6–7	7	10	9
Glutamic acid	18	15–16	17	16	39	36
Proline	5	3	4	4	3	3
Glycine	6	4–5	4–5	3–4	13–14	13
Alanine	3	3	5	2–3	17	16–17
Half-cystine	0	0	0	0	2	ND
Valine	3	4	3	4	5	5
Methionine	0	0	0	0	7	6
Isoleucine	2	4	3	2	11	11
Leucine	14	11	10	10	29	27–28
Tyrosine	1	1	1	1	8	6
Phenylalanine	5	4	5	6	13–14	13
Tryptophan	0	0	0	0	2	ND
Approx. MW	9700	9100	8800	8900	27 000	27 000

Chick intestinal CaBP binds alkaline earth cations in the selectivity series, $Ca^{2+} > Sr^{2+} > Ba^{2+} > Mg^{2+}$. In addition to these, a number of other divalent cations bind to the protein as judged by their effectiveness to displace ^{45}Ca from the protein in a competitive binding situation (Ingersoll and Wasserman, 1971). Recent experiments have shown that chick CaBP also complexes La^{3+} and Nd^{3+} with high affinity (Wasserman *et al.*, 1974b). The calcium-binding reaction is inhibited by high concentrations of urea (Ingersoll and Wasserman, 1971) and by lysolecithin (Wasserman 1970); the binding capacity of the protein in these situations can be restored by removal of urea by dialysis in the first case or by sequestering lysolecithin with taurocholate in the second.

Circular dichroism measurements of the chick CaBP showed 30–40% α-helicity, a value not significantly altered by the presence or absence of Ca^{2+} (Ingersoll and Wasserman, 1971). Sulfhydryl groups are apparently not involved in the binding reaction since *N*-ethyl malemide, iodoacetate and β-chloromercuribenzoate were not inhibitory (Ingersoll and Wasserman, 1971).

The protein also displays a high thermal stability since the immunological, electrophoretic and calcium-binding characteristic were not altered by heat treatment up to 80°C (Bredderman and Wasserman, 1974).

The CaBP found in chick kidney and uterus (shell gland) appear to be identical to that present in intestinal mucosa, as assessed by electrophoretic mobility on acrylamide gels, by cross-reactivity with antiserum prepared against intestinal CaBP, and molecular size (Fullmer *et al.*, 1976; Lippiello and Wasserman, 1975; Corradino *et al.*, 1968). The amino acid composition of the uterus and intestinal protein are essentially identical (Table 4).

The intestinal calcium-binding proteins from the rat, pig and human have been examined by Hitchman and Harrison (1972) and were estimated to be somewhat smaller than 13 000 Daltons. A value has been reported for the molecular weight for the rat intestinal CaBP of 13 000 and 8300 as measured by gel filtration and by sedimentation ultracentrifugation measurements, respectively, implying that the protein is ellipsoidal in shape (Drescher and DeLuca, 1971a).

There is now convincing evidence for the existence of two calciferol-dependent calcium-binding proteins of different molecular weight in rat intestine (Moriuchi *et al.*, 1975). The starting material was heat-treated (60°C, 5 min) supernatants of mucosal homogenates from the duodenum, jejunum and ileum. Separation of proteins by molecular size was carried out by gel filtration chromatography and two different procedures were used for measuring calcium-binding activity of the various fractions. One procedure was a modification of the competitive ion-exchange technique in which resin and binding protein compete for added ^{45}Ca. The other was the use of ^{45}Ca equilibrated columns and determining the enhancement of ^{45}Ca levels in specific fractions above basal levels. Two calciferol-responsive binding peaks could be identified, one of apparent molecular weight of 12 500 and the second with an apparent molecular weight of 27 000. An interesting feature of this important study was, first, that the 27 000 molecular weight protein bound ^{45}Ca on the equilibrated column but showed little binding activity when assayed by the ion-exchange method. The 12 000 molecular weight protein bound ^{45}Ca when assayed by either procedure. Another interesting feature was that the smaller CaBP predominated in the duodenum whereas it occurred in lower concentration in jejunum, and was virtually absent in the ileum. The larger CaBP was present in both ileum and jejunum, and virtually absent from the duodenum. Previous reports, except that from this group (Ooizumi *et al.*, 1970), gave a molecular weight of rat intestinal protein of about 12 000–13 000 (Schachter, 1970; Drescher and DeLuca, 1971b; Hitchman and Harrison, 1972). The newly uncovered rat CaBP of 27 000 molecular weight was apparently not detected by the other groups because of the insensitivity of the usual assay for calcium-binding activity as applied to this protein. These results of Moriuchi *et al.* (1975) were construed to suggest that these two CaBPs serve different functions in the calcium absorptive mechanism. Because of specificity of location, it was suggested that the small CaBP was involved in active transport (duodenal location) and the larger CaBP was involved in passive diffusion (jejunal and ileal location).

A somewhat similar pattern emerged in discerning the intestinal site of location of bovine CaBP, as shown in Fig. 5. Bovine CaBP (MW 11 000) was found primarily in the proximal part of the small intestine and not present in the lower ileum, whereas binding activity was present throughout the intestine. Although not investigated in detail as yet, the binding activity in the distal intestine could be due to another binding protein not immunoreactive with antisera prepared against the 11 000 MW bovine CaBP.

Two intestinal CaBPs have been identified by Alpers and coworkers (1972) in the human duodenum which were of similar size of 20 000–25 000 molecular weight and were reported to contain no phosphate or carbohydrate groups. In contrast Piazolo *et al.* (1971) reported that the binding proteins in human duodenum and kidney were estimated to be somewhat larger than 21 500 molecular weight. Others have claimed the isolation of human kidney CaBP in purified form, which exhibited a molecular size of 27 000 molecular weight in agreement with the value of 28 000 obtained in this laboratory (Morrissey and Rath, 1974).

We have recently completed a comparative evaluation of some of the properties of intestinal CaBPs from several species, including the cow, horse, pig, guinea pig and chick (Fullmer and Wasserman, 1975). CaBPs from these five species were isolated and characterised by identical procedures. Amino acid compositional analyses (Table 4) established the similarity of the mammalian proteins which all possessed one tyrosine residue and were devoid of histidine, cystine, methionine, tryptophan and, with the exception of the porcine CaBP, arginine. The calculated minimum molecular weights for the mammalian CaBPs on the basis of amino acid analyses were about 9000, and the analogous chick protein, about 27 000. Molecular size estimates by gel filtration were 11 000 for the mammalian proteins and 28 000 for the chick CaBP.

The properties of the porcine intestinal calcium-binding protein have been investigated in detail by Dorrington and coworkers (1974) who found that the amino acid composition of their protein preparation was almost identical to that of our preparation as shown in Table 4, and to possess a minimum molecular weight of 9000 as estimated from its composition. No phosphate, glucosamine or galactosamine were detected.

It was also reported by Dorrington *et al.* (1974) that removal of bound calcium from the molecule markedly decreased the circular dichroism spectrum in the tyrosine band at 276 nm. The ultraviolet absorbance of the

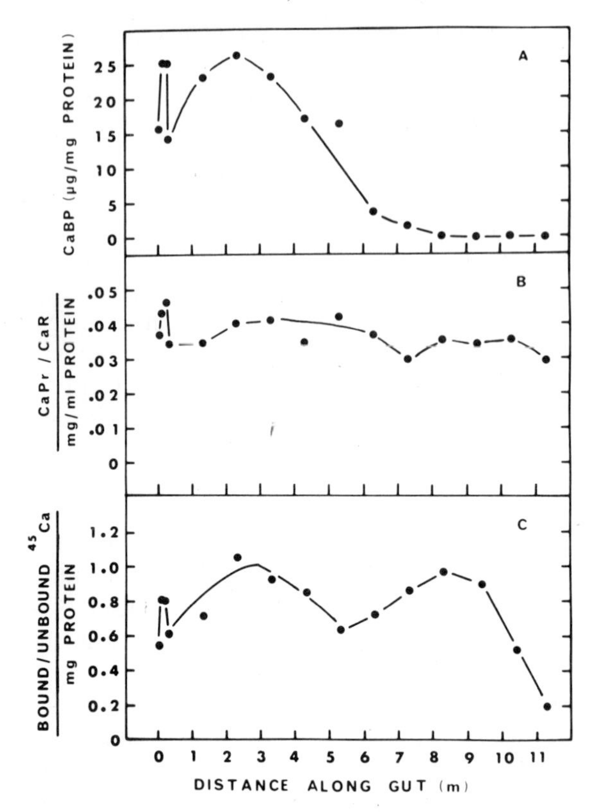

Fig. 5. Bovine calcium-binding protein and calcium-binding activity of intestinal mucosal supernates from various segments of calf intestine. Calcium-binding protein A detected by electroimmunoassay; calcium-binding activity by Chelex-100 assay B; and calcium-binding by equilibrium dialysis procedures C. CaPr/CaR is the ratio of Ca bound to protein vs Ca-bound to the Chelex-100 resin

tyrosyl residue was also altered in the presence of calcium. This perturbance of the spectrum of the tyrosyl residue suggests this residue to be close to a calcium binding site, if not actually constituting one of the ligands.

During the isolation of bovine intestinal calcium-binding protein, the molecule undergoes alterations resulting in the appearance of multiple forms which are easily distinguished from one another by acrylamide gel electrophoresis (see Fig. 6). These forms, originally designated as the Major, Minor A and Minor B components, in order of increasing anodal electrophoretic migration rates, differ only slightly or not at all in amino acid composition, molecular size, calcium-binding activity and immunological reactivity (Fullmer and Wasserman, 1973).

The bovine CaBP Major component has been shown to be the native protein molecule and is converted, during prolonged storage at 4°C, to a mixture of the Minor A and Minor B components. These alterations are apparently irreversible and the products so formed are not susceptible to further change under similar conditions (Fullmer and Wasserman, 1973). The existence of multiple forms is not unique to the bovine CaBP, and similar occurrences have been noted for the CaBPs in the porcine (Hitchman and Harrison, 1972), canine (Alpers *et al.*, 1972) and other species (Fullmer and Wasserman, unpublished observations).

Along another avenue of investigation, it was reported (Fullmer and Wasserman, 1973) that the calcium-binding activity of partially-purified preparations of bovine CaBP was rapidly eliminated following incubation with pronase, but was completely resistant to tryptic digestion. Detailed studies (Fullmer *et al.*, 1975) carried out in conjunction with peptide mapping experiments established that resistance to tryptic hydrolysis was a function of

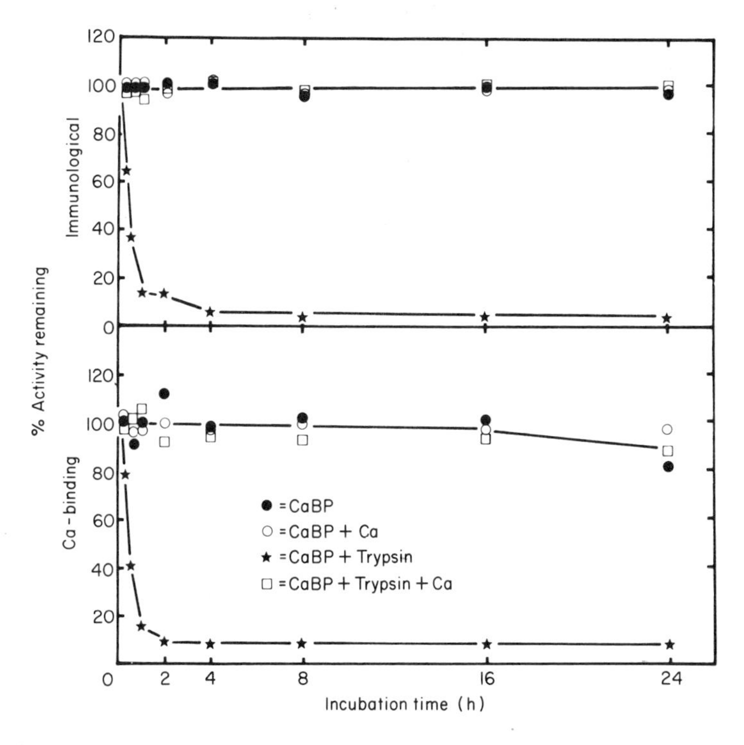

Fig. 6. The effect of 1 mM added calcium on the tryptic degradation of bovine intestinal calcium-binding protein. Immunological and calcium-binding activity expressed as % activity remaining relative to zero time control value. (Taken from Fullmer *et al.*, 1975)

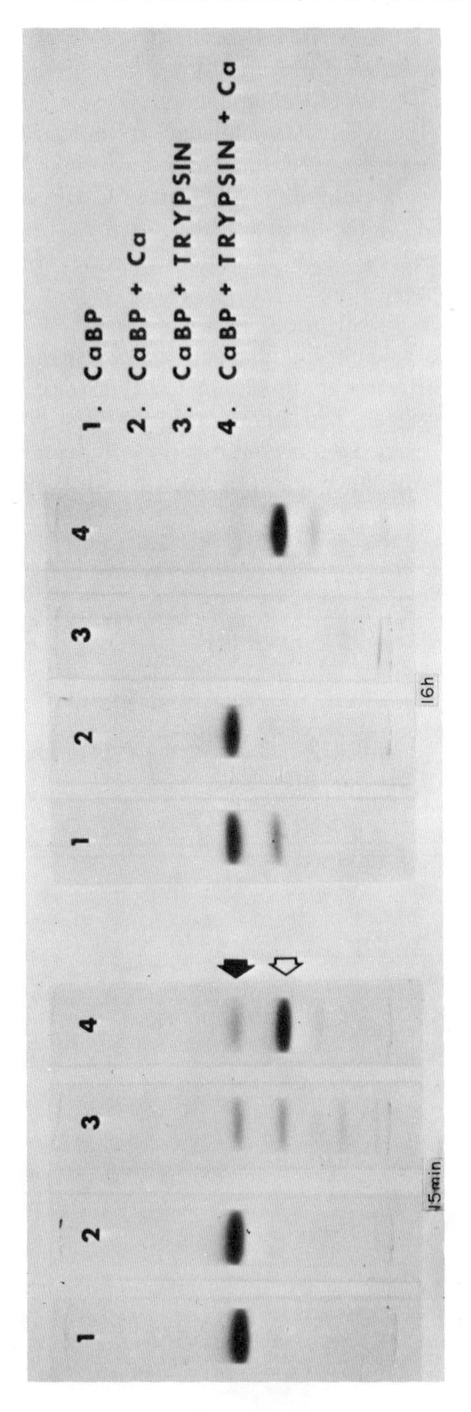

Fig. 7. Results of analytical disc gel electrophoresis performed on samples from the tryptic digestion of bovine calcium-binding protein in the presence and absence of 1 mM added $CaCl_2$ at 38°C for 15 min and 16 h. Open and closed arrows indicate positions of bands identified tentatively as major and minor A components, respectively. Electrophoresis was toward the anode (bottom)

protein-bound calcium. Native bovine CaBP, free of bound calcium, was incubated in the presence and absence of trypsin and 1 mM $CaCl_2$ at 37°C (pH 8.1). At various times, samples were removed and analysed for calcium-binding activity, immunological reactivity and electrophoretic properties. The results (Figs 6 and 7) showed that the native CaBP, incubated with trypsin but without calcium, was rapidly hydrolysed to the constituent peptides with concomitant loss of calcium-binding activity, immunological reactivity and protein-staining bands on acrylamide gels. Samples incubated in an identical fashion with the addition of 1 mM $CaCl_2$ retained complete activity, but exhibited altered electrophoretic properties. Over the time course of the experiment, the protein-staining band corresponding to the native CaBP (Major component) disappeared and was replaced by new bands corresponding in position to the Minor A and (to a lesser extent) the Minor B components.

Bovine CaBP binds cations other than Ca^{2+} with varying affinities. As shown in Fig. 8, a relationship between ionic radius and capacity of a particular cation to displace tracer ^{45}Ca from the protein is evident and yields

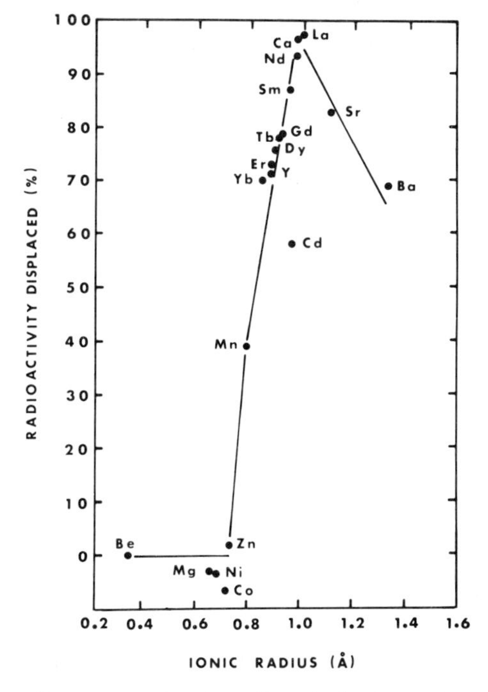

Fig. 8. The relative effectiveness of various di- and trivalent cations in displacing ^{45}Ca from bovine intestinal calcium-binding protein by equilibrium dialysis techniques. In all cases, 1×10^{-5} M $CaCl_2$ and 1×10^{-3} M of the indicated cations (as chloride salts) were present

a pattern similar to that obtained with chick CaBP (Bredderman and Wasserman, 1974). This suggests that those cations with ionic radii close to that of Ca^{2+} bind avidly and this undoubtedly bears on the effective dimensions of the 'cavity' of the binding site.

IX Amino Acid Sequence of Bovine Calcium-Binding Protein

Amino acid sequence studies (Fullmer and Wasserman, 1978) have been undertaken in an effort to establish the chemical differences existing among the various bovine CaBP components. End group determinations by the dansyl chloride procedure (Gray, 1972) have established that the NH_2-terminus of the native protein is blocked, while the Minor A and Minor B components show the presence of bis-DNS-lysine and DNS-serine, respectively. In addition, the three components have been subjected to direct automated Edman degradation in a Beckman Model 890C sequencer, using the DMAA (*N*,*N*-dimethyl-*N*-allylamine)-peptide program. Residues from each cycle were determined as the PTH (phenylthiohydantoin) derivatives by gas-liquid chromatography and thin layer chromatography on polyamide layers. All residues were also identified by amino acid analysis, following back hydrolysis in 6 N HCl at 120°C for 24 hours. No sequence was obtained for the native bovine CaBP (Major component), confirming the existence of an NH_2-terminal blocking group. The Minor A and Minor B components, on the other hand, produced unambiguous sequences for at least 30 cycles. These sequences differed from each other only by the absence of the NH_2-terminal lysine in the Minor B component (Fig. 9).

The absence of tryptophan and histidine and the presence of a single tyrosine in the bovine CaBPs permitted use of the highly specific *N*-bromosuccinimide (NBS) oxidation as a means of peptide cleavage at the tyrosine residue (Ramachandran and Witkop, 1967). NBS oxidation allowed for circumvention of the blocking group in the native protein, as well as extended sequence determination of the Minor A and Minor B components. The three components were incubated in 50% acetic acid containing a 10-fold molar excess of NBS at room temperature for 16 hours, and the cleavage mixtures separated on a column of Sephadex G-50 medium (1.5 cm × 85 cm) equilibrated with 5% acetic acid. Column fractions were analysed for ultraviolet absorbance (279 nm) and fluorescence after reaction with Fluram (Hoffmann-LaRoche, Inc.). Two peptides, one large and one small, were easily separated by this procedure for each of the three bovine CaBPs.

Amino acid compositional analyses of the smaller NBS fragments from the three components showed these to be NH_2-terminal with compositions of the

```
                                                        NBS
Minor A:                5                10              ↓  15
  LYS-SER-PRO-GLU-GLU-LEU-LYS-GLY-ILE-PHE-GLU-LYS-TYR-ALA-ALA-LYS-GLU-
                                                              20
                                                   GLY-ASP-PRO-ASN-GLN-LEU-SER-

Minor B:
  SER-PRO-GLU-GLU-LEU-LYS-GLY-ILE-PHE-GLU-LYS-TYR-ALA-ALA-LYS-GLU-GLY-ASP-
                                                           PRO-ASN-GLN-LEU-SER-

Major:
  (BG,ALA,LYS,LYS,SER,PRO,GLU,GLU,LEU,LYS,GLY,ILE,PHE,GLU,LYS)TYR-ALA-ALA-LYS-
                                               GLU-GLY-ASP-PRO-ASN-GLN-LEU-SER-

25                  30                  35                  49
LYS-GLU-GLU-LEU-LYS-LEU-LEU-LEU-GLN-THR-GLU-PHE-PRO-SER-LEU-LEU-LYS-GLY-PRO-LYS-
GLU-GLU-LEU-LYS-LEU-LEU-LEU-GLN-THR-GLU-PHE-PRO-SER-LEU-LEU-LYS-GLY-PRO-LYS-GLU-
GLU-LEU-LYS-LEU-LEU-LEU-GLN-THR-GLU-PHE-PRO-SER-LEU-LEU-LYS-GLY-PRO-
```

Fig. 9. Partial amino acid sequence of the three bovine calcium-binding proteins

Minor A and Minor B components corresponding exactly to the compositions derived from the sequencing studies (residues 1–12 for the Minor A and 1–11 for the Minor B). The composition of the small NBS fragment generated from the native CaBP was identical to that of the Minor A component, with the addition of 1 lysine and 1 alanine residue (Table 5).

Table 5. Amino acid compositions of the *N*-terminal NBS peptides from bovine CaBPs

	Native	Minor A	Minor B
LYS	3.6	2.8	2.1
SER	1.0	0.9	0.8
GLU	3.0	3.0	2.8
PRO	0.9	1.0	0.8
GLY[a]	1.0	1.0	1.0
ALA	0.5	0.1	0
ILE	0.9	0.9	0.8
LEU	1.0	1.0	0.9
TYR[b]	—	—	—
PHE	0.8	0.9	0.9

[a] Number of residues computed on the basis of 1-glycine
[b] *C*-terminal tyrosine assumed for all peptides but destroyed during NBS reaction

The larger (COOH-terminal)NBS fragments from the three components all produced NH_2-terminal alanine following dansylation. Automated sequence determination established identical sequences for the three bovine CaBPs from the point of NBS cleavage and for at least an additional 30 residues, extending the total sequences to 43 residues.

The results of all sequence and compositional data are summarised in Fig. 9. While the sequence of the NH_2-terminus of the native CaBP (Major component) has not been conclusively established, it is reasonable to assume sequence identity with the Minor A component, for the most part. The additional one alanine and one lysine residue probably appear immediately following the blocking group in the native protein. This lysine-lysine configuration would explain the appearance of the Minor A and Minor B components following limited tryptic hydrolysis, as is the case when calcium is bound to the protein. Protection against total tryptic digestion of CaBP, with consequent loss of calcium-binding activity and immunological reactivity, is conferred upon the molecule by bound calcium, presumably via alteration of the three-dimensional structure in which the 11 'internal' lysine residues are masked from attack by trypsin. In the presence of bound calcium the only substantial points available for cleavage are those immediately adjacent to the lysine residue at position 1 of the Minor A component (see Fig. 9).

The observed charge differences as visualised by electrophoresis are easily explained on the following basis. Conversion of the native CaBP to the Minor A component results in the loss of one ε-amino charge ($pK_a = 10.53$) with the imposition of an additional α-amino charge ($pK_a = 8.95$), while conversion to the Minor B component results in the complete loss of an ε-amino charge.

The amino acid sequence of porcine intestinal CaBP has recently been reported (Hofmann *et al.*, 1977) and bears remarkable resemblance to the bovine CaBP. Comparison of the first 51 residues of each indicates only 6–8 residue differences, each of which can be accounted for by single-base changes within each codon. These results clearly confirm that the previously published bovine sequence (Huang *et al.*, 1975) is incorrect.

X Crystallisation of Bovine Calcium-Binding Protein

Bovine CaBP (Minor A form) was recently crystallised in the presence of high concentrations of ammonium sulphate over a pH range of 6.0 to 8.8 (Moffat *et al.*, 1975). Below pH 7.5, the crystals were primarily thin plate-like and proved too fragile for x-ray analysis. Above pH 7.5, long prisms of usable dimensions predominated. The diffraction pattern that extended to about 1.5 Å resolution indicated that the crystals are orthorhombic with unit cell dimensions of: $a = 56.3 \pm 0.2$, $b = 43.0$ and $c = 29.4 \pm 0.15$ Å, yielding a volume of 71 200 $Å^3$. Upon further analysis, the unit cell was found to contain 4 asymmetrical units, with one molecule constituting one asymmetrical unit. The space group was $P2_12_12$.

XI Comparative Immunological Aspects of Calcium-Binding Protein

Antisera has been prepared against intestinal CaBP from the guinea pig, chick and bovine. The reactivity of these antisera with various tissue extracts and purified CaBPs from different species has been investigated to a limited extent and this information is summarised in Table 6. With the chick CaBP antiserum, cross-reactivity was noted with purified CaBPs or crude tissue preparations from chick kidney and brain, and laying hen uterus. Also this same antisera gave precipitin lines with turtle intestine, rat brain and kidney, bovine brain, and human kidney. Where determined, these cross-reacting proteins were shown to be of the same molecular size as chick intestinal CaBP, i.e. about 28 000.

The antisera against the mammalian intestinal CaBPs (molecular weight 11 000) appeared to be relatively species specific in that guinea pig antisera reacted with material from guinea pig intestine and kidney, and not against other 11 000 molecular weight CaBPs in cow intestine and kidney, pig intestine and rat intestine. No reactivity against the 28 000 molecular weight chick CaBP was observed. Antisera against bovine intestinal CaBP (molecular weight 11 000) reacted only with material from bovine intestine and kidney.

It has been reported, however, that antisera against human kidney CaBP (molecular weight 28 000) reacted both with material from human kidney and human intestine, as well as that from rat kidney and pancreas, and chick kidney (Morrissey *et al.*, 1975).

From the information just described, some interesting patterns and subpatterns seem to emerge, although more data are required to verify these relationships. It appears that the avian species and those lower on the evolutionary scale (amphibian) have an intestinal CaBP molecular weight of about 28 000. The prominent mammalian intestinal CaBPs thus far studied appear to have a molecular weight of about 11 000, i.e. less than one-half that of the chick protein. The molecular size of kidney CaBP varies with species, some having a CaBP similar in size to the mammalian intestinal CaBP (guinea pig, cow) and others, with a protein similar in size to the chick intestinal protein (rat, human). The brain CaBP of both avian and mammalian species appears, with only limited data, to be of the 28 000 molecular weight variety.

Thus, the indication is that intestinal CaBP seems to have been modified during evolution, yielding a protein of less than one-half the size of the chick protein. In the kidney, one of two courses took place – either the 28 000 molecular weight type persisted from avian to mammalian species or the 11 000 molecular weight type evolved. The reason for the apparent difference in the nature of the kidney protein during evolution is certainly not apparent at this time. Also it seems that the antisera produced against the different mammalian intestinal CaBPs are quite species specific, despite similar amino acid content (Table 4).

If this same pattern of antigenic reactivity and molecular size holds as more information becomes available, it would suggest that the larger CaBP represents, evolutionarily speaking, a more primitive type of intestinal protein, whereas the more highly evolved smaller variety is capable of functioning at $\frac{1}{2}$ to $\frac{1}{3}$ the molecular size. It will also be of interest to elucidate the reason for the continued presence of a more primitive type of CaBP in the brain and kidney of some species. However, the recent studies of Moriuchi *et al.* (1975) suggesting that rat intestine has a 12 500 molecular weight CaBP and a 27 000 molecular weight CaBP, both of which are calciferol-dependent, might bear on the aforementioned hypothesis.

Table 6. Antigenic reactivity of CaBP[a]

CaBP present in:	Approx. MW	Antiserum prepared against CaBP isolated from:[b] Chick intestine (MW 28 000)	Guinea pig intestine (MW 11 000)	Bovine intestine (MW 11 000)	Human kidney (MW 28 000)[e]
Chick					
intestine	28 000	+	−	−	ND
kidney	28 000	+	−	−	+
uterus	28 000	+	−	−	ND
brain	28 000	+	−	−	ND
Turtle					
intestine	28 000	+	ND	−	ND
Rat					
intestine	11 000	−	−	−	ND
kidney	28 000	+	ND	−	+
brain	?	+	ND	−	ND
pancreas	?	ND	ND	ND	+
Guinea pig					
intestine	11 000	−	+	−	ND
kidney	11 000	−	+	−	ND
Cow					
intestine	11 000	−	−	+	ND
kidney	11 000	−	−	+	ND
brain	?	+	ND	−	ND
testes[c]	11 000	−	ND	−	ND
Pig					
intestine	11 000	−	−	−	ND
kidney	?	ND	ND	−	ND
Human					
intestine	12 000[d]	−	ND	−	+
kidney	28 000[f]	+	−	−	+

[a] (+) indicates a positive precipitin reaction, (−) indicates no immunological reaction, and ND indicates no data available

[b] All antisera was prepared in rabbits in this laboratory except the data for antisera against human kidney which was from Morrissey *et al.* (1975) and personal communication with R. L. Morrissey

[c] A purified sample of calcium-binding protein (CBP-11) was kindly supplied by F. Siegel, University of Wisconsin

[d] From Hitchman and Harrison (1972)

[e] From Morrissey and Rath (1974)

[f] Fullmer and Wasserman (unpublished)

XII *In Vitro* Synthesis of Calcium-Binding Protein by Intestinal Tissue and Intestinal Cells

Organ Culture. Embryonic chick intestine, as mentioned previously, is devoid of CaBP until the day of hatching. This represented a suitable tissue to culture for the purpose of studying CaBP synthesis under controlled conditions. The advantage of such an *in vitro* culture system is the absence of exogenous factors that might affect the metabolism and behaviour of the tissue, except those present in the tissue itself or supplied in the incubation medium.

The maintenance of embryonic chick intestine in organ culture was successfully accomplished, and the cultured intestine responded to exogenous cholecalciferol or its metabolites by synthesising CaBP and increasing its capacity to accumulate and transport calcium (Corradino and Wasserman, 1971b; Corradino 1973a, c). Using this system, it was also observed that cholecalciferol or metabolites, either directly or indirectly, increased tissue cyclic adenosine-3′, 5′-phosphate (cAMP) levels (Corradino, 1974). The stimulation of the adenylate cyclase system appears to occur prior to the synthesis of CaBP or enhanced ^{45}Ca uptake. However, a puzzling aspect is that cAMP levels decrease to base line concentrations before increasing again as CaBP appears and ^{45}Ca transport is enhanced. Another observation of interest is that dibutyryl cAMP, when added to the culture system, enhances ^{45}Ca transport without inducing the formation of CaBP.

It should also be emphasised that experience with the organ culture system is that the appearance of CaBP always coincides, in time, with an increase in the Ca transport mechanism. This is commensurate with observations made *in vivo*. In addition, the organ culture technique proved useful in assessing the effect of exogenous CaBP on calcium transport by the embryonic intestine. When highly purified CaBP is added to the culture medium, a significant increase in calcium transport occurs, providing direct evidence for a role of the protein in calcium translocation (Corradino *et al.*, 1976).

Isolated Epithelial Cells. Procedures have become available for the isolation of viable intestinal cells, such as those described by Kimmich (1970) and Perris (1966). Using these techniques, Freund and Bronner (1975b) obtained cells from rats that were vitamin D-replete or vitamin D-deficient. It was clearly demonstrated that the uptake of calcium by the isolated cells derived from vitamin D-replete animals was significantly greater than those that were vitamin D-deficient. More importantly, the addition of 1,25-dihydroxycholecalciferol to the incubation medium containing rachitic cells for a 90 minute period yielded a similar enhancement of ^{45}Ca uptake as compared to the controls. A search was made for the presence of CaBP in the intestinal cells incubated with the hormone. Fractionation of supernatants from homogenates of the cells revealed that the vitamin D-deficient material was devoid of CaBP but, those incubated in the presence of 1,25-dihydroxy-cholecalciferol, contained CaBP. Thus, within the period of incubation, the isolated vitamin D-deficient cells were capable of responding to the vitamin D_3 metabolite, both with respect to ^{45}Ca uptake and CaBP formation, and this constitutes further evidence for a role of CaBP in calcium absorption.

XIII Function of Vitamin D-Dependent Calcium-Binding Protein

The evidence documented herein and elsewhere (Wasserman and Corradino, 1973) shows a high correlation, with minimal exceptions, between calciferol-dependent CaBP and the process of calcium transport across the intestine. A reasonable inference would be that CaBP is intimately involved in the calcium transport mechanism, although several investigations and other information suggest that other factors are involved that might be limiting under certain conditions (Wasserman *et al.*, 1977; Wasserman and Feher, 1977; Wilson and Lawson, 1977; Zolock *et al.*, 1977). Unfortunately, information on critical points of CaBP behaviour and properties has not been attained or is controversial, which makes the task of reasonable modelling very difficult at the present time. Complicating the situation is the stimulation of two types of transport processes by calciferol: diffusion and active transport. Is CaBP involved with both the energy-dependent and energy-independent processes of translocation, or one of these?

Investigations on the localisation of CaBP by immunohistochemical methodology has been referred to before. This information is now summarised in Table 7 and, from a cursory glance, the diverse nature of the findings are immediately apparent. This is undoubtedly due to the source of the protein from which the antisera were produced and the different species used. In chick duodenum, intestinal CaBP was found primarily in the goblet cells and at the brush border by Taylor and Wasserman (1970a); in goblet cells, brush border region and basement membrane area of human duodenum by Piazolo *et al.* (1974); not in the human duodenum, but at the basal and lateral membranes and the basement membrane of human jejunum by Morrissey *et al.* (1975). Both of the studies in man were done with antisera produced against CaBP isolated from human kidney and not from the intestine. More extensive investigations are required for confirmational purposes but the above comments and data indicate some of the confusion surrounding an important aspect of this protein.

A point that is difficult to reconcile with any proposal involving a direct membrane interaction of CaBP is its solubility properties. Unlike *bona fide* membrane proteins, such as the Na, K-ATPase, CaBP is almost quantitatively released from the intestinal mucosa upon simple homogenisation in aqueous buffers. However, recent data indicate that about 5–10% of intestinal CaBP is bound to cellular elements, possibly membranous structures (Feher and Wasserman, 1976). This bound CaBP is released by Triton X-100 and certain other reagents, and appears to be identical to the soluble form by several criteria. Although present in small proportion to the total CaBP, it could have

Table 7. Summary of histological localisation of CaBP in various species[a]

Species	Source of CaBP for antibody production	Tissue studied	Localisation	References
Chick	Chick intestine	Duodenum	Goblet cells Brush border region	Taylor and Wasserman, 1970a
Chick	Chick intestine	Kidney	Distal tubule	Lippiello, 1974
Laying hen	Chick intestine	Uterus	Tubular gland cells	Lippiello and Wasserman, 1975
Human	Human kidney	Duodenum	Goblet cell Brush border region Basement membrane	Piazolo *et al.*, 1974
Human	Human kidney	Duodenum	Negative	Morrissey *et al.*, 1975
Human	Human kidney	Jejunum	Lateral and basal membranes	Morrissey *et al.*, 1975
Several[b] species	Human kidney	Pancreas	Islet cell (cytoplasm)	Morrissey *et al.*, 1975

[a] Species included human, monkey, dog, rat, mouse and chick, all presumably displaying the same pattern

[b] Species included cat, dog, rat, mouse and chick, presumably displaying the same pattern

physiological significance and possibly suggests an interaction with membranous components of the cell by even the more readily solubilised form. An interaction of CaBP with membranes is also suggested by the ability of a naturally-occurring phospholipid, lysolecithin, to bind to CaBP and, in so doing, alter its electrophoretic mobility and calcium-binding affinity (Wasserman, 1970). Further, Hamilton and Holdsworth (1970) demonstrated that CaBP enhanced the release of ^{45}Ca from mitochondria pre-loaded with the isotope *in vivo*. Their conditions were such that the high affinity sites of CaBP were saturated. This effect of the protein on mitochondria could be due to the complexation of calcium by the low affinity sites ($k_a \sim 10^2 - 10^3$ M^{-1}) or a direct effect on the mitochondrial membrane. The former possibility is probably unlikely since presumably the intracellular [Ca^{+2}] is maintained in the order of 10^{-5} to 10^{-6} M, concentrations at which the lower affinity binding sites of CaBP would be ineffective. As part of their thesis, Hamilton and Holdsworth (*loc. cit.*) suggested that the mechanism of CaBP action was to enhance the turnover of mitochondrial calcium and, as a consequence, increase the translocation of calcium. Whether or not this proposal has validity, these results do indicate a possible membrane effect of the protein.

The possibility that calcium moves across the intestine in 'packets' was suggested from the electron prode analysis of Warner and Coleman (1975).

Calcium was observed to be concentrated in the supranuclear region of the cell and in the intercellular region. Using histological techniques a greater number of apical pits and vesicles have been observed in chick intestine cells after repletion by cholecalciferol, which apparently paralleled calcium absorption and CaBP synthesis (Jande and Brewer, 1974). Since endocytosis requires absorption of substrate to the membrane and energy source, it was proposed that CaBP might constitute the absorption site, and Ca-ATPase and/or alkaline phosphatase (with ATP) providing the energy source.

Thermodynamic arguments previously made (Wasserman and Taylor, 1969) supported the concept that Ca^{+2}, when present in the intestinal lumen in high concentration, is quite possibly absorbed via the shunt path, i.e. the intracellular route. It was then reported that the absorption of La^{+3} is influenced by cholecalciferol (Wasserman *et al.*, 1974b). Since La^{+3} does not traverse biological membranes (or only minimally), this was construed as indicating that cholecalciferol might influence the Ca^{+2} permeability of the tight junction.

Mention should be made of the vitamin D-dependent calcium-binding complex identified recently in rat intestinal mucosa by Kowarski and Schachter (1975). This complex was present in the particulate fraction of isolated brush borders and varied with the capacity of the intestine to transport calcium under different physiological and nutritional conditions. It was of interest to note from their study that the concentrations of the calcium-binding complex in the intestine occurred in almost a one to one relationship with the concentration of soluble CaBP. This suggests some relationship between these two calcium-binding activities and is reminiscent of the bound form of CaBP referred to previously (Feher and Wasserman, 1976). Also Moriuchi (1975) observed that the electrophoretic mobility of alkaline phosphatase (Ca-ATPase) brush borders from rachitic chicks was modified on SDS gels by the administration of 1,25-dihydroxycholecalciferol. Because the estimated molecular weight difference between the rachitic and the 1,25-dihydroxycholecalciferol-sensitive enzyme was 30 000 Moriuchi (1975) suggested that CaBP (MW: 28 000) might constitute part of the phosphatase complex after repletion. This is an intriguing possibility requiring verification; a manifestation of this proposed interaction might be the conferring of calcium-sensitivity to the enzyme and/or an enhanced calcium transport capacity to the brush border membrane. However, a unifying concept regarding CaBP, alkaline phosphatase and the calcium-binding complex in calcium absorption is not yet justified since Kowarski and Schachter (1975) provide evidence that the enzyme varies differently from that of the two calcium-binding activities in different situations, and Norman (1974) reported that alkaline phosphatase activity, after 1,25-dihydroxycholecalciferol treatment of rachitic chicks, increases in activity sometime later than the calcium absorptive process increases. Thus, a model incorporating these macromolecules in calcium transport by the intestine is premature.

As can be gathered from the foregoing, the exact molecular basis of CaBP action on intestinal transport has not yet been achieved. Hopefully, a fuller understanding of the molecular properties of this very interesting molecule, its exact localisation, and its exact interaction with other intestinal moieties will aid in deciphering its action.

References

Alpers, D. H., Lee, S. W. and Avioli, L. V. (1972). *Gastroenterology* **62**, 559.
Arnold, B. M., Kovacs, K. and Murray, T. M. (1976). *Digestion* **14**, 77.
Bar, A., Dubrov, D., Eisner, U. and Hurwitz, S. (1976). *Poultry Sci.* **55**, 622.
Bar, A. and Hurwitz, S. (1973). *Comp. Biochem. Physiol.* **45A**, 579.
Bar, A. and Wasserman, R. H. (1974). *J. Nutr.* 104, 1202.
Bauman, V. K., Valinience, M. Y. and Pastuhob, M. V. (1972). *Proc. Latvian Acad. Sci.* **294**, 133.
Bredderman, P. B. and Wasserman, R. H. (1974). *Biochemistry* **13**, 1687.
Bronner, F. and Freund, T. (1975). *Amer. J. Physiol.* **229**, 689.
Brumbaugh, P. F. and Haussler, M. R. (1973). *Biochem. Biophys. Res. Comm.* **51**, 74.
Chapman, M. (1974). M. S. Thesis, Cornell University, Ithaca, New York.
Corradino, R. A. (1973a). *J. Cell Biol.* **58**, 64.
Corradino, R. A. (1973b). *Nature* (London) **243**, 41.
Corradino, R. A. (1973c). *Science* **179**, 402.
Corradino, R. A. (1974). *Endocrinol.* **94**, 1607.
Corradino, R. A., Taylor, A. N. and Wasserman, R. H. (1969). *Fed. Proc.* **28**, 760.
Corradino, R. A., Fullmer, C. S. and Wasserman, R. H. (1976). *Arch. Biochem. Biophys.* **174**, 738.
Corradino, R. A. and Wasserman, R. H. (1974). *Nature* (London) **252**, 716.
Corradino, R. A. and Wasserman, R. H. (1971a). *Biophysical Soc. Abstracts* **11**, 15.
Corradino, R. A. and Wasserman, R. H. (1971b). *Science* **172**, 731.
Corradino, R. A., Wasserman, R. H., Pubols, M. H. and Chang, S. I. (1968). *Arch. Biochem. Biophys.* **125**, 378.
Dorrington, K. J., Hui, A., Hofmann, T., Hitchman, A. J. W. and Harrison, J. E. (1974). *J. Biol. Chem.* **249**, 199.
Drescher, D. and DeLuca, H. F. (1971a). *Biochemistry* **10**, 2308.
Drescher, D. and DeLuca, H. F. (1971b). *Biochemistry* 10, 2302.
Emtage, J. S., Lawson, D. E. M. and Kodicek, E. (1974a). *Biochem. J.* **140**, 239.
Emtage, J. S., Lawson, D. E. M. and Kodicek, E. (1974b). *Biochem. J.* **144**, 339.
Feher, J. J. and Wasserman, R. H. (1976). *Fed. Proc.* **35**, 339.
Freund, T. and Bronner, F. (1975a). *Amer. J. Physiol.* **228**, 861.
Freund, T. and Bronner, F. (1975b). *Science* **190**, 1300.
Fullmer, C. S., Brindak, M. E., Bar, A, and Wasserman, R. H. (1976). *Proc. Soc. Exptl. Biol. Med.* **152**, 237.
Fullmer, C. S. and Wasserman, R. H. (1973). *Biochim. Biophys. Acta.* **317**, 172.
Fullmer, C. S. and Wasserman, R. H. (1975). *Biochim. Biophys. Acta* **393**, 134.
Fullmer, C. S. and Wasserman, R. H. (1978). In preparation.
Fullmer, C. S., Wasserman, R. H., Hamilton, J. W., Huang, W. Y. and Cohn, D. V. (1975). *Biochim. Biophys. Acta.* **412**, 1075.

Gray, W. R. (1972). *In* 'Methods in Enzymology' (Ed. C. H. W. Hirs and S. N. Timasheff) Vol. XXV, p. 121, Academic Press, New York.

Hamilton, J. W. and Holdsworth, E. S. (1970). *Biochem. Biophys. Res. Comm.* **40**, 1325.

Harmeyer, J. and DeLuca, H. F. (1969). *Arch. Biochem. Biophys.* **133**, 247.

Harrison, J. E., Hitchman, A. J. W. and Brown, R. G. (1975). *Can. J. Physiol. Pharmacol.* **53**, 144.

Helmke, K., Ferderlin, K., Piazolo, P., Stroder, J., Jeschke, R. and Franz, H. E. (1974). *Gut* **15**, 875.

Hermsdorf, C. L. and Bronner, F. (1975). *Biochim. Biophys. Acta* **379**, 553.

Hitchman, A. J. W. and Harrison, J. E. (1972). *Can. J. Biochem.* **50**, 758.

Hitchman, A. J. W., Kerr, M. K. and Harrison, J. E. (1973). *Arch. Biochem. Biophys.* **155**, 221.

Hofmann, T., Kawakami, M., Morris, H., Hitchman, A. J. W., Harrison, J. E. and Dorrington, K. J. (1977) *In* 'Calcium-Binding Proteins and Calcium Function' (Ed. R. H. Wasserman) p. 373, Elsevier-North-Holland, New York.

Huang, W. Y., Cohn, D. V., Hamilton, J. V., Fullmer, C. S. and Wasserman, R. H. (1975). *J. Biol. Chem.* **250**, 7647.

Hurwitz, S., Bar, A. and Meshorer, A. (1973). *Poultry Science* **52**, 1370.

Ingersoll, R. J. and Wasserman, R. H. (1971). *J. Biol. Chem.* **246**, 2808.

Jande, S. S. and Brewer, L. M. (1974). *Z. Anat. Entwickl-Gesch.* **144**, 249.

Kallfelz, F. A., Taylor, A. N. and Wasserman, R. H. (1967). *Proc. Soc. Exptl. Biol. Med.* **125**, 54.

Kimmich, G. A. (1970). *Biochemistry* **9**, 3659.

Kowarski, S. and Schachter, D. (1975). *Amer. J. Physiol.* **229**, 1198.

Lawson, D. E. M. and Emtage, J. S. (1974). *Vitam. Horm.* **32**, 277.

Lippiello, L. (1974). Ph.D. Thesis. Cornell University, Ithaca, New York.

Lippiello, L. and Wasserman, R. H. (1975). *J. Histochem. Cytochem.* **23**, 111.

MacGregor, R. R., Hamilton, J. W. and Cohn, D. V. (1971). *Clin. Orthop.* **78**, 83.

Menczel, J., Eilon, G., Steiner, A., Karaman, C., Mor, E. and Ron, A. (1971). *Israel J. Med. Sci.* **7**, 396.

Moffat, K., Fullmer, C. S. and Wasserman, R. H. (1975). *J. Mol. Biol.* **97**, 661.

Moriuchi, S. (1975). *Metabolism* (Tokyo) **12**, 1375.

Moriuchi, S. and DeLuca, H. F. (1974). *Arch. Biochem. Biophys.* **164**, 165.

Moriuchi, S., Yamanouchi, T. and Hosoya, N. (1975). *J. Nutr. Sci. Vitaminol.* **21**, 251.

Morrissey, R. L. and Rath, D. F. (1974). *Proc. Soc. Exptl. Biol. Med.* **145**, 699.

Morrissey, R. L., Bucci, T. J., Empson, R. N. Jr. and Lufkin, E. G. (1975). *Proc. Soc. Exptl. Biol. Med.* **149**, 56.

Morrissey, R. L., Empson, R. N., Zolock, D. T., Bikle, B. D. and Bucci, T. J. (1978). *Biochim. Biophys. Acta* **538**, 34.

Murray, T. M., Arnold, B. M., Kuttner, M., Kovacs, K., Hitchman, A. J. W. and Harrison, J. E. (1975). *In* 'Calcium Regulating Hormones' (Ed. R. V. Talmage, M. Owen and J. A. Parsons) p. 371, Excerpta Medica, Amsterdam.

Murray, T. M., Arnold, B. M., Tam, W. H., Hitchman, A. J. W. and Harrison, J. E. (1974). *Metabolism* **23**, 829.

Norman, A. W. (1974). *Vitam. Horm.* **32**, 325.

Oku, T., Shimura, F., Moriuchi, S. and Hosoya, N. (1975). Proc. 10th International Congress of Nutrition, Kyoto.

Oldham, S. B., Fischer, J. A., Shen, L. H. and Arnaud, C. D. (1974). *Biochemistry* **13**, 4790.

Omdahl, J. L. and DeLuca, H. F. (1973). *Physiol. Rev.* **53**, 327.

Ooizumi, K., Moriuchi, S. and Hosoya, N. (1970). *J. Vitaminol.* 16, 228.
Perris, A. D. (1966). *Can. J. Biochem.* **44**, 687.
Piazolo, P., Schleyer, M. and Franz, H. E. (1971). *Hoppe-Seyler's Z. Physiol. Chem.* **352A**, 1480.
Piazolo, P., Schleyer, M., Helmke, K. and Franz, H. E. (1974). *In* 'Calcium Binding Proteins' (Ed. W. Drabikowski, H. Strzelecka-Golaszewska, E. Carafoli) p. 791, PWN-Polish Scientific Publishers, Warsaw.
Ramachandran, L. K. and Witkop, B. (1967). *In* 'Methods in Enzymology' (Ed. C. H. W. Hirs) Vol. XI, p. 283, Academic Press, New York.
Reynolds, R. D., Knutson, J. C. and DeLuca, H. F. (1975). *Fed. Proc.* **34**, 893.
Sands, H. and Kessler, R. H. (1971). *Proc. Soc. Exptl. Med.* **137**, 1267.
Schachter, D. (1970). *In* 'Fat Soluble Vitamins' (Ed. H. F. DeLuca and J. W. Suttie) p. 55, University of Wisconsin Press, Madison, U.S.A.
Taylor, A. N. (1974a). *Arch. Biochem. Biophys.* **161**, 100.
Taylor, A. N. (1974b). *Fed. Proc.* **33**, 1551.
Taylor, A. N. and McIntosh, J. E. (1977). *In* 'Vitamin D: Biochemical, Chemical and Clinical Aspects Related to Calcium Metabolism' (Ed. A. W. Norman) p. 303, De Gruyter, Berlin.
Taylor, A. N. and Wasserman, R. H. (1969). *Fed. Proc.* **28**, 1834.
Taylor, A. N. and Wasserman, R. H. (1970a). *J. Histochem. Cytochem.* **18**, 107.
Taylor, A. N. and Wasserman, R. H. (1970b). *Fed. Proc.* **29**, 368.
Taylor, A. N. and Wasserman, R. H. (1972). *Amer. J. Physiol.* **223**, 110.
Taylor, A. N., Wasserman, R. H. and Jowsey, J. (1968). *Fed. Proc.* **27**, 675.
Tsai, H. C. and Norman, A. W. (1973). *J. Biol. Chem.* **248**, 5967.
Warner, R. R. and Coleman, J. R. (1975). *J. Cell Biol.* **64**, 54.
Wasserman, R. H. (1970). *Biochim. Biophys. Acta* **203**, 176.
Wasserman, R. H. and Corradino, R. A. (1973). *Vitam. Horm.* **31**, 44.
Wasserman, R. H., Corradino, R. A., Fullmer, C. S. and Taylor, A. N. (1974a). *Vitam. Horm.* **32**, 299.
Wasserman, R. H., Corradino, R. A. and Krook, L. P. (1975). *Biochem. Biophys. Res. Comm.* **62**, 85.
Wasserman, R. H., Corradino, R. A. and Taylor, A. N. (1968). *J. Biol. Chem.* **243**, 3978.
Wasserman, R. H., Corradino, R. A., Feher, J. J. and Armbrecht, H. J. (1977). *In* 'Vitamin D: Biochemical, Chemical and Clinical Aspects Related to Calcium Metabolism' (Ed. A. W. Norman) p. 331, De Gruyter, Berlin.
Wasserman, R. H. and Feher, J. J. (1977). *In* 'Calcium-Binding Proteins and Calcium Function' (Ed. R. H. Wasserman) p. 293, Elsevier-North-Holland, New York.
Wasserman, R. H. and Taylor, A. N. (1971). *Proc. Soc. Exptl. Biol. Med.* **136**, 25.
Wasserman, R. H. and Taylor, A. N. (1969). *In* 'Mineral Metabolism' (Ed. C. L. Comar and F. Bronner) Vol. 3, p. 321, Academic Press, New York and London.
Wasserman, R. H. and Taylor, A. N. (1966). *Science* **152**, 791.
Wasserman, R. H., Taylor, A. N. and Lippiello, L. (1974b). *In* 'Calcium Metabolism, Bone and Metabolic Bone Diseases' (Ed. F. Kuhlencordt and H.-P. Kruse) p. 87, Springer-Verlag, Berlin.
Wilson, P. W. and Lawson, D. E. M. (1977). *Biochim. Biophys. Acta* **497,** 805.
Zolock, D. T., Morrissey, R. L. and Bikle, D. D. (1977). *In* 'Vitamin D: Biochemical, Chemical and Clinical Aspects Related to Calcium Metabolism' (Ed. A. W. Norman) p. 345, De Gruyter, Berlin.

5 Biochemical Responses of the Intestine to Vitamin D

D. E. M. LAWSON

I Introduction

There is a general acceptance that one, if not the sole effect of vitamin D is to contribute, along with parathyroid hormone and calcitonin, to the maintenance within quite narrow limits, of plasma calcium concentrations. This effect of the vitamin is achieved through the hormonal metabolite 1,25-dihydroxycholecalciferol which regulates calcium movements across the mucosal cells of the intestine and the renal tubular cells and regulates also the mobilisation of calcium from bone. Over the last ten years, several findings have been made which have provided a firm basis for the biochemical investigations into the mechanisms by which this regulation is achieved in these tissues. For a number of reasons, most of the studies have been concerned with the changes in the metabolic reactions in the intestine which are affected by vitamin D in the belief that the action of the hormone will be similar in principle in all the tissues in which it is effective. Notable among these reasons is the fact that the action of the vitamin in the intestine, i.e. stimulation of calcium absorption, can be readily observed and has an obvious relationship to the overall function of this tissue. In addition, the variety of cells within the intestine is limited, and there are well described techniques for the isolation of their intracellular structures. Some of the early investigations drew their inspiration from studies of the biochemical function of the water soluble vitamins, and considered a co-factor role for vitamin D (Zetterstrom, 1951). Somewhat later the first reports appeared of the changes in the activity of several intestinal enzymes, including alkaline phosphatase, Ca/Mg-ATPase, and phytase.

The present era of research into the biochemistry of vitamin D began with the availability of a radioactive form of the vitamin, thereby allowing its metabolism to be followed and the intracellular distribution of the metabolites to be established. These studies showed that vitamin D was simply a precursor of a steroid hormone, 1,25-dihydroxycholecalciferol, which was accumulated in the nuclei of the target cells. As with the other steroid hormones the study of the proteins in plasma and tissues which can specifically bind this new hormone and its biosynthetic precursors, became of importance in understanding the function of 1,25-dihydroxycholecalciferol. Thus a comparison has been made of these proteins from the various sites at which they are found. It was also established that the action of vitamin D could be prevented by antibiotics which inhibit RNA synthesis and this, with the discovery of the vitamin D-dependent calcium-binding protein, suggested that 1,25-dihydroxycholecalciferol regulates the transcription of the gene for this protein.

This chapter reviews the evidence in favour of this view, and shows that there is an obligatory requirement for 1,25-dihydroxycholecalciferol in the synthesis of messenger RNA for calcium-binding protein, and also discusses the evidence for additional actions of the hormone in the intestine.

II Intracellular Distribution of Cholecalciferol and Metabolites in Target Tissues

The first preparations of radioactive cholecalciferol, whether labelled with ^{14}C or ^{3}H, were of low specific activity, and consequently non-physiological doses were used in studies of the metabolism of the vitamin and its localisation within cells (Kodicek, 1962; Norman and DeLuca, 1964). Eventually tritium labelled cholecalciferol was produced of sufficiently high specific activity to enable these types of studies to be carried out with doses similar to the daily requirements of the animal (Neville and DeLuca, 1966). The accumulation of radioactivity in the target tissues of the vitamin such as intestine, bone and kidney then became apparent. The earlier studies had not shown any specific accumulation of radioactivity within the intracellular fractions of these tissues, with the radioactivity being almost uniformly distributed between the nuclear, mitochondrial and microsomal fractions. In subsequent experiments, in which physiological doses of cholecalciferol were administered to rats and chicks, a high proportion (50%) of the total intestinal radioactivity was found in the cell fraction sedimented by centrifugation at 800 g. This fraction contained nuclei, brush borders and cell debris. Because of the findings with actinomycin D, efforts were concentrated on isolating pure intestinal nuclei and as expected, they showed that intestinal nuclei can accumulate metabolites of cholecalciferol (Haussler and Norman, 1967; Stohs and DeLuca, 1967; Lawson *et al.*, 1969a).

In a number of experiments carried out since this time, metabolites of cholecalciferol have never been found in any pure brush border preparation from mucosa of chick intestine (Lawson, unpublished observations). An indication of the importance of the nuclear sites for the biological function of the vitamin in the intestine was provided by Stohs and DeLuca (1967), who showed that they could be saturated by the administration of large doses of the vitamin and of dihydrotachysterol-2 but not by the biologically inactive 7-dehydrocholesterol.

At first the identity of the nuclear radioactivity was unclear with claims that it was due to cholecalciferol itself (Haussler and Norman, 1967) and then that it was due to the 25-hydroxy-metabolite (Stohs and DeLuca, 1967). The use of [4-^{14}C,1-^{3}H]cholecalciferol in studies of the metabolism of the vitamin showed that the nuclear radioactivity was not due to 25-hydroxycholecalciferol but rather to a more polar substance, which was labelled only with ^{14}C, the tritium having been replaced in the formation of the metabolite (Lawson *et al.*, 1969a). This polar metabolite was subsequently identified as 1,25-dihydroxycholecalciferol (Holick *et al.*, 1971; Lawson *et al.*, 1971a; Norman *et al.*, 1971). Following the administration of a physiological dose of radioactive cholecalciferol to rachitic animals, the major metabolite in the intestine is 1,25-dihydroxycholecalciferol and it accounts for 97% of the nuclear radioactivity. At higher dose levels or in normal chicks, cholecalciferol and its 25-hydroxy-metabolite are bound to intestinal nuclei but at a different site (i.e. nuclear membranes) to that at which the 1,25-dihydroxylated metabolite is located (see Section III).

After a physiological dose of cholecalciferol to chicks, only a small proportion of the total content of intestinal metabolites was found in the mitochondrial and microsomal fractions (Lawson *et al.*, 1971b). The mitochondrial fraction appears to have some capacity to accumulate the 25-hydroxy-metabolite, although this substance is also present in all fractions.

Cholecalciferol itself was present in all cell fractions except the cytoplasmic component. In the case of the two other major target tissues of cholecalciferol, i.e. kidney and bone, the intracellular distribution of the metabolites within them appears to be similar to that in the intestine in that the hormone is accumulated in the cell nuclei (Lawson *et al.*, 1971b; Weber *et al.*, 1971). It is worth pointing out that although an effect of the vitamin on kidney and bone has been described, there is no clear indication as to the identity of the cells in these tissues in which the hormone is concentrated.

III Localisation of 1,25-Dihydroxycholecalciferol within Intestinal Nuclei

Although there is general agreement that 1,25-dihydroxycholecalciferol is accumulated in the nuclei of the target tissues, there is still some controversy as to the intranuclear location of this metabolite. The nuclear membrane was one of the first suggestions for the location of the hormone, since its removal with Triton X-100 or with citric acid was associated with a loss of 60–80% of the nuclear hormone content (Stohs and DeLuca, 1967). However, although Triton X-100 denudes the nuclei of the membrane, this detergent has deleterious effects on the chromatin component and thus loss of the hormone from the nuclei cannot be ascribed to removal of the membrane. In addition, nuclear membranes from chick intestine have been isolated and analysed for cholecalciferol metabolites (Lawson and Wilson, 1974). Using rachitic chicks and a dose of cholecalciferol (2.5 μg), sufficient to saturate the intestine with 1,25-dihydroxycholecalciferol, it was found that the nuclear membranes did contain metabolites of the vitamin, but 75% of the total metabolite content of this fraction was due to cholecalciferol and its 25-hydroxy metabolite. At lower doses of cholecalciferol (0.5 μg), only the hormone itself was found in the nuclei, and of this material, only about 1% was associated with the isolated nuclear membranes.

The other suggested site for the intranuclear localisation of the hormone is chromatin (Haussler *et al.*, 1968), but as with the nuclear membranes, subsequent investigations have failed to confirm the original report. The problem arises partly from lack of agreed methods for the preparation of chromatin and partly from a lack of accepted criterion as to the nature of chromatin.

The original report of Haussler *et al.* (1968) described a method for chromatin preparation which resulted in about 70% of the nuclear 1,25-dihydroxycholecalciferol being associated with this fraction. However, as first shown by Chen *et al.* (1970), this chromatin preparation contains a high proportion of nuclear membranes, and in our hands appears to consist more of damaged nuclei than of homogeneous sheets of DNA (Lawson and Wilson, 1974). The object of the procedures used in the preparation of chromatin is not only the removal of the nuclear membranes, but also of nuclear proteins not firmly attached to the DNA. Chromatin can be solubilised by shearing and re-precipitated by adjusting the ionic concentration (Dingman and Sporn, 1964) and such a procedure will establish which proteins are truly associated with the DNA. On applying this procedure to the preparation of chromatin from the intestine of rachitic chicks dosed with radioactive cholecalciferol, a loss of radioactivity was observed at each stage. It can be concluded therefore that although 1,25-dihydroxycholecalciferol is contained within the nuclei, it is not bound to a protein which is closely associated with the DNA. Similar results were obtained with chromatin isolated from bone and kidney. The use of alternative methods of chromatin preparation such as that of Marushige and Bonner (1966) gave essentially the same result. Other investigators have found proportions of 1,25-dihydroxycholecalciferol associated with intestinal chromatin which are intermediate between the two values discussed above (Chen and DeLuca, 1973). Most interestingly, it was reported that over 35% of the nuclear radioactivity was either extranuclear or loosely bound to the nuclei and could be recovered associated with a lipoprotein fraction.

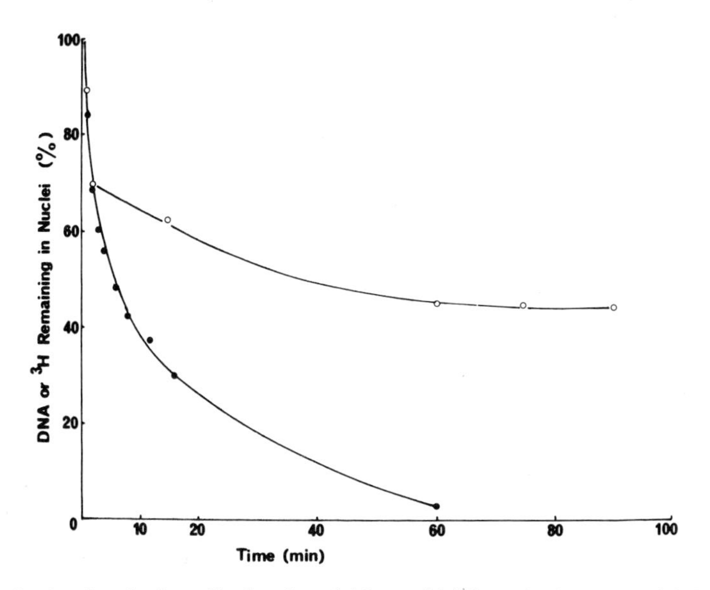

Fig. 1. *In vitro* incubation of isolated nuclei from chick intestinal mucosa with DNase. Nuclei were isolated from intestinal mucosa of rachitic chicks which had received [1,2-^{3}H]cholecalciferol (2.5 μg) and incubated at 37°C with DNase. The amount of DNA and ^{3}H remaining in the nuclear pellet was followed over 90 min. ○, ^{3}H radioactivity; ●, DNA

A possible explanation for the differences reported by these three groups is suggested by the investigations made to explain an observation found repeatedly in this laboratory of a two-fold variation in the level of labelled 1,25-dihydroxycholecalciferol present in nuclei isolated from the intestine of rachitic birds dosed with radioactive cholecalciferol (Lawson and Wilson, 1974). In addition incubation of these nuclei in 0.32 M sucrose in Tris buffer containing 25 mM K^+ and 5 mM Mg^{2+} resulted in a further 24% loss of nuclear radioactivity over 20 min. Although phospholipase, hyaluronidase and RNase released very little of the hormone from intestinal nuclei, significant amounts were released by DNase. The release of the hormone by the DNase was very rapid for 15 min, but appeared to stop after 60 min although DNA hydrolysis was completed by this time (Fig. 1 and Stohs and DeLuca, 1967). As discussed in Section IVE it is now known that nuclear 1,25-dihydroxycholecalciferol is bound to acidic proteins and this protein-hormone complex exists either bound to DNA or free within the nucleoplasm. This latter form may be released under the conditions in which nuclei are normally kept and any damage to the nuclear membrane as would be caused by hydrolysis of the DNA would accelerate this release. The unbound form of the hormone-nuclear protein complex would be released rapidly and the DNA bound form more slowly. Such a situation would explain the variable amounts of hormone observed in the nuclei and the differing recoveries of the hormone in the isolated chromatin.

IV Binding Proteins in Tissues for Cholecalciferol and Metabolites

A PLASMA CHOLECALCIFEROL-BINDING PROTEINS

In common with most other steroids, cholecalciferol and its metabolites circulating in plasma, except perhaps 1,25-dihydroxycholecalciferol, are protein bound. The vitamin activity associated with the various protein fractions was detected in the original observations by standard bioassay procedures and assumed to be due to calciferol (Thomas *et al.*, 1959; see also Crousaz *et al.*, 1965). In later studies, radioactive cholecalciferol was used to investigate this association but in either type of study, both the vitamin D activity and the radioactivity were associated with one of the components of the α-globulin fraction, although occasionally a portion of the steroid has been found with the albumin fraction (Chalk and Kodicek, 1961; Chen and Lane, 1965). Subsequent investigations took a more dynamic approach by following the distribution of radioactivity on the various plasma protein fractions at time intervals after the administration of low doses of radioactive cholecalciferol to rats (Rikkers and DeLuca, 1967). This latter study showed that the association of cholecalciferol with plasma lipoproteins as occasionally observed in the past occurred only at short time intervals after dosing. There was an increasing association of radioactivity with the proteins of the α-globulin fraction, rising from 5% at 0.5 h to a maximum of 8% at 24 h. Similar findings have been reported on the distribution of cholecalciferol on the protein fractions of baboon plasma (Rosenstreich *et al.*, 1971). Following the demonstration that the major form of vitamin D activity in plasma is 25-hydroxycholecalciferol, it was shown that the α-globulin fraction of animals contains a protein with a high affinity specifically for the 25-hydroxy-metabolite.

Specific binding proteins for cholecalciferol itself have been found in the plasma of only a few species of birds (Edelstein *et al.*, 1973; Hay, 1975) and so far there has been no reported instance of their presence in tissues. The search for such binding proteins is hindered by the relative insolubility of the vitamin in aqueous solutions and the resulting tendency of this steroid to form micelles or adhere to the surface of the apparatus. Consequently it has not been possible to construct displacement curves for cholecalciferol with potential

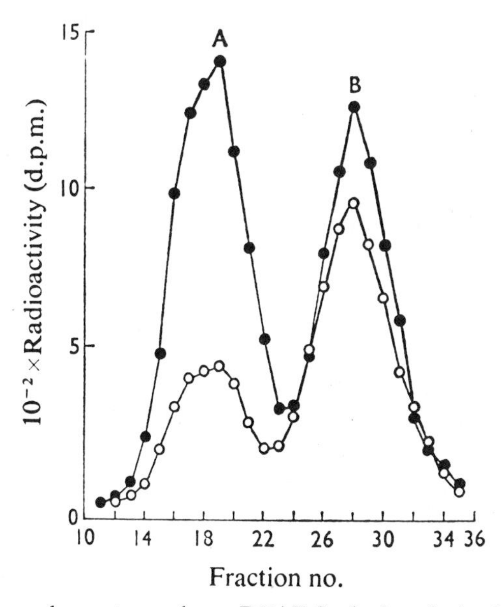

Fig. 2. Ion exchange chromatography on DEAE-Sephadex of mixed samples of serum of chicks given a dose of either [26-^{3}H]25-hydroxycholecalciferol (0.5 μg) or [4-^{14}C]cholecalciferol (2.5 μg). The serum was chromatographed on Sephadex G-200 and this was followed by ion-exchange chromatography. 2.5 ml fractions were collected and the gradient was 0–0.3 M NaCl in 0.02 M sodium phosphate buffer, pH7.6. ○, ^{14}C radioactivity; ●, ^{3}H radioactivity; A, 25-hydroxycholecalciferol-binding protein; B, cholecalciferol-binding protein

binding proteins as the usual techniques for the separation of protein bound cholecalciferol from the unbound or free form are ineffective. Nevertheless, it does seem that birds contain a cholecalciferol-binding protein in their circulation and a similar claim has subsequently been made for human plasma (Belsey *et al.*, 1974a). The plasma proteins of chicks can be fractionated by chromatography on DEAE-Sephadex to give two protein fractions with binding activity *in vitro* for both cholecalciferol and its 25-hydroxy-metabolite. However, experiments on the metabolism *in vivo* of [4-^{14}C] cholecalciferol and [26-^{3}H] 25-hydroxycholecalciferol showed that one of these proteins was primarily responsible for the transport of the vitamin in chick plasma and presumably the other protein is a specific carrier for the 25-hydroxy-metabolite (Edelstein *et al.*, 1973). Thus some 8 h after the administration to rachitic chicks of these labelled steroids, one plasma protein (A, Fig. 2) contained primarily ^{3}H with only a small quantity of ^{14}C present due to [^{14}C] 25-hydroxycholecalciferol formed from the administered ^{14}C labelled vitamin. Consequently all the labelled cholecalciferol in chick plasma was associated with peak B. [^{3}H] 25-Hydroxycholecalciferol was found associated with both proteins but since they both have a high affinity for this metabolite, it may have become distributed between the two proteins during analysis. These two chick plasma proteins have been isolated and purified; the molecular weight of the cholecalciferol-binding protein was found to be 60 000 and the sedimentation constant to be 3.5S.

The function of this binding protein has recently been established by Fraser and Emtage (1976). In the absence of any regulatory mechanism it would be expected that the pattern of metabolites of cholecalciferol in eggs would reflect the pattern in the hen plasma. However, egg yolk primarily contains cholecalciferol with only a small quantity of the 25-hydroxy-metabolite. In addition the plasma cholecalciferol-binding protein is present in the yolk but not the 25-hydroxycholecalciferol binding protein. An association of the cholecalciferol-binding protein with the egg yolk protein, particularly phosvitin, in the plasma was also observed and Fraser and Emtage have suggested that the cholecalciferol was accumulated by the egg through an association of its specific binding protein with the yolk protein in the formation of the egg.

B PLASMA 25-HYDROXYCHOLECALCIFEROL-BINDING PROTEIN

The levels of plasma 25-hydroxycholecalciferol are related primarily to the intake of cholecalciferol whether this intake is derived from the diet or sunlight. However, at intakes generally prevailing for man the majority of the biological activity in plasma is attributable to 25-hydroxycholecalciferol and as explained in the previous section this metabolite is associated in animals with the plasma globulins (but see Section IVB3). Reports have appeared of the characteristics of these binding proteins in the plasma of a number of species with claims for the purification and partial purification of the binding proteins from man and chick respectively. There is only one binding protein in the plasma of mammals and, except in a very few species, the electrophoretic mobility is that of an α-globulin. The best estimates of the concentration of this protein in human plasma (250–500 μg/ml) are such that at 25-hydroxycholecalciferol levels generally found (less than 50 μg/ml, depending on the nationality of the people being surveyed), only 2% of the binding sites on this protein are occupied by the metabolite. Even when allowances are made for the other metabolites of cholecalciferol in plasma and for the higher levels of 25-hydroxycholecalciferol which can on occasion be found there still remains a very high 25-hydroxycholecalciferol carrying capacity apparently unused. This observation is one of the more puzzling features of the plasma 25-hydroxycholecalciferol-binding protein.

Nevertheless this binding protein is typical of those in the general class of steroid binding proteins. The uptake of the steroid by the protein is rapid and saturable, and the association constant indicates that high affinity sites are involved. The features of the steroid molecules which are necessary for binding activity have been recorded (Belsey *et al.*, 1974a). The three double bonds of the molecule are essential with the C-7,8 and C-10,19 bonds being *cis* to the C-5,6 double bond. A hydroxyl group at C-25 is also required but binding activity is only slightly reduced by the presence of other hydroxyl groups at adjacent carbon atoms such as in 24,25- and 25,26- dihydroxy-cholecalciferol (Fig. 3).

The binding protein from rat plasma has been used by several groups to develop a standard competitive protein binding assay for 25-hydroxycholecalciferol (Belsey *et al.*, 1971; Edelstein *et al.*, 1974; Preece *et al.*, 1974). For the most accurate estimation of the plasma 25-hydroxycholecalciferol levels it is necessary to isolate the steroid by appropriate chromatographic procedures but recently methods have been described which omit this step (Belsey *et al.*, 1974b; Garcia *et al.*, 1976). These later methods give only an approximate value for 25-hydroxycholecalciferol levels since they measure other dihydroxy-metabolites of cholecalciferol but they may be of value in large scale surveys for assessment of vitamin D status.

A summary of the characteristics of the 25-hydroxycholecalciferol binding proteins in plasma of various species is presented in the following sections.

1. *Man.* The first attempt to characterise a plasma carrier protein for cholecalciferol from animal plasma was made by Peterson (1971) before it was appreciated that 25-hydroxycholecalciferol was the major form of vitamin D activity in plasma. Starting with 30 litres of outdated human plasma, he

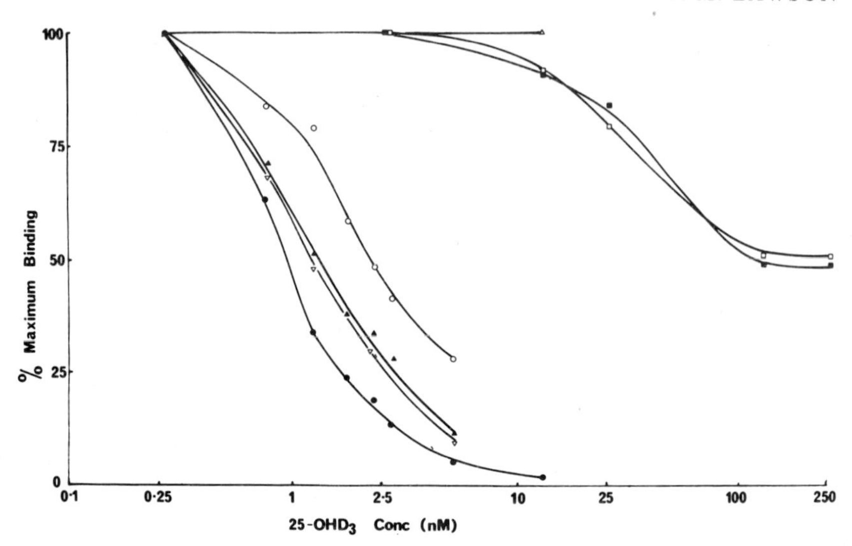

Fig. 3. Competition for the 25-hydroxycholecalciferol binding sites on rat plasma proteins by metabolites of cholecalciferol (D. E. M. Lawson, unpublished observations). Diluted plasma was incubated with [^{3}H]25-hydroxycholecalciferol and increasing amounts of steroids and the bound steroid separated from the free by dextran-coated charcoal; ●, 25-hydroxycholecalciferol; ▽, 24,25-dihydroxycholecalciferol; ▲, 25,26-dihydroxycholecalciferol; ○, 25-hydroxy-27-norcholecalciferol; △, 25-hydroxyisotachysterol; 25,-hydroxy-5,6-transcholecalciferol; ■, 1-hydroxycholecalciferol; □, cholecalciferol

isolated by a succession of standard procedures a total of 7.2 mg of purified cholecalciferol-binding protein (approximate recovery of 10%). The calciferol-binding protein was followed throughout these procedures by labelling the protein with a small quantity of ^{14}C-cholecalciferol. Although a high degree of purification was achieved by these column chromatographic procedures, the preparation was resolved by polyacrylamide electrophoresis into two components only one of which had ^{14}C-cholecalciferol attached. Peterson concluded that he was dealing with only one protein since addition of cholecalciferol to the protein in the band which did not have ^{14}C attached to it caused its electrophoretic mobility to become identical to that of the ^{14}C-labelled protein. In addition immunological techniques showed the two proteins to have antigenic determinants in common. The molecular weight of the isolated protein was established by three distinct methods and gave an average value of 52 300 and the sedimentation constant was found to be 3.8S. The electrophoretic mobility was similar to that of an α_1 globulin. Other estimates have been made of the physical properties of the binding protein in human plasma, but using labelled 25-hydroxycholecalciferol to identify the carrier protein. A molecular weight of 50 000–60 000 has been reported (Smith and Goodman, 1971) which is within the range reported by Peterson for his protein, but the electrophoretic mobility was faster than albumin. On the other hand Haddad and Chyu (1971) found the molecular weight to be 40 000–45 000, the electrophoretic mobility to be that of an α-globulin and the sedimentation constant to be 3.1S.

An interesting development in the characterisation of the binding protein was recently reported by Daiger *et al.* (1975). Substantial information has been provided by these investigators that the calciferol-binding protein of plasma is identical with group-specific component (Gc) proteins. The protein preparation isolated by Peterson was reported not to contain Gc protein although the electrophoretic mobility and the behaviour in various chromatographic systems of the two proteins was found to be similar. A physiological role for the Gc protein has not so far been proposed, and although most information on this protein comes from studies made with human plasma a similar protein has been reported in other species. Two alleles, Gc^1 and Gc^2 for these proteins are found in all human populations, with a frequency of 0.75 for Gc^1 and 0.25 for Gc^2. The products of the two alleles, proteins Gc1 and Gc2, can be separated electrophoretically and in one study the proteins were found in 75 000 individuals. Using electrophoretic techniques developed for the separation of the Gc1 and Gc2 proteins, Daiger and coworkers found that the proteins of human plasma which had been labelled *in vitro* with ^{14}C cholecalciferol could be separated into two components. Examination of the number and electrophoretic mobility of the proteins containing the ^{14}C-cholecalciferol in the plasma of 80 Caucasians showed three distinct patterns. In some persons two ^{14}C labelled protein bands were observed while in others only one of these two bands was present. The calciferol-binding genotype for this group of people can be determined if the pattern is assumed to be due to two homozygotes and a single heterozygote for a two allele autosomal locus (Daiger *et al.*, 1975). The gene frequencies were found to be 0.73 and 0.27 and as for Gc proteins the allele coding for the electrophoretically faster protein was the more common. Support for the identical nature of the Gc protein and the cholecalciferol-binding protein was provided by radioprecipitation and immunoelectrophoretic techniques.

Although most of the experiments reported by Daiger *et al.* (1975) were carried out using ^{14}C-cholecalciferol these investigators did show that the use of tritium labelled 25-hydroxycholecalciferol also resulted in an association of the radioactivity with the Gc protein. The similarity in gene frequency studies for the calciferol-binding protein and for Gc protein coupled with the immunological cross-reaction between the anti-Gc protein and the calciferol-binding proteins provide strong evidence that the two proteins are identical. On the other hand the claim by Peterson (1971) to have removed the Gc protein in his preparation makes these two reports difficult to reconcile. Nevertheless subsequent investigations have isolated and characterised the 25-hydroxycholecalciferol-binding protein and compared it to the known characteristics of Gc protein (Bouillon *et al.*, 1976; Imawari *et al.*, 1976). The evidence is becoming convincing that the well-known plasma Gc protein is the carrier for these steroids. It is perhaps worth noting at this point that Belsey *et al.* (1974a) have claimed that human plasma contains two binding proteins for cholecalciferol but only one for its 25-hydroxylated-metabolite. Using lipoprotein free plasma they have resolved the cholecalciferol-binding proteins into two components on both gel-electrophoresis and gel-filtration chromatography. One of these proteins with an electrophoretic mobility similar to albumin could bind the vitamin but not its metabolite whereas the other protein with α-globulin mobility bound both steroids.

2. *Chick*. The only other binding protein from plasma for which physical properties have been reported is that from chick (Edelstein *et al.*, 1972, 1973). The 25-hydroxycholecalciferol-binding protein from the plasma of this species has been purified using standard procedures. The protein has a molecular weight of approximately 54 000, a sedimentation constant of 3.5S and an electrophoretic mobility similar to that of the β-globulins. The association constant for the reaction of this protein with the 25-hydroxy-metabolite was 3×10^8 M^{-1}.

It is of course well known that ergocalciferol is much less potent than cholecalciferol in preventing or curing rickets in chicks. The reported values for the relative potencies of these two forms of vitamin D activity range from 1 to 10% (Chen and Bosman, 1964; Hibberd and Norman, 1969). Part of the reason for the relative ineffectiveness of ergocalciferol may lie in the observation reported by Belsey *et al.* (1974c) that 15 times more 25-hydroxyergocalciferol than 25-hydroxycholecalciferol was required to effect 50% displacement of tritiated 25-hydroxycholecalciferol from the plasma-binding protein. These authors suggest that the lower affinity of protein for ergocalciferol and its metabolite may result in a lowered efficiency of the hepatic and renal hydroxylation reactions. Whatever the reason for the relative ineffectiveness of ergocalciferol in chicks similar observations have been made on the relative affinities of these two forms of vitamin D for the binding protein from the plasma of the new world monkeys. This species of animal also responds poorly to ergocalciferol (Hunt *et al.*, 1967).

3. *Other Species*. 25-Hydroxycholecalciferol-binding proteins have been recognised in the plasma of a wide range of species (Edelstein *et al.*, 1973; Belsey *et al.*, 1974a), with the particularly extensive series reported by Hay (1975) and Hay and Watson (1976a, b). In species such as rat, pig and old-world monkeys (Erythrocebus patas) it seems clear that a single protein carries both cholecalciferol and its 25-hydroxy-metabolite (Edelstein *et al.*,

1973). Two groups of rats were injected with either ^{14}C cholecalciferol or [26-^{3}H] 25-hydroxycholecalciferol and the plasma obtained when both the vitamin and its metabolite were bound to the plasma proteins. After fractionating the protein by either gel filtration chromatography, or gel electrophoresis only a single peak of radioactivity was observed with a constant $^{3}H/^{14}C$ ratio throughout the peak (Edelstein *et al.*, 1973).

The binding protein from plasma of most animals has the electrophoretic mobility of an α-globulin, but there are at least seven exceptions in which the 25-hydroxycholecalciferol carrier is either albumin or a protein with very similar properties to albumin. The plasma protein with which the 25-hydroxycholecalciferol associates could not be separated from albumin by either gel filtration chromatography, ion exchange chromatography or iso-electric focusing (Edelstein *et al.*, 1973; Hay, 1975). In addition to the three species of new-world monkeys which use albumin or an albumin like protein as the carrier there are also four other species namely the African elephant (*Loxodonea africana*), the Indian elephant (*Elephas maximus*), the Pacific Dolphin (*Delphinus bairdi*) and the killer whale (*Orcinus orca*).

Birds show the largest variation in the class of protein used as a carrier for 25-hydroxycholecalciferol (Table 1) since proteins with the mobility of α- and β-globulins and of albumin are used by some species of birds. However, only three species of bird resemble the domestic chicken (*Gallus gallus*) in having two proteins, both with β-globulin mobility, as carriers for these steroids. Proteins showing the mobility on gel electrophoresis of α-globulins are used by the widest range of species from boney fish, including coelocanth, to reptiles, birds and mammals (61 species from 14 mammalian orders). The last type of binding protein for 25-hydroxycholecalciferol which has been recognised is

Table 1. Classes of vertebrate 25-hydroxycholecalciferol-binding proteins

Species	Electrophoretic mobility
Fish	
cartilagenous	Lipoproteins (4)
bony	α-Globulin (18)
Amphibia	Lipoproteins (12)
Reptiles	α-Globulin (5)
Birds	α-(3) and β-Globulins (12)
	Albumin (4)
Mammals	α-Globulin (65)
	Albumin (7)

Figures in parentheses indicate the number of species in each class (taken from Hay and Watson, 1975)

lipo-protein, an observation first made with the toad (*Xenopus laevis*). The use of these rather non-specific proteins as carriers for 25-hydroxycholecalciferol extends to other amphibians and to at least 3 cartilagenous fish (Hay and Watson, 1976a, b).

C PLASMA 1,25-DIHYDROXYCHOLECALCIFEROL-BINDING PROTEIN

Good evidence for a specific plasma protein with a high affinity for 1,25-dihydroxycholecalciferol has been difficult to find (Lawson, unpublished). Plasma has been incubated with tritiated 1,25-dihydroxycholecalciferol to allow the steroid to interact with the proteins which have then been fractionated by a number of techniques including gel electrophoresis, ion exchange chromatography and sucrose gradient centrifugation. In all cases the protein to which the radioactivity was bound could not be separated from the 25-hydroxycholecalciferol-binding protein. Similar results were obtained with plasma from rats injected with labelled cholecalciferol, i.e. binding of the hormone to the plasma proteins occurred *in vivo* during or immediately after its formation. Since it seemed possible that the α-globulin with 25-hydroxycholecalciferol binding activity was also the carrier for the hormone the binding characteristics of the protein for these two steroids have been compared.

The protein fraction from rat plasma with binding activity for the calciferol metabolites was partially purified, and shown to bind up to two hundred times more of the 25-hydroxy-metabolite than of the hormone per unit weight of protein. The protein fraction shows saturable binding activity for 25-hydroxycholecalciferol but not for the hormone. In addition the K_a for the reaction of the protein with 25-hydroxycholecalciferol was $9 \times 10^{10} \mathrm{M}^{-1}$ whereas with 1,25-dihydroxycholecalciferol the K_a was $5 \times 10^{7} \mathrm{M}^{-1}$. In competition experiments the hormone could not displace the 25-hydroxy-cholecalciferol from its binding sites on the protein but interestingly the latter metabolite could not displace the hormone either. Accordingly 1-25-dihydroxycholecalciferol does not bind to the 25-hydroxycholecalciferol binding sites on this protein and indeed the low K_a and lack of saturable binding activity suggests that this protein is not a carrier protein for the hormone even if it is the protein on which the hormone is found when plasma proteins are fractionated. Attempts to show by the equilibrium dialysis technique that the 1,25-dihydroxycholecalciferol in plasma is protein bound have been unsuccessful since at the end of the dialysis procedure the hormone is always found attached to the dialysis bag or membrane. Other means are therefore required to show that 1,25-dihydroxycholecalciferol in plasma is protein bound.

D TISSUE 25-HYDROXYCHOLECALCIFEROL RECEPTOR PROTEINS

Evidence has been accumulating over the past ten years that in almost all steroid hormone sensitive systems the response to the hormone requires the presence of a cytoplasmic binding protein, frequently referred to as a receptor protein. It was therefore somewhat surprising to find binding activity for 25-hydroxycholecalciferol in the cytoplasm of tissues in spite of the lack of evidence that this steroid has a function of its own in these tissues (Lawson and Emtage, 1975; Haddad and Birge, 1975; Lawson *et al.*, 1976). Proteins have been recognised as the source of this binding-activity and can be found in all cell types and in plasma of both rachitic and normal chicks and rats. The only

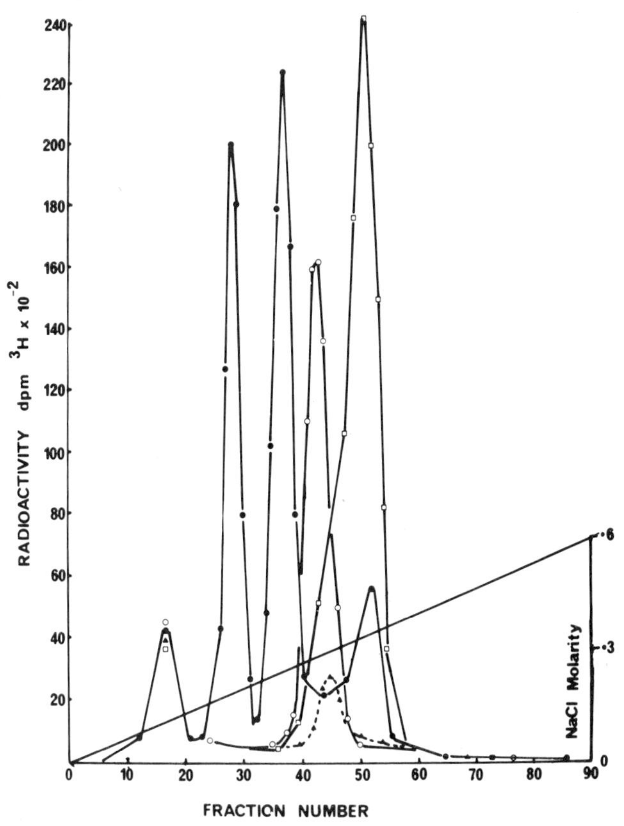

Fig. 4. Chromatography on DEAE-Sephadex of cytosols of chick tissues after incubation with [26-^{3}H] 25-hydroxycholecalciferol. The tissue cytosols (0.2 μg of protein) were incubated with 2.7×10^{-10} M [26-^{3}H]25-hydroxycholecalciferol and the unbound steroid removed with dextran-coated charcoal. ●, serum; ▲, mucosa; ○, muscle; □, skin.

cell type which does not seem to possess these receptor proteins is the erythrocyte. The physical properties of these binding proteins showed them to be quite distinct from the other binding proteins for the metabolites of cholecalciferol which have been described, namely the plasma 25-hydroxycholecalciferol-binding protein and the binding protein in tissues for 1,25-dihydroxycholecalciferol. The evidence for this view is based on the behaviour of these proteins on ion-exchange chromatography, gel-electrophoresis and sucrose gradient centrifugation. Some of the properties of these binding proteins from various sources are recorded in Table 2. It is not yet clear, however, whether the same binding protein for 25-hydroxycholecalciferol is present in all the tissues as there are some minor differences in the chromatographic profiles obtained when cytosols from various tissues with bound tritiated 25-hydroxycholecalciferol were fractionated separately on DEAE-Sephadex (Fig. 4). These differences are insufficient, however, to effect a separation by this system of a mixture of these binding proteins. The interaction of the 25-hydroxycholecalciferol with the tissue cytosols was found to consist of an initial uptake of the steroid for 15–20 min, followed by a slower uptake, until by 60 min the maximum amount of steroid had been bound. Analysis of this interaction showed that the binding protein was saturable at relatively low concentrations of steroid. More detailed analysis established that in some tissues, for example muscle, skin and kidney, the

Table 2. Some characteristics of the binding proteins for calciferol and metabolites in some tissues of chicks and rats

	Chick				Rat		
	Plasma		Tissues	Intestine	Plasma	Tissues	Intestine
	D^3	25-OHD_3	25-OHD_3	1,25-$(OH)_2D_3$	25-OHD_3	25-OHD_3	1,25-$(OH)_2D_3$
Ka	–	3×10^{8}[a]	2.5×10^{9}[b]	1.5×10^{9}[d]	8×10^{9}[e]	7.2×10[h]	N.D.
S	3.5– 4.0[a]	3.5–4.0[a]	5.0[b]	3.5[d]	4.0[f]	6.0[h]	5.0[c]
M.W.	60 000[a]	54 000[a]	N.D.	47 000[g]	52 000[f]	N.D.	76 000[c]
E.M.	1.0[a]	0.8[a]	0.65[e]	N.D.	1.0[b]	0.8[b]	N.D.

This information is taken from the following publications:
[a] Edelstein *et al.*, 1973
[b] Lawson *et al.*, 1976. [c] Frolick and DeLuca, 1976
[d] Lawson and Wilson, 1974
[e] Lawson, unpublished observations
[f] Botham and DeLuca (1976) on the basis that this protein is indistinguishable from the inhibitor of the kidney 1-hydroxylase (chapter 2, 11B)
[g] Brumbaugh and Haussler, 1975
[h] Haddad and Birge, 1975
N.D., not determined
E.M., electrophoretic mobility

Table 3. Association constants of 25-hydroxycholecalciferol-binding protein in rat and chick tissues

Tissue	Chick	Rat
	Assoc. Constant ($M^{-1} \times 10^9$)	Assoc. Constant ($M^{-1} \times 10^9$)
Plasma (A)	0.43	7.2
(B)	0.30	—
Intestine	3.05	3.1
Liver	3.45	2.2
Kidney	3.57	1.1
Muscle	4.58	1.7
Skin	2.83	1.0
Spleen	2.50	—
Eye	2.13	—
Pancreas	4.61	—
Brain	4.38	—
Bone	—	4.0

The proportion of [26-^{3}H] 25-hydroxycholecalciferol bound by the proteins of the tissue cytosols in the presence of increasing amounts of the steroid was measured and the displacement curves analysed (Lawson *et al.*, 1976)

interaction primarily involved high affinity sites whereas with other tissues, such as intestine and liver both high and low affinity sites were involved. The association constant for the reaction between 25-hydroxycholecalciferol and the high affinity sites in the chick tissues varied between $2\text{–}5 \times 10^9\ M^{-1}$ (Table 3).

The features of the steroid molecule necessary for binding to these proteins have been examined by comparing the displacement of tritiated 25-hydroxycholecalciferol effected by various analogues of cholecalciferol. Binding activity was virtually lost by the removal of the hydroxyl group at C-25, but it was almost unaffected by insertion of another hydroxyl group at an adjacent carbon atom, as in the compounds 24,25- and 25,26-dihydroxycholecalciferol. The configuration of the double bond system also seems to be critical in that 5,6-*trans* cholecalciferol, isocholecalciferol and isotachysterol$_3$ had very little replacement activity. It seems clear from these studies that all tissues of both rats and chicks contain a protein distinct from 1,25-dihydroxycholecalciferol receptor protein and which, although it has a high affinity for 25-hydroxycholecalciferol, is nevertheless not the binding protein in plasma for this metabolite (Section IVB). But whether 25-hydroxycholecalciferol is the specific ligand for this protein under physiological conditions is still an open question. The existence of this receptor protein raises stimulating questions as to its function. The presence in virtually all tissues of such a receptor for 25-hydroxycholecalciferol or a metabolite of a similar chemical structure implies that the steroid affects a process common to all cells. As the binding protein is present in the cell nuclei it appears that the function of this ligand, as with other steroids, may be to regulate the synthesis of tissue specific proteins. Such a protein may possibly be involved in regulating aspects of calcium metabolism which are a feature of all cells. The binding proteins ubiquitous nature implies a role for the ligand in a more general aspect of cell metabolism than it has been customary to associate with the function of calciferol.

E INTESTINAL 1,25-DIHYDROXYCHOLECALCIFEROL RECEPTOR PROTEINS

As expected from the hormonal nature of 1,25-dihydroxycholecalciferol, binding proteins for this steroid have been found in the cytoplasm and nuclei of intestinal cells (Haussler and Norman, 1969; Tsai and Norman, 1973; Brumbaugh and Haussler 1973; Lawson and Wilson, 1974; Oku *et al.*, 1974). At present there are no reports on these receptors in other target tissues such as kidney and bone.

The receptor proteins for the other steroid hormones have been the subject of much investigation and their physical characteristics and their properties in different systems have been well described (e.g. Liao, 1975). In the majority of cases the cytoplasmic protein with a high affinity for the hormone can, under the appropriate conditions, undergo a conformational change so as to produce a protein, recognisable by its smaller sedimentation constant, which is indistinguishable from the receptor protein in the target tissue nuclei. This reversible conversion between the form of the receptor in the cytoplasm and the form in the nucleus, can be effected *in vitro* by altering the concentration of KCl in the system. It appears that in the cell the transfer of the steroid hormone into the nucleus involves the uptake of the cytoplasmic protein-hormone complex with the simultaneous transformation of the protein component into the nuclear form. This mechanism, by which the nuclei takes up the hormone, is often a temperature dependent process.

The nuclear receptors for 1,25-dihydroxycholecalciferol in the intestine can be solubilised by extracting nuclear fractions with buffers containing up to 0.6 M KCl. Such an extract shows saturable binding activity for 1,25-dihydroxycholecalciferol when incubated with the hormone *in vitro* (Lawson and Emtage, 1974; Lawson and Wilson, 1974). For such a nuclear extract to show binding activity for a steroid hormone is unusual since in almost all other systems binding of the hormone by the nuclear components is only apparent when the nuclei are incubated with hormone in the presence of the cytoplasmic receptor. Nevertheless this particular nuclear component showing binding activity for 1,25-dihydroxycholecalciferol seems to have the characteristics expected of one which is involved in the physiological response of the intestine to the hormone. Its macromolecular nature was shown by its behaviour on gel filtration chromatography, its precipitation with ammonium sulphate and position after centrifugation through a sucrose gradient. In addition its protein nature was indicated by loss of binding activity following treatment with proteolytic enzymes whereas RNase and DNase had no effect on binding activity. It has also been observed that the sedimentation constant for the binding protein in the nuclear extract is the same as the protein to which the hormone is bound *in vivo*. Other features of the nuclear receptor protein which indicate its physiological importance include its high affinity for the hormone ($K_a 1.5 \times 10^9$ M^{-1}) and analysis of this binding activity showed that the number of sites in the intestinal nuclei due to this high affinity receptor is sufficient to bind the hormone up to a concentration of 2.4 pmoles/g of tissue. This is the amount of hormone bound to the receptor when saturated and is close to the maximum amount of 1,25-dihydroxycholecalciferol which the intestinal nuclei can accumulate *in vivo*. A further indication of the importance of this type of receptor in the physiological response to the hormone is provided by the finding of a similar binding activity in extracts of kidney nuclei but such activity was not found in extracts of liver and muscle nuclei.

Other investigations have taken the more traditional approach and studied the binding of the hormone to the nuclei in the presence of the cytoplasm. The importance of the cytoplasmic component in the transfer of the hormone to the nucleus was established in experiments such as those by Tsai and Norman (1973) and Brumbaugh and Haussler (1974). Intestinal nuclei in the presence of cytosols from liver, kidney and spleen take up 44% of that accumulated in the presence of intestinal cytosols. This transfer is temperature dependent (Fig. 5). On incubating intestinal tissue with the hormone for 40 min at 0°C approximately 75% of the 1,25-dihydroxycholecalciferol is in the cytosol but on raising the temperature to 37°C only 50% of the hormone is in the cytosol fraction and after 30 min over 80% has been accumulated by the nuclei.

Evidence from experiments similar to those applied to the nuclear receptor showed that the cytoplasmic component with a high affinity for the 1,25-dihydroxycholecalciferol was also a protein. The association constant for this component is also 10^9 M^{-1}. Interestingly the sedimentation constant of both the nuclear and cytoplasmic receptors are the same and this may explain why the nuclear protein can bind the hormone *in vitro* since the uptake by the nuclei does not involve a conformational change of a receptor–protein–hormone complex.

A number of studies have considered the specificity of these receptors for

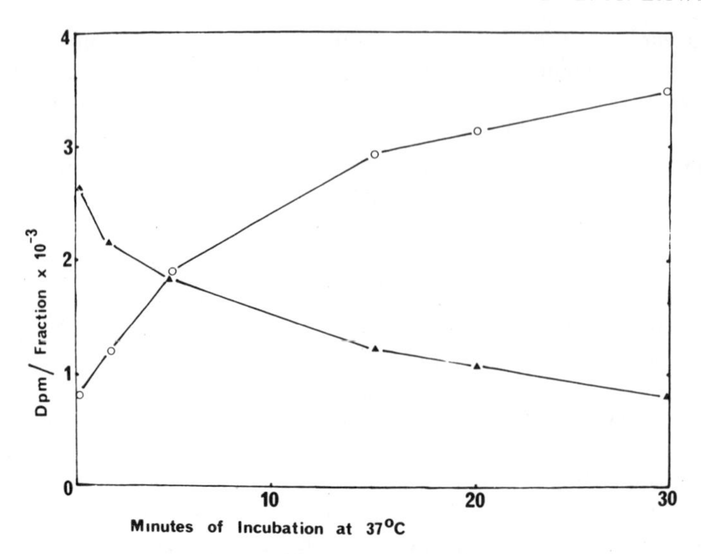

Fig. 5. Transfer of 1,25-dihydroxycholecalciferol from cytosol to nuclei at 37°C. Chick intestines were incubated with the hormone (120 pmoles) at 0°C for 40 min and then transferred into hormone-free medium at 37°C. At time intervals thereafter radioactivity in the cytosol and chromatin fractions was measured. ▲, cytosol radioactivity; ○, chromatin radioactivity (Brumbaugh and Haussler, 1974)

steroids of the calciferol type. The extent to which the features of the cholecalciferol molecule influence the binding affinity of the hormone with the cytoplasmic receptor is not as absolute as expected from the observation that 25-hydroxycholecalciferol is inactive in anephoric rats. Part of the problem in examining the specificity of the cytoplasmic receptor for 1,25-dihydroxycholecalciferol is the presence of an excess of the 25-hydroxycholecalciferol receptor. However, when care is taken to examine only the binding to the cytoplasmic 1,25-dihydroxycholecalciferol receptor, the importance of a C-25-hydroxyl-group and of an intact tri-ene system was apparent (Brumbaugh and Haussler, 1974). Recently a study of the ability of a wide range of different secosteroids to compete with 1,25-dihydroxycholecalciferol for the high affinity binding sites in the nuclei has been published (Procsal *et al.*, 1975).

V Response of Intestinal Protein Synthesis to Cholecalciferol Metabolites

A INTRODUCTION

There are a number of pieces of evidence that the action of calciferol in the intestine is explicable in the main on the basis of an effect of 1,25-

dihydroxycholecalciferol on DNA transcription in the intestinal nuclei. Thus in rachitic animals dosed with radioactive cholecalciferol the majority of the radioactivity in the intestine is 1,25-dihydroxycholecalciferol and in normal animals approximately 30% of the substances derived from calciferol in the intestine is due to the hormone. Furthermore, the 1,25-dihydroxycholecalciferol is accumulated in the nuclei of the intestine and its action can be prevented by inhibitors of protein synthesis particularly actinomycin D and α-amanitin. 1,25-Dihydroxycholecalciferol is the most potent of the substances so far recognised to be able to stimulate calcium transport and in addition it has the most rapid onset of action. Nephrectomised animals or animals dosed with Sr^{2+} cannot produce 1,25-dihydroxycholecalciferol from its biosynthetic precursors and consequently, the stimulation of calcium absorption observed after cholecalciferol administration is not apparent. In contrast there are other conditions such as a low calcium diet, which result in a stimulation of 1,25-dihydroxycholecalciferol production and thereby an increase in the proportion of dietary calcium absorbed. The following section reviews the progress which has been made in the attempts to describe the molecular basis of the action of 1,25-dihydroxycholecalciferol in the intestine.

B RNA TURNOVER AND RNA POLYMERASE ACTIVITY

Actinomycin D binds to the guanine residue of DNA providing it is in a helical configuration, thereby inhibiting all DNA-dependent RNA synthesis. Other antibiotics are known which prevent the synthesis of specific types of RNA, in particular α-amanitin which prevents the synthesis specifically of messenger RNA. Neither of these inhibitors allows the intestine and/or the bone to respond to cholecalciferol (Eisenstein and Passavoy, 1964; Zull *et al.*, 1965; Norman, 1965; Corradino, 1973). Following the discovery of 1,25-dihydroxycholecalciferol and its synthesis in the kidney, there has been some controversy as to whether this inhibition is at the site of synthesis of the hormone or at its site of action. Reports have appeared showing that actinomycin D treatment decreased the intestinal level of 1,25-dihydroxycholecalciferol by 84% in rats and 50% in birds (Tanaka and DeLuca, 1971; Gray and DeLuca, 1971). Other tissues were similarly affected. In addition it was claimed that actinomycin D did not inhibit the 1,25-dihydroxycholecalciferol-stimulated calcium absorption in rat intestine (Tanaka *et al.*, 1971). Other groups, however, have not been able to confirm either of these findings, at least in the chick (Tsai *et al.*, 1973; Lawson and Emtage, 1974; see also chapter 3, III). In this species the evidence presently available seems to convincingly show that at least one action of 1,25-dihydroxycholecalciferol is to regulate the transcription of that portion of intestinal DNA containing the code for calcium-binding protein (CaBP) and the studies on the relationship of cholecalciferol and its 1,25-dihydroxy-metabolite with intestinal RNA is consistent with this view. The total amount of intestinal RNA is unaffected by the vitamin D-status of the birds, being approximately 9 mg/g of the tissue. However, there is an increased incorporation of [5-^{3}H] orotic acid and of ^{3}H-uridine into RNA in response to cholecalciferol (Norman, 1966; Lawson *et al.*, 1969b) and in response to 1,25-dihydroxycholecalciferol (Tsai *et al.*, 1973). Although the effect of antibiotics in the rat on 1,25-dihydroxycholecalciferol activity is not consistent with an effect on RNA synthesis there is nevertheless an increased incorporation of [8-^{3}H] orotic acid into rat intestinal RNA (Stohs *et al.*, 1967).

An increase in RNA polymerase activity might be expected to accompany this increased incorporation of nucleotide precursors into RNA although as there is no net synthesis of RNA and as the earliest response to the vitamin involves *de novo* synthesis of only one or two proteins, such an increase might be marginal and involve only the DNA-dependent RNA polymerase II. Only this latter polymerase synthesises messenger RNA, polymerase I being responsible for the synthesis of ribosomal RNA. The first measurement of the variations in the activity of this enzyme in response to cholecalciferol seemed to show a small decrease in activity of both polymerase I and II (Lawson *et al.*, 1969b; Iotoya *et al.*, 1971). Subsequently diurnal variations in the activity of both RNA polymerase I and II were shown (Glasser and Spellsburgh, 1972),

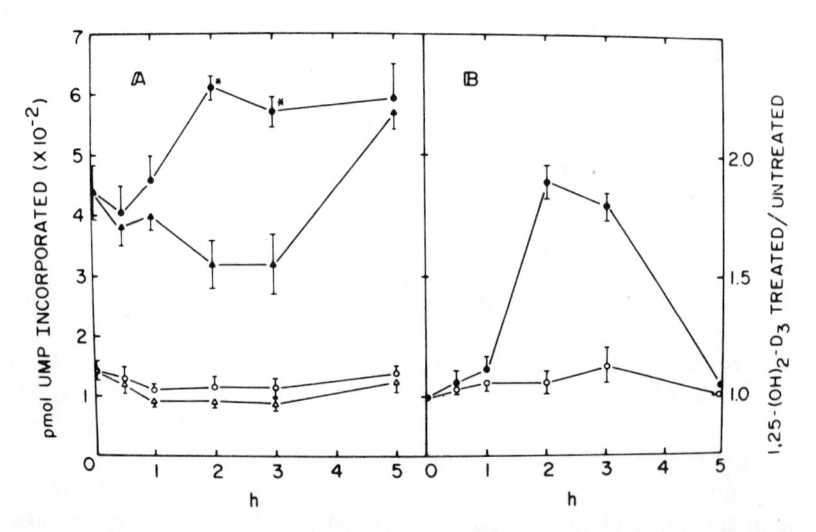

Fig. 6. Time course of activity of chick intestinal RNA polymerase I and II after oral 1,25-dihydroxycholecalciferol (0.27 μg). A, Activity of RNA polymerase I of sterol-treated (○—○) and rachitic (△—△) and for polymerase II on sterol-treated (●—●) and rachitic (▲—▲) birds. B, Ratio of enzyme II (●—●) and emzyme I (○—○) for hormone-treated birds to non-treated controls (Zerwekh *et al.*, 1974)

allowance for which revealed a two-fold stimulation in RNA polymerase II but not polymerase I in response to the hormone (Zerwekh *et al.*, 1974). This stimulation was observed within 2–3 h after a dose of 0.27 μg of 1,25-dihydroxycholecalciferol and the enzyme activity had returned to normal values by 5–9 h after dosing with hormone (Fig. 6). These results are consistent with an effect of 1,25-dihydroxycholecalciferol on messenger RNA formation in intestinal mucosal cells.

C CALCIUM-BINDING PROTEIN: ITS SYNTHESIS ON INTESTINAL POLYSOMES AND CHARACTERISATION OF ITS mRNA

Undegraded polysomes can be isolated from the intestine providing that appropriate inhibitors of the potent intestinal RNase, such as heparin and rat liver cell sap, are included in the homogenisation buffers. The preparation

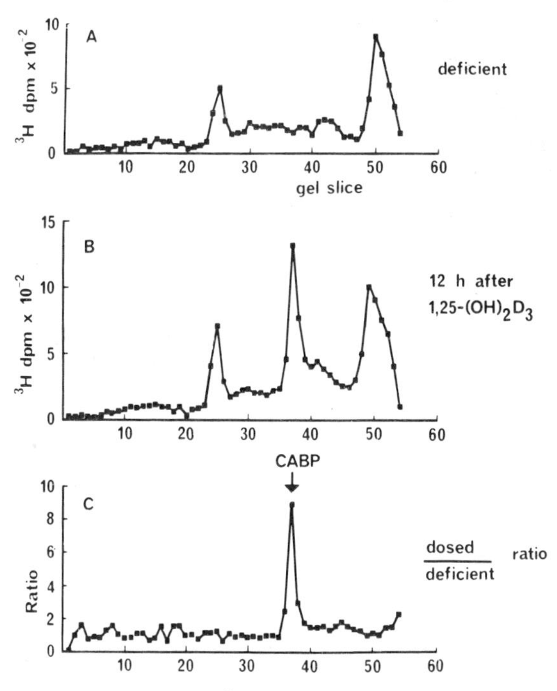

Fig. 7. SDS-gel electrophoreses of ^{3}H-polypeptides synthesised by the wheat germ system primed with intestinal polysomal RNA. For technical details see Spencer *et al.* (1976). Immunoprecipitates were prepared of the newly synthesised proteins with CaBP antiserum before electrophoresis. Pattern of ^{3}H proteins synthesised by RNA from rachitic chicks, A and from chicks treated with 125 ng of hormone, B. Ratio of ^{3}H in slices of gel B to that in equivalent slices of gel A is given, C

obtained consists mainly of large polysomes with a peak of 11–12 ribosomes per polysome and the addition of necessary factors can cause completion and release of the partially completed polypeptide chains on these polysomes. Although a thorough study has not been carried out it seems that the yield and size of the polysome preparation is not affected by the vitamin D-status of the birds. The synthesis of CaBP by the polysomes from vitamin D-replete birds has been examined using antisera raised against pure CaBP. At 72 h, after 5 μg of cholecalciferol, approximately 5–7% of the total protein synthesised by intestinal polysomes was immunologically identified as CaBP, whilst polysomes from the intestines of vitamin D-deficient chicks did not show any synthesis of this protein (Emtage *et al.*, 1974a). Since in this experiment only the polysomes came from the chick intestine the effect of cholecalciferol in the chick cannot be on tRNA or other essential factors of the cell sap or on the conversion of an inactive precursor of calcium binding protein to an activated form as was suggested for the rat (Drescher and DeLuca, 1971).

Consequently polysomal RNA was examined for the presence of messenger activity for CaBP using both the rabbit reticulocyte lysate system and the wheat germ extract system (Fig. 7) both of which can translate exogenous messenger RNA. As a result of such studies messenger RNA for CaBP has been found in the intestines of cholecalciferol dosed and 1,25-dihydroxycholecalciferol-dosed birds but not in the intestines of rachitic animals (Emtage *et al.*, 1973; Spencer *et al.*, 1976). This messenger RNA was found associated with the larger intestinal polysomes containing between 11 and 14 ribosomes. From the molecular weight of chick intestinal CaBP (27 500) it was expected that the protein would be synthesised on polysomes containing six to eight ribosomes. Although it is known that more nucleotides are present in messenger RNA than are necessary for the synthesis of the protein concerned, in particular a large polyA sequence, the difference in this case between the observed size of the messenger and that expected on theoretical grounds, seems greater than imagined. One possible explanation, of course, is that CaBP is synthesised as a larger molecule which is cleaved after or during synthesis to yield the active form. At present attempts to detect such a phenomenon have been unsuccessful irrespective of whether the CaBP was synthesised in a cell free system or in whole intestinal cells and it therefore appears that the chick does not synthesise a stable precursor of CaBP (Fig. 7). In addition the CaBP messenger RNA has been isolated and partially characterised. The molecular weight of 700 000 is larger than expected for a protein of the size of intestinal CaBP even when allowance is made for a polyA tract (Spencer *et al.*, 1976). The conclusion from these studies therefore is that the synthesis of CaBP in response to 1,25-dihydroxycholecalciferol occurs through the *de novo* production of messenger RNA for this protein. Since the hormone is accumulated on specific receptor proteins in the intestinal nuclei it seems reasonable to conclude that the hormone regulates either the synthesis of the messenger or its release into the cytoplasm.

D RELATIONSHIP BETWEEN CALCIUM ABSORPTION AND CALCIUM-BINDING PROTEIN SYNTHESIS

Consideration has also been given to the sequence of events following the entry of 1,25-dihydroxycholecalciferol into the mucosal cell and whether the appearance of CaBP in the cell is correlated with the consequent stimulation of calcium absorption (Emtage *et al.*, 1974b). Following the administration of cholecalciferol to rachitic animals, 1,25-dihydroxycholecalciferol was found in the plasma within 30 min and in the intestine within an hour, reaching a maximal intestinal concentration after approximately a further 7 h (Fig. 8). From the first appearance of 1,25-dihydroxycholecalciferol into the intestinal nuclei there was a lag of some 5–6 h before the translation of messenger RNA for CaBP was detected and then a further 5 h elapsed before the protein was observed in the cytoplasm. At this time, some 12 h after the vitamin had been administered, the first increase in calcium transport was detected suggesting a causal relationship between the appearance of the protein in the intestinal cytoplasm in response to cholecalciferol and the ability of the tissue to absorb calcium. This correlation between the changes in calcium absorption and CaBP levels has been observed in chicks whenever CaBP levels have been measured immunologically (Wasserman *et al.*, 1974), but not by the chelex assay (Harmeyer and DeLuca, 1969).

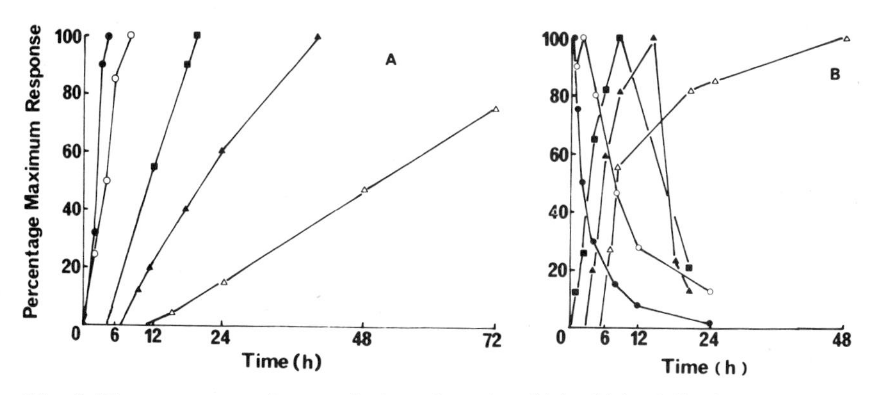

Fig. 8. Time sequence of events in intestine of rachitic chicks following a dose of cholecalciferol (5 μg, A) or its 1,25-dihydroxy-metabolite (125 ng, B). Details are to be found in references quoted; ●, Plasma 1,25-dihydroxycholecalciferol levels; ○, Intestinal 1,25-dihydroxycholecalciferol levels (Lawson *et al.*, 1969a; Lawson and Emtage, 1974.) ▲, CaBP mRNA activity; △, Intestinal CaBP; ■, ^{45}Ca absorption (Emtage *et al.*, 1974b; Spencer *et al.*, 1975)

As a consequence of the continuous production of 1,25-dihydroxycholecalciferol there is a continuing formation of all vitamin D-dependent factors, so that there is some difficulty in analysing the type of substances synthesised and in establishing the order in which they are formed. Following 1,25-dihydroxycholecalciferol administration the changes in calcium absorption and CaBP synthesis are much more rapid than after a dose of the vitamin. Thus translation of messenger RNA for CaBP can be observed within two hours of the administration of the hormone and again statistically significant changes in calcium absorption occurred only when CaBP was being synthesised (Fig. 8). But in this instance whereas calcium transport increased rapidly the formation of CaBP proceeded quite slowly for the first 1.5–2 h and not unexpectedly the levels of CaBP produced during this earlier period could not be detected by immunological methods (Spencer *et al.*, 1975). Consequently it appears that a situation has been found in which it is possible to see an increase in calcium absorption in response to the hormone in the absence of all but a trace of CaBP. Only when calcium transport had been proceeding for about 4 h and had reached about half its maximum value did CaBP synthesis increase rapidly. This observation together with the large size of the CaBP synthesising polysomes indicated that factors exist to regulate CaBP synthesis either by increasing the amount of intestinal messenger RNA or the rate at which it is translated.

The first time interval at which CaBP could be detected (1 μg/g of tissue) was at 6 h after hormone dosage and the levels continue to rise until some time after 24 h. The response of calcium absorption to 1,25-dihydroxycholecalciferol declines after reaching a maximum at 8–10 h so that by 24 h calcium absorption is only a little above that in the untreated bird thus conclusively showing that the effect of the hormone in the intestine is not only on production of CaBP. The process of calcium absorption requires other vitamin D-dependent factors in addition to CaBP. The identity of these factors is not at present known but obvious possibilities are cAMP (chapter 4, XIII) and other vitamin D-dependent proteins (Section VII). The concentration of 1,25-dihydroxycholecalciferol also declines rapidly after the maximum levels are reached and as shown in Fig. 8 this decline parallels that occurring in calcium absorption suggesting that the factors involved have a high turnover rate.

The synthesis of CaBP on intestinal polysomes also falls rapidly as a consequence of the decrease in the nuclear level of 1,25-dihydroxycholecalciferol and the cessation of messenger RNA production. It is interesting that the half-life of the messenger (about 3–4 h) is relatively short for a eukaryotic cell. Polysomal synthesis of CaBP stops about 24 h after a dose of the hormone which is just prior to the time at which maximum levels of the protein can be detected in the intestine. The observation is consistent with the view that the appearance of messenger RNA for CaBP in the cytoplasm requires the continuing presence of 1,25-dihydroxycholecalciferol in the intestinal nuclei and implies that the hormone has a direct effect on messenger RNA formation. Once CaBP has been produced, however, it is stable and has a turnover time similar to that of the mucosal cell. Thus by 96 h, which is the life of the mucosal cell, CaBP is no longer detectable in the intestine. This slow turnover time of CaBP may explain the finding that CaBP is detectable in the brain, and to a lesser extent kidney, of the rachitic animal (Taylor, 1974). Once the brain is formed, of course, new cells are no longer produced and renal cells have a very much longer half-life than intestinal cells, and thus in rachitic animals CaBP will be detectable at these sites for some considerable time after it has disappeared from the intestine.

E 'IN VITRO' SYNTHESIS OF CALCIUM-BINDING PROTEIN AND INTESTINAL MEMBRANE PROTEIN

The question of whether other proteins in addition to CaBP are involved in calcium absorption is one which must be answered before any understanding of intestinal calcium transport can be achieved. The only proteins with this role which it is possible to recognise at present are those whose synthesis is enhanced by cholecalciferol. The results of two experiments demonstrating the stimulation by cholecalciferol and its 1,25-dihydroxy-metabolite of CaBP synthesis in intestinal slices of chicks are shown in Fig. 9. Polyacrylamide gel electrophoretic analysis of the cytoplasmic proteins at any time interval after either steroid has shown that the synthesis has been stimulated of only one protein in this fraction. On the basis of its electrophoretic properties and reaction with CaBP antisera this protein has been characterised as CaBP. The

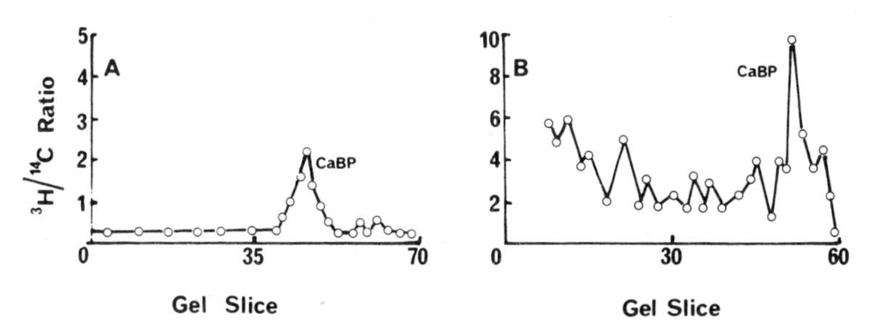

Fig. 9. Comparison of intestinal cytoplasmic proteins synthesised *in vitro* in response to A, cholecalciferol (5 μg) or to B, 1,25-dihydroxycholecalciferol (125 ng). Slices from rachitic chicks were incubated with ^{14}C-leu and those from treated chicks with ^{3}H-leu. Mixed samples of the ^{3}H and ^{14}C labelled cytoplasmic proteins were fractionated by SDS gel electrophoresis and the proportion of ^{3}H: ^{14}C measured. An increase in ratio indicates protein synthesised in response to either the vitamin or the hormone

changes in the rate of CaBP synthesis in the intestinal slices system mirror those found in the polysomal system (see Section VD), e.g. synthesis of CaBP was first observed 12 h after cholecalciferol and 3 h after the hormonal metabolite (Lawson and Wilson, unpublished observations).

In recent studies the synthesis by intestinal slices of microvillar proteins in response to 1,25-dihydroxycholecalciferol has been examined in a similar manner. Within one hour of the administration of the hormone more than one newly synthesised protein was detected in the microvillar fraction of the mucosal cells. Preliminary analysis has shown the presence of at least two protein sub-units of the brush border membranes, the molecular weight of one being approximately 45 000 and of the other about 84 000. These two proteins appear not to be related to one another. The synthesis of the smaller one increases more rapidly after 1,25-dihydroxycholecalciferol than the larger protein and the peak concentration of the smaller protein is reached about 4 h after a dose of the hormone, whereas the peak concentration of the larger is reached after 6 h (Fig. 10). The presence of the smaller and larger proteins in the intestinal slices cannot be detected 10 h and 21 h after the hormone respectively. The correlation between the appearance and disappearance of the larger protein with the changes in calcium absorption in the intestine of rachitic chicks in response to 1,25-dihydroxycholecalciferol is striking.

VI Miscellaneous Responses of the Intestine to Cholecalciferol

A ALKALINE PHOSPHATASE/Ca-ATPase

It has been known for many years that alkaline phosphatase activity in the intestine is related to the cholecalciferol status of the animal (Pileggi *et al.*, 1955), rachitic animals having lower levels of activity than normal. In addition changes in intestinal alkaline phosphatase activity of rachitic animals repleted with cholecalciferol paralleled the changes in calcium absorption (Haussler *et al.*, 1970; Norman *et al.*, 1970). However, the physiological significance of alkaline phosphatase has been difficult to appreciate since the pH optimum (9.5) is so far removed from neutrality and a specific substrate has not been recognised. However, the activity of Ca^{2+}-stimulated ATPase is also dependent upon cholecalciferol (Melancon and DeLuca, 1970) and it has been suggested that the ATPase activity and alkaline phosphatase activity of intestinal membranes are properties of the same enzyme protein complex. Thus it has been claimed that the activities of the two enzymes are similarly affected by heat, disphosphonates and variations in dietary calcium levels (Russell *et al.*, 1972) and by inhibitors of alkaline phosphatase (Haussler *et al.*, 1970).

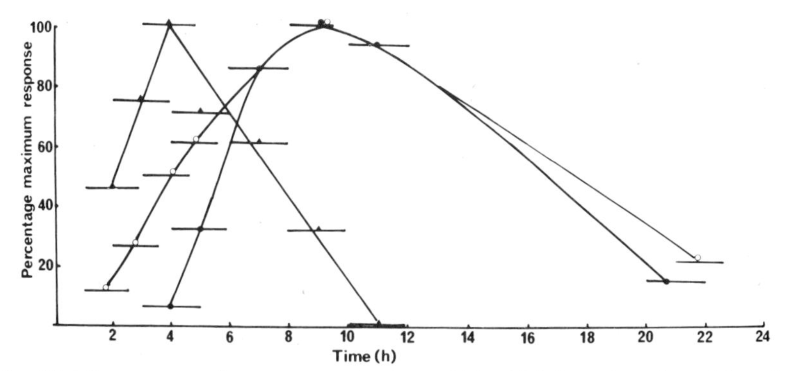

Fig. 10. Time course of some events in the rachitic chick intestine after 125 ng 1,25-dihydroxycholecalciferol. ●, 84 000 molecular weight membrane protein synthesised in response to the hormone; ▲, 45 000 molecular weight membrane protein synthesised in response to the hormone; ○, ^{45}Ca absorption

However, a more detailed analysis of the characteristics of these two enzymes has caused other investigators to reach the contrary conclusion (Felix and Fleisch, 1974; Wass and Butterworth, 1972). In addition there are now several pieces of evidence that alkaline phosphatase activity is not involved in the response of the intestine to cholecalciferol. Although calcium is absorbed in the duodenal, jejunal and ileal regions of the intestine there is only a trace of alkaline phosphatase activity in the ileum. The adaptive response of the intestine to calcium deprivation is seen throughout the whole of the small intestine but alkaline phosphatase is increased in the duodenum only (Krawitt *et al.*, 1973). Histochemical methods showed alkaline phosphatase to be located in the microvillar and in the baso-lateral membrane of the duodenum and in the microvillar region of the jejunum but not present at all in the ileum (Ono, 1974). Other evidence against a role for alkaline phosphatase in cholecalciferol-stimulated calcium absorption includes the acute effect of diphenylhydantoin. This substance can under the appropriate conditions inhibit alkaline phosphatase at the same time as stimulating both calcium absorption and Ca-ATPase (DeWolff, 1975). Finally, the increase in alkaline phosphatase activity in the intestine of rachitic chicks in response to 1,25-dihydroxycholecalciferol is much slower than the increase in calcium absorption (chapter 3 II).

Changes in Ca-ATPase in response to cholecalciferol have not been as frequently studied as those in alkaline phosphatase so that there is no description yet of the changes in activity of this enzyme in response to 1,25-dihydroxycholecalciferol. In response to the vitamin itself Ca-ATPase increases at a similar rate to calcium absorption. The effectiveness compared with calcium of other ions such as Sr^{2+}, Be^{2+}, Mn^{2+} in stimulating this ATPase correlates with the effect of cholecalciferol in stimulating the absorption of these ions. This enzyme deserves more consideration for a role in calcium absorption than it has so far been given.

B LIPID TURNOVER

There have been many attempts over the years to show that movement of cations across membranes involves the phospholipid components and that calciferol functions by influencing the rate of turnover of the phosphate moiety of these substances (Woolley and Campbell, 1962; Hokin and Hokin, 1964). One of the responses of rachitic rats to cholecalciferol is an increased incorporation of ^{32}P in phospholipids (Thompson and DeLuca, 1964). A report by Goodman *et al.* (1972) has recently tried to revive interest in these components to explain calcium absorption. Cholecalciferol was observed to bring about a decrease in the molar ratio of cholesterol: phospholipid due to an increase in phospholipid levels. The proportion of fatty acids in both phospholipids and cholesterol esters is also affected by treatment with cholecalciferol. Although these changes must alter the physical state of the membrane it is not apparent how this could affect calcium absorption. There is a lack of specificity in these effects since not only are the phospholipids of all membrane types affected but there is also no tissue specificity in these changes (Hosoya *et al.*, 1964a, b). In all probability the changes reflect concomitant changes in the protein components of the membranes (Tata, 1967).

VII Summary

Much can be learned about the biochemical aspects of 1,25-dihydroxycholecalciferol function from the studies carried out with the other steroid hormones since a large body of information and experience is available which can serve to support the findings with 1,25-dihydroxycholecalciferol and indicate the most rewarding direction for future studies. Investigations with the other hormones suggest that specific binding proteins in plasma are not essential for the biochemical action of a steroid hormone and that some steroids at least are able to be transported in the circulation without the aid of such a protein. With regard to the calciferol series of compounds, the plasma protein in animals with a high affinity for 25-hydroxycholecalciferol is able to bind cholecalciferol itself and all its metabolites so that it is incorrect to think of it only as a 25-hydroxycholecalciferol-binding protein. Nevertheless its role is most probably that of providing a special pool of vitamin D-activity which may be of value in certain circumstances to regulate the metabolism of the vitamin and its metabolites. A function for the 25-hydroxycholecalciferol-binding protein in the tissues is even more difficult to envisage because of its apparent ubiquitous nature, its high concentration and lack of a function which can be ascribed to 25-hydroxycholecalciferol. In addition the identity of the true ligand for this binding protein is not known and once again it would be wrong at this stage to regard it solely as a 25-hydroxycholecalciferol-binding protein.

The 1,25-dihydroxycholecalciferol-binding proteins in tissues are in a different category, however, and by inference from the findings with the other steroids, can be expected to be essential for expression of the biological activity of the hormone. The cytoplasmic protein confers the property of tissue specificity associated with a hormone and its role is to transfer the steroid into the nucleus. At this site the hormone in conjunction with the nuclear receptor regulates the transcription of specific portions of the target cell genome. Perhaps the system about which most is known is the regulation of ovalbumin synthesis by oestrogens (Harris *et al.*, 1976).

There is now convincing evidence that the only calciferol metabolite able to regulate calcium absorption is 1,25-dihydroxycholecalciferol. The time scale of some of the changes in the intestine following the administration of either cholecalciferol or its hormonal metabolite is now known and attempts have been made to correlate these changes with the increase in calcium absorption. There is a clear cut early effect of 1,25-dihydroxycholecalciferol on RNA metabolism in intestinal mucosa and it has been possible to show that a component of these changes involves the messenger RNA for CaBP. The presence of CaBP in the intestine is primarily dependent upon the presence of 1,25-dihydroxycholecalciferol in the nucleus and as a result of the activity of the hormone at this site an increase in CaBP messenger RNA activity in polysomes can be observed. However, CaBP's slow turnover and its appearance in the intestine after calcium absorption can be detected show that whatever function CaBP may have in this process other factors are also involved. The two 1,25-dihydroxy-cholecalciferol-stimulated membrane proteins are possibilities for such factors. The biochemical evidence on the size of the CaBP messenger RNA product, summarised here, and recent cytological evidence on CaBP location (Arnold *et al.*, 1976) suggest that this protein is present in the intestinal cytoplasm, a finding with implications for CaBP's function (but see chapter 4). The extent to which these findings, made using chick intestine, apply in mammalian species is uncertain (Freund and Bronner, 1975).

The question has also to be considered whether the role of 1,25-dihydroxycholecalciferol in the intestine is entirely explicable on the basis of an effect of gene transcription. Its absence from the plasma membrane suggests that any action at this site involving for example cAMP or possibly lipid metabolism is secondary to some of the more fundamental effects.

References

Arnold, B. M., Kovacs, K. and Murray, T. M. (1976). *Digestion* **14**, 77.

Belsey, R. E., DeLuca, H. F. and Potts, J. T. (1971). *J. Clin. Endocrinol. Metab.* **33**, 172.

Belsey, R. E., Clark, M. B., Bernat, M., Glowacki, J., Holick, M. F., DeLuca, H. F. and Potts, J. T. (1974a). *Amer. J. Med.* **57**, 50.

Belsey, R. E., DeLuca, H. F. and Potts, J. T. (1974b). *J. Clin. Endocrinol. Metab.* **38**, 1046.

Belsey, R. E., DeLuca, H. F. and Potts, J. T. (1974c). *Nature* (London) **247**, 208.

Bouillon, R., van Baelen, H., Rombants, W. and DeMoor, P. (1976). *Europ. J. Biochem.* **66**, 285.

Botham, K. M., Ghazarian, J. G., Kream, B. E. and DeLuca, H. F. (1976). *Biochemistry*, **15**, 2130.

Brumbaugh, P. F. and Haussler, M. R. (1973). *Biochem. Biophys. Res. Commun.* **51**, 74.

Brumbaugh, P. F. and Haussler, M. R. (1974). *J. Biol. Chem.* **249**, 1251.

Brumbaugh, P. F. and Haussler, M. R. (1975). *J. Biol. Chem.* **250**, 1588.

Chalk, K. J. I. and Kodicek, E. (1961). *Biochem. J.* **79**, 1.

Chen, P. S. and Bosman, H. (1964). *J. Nutr.* **83**, 133.

Chen, P. S. and Lane, K. (1965). *Arch. Biochem. Biophys.* **112**, 70.

Chen, T. C. and DeLuca, H. F. (1973). *J. Biol. Chem.* **248**, 4890.

Chen, T. C., Weber, J. C. and DeLuca, H. F. (1970). *J. Biol. Chem.* **245**, 3776.

Corradino, R. A. (1973). *Nature* (London) **243**, 41.

Crousaz, P. De, Blane, B. and Antener, I. (1965). *Helv. Odontol. Acta* **9**, 151.

Daiger, S. P., Schanfield, M. S. and Cavalli-Sporza, L. L. (1975). *Proc. Natl. Acad. Sci. U.S.* **72**, 2076.

DeWolff, F. A. (1975). *Eur. J. Pharm.* **33**, 71.

Dingman, C. W. and Sporn, M. B. (1964). *J. Biol. Chem.* **239**, 3483.

Drescher, D. and DeLuca, H. F. (1971). *Biochemistry* **10**, 2308.

Edelstein, S., Lawson, D. E. M. and Kodicek, E. (1972). *Biochim. Biophys. Acta* **270**, 570.

Edelstein, S., Lawson, D. E. M. and Kodicek, E. (1973). *Biochem. J.* **135**, 417

Edelstein, S., Charman, M., Lawson, D. E. M. and Kodicek, E. (1974). *Clin. Sci. Mol. Med.* **46**, 231.

Eisenstein, R. and Passavoy, M. (1964). *Proc. Soc. Exp. Biol. Med.* **117**, 77.

Emtage, J. S., Lawson, D. E. M. and Kodicek, E. (1973). *Nature* (London) **246**, 100.

Emtage, J. S., Lawson, D. E. M. and Kodicek, E. (1974a). *Biochem. J.* **140**, 239.

Emtage, J. S., Lawson, D. E. M. and Kodicek, E. (1974b). *Biochem. J.* **144**, 339.

Felix, R. and Fleisch, H. (1974). *Biochim. Biophys. Acta* **350**, 84.

Freund, T. and Bronner, F. (1975). *Science* **190**, 1200.

Fraser, D. R. and Emtage, J. S. (1976). *Biochem. J.* **160**, 671.

Frolick, C. A. and DeLuca, H. F. (1976) *Steroids* **27**, 433.

Garcia, B. G., Peytremann, A., Courvaoiser, B. and Lawson, D. E. M. (1975). *Clin. Chem. Acta* **68**, 99.

Glasser, S. R. and Spellsburgh, T. C. (1972). *Biochem. Biophys. Res. Commun.* **47**, 951.

Goodman, D. B. P., Haussler, M. R. and Rasmussen, H. (1972). *Biochem. Biophys. Res. Commun.* **46**, 80.

Gray, R. W. and DeLuca, H. F. (1971). *Arch. Biochem. Biophys.* **145**, 276.

Haddad, J. G. and Chyu, K. J. (1971). *Biochim. Biophys. Acta* **248**, 471.

Haddad, J. G. and Birge, S. J. (1975). *J. Biol. Chem.* **250**, 299.

Harmeyer, J. and DeLuca, H. F. (1969). *Arch. Biochem. Biophys.* **133**, 247.
Harris, S. E., Schwartz, R. J., Tsai, M. J. and O'Malley, B. W. (1976). *J. Biol. Chem.* **251**, 524.
Haussler, M. R. and Norman, A. W. (1967). *Arch. Biochem. Biophys.* **118**, 145.
Haussler, M. R. and Norman, A. W. (1969). *Proc. Natl. Acad. Sci. U.S.* **62**, 155.
Haussler, M. R., Myrtle, J. F. and Norman, A. W. (1968). *J. Biol. Chem.* **243**, 4055.
Haussler, M. R., Nagode, L. A. and Rasmussen, H. (1970). *Nature* (London) **228**, 1199.
Hay, A. W. M. (1975). *In* 'Calcium Regulating Hormones' (Ed. R. V. Talmage, M. Owen and J. A. Parsons) p. 405. Excerpta Medica, Amsterdam.
Hay, A. W. M. and Watson, G. (1976a). *Comp. Biochem. Physiol.* **53B**, 163.
Hay, A. W. M. and Watson, G. (1976b). *Comp. Biochem. Physiol.* **53B**, 167.
Hibberd, K. A. and Norman, A. W. (1969). *Biochem. Pharmacol.* **18**, 2347.
Hokin, M. R. and Hokin, L. E. (1964). *In* 'The Metabolism and Physiological Significance of Lipids' (Ed. R. M. C. Dawson and D. N. Rhodes) p. 423. John Wiley & Sons Ltd., London.
Holick, M. F., Schnoes, H. K., DeLuca, H. F., Suda, T. and Cousins, R. J. (1971). *Biochemistry* **10**, 2799.
Hosoya, N., Fijimori, A. and Watanabe, T. (1964a). *J. Biochem.* **56**, 613.
Hosoya, N., Watanabe, T. and Fujimori, A. (1964b). *Biochim. Biophys. Acta* **84**, 770.
Hunt, R. D., Garcia, F. G., Hegsted, D. M. and Kaplinsky, N. (1967). *Science* **157**, 943.
Imawari, M., Kida, K. and Goodman, D. S. (1976). *J. Clin. Invest.* **58**, 514.
Iotoya, N., Moriuchi, S., Takase, S. and Hosoya, N. (1971). *J. Vitaminol.* (Kyoto) **17**, 73.
Kodicek, E. (1962). *In* 'The Transfer of Calcium and Strontium across Biological Membranes' (Ed. R. W. Wasserman) p. 185. Academic Press, New York and London.
Krawitt, E. L., Stubbert, P. A. and Ennis, P. H. (1973). *Amer. J. Physiol.* **224**, 548.
Lawson, D. E. M. and Emtage, J. S. (1974). *In* 'The Metabolism and Function of Vitamin D' (Ed. D. R. Fraser) p. 75. The Biochemical Soc., London.
Lawson, D. E. M. and Emtage, J. S. (1975). *In* 'Calcium Regulating Hormones' (Ed. R. V. Talmage, M. Owen, J. A. Parsons) p. 330. Excerpta Medica, Amsterdam.
Lawson, D. E. M. and Wilson, P. W. (1974). *Biochem. J.* **144**, 573.
Lawson, D. E. M., Wilson, P. W. and Kodicek, E. (1969a). *Biochem. J.* **115**, 269.
Lawson, D. E. M., Wilson, P. W., Barker, D. C. and Kodicek, E. (1969b). *Biochem. J.* **115**, 263.
Lawson, D. E. M., Fraser, D. R., Kodicek, E., Morris, H. P. and Williams, D. H. (1971a). *Nature* (London) **230**, 228.
Lawson, D. E. M., Pelc, B., Bell, P. A., Wilson, P. W. and Kodicek, E. (1971b). *Biochem. J.* **121**, 673.
Lawson, D. E. M., Charman, M., Wilson, P. W. and Edelstein, S. (1976). *Biochim. Biophys. Acta.* **437**, 403.
Liao, S. (1975). *Inter. Rev. Cytol.* **41**, 87.
Marushige, K. and Bonner, J. (1966). *J. Mol. Biol.* **15**, 160.
Melancon, M. J. and DeLuca, H. F. (1970). *Biochemistry* **9**, 1658.
Neville, P. F. and DeLuca, H. F. (1966). *Biochemistry* **5**, 2201.
Norman, A. W. (1965). *Science* **149**, 184.
Norman, A. W. (1966). *Biochem. Biophys. Res. Commun.* **23**, 335.
Norman, A. W. and DeLuca, H. F. (1964). *Arch. Biochem. Biophys.* **107**, 69.

Norman, A. W., Mircheff, A. K., Adams, T. H. and Spielvogel, A. (1970). *Biochim. Biophys. Acta* **215**, 348.
Norman, A. W., Myrtle, J. F., Midgett, R. J., Nowicki, H. G., Williams, V. and Popjak, G. (1971). *Science* **173**, 51.
Oku, T., Ooizumi, K. and Hosoya, N. (1974). *J. Nutr. Sci. & Vitaminol.* **20**, 9.
Ono, K. (1974). *Acta Histochem.* **51**, 124.
Peterson, P. A. (1971). *J. Biol. Chem.* **246**, 7748.
Pileggi, V. J., DeLuca, H. F. and Steenbock, H. (1955). *Arch. Biochem. Biophys.* **58**, 194.
Preece, M. A., O'Riordan, J. L. H., Lawson, D. E. M. and Kodicek, E. (1974). *Clin. Chem. Acta* **54**, 235.
Proscal, D. A., Okamura, W. H. and Norman, A. W. (1975). *J. Biol. Chem.* **250**, 8382.
Rikkers, H. and DeLuca, H. F. (1967). *Amer. J. Physiol.* **213**, 380.
Rosenstreich, S. J., Volwiler, W. and Rich, C. (1971). *Amer. J. Clin. Nutr.* **24**, 897.
Russell, R. G. G., Monod, A., Bonjour, J. P. and Fleisch, H. (1972). *Nature* (London) **240**, 126.
Smith, J. E. and Goodman, D. S. (1971). *J. Clin. Invest.* **50**, 2159.
Spencer, R., Charman, M., Wilson, P. and Lawson, D. E. M. (1975). *Nature* (London) **263**, 161.
Spencer, R., Charman, M., Emtage, J. S. and Lawson, D. E. M. (1976). *Europ. J. Biochem.* **71**, 399.
Stohs, S. J. and DeLuca, H. F. (1967). *Biochemistry* **6**, 3338.
Stohs, S. J., Zull, J. E. and DeLuca, H. F. (1967). *Biochemistry* **6**, 1309.
Tanaka, Y. and DeLuca, H. F. (1971). *Proc. Natl. Acad. Sci. U.S.* **68**, 605.
Tata, J. R. (1967). *Nature* (London) **213**, 566.
Taylor, A. N. (1974). *Arch. Biochem. Biophys.* **161**, 100.
Tanaka, Y., DeLuca, H. F., Omdahl, J. and Holick, M. F. (1971). *Proc. Natl. Acad. Sci. U.S.* **68**, 1286.
Thomas, W. C., Morgan, H. G., Connor, T. B., Haddock, L., Bills, C. E. and Howard, J. E. (1959). *J. Clin. Invest.* **38**, 1078.
Thompson, V. W. and DeLuca, H. F. (1964). *J. Biol. Chem.* **239**, 984.
Tsai, H. C. and Norman, H. W. (1973). *J. Biol. Chem.* **248**, 5967.
Tsai, H. C., Midgett, R. J. and Norman, A. W. (1973). *Arch. Biochem. Biophys.* **157**, 339.
Wass, M. and Butterworth, P. J. (1972). *Biochim. Biophys. Acta* **290**, 321.
Wasserman, R. H., Taylor, A. N. and Fullmer, C. S. (1974). *In* 'The Metabolism and Function of Vitamin D' (Ed. D. R. Fraser) p. 55. The Biochemical Soc., London.
Weber, J. C., Pons, V. and Kodicek, E. (1971). *Biochem. J.* **125**, 147.
Woolley, D. W. and Campbell, N. K. (1962). *Biochim. Biophys. Acta* **57**, 384.
Zerwckh, J. E., Haussler, M. R. and Lindell, T. J. (1974). *Proc. Natl. Acad. Sci. U.S.* **71**, 2337.
Zetterstrom, R. (1951). *Nature* (London) **167**, 409.
Zull, J. E., Czarnoswka-Misztal, E. and DeLuca, H. F. (1965). *Science* **149**, 183.

6 Histological Aspects of the Relationship between Vitamin D and Bone

JEAN E. AARON

I Introduction

The association between vitamin D and bone has a long history, but controversy persists as to the precise nature of their relationship. The experiments of Barnicot (1951) *in vivo* and subsequent studies *in vitro* (Trummel *et al.*, 1969; Reynolds *et al.*, 1973; Atkins and Peacock, 1974) have established that certain metabolites of cholecalciferol are potent stimulators of bone resorption in a manner reminiscent of parathyroid hormone. High doses of calciferol also undoubtedly produce direct and destructive effects in man. However, the mode of action of the hormone (as it has now become) on cell metabolism and its possible effect on bone formation in general and calcification in particular, is far from clear. The resolution of the problem requires a better understanding of the functioning of bone and of the bone cell in relation to its environment, since bone is not a static arrangement of mineral and matrix, but is subject to constant cellular exchange. The importance of calciferol in maintaining calcium and phosphate levels in the blood is well recognised, but these are only two items in an extensive shopping list demanded by active bone cells, whose internal environments are dictated by their own needs and as such are only distantly related to that of their surrounding fluids. This chapter describes some aspects of normal bone, its origins and the changes which occur in vitamin D deficiency. The cytology of bone resorption is considered elsewhere (Aaron, 1976a).

II History of the Histological Approach to Osteomalacia and Rickets

The increasing incidence of pathological changes in the skeleton characteristic of osteomalacia and rickets, and now attributable to a deficiency of vitamin D, stimulated early authors to study the inexplicable condition which in 1868 was affecting one third of the school children of London (Gee, 1868). While the term 'osteomalacia' derives from the Latin for soft bones, the origin of the name 'rickets' is more obscure. Suggestions include its adoption from a Dorchester colloquialism 'to rucket' meaning to breathe laboriously; from the Norman word 'riquets' for a hunchback; from the Old English 'Wrygates' implying a crooked gait; from the Anglo-Saxon 'rieg' meaning a protuberance, from 'wrick' meaning twist; or from the surname of a West Country doctor who successfully treated the condition (see Ell, 1972). Whistler (translated by Smerdon, 1950) in 1645 described the disease as 'most frequent in the ranks of the highest citizens, next amongst the dregs of the populace', a statement borne out in part by the documentation of the disease in two members of the royal family. The illness of Charles, Duke of Albany and future king of England, from 1600 to 1612 is considered by Keevil (1954) as due to rickets. His evidence is gleaned from the papers of Dr Henry Atkins, who reported to James I in 1604 on the health of Charles '(the) joynts of his knees, hips and ankles being great and loose are not yet closed and knit together as it happeneth to many in their tender years . . .'. Burland (1918) also described the diagnosis of rickets as beyond question in an analysis of the exhumed remains of Charles' daughter, the Princess Elizabeth, who had died in 1650.

The spread of the 'Englische Krankheit' throughout Northern Europe prompted Glisson and a group of Fellows of the College of Physicians of London to form a committee to investigate the disease. The result was the publication in 1650 of a book 'De rachitide sive morbo puerili' (Clarke, 1962). However, five years earlier, a young English student of medicine, Daniel Whistler, had written a dissertation on the same topic (see Smerdon, 1950). This received little attention at the time and was regarded with disfavour some years later when its author was accused of having stolen material from the more learned group. Nonetheless, his document has now assumed an historically interesting position. In his thesis Whistler drew attention to the observations of an earlier unnamed scholar who had described an 'excessive density or imporosity' of bone in rickets, particularly at the centre of the shaft, and 'less dense, spongier and more porous parts' at either end. About this Whistler comments 'Clearly the middle of the shaft of the bone is harder, not simply denser, than the ends: the ends are fundamentally softer parts of the bone'. After scraping away the periosteum he noted larger and more numerous veins and arteries in the region of the epiphyses. These, he considered, transported the nutritive fluid, and it was an 'exudate' of this which accumulated in the joints and caused their swelling. The prevalence of the disease in children who 'stuffed themselves with meat before they had any teeth', and its absence from those who drank milk did not escape his attention, nor did the prophylactic benefits derived from the 'penetrating and unobstructive' milk produced by wet nurses with red hair ('a sign of warmth'). The macroscopic observations made by Whistler were continued by other authors, such as Locke (see Dewhurst, 1962) who in 1666 described after a post-mortem examination 'knobs on the sides of the ribs, which upon opening we found to be just where the band of the ribs ends and the cartilages begin and to that place the ribs seem to grow too much inward but at the knobs they began to bud more outward'.

There was little refinement of these preliminary observations, however, for almost two hundred years. This is understandable when considered in the context of contemporary technical innovation. For instance, it was not until 1858 that the use of carmine, one of the earliest histological stains, was described by Gerlach. In addition, the technique of paraffin embedding, which enabled the preparation of large numbers of thin sections of soft tissues, was not developed by Klebs until 1869. It was, however, the contributions of Virchow which provided fresh impetus to the subject, with his analysis in 1853 of the microscopy of the disease. He described the abnormal proliferation of the preosteoid cartilage (having introduced the term 'osteoid' two years earlier) and attributed the pronounced curvature of the bones to incomplete fracturing. According to the interpretation of his manuscript by Ackerknecht (1953), he considered that none of the existing bone 'softened' in rickets, only 'hardening' of new parts was retarded. (This is at variance with the translation by Chance in 1860, where uncalcified bone in osteomalacia is apparently described as due to the leaching action of blood on previously normal bone, see Wilson *et al.*, 1966.) Virchow did believe, however, that osteomalacia and rickets were separate conditions.

Pommer, in 1885, was stimulated to pursue the histology further, confirming and extending observations by Virchow and by Müller, who in 1858 had described the zone of provisional calcification in prerachitic and postrachitic cartilage. The drawings of Pommer (Figs. 1 and 2) are today a testament to his insight and a tribute to the skill of their engraver, E. A. Funke of Leipzig. He described the pathologic lesion as one of accumulating osteoid tissue which had failed to mineralise, but he considered this the cause of the problem, rather than the effect (see Stein *et al.*, 1955). He recognised rickets and osteomalacia as aspects of a common disease, so rectifying Virchow's misconception. Further details of the condition were supplied by Cohnheim (1889) who agreed with Pommer's conclusions, by von Recklinghausen

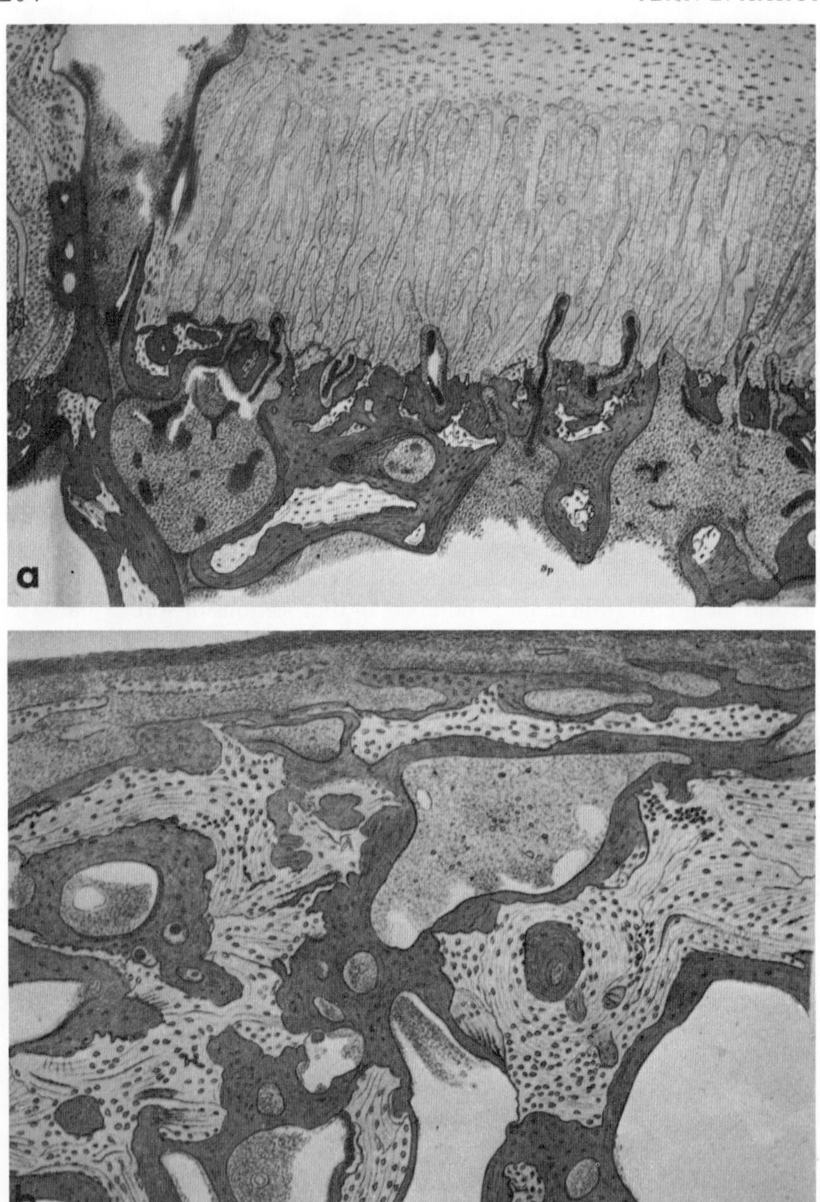

Fig. 1. Drawings from 'Osteomalazie und Rachitis' by Gustav Pommer, 1885, etched by E. A. Funke showing (a) features of rickets in the region of the epiphyseal plate, and (b) the extensive osteoid tissue characteristic of osteomalacia

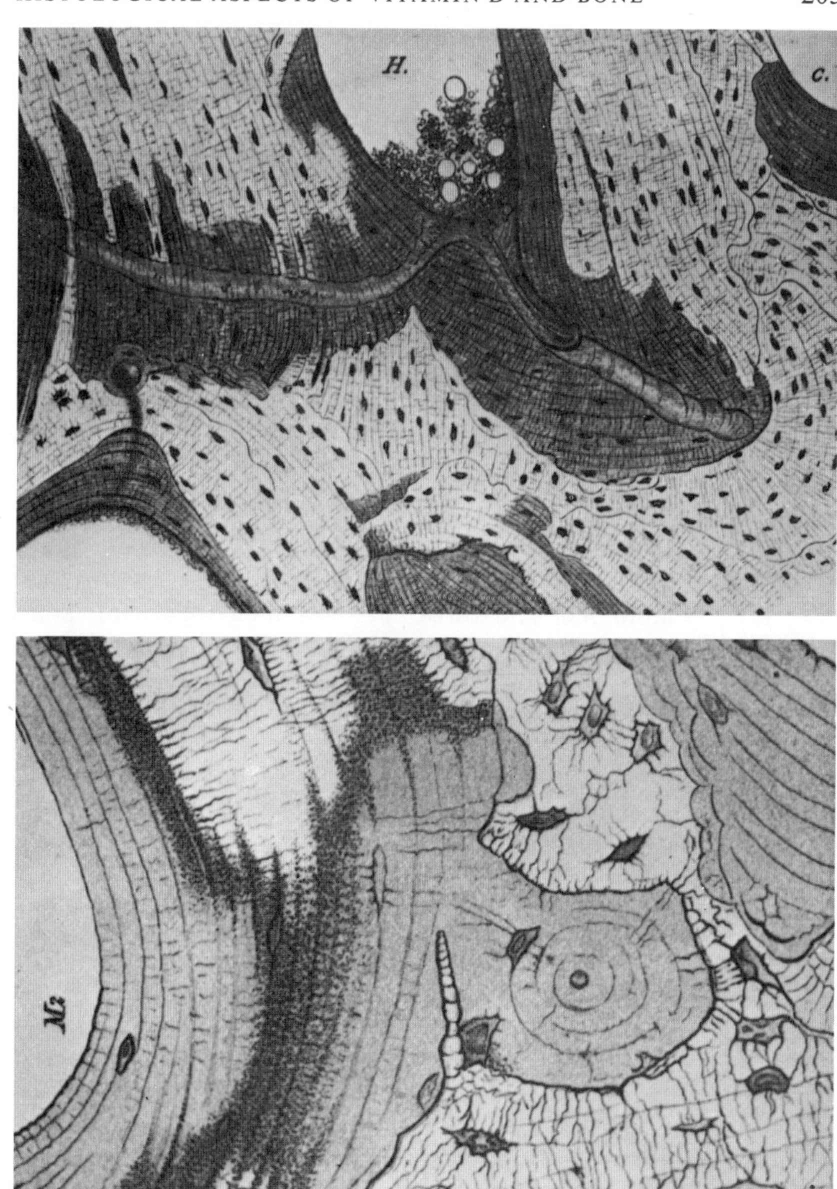

Fig. 2. Drawings from 'Osteomalazie und Rachitis' by Gustav Pommer, 1885, etched by E. A. Funke showing details of the mineralised and unmineralised regions in osteomalacic bone

(1910), who apparently maintained that the presence of osteoid tissue was the result of withdrawal of mineral from calcified bone (see Raina, 1972), and by Looser (1908) who characterised 'Looser zones', features of osteomalacia usually recognised radiographically as united but uncalcified pseudofractures. Looser however, did not associate their origin with fracture but described them as zones of transformation or 'umbauzonen' where a slow progressive formation of callus took place inside the lamellar bone, brought about by 'mechanical irritation due to strain' and by 'small local infarctions' (see Albright *et al.*, 1946). He noted their occurrence in specific parts of the skeleton and their symmetrical distribution, which he attributed to the equal nature of stress as opposed to trauma.

Without the aid of modern techniques and despite the encroaching folklore, the early authors provided a remarkable basis for a histological understanding of osteomalacia and its implications. The microradiography, autoradiography and electron microscopy of today are seals of respect for these beginnings.

III Histological Features of Osteomalacia and some Problems Associated with its Definition

Rickets and osteomalacia are the juvenile and adult forms of a single group of disorders characterised by deficient mineralisation of bone and cartilage. Rickets appears during growth because of its effect on the epiphyses (Fig. 3) where the maturation of the cartilage cells (but not their proliferation) is retarded, such that this zone becomes abnormally wide (Fig. 1). At the same time, the chondrocytes are displaced from their characteristic alignment in columns, the penetration of blood vessels from the marrow cavity is disorderly and no longer takes place along a defined front, osteoid accumulates in the metaphyses and osteoclastic remodelling is delayed (Collins, 1966; Kember, 1971 and Aaron, 1976a for details of the normal structure and development of this region). Osteomalacia is the same condition in the mature skeleton when the epiphyses have closed. The nomenclature was first coined simply to describe the softness of severely diseased bone, but the increasing number of histological variables now measured has given rise to a variety of diagnostic definitions, which are the subject of some disagreement. The controversy concerns the adoption of the term 'osteomalacia' to include diseases of widely diverse etiology, but with a similar bone pathology to that produced by vitamin D-deficiency. In addition the contribution to the histological changes of secondary events such as hyperparathyroidism, is often not clear. Finally, for every case of severe clinically evident osteomalacia, there are others with milder deficiency and sub-clinical levels of the disease (Aaron *et al.*, 1974a, b)

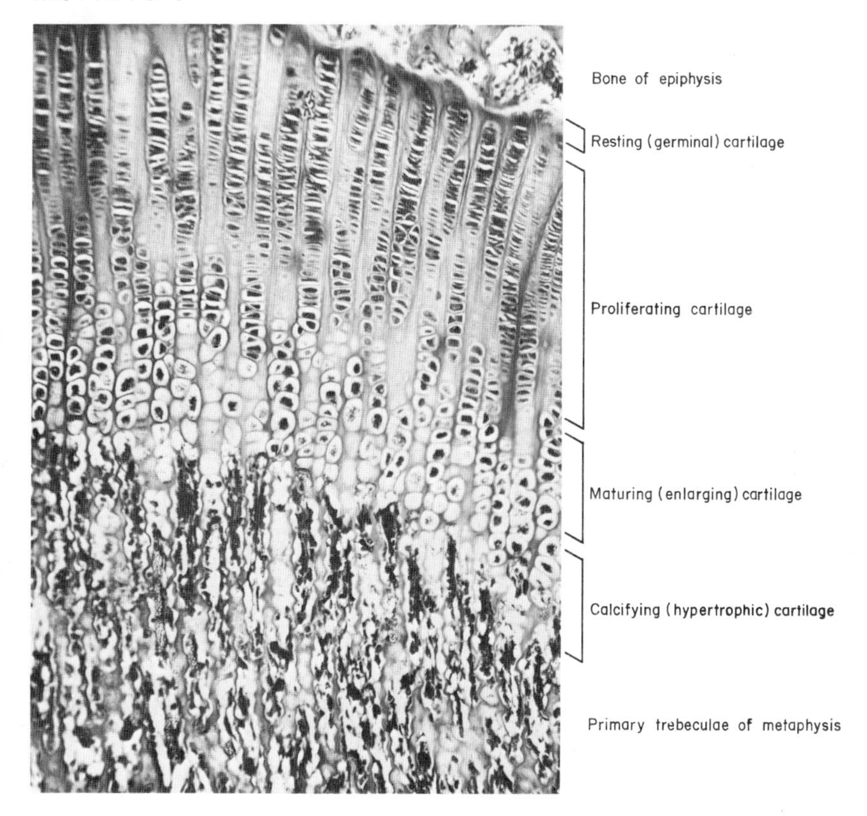

Fig. 3. Epiphyseal cartilage from the tibia of a growing rabbit showing the four characteristic regions. The resting zone (narrow in this instance) anchors the epiphyseal cartilage to the bone of the epiphysis. The flat, dividing chondrocytes of the proliferating zone are arranged in regular columns (or less regular clusters, depending upon the part of the skeleton and the species). The large, round cells of the maturing cartilage synthesise alkaline phosphatase, accumulate glycogen and become hypertrophic. With calcification, the thin horizontal partitions between the chondrocytes disintegrate, leaving the thicker vertical partitions as structures upon which the primary trabeculae of the metaphysis are deposited. Blood vessels approach from the metaphysis. ×100 (Based upon Little, 1973)

which can only be determined histologically. Perhaps these should be dismissed as abnormalities of academic interest only. On the other hand their long term implications for the functioning of bone (and other tissues) are not understood and any significance they might have for the progress of other metabolic diseases is not yet established. Present debates illustrate the uncertainty still surrounding the development of osteomalacia, and some consideration of the present position is therefore important.

A OSTEOMALACIA, DEFICIENT MINERALISATION VERSUS HALISTERESIS

Arguments about the histology of osteomalacia began with its earliest documentation. Pommer (1885; cited by Nordin and Smith, 1967) was one of the first to conclude that the extensive osteoid characteristic of the condition arose from a failure to mineralise new bone, rather than the withdrawal of mineral from previously calcified tissue. He formed this opinion for several reasons, one of them being the difference between the appearance of osteomalacic bone and bone demineralised *in vitro*, and another being the abrupt transition from osteoid to fully mineralised bone. His proposal was contrary to the widely accepted hypothesis of 'halisteresis' which had been introduced by Kilian in 1857, but which was diminished by both the failure to find 'free acid in the medulla of the affected bones' (Cohnheim, 1889) and by the theory of osteoclasis. Recently, after prolonged neglect, limited interest in halisteresis is returning with descriptions not only of a specific demineralisation in relation to osteocytes (Juster *et al.*, 1967), and possibly in relation to cement lines (Jowsey, 1963), but also of a more general process taking place along the surface of trabeculae (Bohatirchuk and Jeletzky, 1971; Aaron, 1976a). Moreover when trabecular bone is etched *in vitro* with 10% ethylenediaminetetracetic acid (EDTA) demineralisation takes place in a different manner from that described *in vitro* by Pommer, who apparently used hydrochloric acid. The removal of mineral by EDTA from some surfaces and not from others, together with the abrupt nature of the transition zone between the demineralised and the fully mineralised regions produces an image reminiscent of the appearance and distribution of osteoid. Clearly, a number of factors have to be considered before any conclusion can be drawn, but it is many years since Pommer conducted his experiments and a reappraisal of this aspect of his work may be useful.

Present evidence may cast doubts upon the assumption that *all* regions of osteoid-like material are invariably sites of matrix apposition, but until the extent of any demineralisation is known and its precise mechanism understood, opinion will remain firmly on the side of Pommer in favour of a failure in mineralisation as the most significant factor in osteomalacia.

B OSTEOMALACIA AND THE ACCUMULATION OF OSTEOID TISSUE

The layers of uncalcified bone matrix characteristic of sites of apposition (Fig. 4) illustrate the dual nature of bone formation, with collagen synthesis and calcification taking place as separate events. The thickness of the osteoid tissue depends upon the degree of separation between the two processes. In

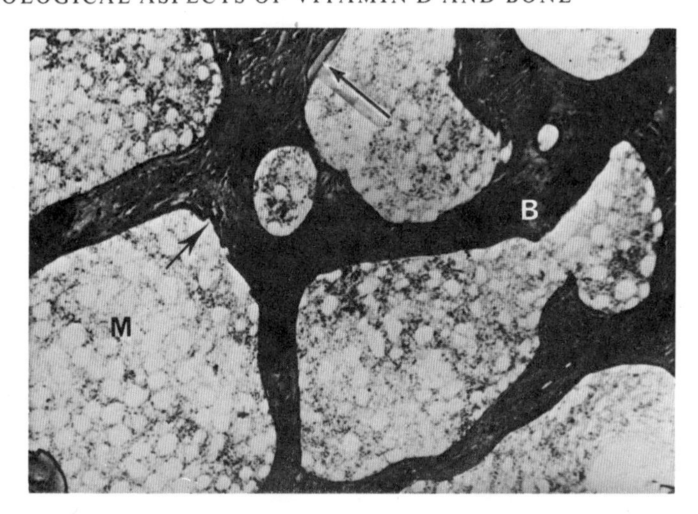

Fig. 4. Trabecular bone from the iliac crest of a normal 41-year-old man. The bony tissue (B) is surrounded by marrow tissue (M). An osteoid border (small arrow) and a resorption cavity (large arrow) are indicated. Undecalcified bone, Goldner stain, ×40

some animals (for example, rat, mouse, pigeon) mineralisation apparently takes place almost immediately after collagen deposition and the osteoid borders are consequently thin. They are so tenuous that McLean and Bloom (1940) were prompted to criticise the idea of osteoid manufacture as a separate stage in bone formation, and concluded that, under optimal conditions of mineral supply, the new matrix calcifies instantly. For them the presence of osteoid tissue signified a mineral deficiency. Whatever the situation in the skeleton of early man might have been, it has been demonstrated both optically and in the electron microscope that in the skeleton of modern man there is a delay of approximately 10 days before calcification takes place. During this time the organic matrix passes through a nonspecific phase, described loosely as a period of 'maturation' (an aspect which will be considered further in another section). Therefore while osteoid in large amounts is a distinctive feature of osteomalacia (Fig. 5), its presence in smaller quantities is a normal part of bone structure, and requires assessment in order to distinguish the normal from the abnormal condition.

1. *Seam Thickness.* The thickness of osteoid borders varies both within and between individuals, and some of the values cited in the literature are shown in Table 1. All these are underestimates of the true fresh hydrated state since there is a shrinkage during the dehydration preceding microscopy. The occurrence of wider seams in osteomalacia has led some authors to use seam thickness as a diagnostic tool (Byers, 1962; Burkhardt and Jowsey, 1966; Olah *et al.*, 1975). Others consider such assessment misleading, since it fails to take

Table 1. Variables used in the diagnosis of osteomalacia

Osteoid volume					Osteoid Borders					Osteoid Borders + osteoblasts				Seam thickness or number of anisotropic bands				Calcification front			
Normal			Om		Normal			Om		Normal		Om		Normal		Om		Normal		Om	
Age	Vol.	Ref.	Vol.	Ref.	Age	%	Ref.	%	Ref.	%	Ref.	%	Ref.	Thick-ness	Ref.	Thick-ness	Ref.	%	Ref.	%	Ref.
<50	0.21	1	>2	9	♂20–30	8.1	12	>27	9	7	16	11	16	4–16	18	15–18	18			<59	9
>50	0.16	1			♀20–30	5.5	12							3–18	19			90–95	21	46	21
<50♂	0.13	2			♂70–80	7.9	12			4.7	17			8.7	20						
<50♀	0.10	2			♀70–80	5.1	12														
>50♂	0.09	2			20–30	4	13														
>50♀	0.09	2			70–80	4	13														
20–30	0.58	3			20–30	13.8	3			5 (20–30)	3	3	3	2.8–16.7	3	50	3				
70–80	0.47	3			70–80	20.5	3			3.5 (70–80)											
♂	0.30	4	♂0.61[m]	4		11–15	14	54.5–98	14									80–86	14	0	14
♀	0.33	4	♀0.83[m]	4																	
	0.9	5	8.9	5				80	5									83	5	1	5
	1.1[a]	6				0–45	6							Bands		Bands					
♂	1.85[a]	7	10–60[a]	10	20–30	11	15	75–100	10					0–3	6	3–12	6	84.6 (20–39)	8	35.8[m]	8
♀	1·05[a]	7			70–80	14	15							0–3	10	3–13	10				
	5.7[a]	8	8.2[a,m]	8	20–39	12	8	36[m]	8					2–3	2			76.4 (60–79)	8	19.2[s]	8
	0–6.85[a]	3	20.9[a,s]	8	60–79	19	8	68[s]	8												

Osteoid volume is as % total sample; osteoid borders is % total surface; seam thickness is in μm; bands is number of anisotropic bands and calcification front is % of osteoid surface
[a] Volume expressed as % of bony tissue only
[m] Mild
[s] Severe
Om Osteomalacia

References: (1) Garner and Ball, 1966; (2) Ellis and Peart, 1972; (3) Merz and Schenk, 1970a; (4) Garrick *et al.*, 1971; (5) Matrajt *et al.*, 1967; (6) Woods *et al.*, 1968; (7) Meunier *et al.*, 1973; (8) Bordier and Tun Chot, 1972; (9) Melvin *et al.*, 1970; (10) Paterson *et al.*, 1968; (11) Morgan *et al.*, 1968; (12) Wakamatsu and Sissons, 1969; (13) Jowsey *et al.*, 1965; (14) Haas *et al.*, 1967; (15) Sissons *et al.*, 1967; (16) Eastwood *et al.*, 1975; (17) Fischer *et al.*, 1970; (18) Frost, 1962; (19) Wilson *et al.*, 1966; (20) Byers, 1962; (21) Frost, 1967

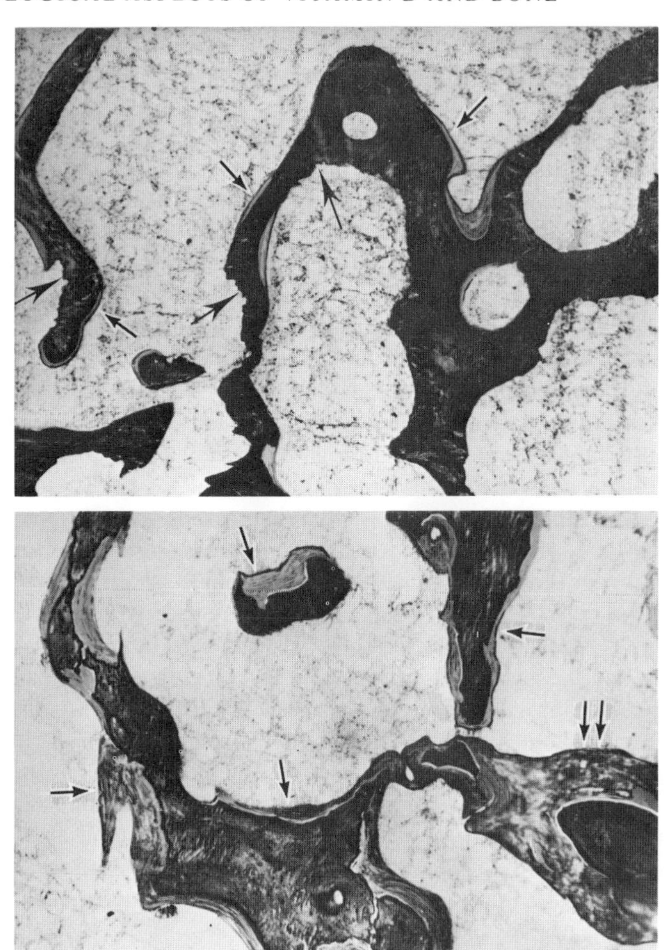

Fig. 5. Trabecular bone from the iliac crest of patients with osteomalacia. Top, osteoid borders (small arrows) of varying thickness are increased in number. Resorption cavities (large arrows) are also extensive implying secondary hyperparathyroidism, 25-year-old man with renal failure. Bottom, wide osteoid borders (arrowed) have extended to cover the majority of trabecular surfaces. Irregular masses of fracture callus (double arrow) are associated with some trabeculae, 45-year-old man with renal failure. Undecalcified bone, Goldner stain, ×40. (Photographs hand-finished to improve the reproduction of this stain in black and white)

into account the obliqueness at which some seams are sectioned. The shape of the haversian canals provides a guide to the plane of sectioning in cortical bone (Wilson *et al.*, 1966) but Woods *et al.* (1968) observed in normal tissue osteoid borders which were 50 μm wide and these were shown to be the product of the tangential plane of sectioning in that region. However, obliqueness of sectioning is quickly recognised in polarised light, when the lamellar organisation is seen as a birefringent series of alternating isotropic and anisotropic bands. Woods *et al.* (1968) and Ellis and Peart (1972) described two or three lamellae in the average seam in human bone, taking a single lamella to include a light and a dark component, each 2 μm wide (Table 1). The width of an individual lamella is generally regarded as relatively constant (although Bonucci *et al.*, 1969 describe wider lamellae in osteomalacia), and therefore any genuine increase in seam thickness is the result of an increase in their number. When a seam is cut obliquely, on the other hand, the individual lamellae appear artifactually wider, but the number remains constant (except when the cut is exactly tangential and the lamellation disappears). Any error in measuring thickness may then be overcome by counting the lamellae and on this basis Woods *et al.* (1968) described an increase in the number of anisotropic bands in a series of patients with osteomalacia (Table 1).

Ellis and Peart (1972) have reported a general decrease in the number of lamellae per seam with age. This is contrary to observations by Frost (1962, later modified by Wilson *et al.*, 1966), but consistent with descriptions by Merz and Schenk (1970a) of a reduction in mean seam thickness (calculated from the volume and the surface extent of osteoid tissue). Unless corrected for, such a reduction with age will tend to mask the earliest stages of osteomalacia in the elderly as it is demonstrated by this method. Frost (1967) has reservations about the importance attached to the seam thickness in diagnosing osteomalacia but for another reason. While acknowledging that abnormally wide seams may be a feature of some types of osteomalacia (and also of some instances of thyrotoxicosis, Wilson *et al.*, 1966), the more common characteristic, he maintains, is not an increase in the normal mean thickness but an increase in the variance (Byers, 1962).

2. *The Surface Extent of Osteoid Tissue*. While an accumulation of osteoid tissue may be due to its increased thickness at sites of apposition as described above, it may also be brought about by an increase in its extension over bone surfaces, and as Woods *et al.* (1968) point out, the two may represent different pathologies. Assessment of the extent of osteoid tissue may be performed in several ways. Villanueva *et al.* (1963) using cortical bone counted the number of osteoid borders in a given field as an index of the activation rate of remodelling regions. This is less useful in trabecular bone where irregularities in a single seam may give the appearance of two separate seams in section. More commonly the proportion of the bone surface covered with osteoid is measured. Such methods are now well documented, and usually employ integrating eyepieces and line sampling procedures (Zeiss, Oberkochen, publication G41-260-e) on large numbers of sections (Aaron, 1976a for

details). The final result is expressed either as a percentage (Matrajt *et al.*, 1967; Wakamatsu and Sissons, 1969; Schenk *et al.*, 1969) or in absolute terms (Sissons *et al.*, 1967; Merz and Schenk, 1970a; Jowsey *et al.*, 1965 and Baylink *et al.*, 1970 using planimetry and map-meter methods).

Osteoid borders may be deposited on smooth or irregular surfaces and, in section, they are 50 μm to several hundred microns in length, tapering at either end. Raina (1972) after examining thin sections (2 μm thick) of undecalcified bone under the optical microscope, came to the interesting conclusion that osteoid tissue covers the entire bone surface, except for areas of active resorption. Even otherwise inactive bone surfaces were found to be covered by a layer of organic material 2 μm or less in width which had similar staining characteristics to osteoid tissue. Clearly, if verified this undermines the significance of all assessments of the surface extent of osteoid seams unless an arbitrary limit is applied. However, the observation has not yet been confirmed at the ultrastructural level, and this is an important omission. It is well established that cells often become enveloped in a layer of organic material of variable thickness which is crucial to their viability (Rambourg and Leblond, 1967). In the absence of ultrastructural evidence, the possibility arises that the spindle-shaped cells lining most bone surfaces are surrounded by such an envelope, which may be thickened along the surface of contact with the bone and may even fuse with the envelopes of neighbouring cells. Such a structure may closely resemble a thin layer of osteoid tissue both histochemically and morphologically and it would require the electron microscope to resolve the truth.

Variations in the quantitative assessment of osteoid tissue may be anticipated from a number of sources. For instance, there is a clear difference between species. There is also a natural variation between individuals which is compounded not only by the use of small samples, and the cyclic nature of remodelling (Frost, 1966), but also by seasonal changes in histological parameters such that osteoid tissue becomes more extensive in the late winter and spring, than during late summer and autumn (Aaron *et al.*, 1974b). In addition it has been well documented (Amprino and Marotti, 1964; Frost, 1969; Van Nguyen and Jowsey, 1970) that some parts of the skeleton remodel more frequently than others, producing regional differences in morphology. To these may be added variations of technique, ranging from the differences in resolution of the histological and microradiographical methodologies, to the differences resulting from individual preferences for thin sections (Merz and Schenk, 1970a use sections 4–6 μm in thickness) or for thick sections (Jowsey *et al.*, 1965 use sections 100 μm in thickness). Also significant is the choice of stain, since they differ in their capacity to demonstrate osteoid, Merz and Schenk (1970a) compared fuchsin-stained ground sections with plastic-embedded microtome sections stained according to the Goldner method and

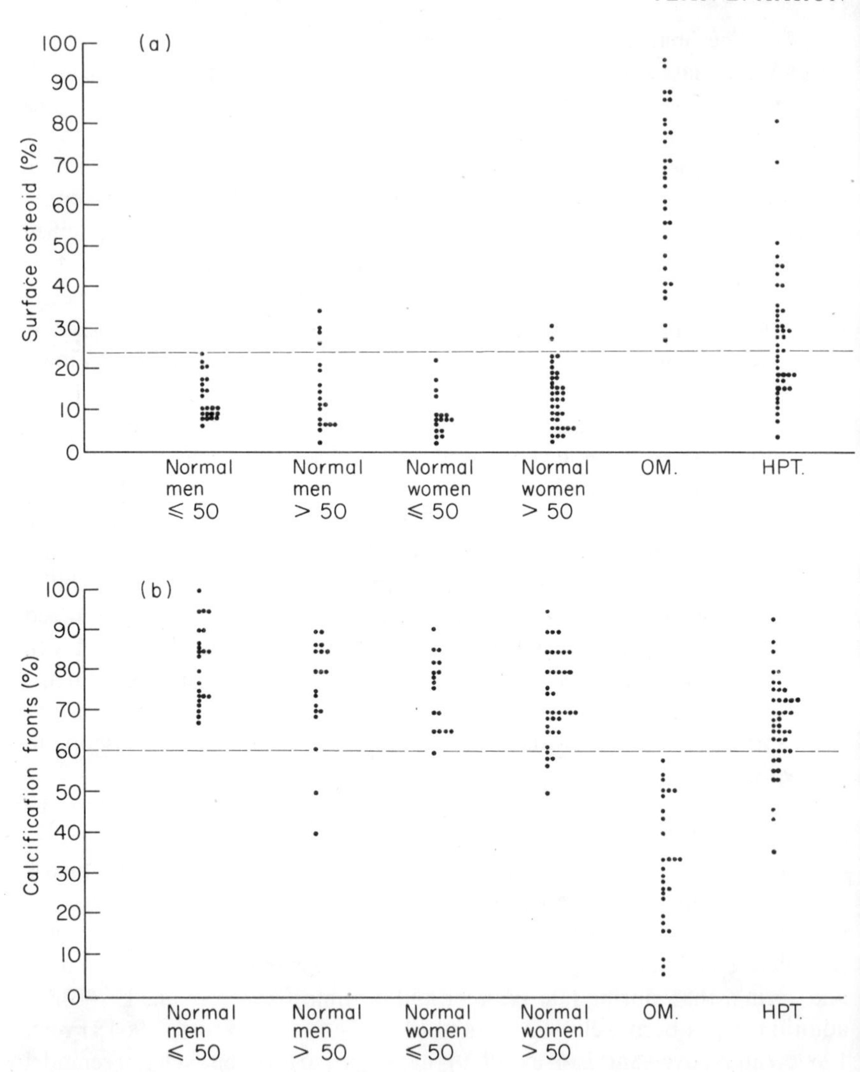

Fig. 6. The percentage of osteoid covered surfaces (a) and the proportion of them having a calcification front (b) in 'normal' males and females obtained at autopsy after sudden death and from patients with nutritional osteomalacia. The dotted lines represent useful, but arbitrary limits of normality. On these criteria, 4 out of the 6 elderly 'normals' with high osteoid values also have poor calcification fronts, implying that they too have mild osteomalacia. A group of patients with primary hyperparathyroidism is included for comparison with a high turnover condition. While the majority of these have normal calcification fronts, despite extensive osteoid, a proportion do have poor calcification fronts and may also be regarded as osteomalacic according to Bordier *et al.* (1973)

found that the colour contrast of the latter enabled thin seams, which otherwise tended to escape detection, to be identified.

Over and above all these sources of variability there is finally diverse opinion as to which osteoid borders are assessed. For instance numbers of seams as thin as 1 μm are described in salicylate-treated rheumatoid arthritis (Wilson *et al.*, 1966) but Woods *et al.* (1968) choose to omit from their measurements uncalcified layers less than 1 μm wide. In our laboratory it has been our constant policy to exclude any osteoid tissues less than 2 μm in thickness, since the significance of seams so thin is not clear, nor are they easily differentiated from the spindle-shaped cells on their surface. The observation of Raina (1972) seems to confirm this view. It is not surprising, however, that the degree of variation between authors using similar material is sometimes wide (Table 1). On the basis of the criterion described above and preparative procedures previously recorded (Aaron, 1976a) the surface extent of osteoid does not exceed 24% in young adult males and is often less than 10% in young females (Fig. 6a). After the age of 50 the values for women tend to rise and more closely resemble those of men. There is however no significant change with time in the normal population as a whole. When the constancy of this expression for osteoid *relative* to the total surface is viewed in the context of the decrease in total cancellous surface which takes place with age, (Sissons *et al.*, 1967; Merz and Schenk, 1970b) a decrease in osteoid tissue in *absolute*

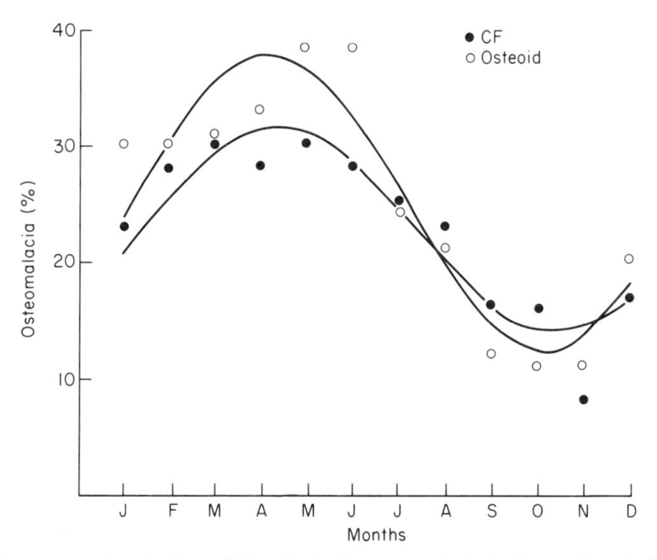

Fig. 7. The seasonal variation of histological osteomalacia in femoral-neck fractures. The percentage of abnormal biopsies, on the basis of either the calcification front (CF) or the relative surface extent of osteoid, increases during the spring and falls during the autumn. (Based upon Aaron *et al.*, 1974b; statistical analysis by Dr D. Marshall)

terms is implied. Further analysis showed this to be the case in the male population (Nordin *et al.*, 1975), though it was less evident among the females. A fall in the absolute amount of osteoid with time is consistent with both the observations of Merz and Schenk (1970a), that the surface extent of osteoblasts falls with age, and with the decrease in the number of lamellae in osteoid borders with age described by Ellis and Peart (1972).

The normal range for osteoid seams from 2–24% of the total surface described above although adopted in an arbitrary manner (Aaron *et al.*, 1974c) is in general agreement with a report by Melvin *et al.* (1970) of an upper limit of 26% (Table 1). Higher values suggest osteomalacia but may occur in other conditions. Out of a total of 95 control subjects only 6 had values greater than 24%, and 4 of these had other features consistent with a deficiency in mineralisation. Relevant to this is the high incidence of osteomalacia among the elderly in Scotland described by Chalmers *et al.* (1967) and confirmed by Exton-Smith (1971). Our own data would suggest that an incidence of osteomalacia of at least 8% is a feature of the 'normal' elderly population (4 out of 55 subjects over the age of 50 years). Furthermore, all 'abnormal' control specimens were obtained in the winter and spring seasons when osteomalacia is apparently most prevalent (Fig. 7; see also Schmorl, 1909). This suggests that the normal range of bone histology in respect of indices of osteomalacia should be established, in Britain at least, in the autumn. It also illustrates the problem of establishing in a statistical manner not only the relative surface extent of osteoid, but also the normal range of any parameter in an ageing population, some of whom may be suffering from the very disease under study (Aaron *et al.*, 1974c).

Some of the interpretations made by Merz and Schenk (1970a) tend to differ from those expressed above. These authors noted in their normal autopsy material an enlargement of the relative area of the trabecular surface occupied by osteoid after the age of forty (confirmed by Bordier and Tun Chot, 1972), a change which, they point out, is consistent with the increased remodelling activity described by Frost (1963) in the rib cortex. However, not only do the seams become increasingly extensive into old age, but also they become thinner and lack the osteoblasts characteristic of seams in younger individuals (see p. 229). Describing these as 'terminal' seams and acknowledging their similarity in some respects to the 'resting' seams of Frost (1960), Merz and Schenk (1970a) attribute their accumulation with time to a delay in mineralisation. This, they regard as a phenomenon of physiological ageing which is separate from osteomalacia.

The idea of an undefined 'physiological ageing phenomenon' raises again the question of exactly how abnormalities in the elderly should be assessed, whether they should be compared with 'normal' old people or 'normal' young people. It also introduces a variable which cannot be appreciated until there is a better understanding of the mechanism of bone mineralisation (see p. 231). For the present, I am inclined to favour the opinion that histological osteomalacia be viewed simply as a delay in mineralisation relative to matrix synthesis from whatever cause.

3. *The Volume of Osteoid Tissue.* Some authors rely on a volumetric assessment of osteoid tissue, Table 1, since it takes into account both the thickness of the osteoid and the length of the trabecular surface it covers. Merz and Schenk (1970a) measure the volume of the osteoid and its surface extent and use the quotient of the two to calculate the mean seam thickness. Derived in this way, they consider that seam thickness represents a true average figure which is more precise than direct measurements of the greatest width, or the determination of the maximum number of lamellae (see p. 209). For my own part, I find this expression of osteoid a useful addition to surface measurements when the degree of osteomalacia is moderate or severe, since it provides a scale for comparing the severity of the condition in those instances where most of the trabeculae are covered by osteoid, such that measurement of length alone cannot grade the development of the disease. I hesitate to depend entirely on osteoid volume however, since when the amount of this tissue is small difficulties arise in its measurement. Yet it is in this region where assessment is important if subclinical degrees of osteomalacia are not to be missed and the situation avoided in which osteomalacia can only be detected histologically when the disease is clinically obvious.

The relative area of any structural component can be measured by point-sampling, using an integrating eyepiece (see Zeiss, Oberkochen, publication G41-260-e). The area so determined provides a basis for comparison and is, at the same time, a valid measure of the relative volume of that component (Delesse, 1848). By superimposing the grid image onto sections of trabecular bone and counting as hits first those points overlying bony tissue, then those points overlying osteoid alone, the percentage area occupied by each can be determined. However, as Merz and Schenk (1970a) point out, the statistical deviation increases for few and for thin seams. It is inevitable when measuring such small volume fractions that the error in the final result will be relatively large (Hennig, 1958; Weibel, 1963). This error can be reduced by using a higher magnification for analysis and an integration eyepiece with a lower grid constant (i.e. a higher number of points), but the method becomes increasingly tedious. Automatic analysis, using image analysing computers would seem to be the answer, and this method is now employed by some authors (Meunier *et al.*, 1973; Faccini *et al.*, 1976). The Quantimet 720, for instance, apparently analyses 500 000 picture-points on the screen in a fraction of a second. Artifactual fringes, however, tend to be displayed at the bone surfaces along the marrow interphase in a manner resembling osteoid tissue and since these are not easily eliminated can create problems in resolving thin borders.

Using such methods, a weak age dependency in the volume of osteoid was reported by Merz and Schenk (1970a; Table 1). This was not observed by either Woods *et al.* (1968) or by Meunier *et al.* (1973), but the latter authors described a difference in this parameter between the sexes, the mean value for men being significantly higher than that for women.

The expression of osteoid in this way allows some appreciation of the proportion of mineralised and unmineralised bony tissue together with the implications this might hold for structural adequacy. In severe osteomalacia, the osteoid encroaches into the marrow spaces such that the marrow cavities become reduced in size and the total volume of bony tissue is considerably increased. At the same time, the volumetric density of calcified tissue may fall as old bone is replaced by slowly mineralising new bone. However, the volumetric density of the calcified bone (in the region of the iliac crest, at least) is frequently not low, but within the *normal* range (Fischer *et al.*, 1970; Stanbury and Lumb, 1967) or even abnormally high (Garner and Ball, 1966). This paradoxical situation in which the amount of calcified bone is maintained or accumulates despite an anticipated diminution in mineralisation, was also noted radiographically by Nordin and Smith (1967) in the spine. One explanation might be that, although the preponderance of evidence suggests that the essential feature of osteomalacia is a failure to calcify new osteoid, matrix apposition and even calcification are proceeding at a higher rate than normal. Such would be consistent with isotope turnover studies (Fraser *et al.*, 1960; Nordin and Smith, 1967). An alternative explanation and one which seems reasonable from a histological point of view is that the retention and accumulation of calcified tissue in such patients is a function of reduced osteoclastic resorption in certain regions. In support of this possibility is the relatively small surface of mineralised bone which remains exposed to the marrow cavity in severe osteomalacia. Osteoid tissue is not normally resorbed by osteoclasts, suggesting that this tissue will afford some protection to the underlying mineralised bone. Conversely resorptive activity in these patients is often high in terms of hydroxyproline excretion, higher than can apparently be accounted for by increased osteocytic osteolysis or by the 'tunnelling' of osteoclasts into the mineralised bone beneath the osteoid. The increasing confinement of osteoclastic resorption to other areas of the skeleton, such as the cortex seems likely. In these regions a lower remodelling rate means that the progress of osteomalacia is slower, and the development of the protective layers of osteoid consequently delayed. Consistent with this is the observation of Nordin *et al.* (1965) that while the spinal density tended to be high for the age of the patient in osteomalacia, the metacarpal cortical thickness was generally low.

Such a theory also implies the retention within the osteomalacic trabeculae of ageing calcified bone which is inaccessible to the normal remodelling activities. The development and proliferation of microfissures resulting from the stresses of daily life might then proceed unchecked and lead to trabecular fragmentation. The excessive callus (Fig. 5b) which is particularly characteristic of defined regions of the osteomalacic vertebra (Aaron, 1976b, 1977) may be a response to these events and a microscopic manifestation of the pseudofracture, that first pathognomonic radiological feature of osteomalacia (Looser, 1920; Milkman, 1930).

4. *The Accumulation of Osteoid and Vitamin D-Deficiency.* The pseudofracture is considered by some authors as the most certain criterion of osteomalacia. In its absence there is no other single clinical, biochemical or radiological characteristic which is reliably diagnostic of the disease. Many factors must be taken into account and increasing importance has therefore been attached to the histology. From this can be derived not only the severity of the condition, but also the sensitivity of the tissue to therapy and the length of treatment before total healing takes place. However, the acceptance of an excess of osteoid in a bone biopsy as the final definition of osteomalacia has been criticised by Morgan *et al.* (1967), who point out that an accumulation of osteoid may be encountered in other disorders such as Paget's disease, hyperparathyroidism (Fig. 6a) and thyrotoxicosis. Consequently these authors have endeavoured to be restrictive in their definition of the disease by including the sensitivity of the condition to vitamin D therapy, adding '. . . we question whether the one term osteomalacia can serve to describe conditions responding to small physiological doses of vitamin D, as well as those requiring large, pharmacological, and even toxic, doses of vitamin D'.

Stanbury (1972) on the other hand opposes the confinement of the term to the osteodystrophy that results from a deficiency of vitamin D and is remedied by its correction since it deprives the expression of much of the significance attached from long histopathological usage. For instance, the so-called vitamin D-resistant osteomalacias, the less common hypophosphatasia (Fraser, 1957), fibrogenesis imperfecta ossium (Baker, 1956) and fluorosis are immediately excluded, although the histological features of defective mineralisation are, in many respects, indistinguishable from those of nutritional deficiency of vitamin D. An approach concerned with the mechanism whereby diverse agents produce the same pathological picture seems the one most in keeping with the time envisaged by Frost (1966) when the practice of classifying these diseases on the basis of responsiveness to vitamin D will be of progressively limited value since their variety will increase with the sophistication of the diagnostic procedures.

C OSTEOMALACIA AND THE CALCIFICATION FRONT

Frost (1966) shares the concern of Morgan *et al.* (1967) and Paterson *et al.* (1968) that a definition with the flexibility to encompass diseases of widely diverse etiology requires modification. At the same time, he prefers to concentrate on the histological manifestations of diminished mineralisation from whatever cause, and objects to the confidence sometimes placed in an assessment of the osteoid tissue as diagnostic of osteomalacia. In his opinion the only approach other than the radiological demonstration of pseudo-fractures that enables osteomalacia to be determined without ambiguity, is the histological analysis of bone after tetracycline labelling. Labelling allows a dynamic interpretation of a static image. Conclusions drawn from the static image alone can be misleading. For instance, patients deficient in vitamin D or with thyrotoxicosis each have too many osteoid borders and may therefore be described as osteomalacic, even though the metabolic disorders are unrelated. Tetracycline enables the two conditions to be separated in terms of the nature of the calcification front and its rate of deposition.

The mineralisation of lamellar bone normally takes place in a well-defined manner at the junction between the bone and the osteoid. This discrete region has been referred to as the 'ligne frontière' (Lacroix, 1954), the 'phosphate ridge' (Johnson, 1964), the 'demarcation line' or 'calcification front' (Matrajt *et al.*, 1967). The different staining characteristics of the calcification front from that of either the osteoid or the mineralised bone have been attributed to changes in the nature of the collagen and in the quantity and nature of the noncollagenous matrix (Thomas, 1961; Johnson, 1964). It is in this region that tetracycline, while failing to complex with the bulk of the bone mineral, is incorporated either by chelation with calcium salts, with some part of the organic matrix or with both (see Kaitila, 1971 for references).

1. *The Calcification Front and Tetracycline Labelling*. The observation that tetracycline antibiotics will deposit *in vivo* at sites of bone formation and can be subsequently studied in undecalcified sections by fluorescence microscopy was described by Milch *et al.* (1957). Fluorescent labels so incorporated provide time markers for the study of growth, turnover and repair of bone and dentin. Not only is the technique safer and more convenient than alizarin (Hoyte, 1968) or heavy metal markers (Schneider, 1968), but it may be used in studies of human bone directly, rather than indirectly via animal models. Tetracycline-based approaches to dynamic studies of bone remodelling have been devised by Frost *et al.* (1960) and Harris *et al.* (1962) and have subsequently been applied in many laboratories (Amprino and Marotti, 1964; Haas *et al.*, 1967) and are now well documented. In principle, doses of tetracycline are administered at recorded time intervals (usually as 2 series of applications, 10 days apart). The position of the calcification front on these occasions appears in section as discrete fluorescent bands, the distance between the bands providing a means of assessing the linear rate at which the calcification front has advanced. This apparently falls persistently with age, in cortical bone at least (from 1.5 μm to 0.7 μm per day, Frost, 1969). A gradient

of activity has been described at the calcification front by Lacroix (1970), mineral deposition taking place more rapidly at the beginning of the mineralisation phase (2 μm per day) than at the end. In addition to such time-related differences, Harris *et al.* (1962) observed variation from region to region in the same bone (Aaron, 1976a for details).

Normally, the majority of the seams are mineralising actively (Table 1) and the calcification front is well defined and takes up tetracycline. Similarly, the extensive osteoid borders associated with those metabolic disorders such as thyrotoxicosis, characterised by a high bone turnover, label with tetracycline in a normal manner. In osteomalacia, on the other hand, only a fraction of the seams are labelled (Frost, 1967), and in some instances no label at all is incorporated (Haas *et al.*, 1967). At the same time, the rate of advance of the calcification front tends to be irregular and generally slower than normal (0.2 μm per day, Frost, 1967). In order that the labels should be adequately separated for measurement Frost (1969) recommends a time interval of three weeks between applications rather than the usual period of ten days. On this basis he described dynamic osteomalacic bone as taking more than three times longer than normal to complete the formation stage of a histologically defined region of remodelling which he has named the Basic Multicellular Unit or BMU (Frost, 1966).

There are difficulties associated with tetracycline labelling. For instance, most of the literature on this subject pertains to cortical bone, and Merz and Schenk (1970a) while not denying the value of tetracycline labelling, have reservations concerning its application to trabecular bone. For stereological reasons, they consider that it provides reliable information about bone formation only within compact bone, being of limited use in cancellous bone because of oblique and tangential sectioning of a proportion of the trabeculae. This problem of oblique sectioning can be overcome to some extent by avoiding those areas where the calcification front is wide and diffuse and by limiting measurements to those regions where the calcification fronts are thin and sharply defined and where an examination of the lamellae in polarised light tends to confirm the absence of obliqueness. But in osteomalacic bone the calcification fronts are often wider and more diffuse in character than normal, making obliqueness difficult to recognise. In addition, systematic labelling with tetracycline can only be carried out in biopsies, and since these are usually taken from patients with skeletal disorders, the difficulty of acquiring comparative, normal, labelled material has to be circumnavigated.

2. *The Calcification Front and Histological Dyes*. A number of authors have investigated the features of the calcification front further by directing attention to dyes with specific staining reactions or affinities for this region (Table 2). Not only do these methods indicate activity at the calcification front, but they also detect changes in its nature, which are the earliest signs of histological

response when nutritional osteomalacia is treated with vitamin D. For instance, the observation of lipid-staining materials in this region (Irving and Wuthier, 1968) is of particular interest, because they are absent in all osteomalacias and are restored, together with their specific histochemical reactivity, by appropriate treatment within seven days (Bordier *et al.*, 1969). The positive lipid reaction is apparently associated with the earliest stage at which calcium and phosphorus combine during calcification (Heeley and Irving, 1973). Such changes allow the information needed to recognise osteomalacia to be obtained without previous tetracycline labelling, which may be inconvenient, even hazardous, in patients with renal failure. Furthermore, since methods involve *in vitro* staining and not *in vivo* labelling, they can be applied to autopsy material, allowing comparison with normal values. The calcification front is usually expressed relative to the osteoid surface (Fig. 6) or total surface using an integrating eyepiece and line-sampling procedures (Aaron, 1976a). While some authors regard the histological demonstration of the calcification front with enthusiasm, others have found the stains fugitive and inconsistent, possibly as a result of varying preparative techniques, and the method of fixation may be critical.

Table 2. Staining and labelling characteristics of the calcification front

Stain or label[a]	Mature bone	Calcification front	Osteoid tissue	Reference
Sudan B	−ve	Black	−ve	Irving (1960)
Osmic acid	Grey	Black	−ve	Johnson (1964)
Toluidine blue	Deep blue	Black	Light blue	Melvin *et al.* (1970)
Solochrome cyanine R	Blue	Purple	Orange	Matrajt and Hioco (1966)
Osteochrome	Green	Brown	Red	Villanueva (1967)
Haematoxylin and eosin	Orange	Purple-brown	Orange	Johnson (1964)
Acridin orange	−ve	Red (UV light)	−ve	Johnson (1964)
Histochemical reaction for sialic acid	−ve	+ve	−ve	Johnson (1964)
Alizarin red S[a]	−ve	Red	−ve	Johnson (1964)
Tetracycline[a]	−ve	Yellow (UV light)	−ve	Milch *et al.* (1957)
^{35}S[a]	−ve	+ve	−ve	Kent *et al.* (1956)
Lead[a] or zinc[a]	−ve	+ve	−ve	Vincent (1963)

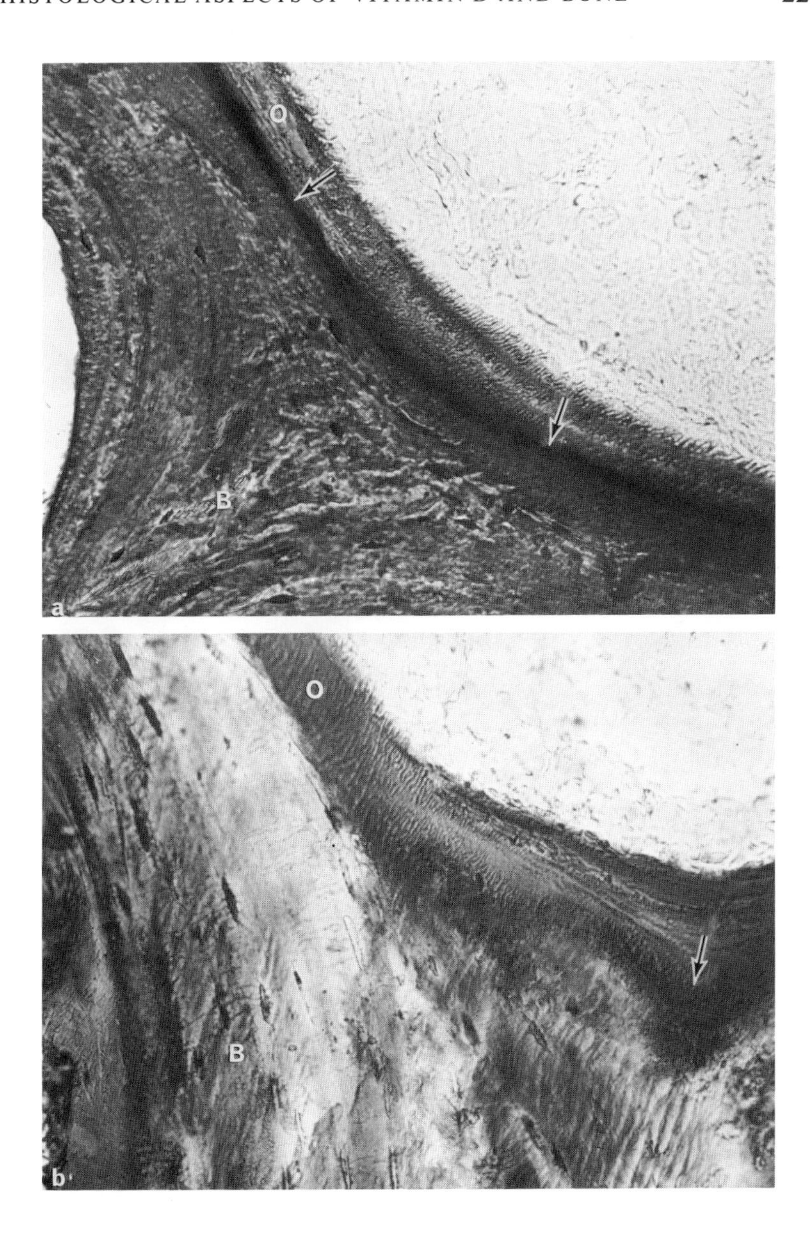

Fig. 8. The calcification front in undecalcified bone from the human iliac crest stained with toluidine blue. (a) The calcification front (arrowed) is normally clearly defined from the osteoid (O) and the mineralised bone (B). (b) In osteomalacia the calcification front (arrowed) is diffuse or absent, $\times 170$

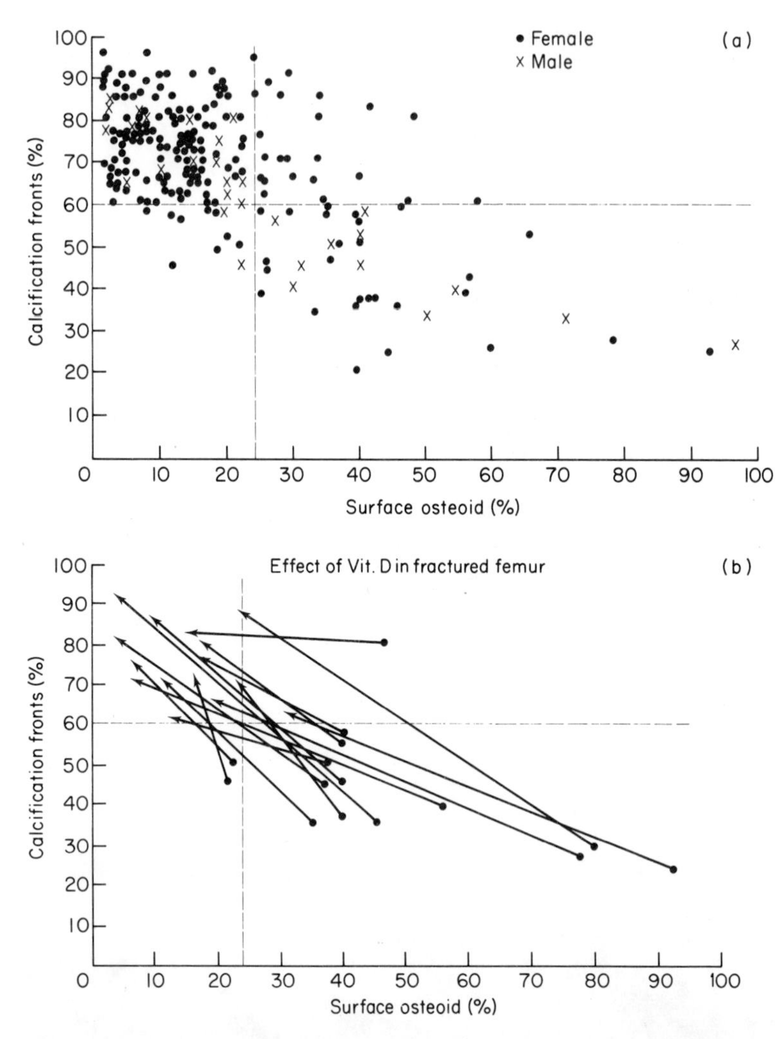

Fig. 9. Relationship between the percentage of osteoid-covered surfaces and the proportion of them having a calcification front in patients with fractures of the proximal femur. The vertical dotted line represents the upper normal limit for surface osteoid. The horizontal dotted line represents the lower normal limit for calcification fronts. (a) On this basis, cases with normal bone histology lie in the top left-hand quadrant; cases with osteomalacia lie in the bottom right-hand quadrant. Those cases in the bottom left and upper right quadrant may represent milder degrees of the disease. (Based upon Aaron *et al.*, 1974a.) (b) Confirming the diagnosis of osteomalacia in a proportion of these patients is the effect of varying doses of vitamin D. All patients treated responded to therapy and their osteomalacia healed (see Gallagher, 1976)

Toluidine blue stain (Fig. 8) is particularly useful in the routine assessment of the calcification front (Figs. 6 and 7) before and after vitamin D therapy (Fig. 9), and according to Bordier and Tun Chot (1972) results correlate well with values obtained from tetracycline labelling (r = 0.92). Using toluidine blue Melvin *et al.* (1970) have derived a number of indices for defining osteomalacia, as follows:

(*i*) more than 2% of the gross volume of cancellous bone is composed of uncalcified osteoid,

(*ii*) some partly calcified osteoid is present.

(*iii*) more than 27% of the total cancellous bone surface is covered with osteoid,

(*iv*) less than 59% of the osteoid surface has a calcification front. In severe osteomalacia all four criteria are satisfied; in milder forms only (*iii*) and (*iv*) may apply.

While the precise figures may be debatable and manipulated statistically, these criteria do seem to represent a good working guide, although they constitute no more than a superficial description of a general syndrome, without commitment to any specific mechanism of development. Inevitably, they will become less important as the present uncertainty about bone metabolism at the cytological level is resolved and a further separation on the basis of pathogenesis is forthcoming.

3. *The Calcification Front and Tetracycline Stain.* While the histological stains described in Table 2 detect activity at the calcification front, most relate to changes in the organic matrix, either in composition, configuration or accessibility. With the exception of haematoxylin and alizarin, none is directly associated with the mineral element and none combines specifically with the calcium phosphate or carbonate complex. They differ in this respect from the tetracycline label. However, it has recently been observed (Aaron and Pautard, 1973a, 1975) that if the customary technique of labelling with tetracycline is replaced by a simple *staining* procedure, in which the specimen is immersed in a solution of the antibiotic, there are differences in the pattern of extracellular staining between normal and pathological states. Analysis by this method offers a means of identifying abnormal behaviour. At the same time, the disposition of the tetracycline binding after staining raises questions about the pathways of calcification in bone and its origins (see p. 243).

When *sections* of bone are stained with tetracycline, the mineralised tissue is fluorescent over its entire surface. But when the sample of bone is treated in *bulk*, before embedding and sectioning, the stain is readily taken up in a regional and discontinuous manner (Fig. 10). Normally, the gross bone mineral has only a dull green autofluorescence, suggesting that the tetracycline-binding site is not accessible in the intact tissue (Fig. 10a, b), although it may become so after damage, or by sectioning. Areas of diffuse

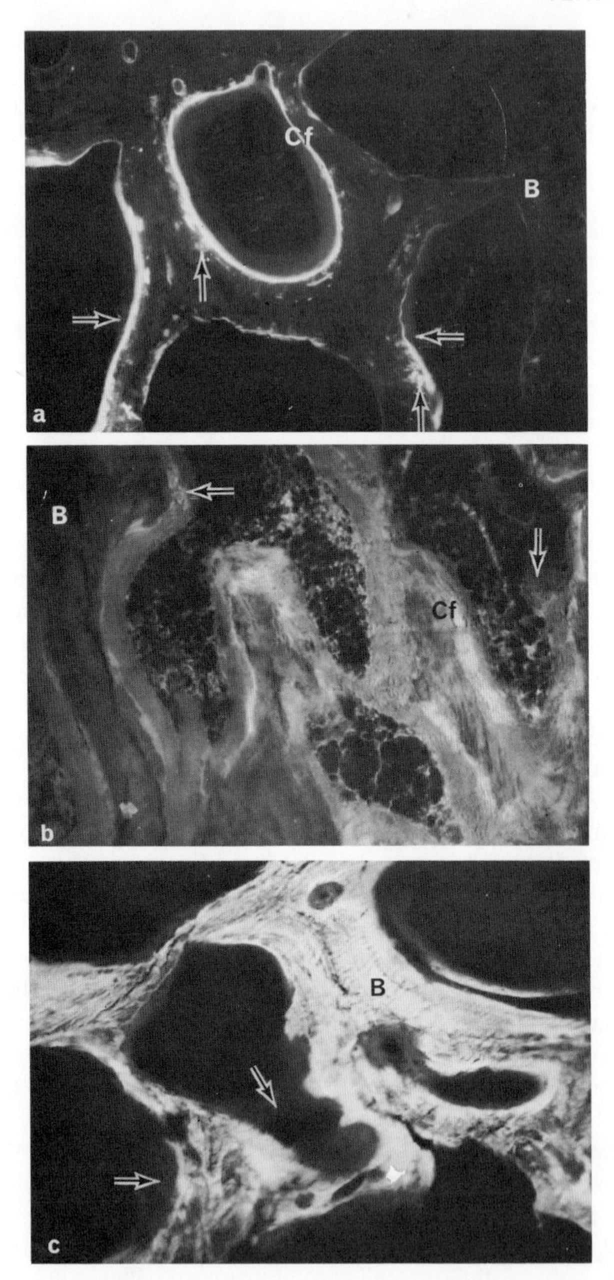
Cf
B
a
B
Cf
b
B
c

fluorescence increase in certain pathological conditions such as renal osteomalacia. In some of these regions the morphology of the osteocytes implies that they are areas of active mineralisation (see p. 243), despite their location within the trabecula at some distance from the surface. In others, anomalies in the way in which the stain complexes with the mineral component suggests important structural arrangements (Fig. 10c). For example, some areas are physically more porous to the stain, apparently as a result of a network of microfissures, which develops in specific trabeculae from time to time (Aaron, 1976b, 1977). In other instances the continued accessibility of 'mature' extracellular mineral to tetracycline stain may imply an abnormality in the 'packaging' of the mineral (see p. 250).

Particularly significant is the affinity of the calcification front for the tetracycline stain, in a manner closely reminiscent of the distribution of the tetracycline label (Fig. 10a). Any differences in this region, either in the intensity of the fluorescence or in its spatial disposition would seem to be largely a matter of concentration and time, since the labelling pattern increasingly resembles the staining pattern as the time between labelling and biopsy is reduced. While the staining technique lacks the time scale conferred by the labelling procedure, it equally lacks the disadvantages of toxicity and the problems in obtaining normal control material as described on p. 221. It compares favourably with other stains in defining the calcification front, and the fluorescent image is probably more sensitive than the tinctorial image, particularly in those circumstances where the calcification front is present, but less well-defined than normal. Such a property is important in osteomalacia where the calcification front is often discontinuous, thin or diffuse (Matrajt *et al.*, 1967). In the most severe degrees of osteomalacia the uptake of tetracycline by the tissue is negligible, implying minimal levels of mineral deposition.

The most significant feature of tetracycline as a histochemical stain, however, undoubtedly lies not so much in its extracellular distribution, but in its characteristic intracellular pattern (see p. 243) and the relationship which

---

Fig. 10. Tetracycline staining of the calcification front in undecalcified bone from the human iliac crest. (a) Bone from a normal 55-year-old male showing tetracycline fluorescence at the calcification front (Cf) and in adjacent osteocytes (vertical arrows). The osteoid tissue (horizontal arrows) and mineralised bone (B) do not stain, but have a dull green autofluorescence. UV light, × 50. (b) Bone from a 33-year-old woman with osteomalacia. Osteoid borders (arrowed) are wide and extensive. Tetracycline staining is diffuse and the calcification front (Cf) is discontinuous or absent. The mineralised bone (B) does not stain. UV light, × 50. (c) Bone from an 83-year-old woman with fractured neck of femur and osteomalacia. Osteoid borders (arrowed) are wide and extensive. The mineralised bone (B) stains densely with tetracycline, indicating some difference in its nature from that of (a) and (b). UV light, × 65

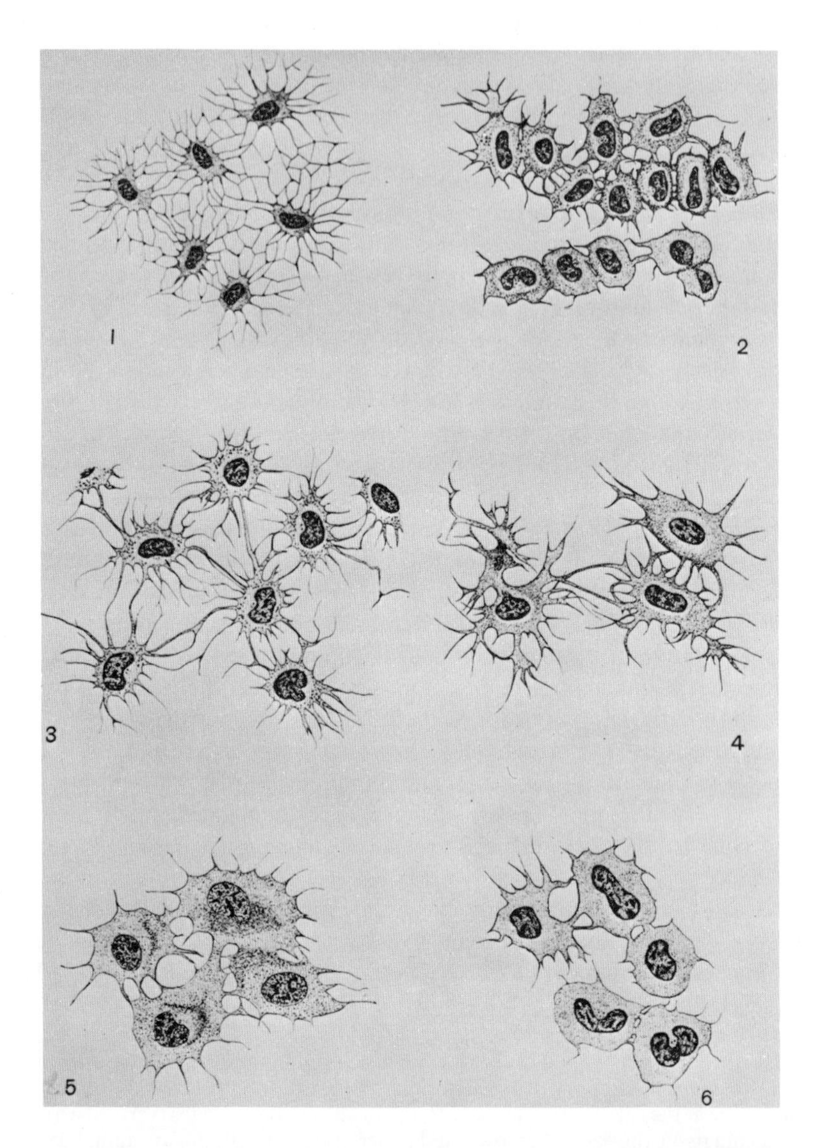

Fig. 11. Camera lucida drawings of cells from ethmoid bone of dog (1) and parietal bone of rat (2–6). Entire bone preserved in 95% alcohol and stained in gentian violet. (From Bast, 1921.) The morphology of 2 and 6 is characteristic of osteoblasts. These occur in layers, usually one cell thick, upon the bone surfaces. They synthesise and export the collagenous osteoid, within which they become embedded and separate from each other (5) as they modulate into osteocytes (1, 3, 4) surrounded by calcified bone

clearly exists between the two. The discussion that follows seeks to show that it is not only the extracellular scene, but also intracellular events which are important to an understanding of calcification and hence of osteomalacia.

D OSTEOMALACIA AND THE OSTEOBLAST

One of the difficulties in trying to rationalise the diverse observations in the literature about the osteoblast and osteomalacia is the variety of the methods applied, with the result that some authors present evidence consistent with decreased bone formation (Canas *et al.*, 1969) while others report that bone formation is increased (see p. 218). However, even when the methodology is similar the results are often open to interpretation. If the premise is accepted that the osteoblast is the bone cell primarily responsible for the development of osteomalacia (either because of a change in its rate of activity or in its number), then it follows that some assessment of the state and distribution of these cells along the osteoid border might be helpful. The morphology of the osteoblast is usually dismissed with no more than a cursory description of its shape and whether it is cuboidal and hence characteristic of the active cell (Fig. 11), or whether it has regressed to the spindle-shape adopted during the 'resting' phase. All bone surfaces, other than those which are resorbing, are generally considered to be lined by one or other of these (Matthews and Martin, 1971; see Aaron, 1976a for details of function). Woods (1976) points out that the cytoplasm of the so-called 'resting' osteoblast is often rich in RNA implying greater synthetic activity than is generally attributed to these cells. In studies of remodelling, however, it is the surface extent of the cuboidal form which is measured, as for surface osteoid tissue using an integrating eyepiece and line-sampling procedures. The results (shown in Table 1) may be expressed relative to the total cancellous surface, or relative to the osteoid surface, or as an absolute value as mm^2/cm^3 total volume of trabecular bone (Merz and Schenk, 1970a). In normal subjects a positive linear correlation between osteoid volume and the extent of osteoblasts has been established by Merz and Schenk (1970a). They further suggest that, since the disappearance of osteoblasts inevitably halts matrix apposition, only their determination can give reliable information about bone formation.

An increase in the surface extent of osteoblasts in anticonvulsant osteomalacia has been described by Eastwood *et al.* (1975). Similarly a feature of skeletal fluorosis which continues to attract attention from a therapeutic standpoint is the apparent tendency for the balance of remodelling to shift towards formation, with an increased surface density of osteoblasts, increased matrix synthesis and the production of wide seams (Olah *et al.*, 1975). Part of the problem in osteomalacia might then be the synthesis of too much osteoid by too many osteoblasts perhaps to compensate for the diminished structural capacity of the mineralised region. The possibility arises that the disease progresses because of an increased requirement for vitamin D, such as Woodhouse *et al.* (1971) and Bordier and Tun Chot (1972) have been investigating in conditions of high bone turnover (see also Fig. 6b).

On the other hand, if it takes each osteoblast longer to manufacture its complement of organic matrix, then an accumulation of these cells would tend to follow with time, and the number of osteoblasts may present a misleading picture of the synthetic activity of the tissue. Consistent with this are the observations of Baylink *et al.* (1970) using cortical bone and an animal model. They observed that in vitamin D-deficient rats the rate of organic matrix formation was 20% less than normal, principally because of changes in the linear rate of matrix apposition, rather than because of changes in the extent of its surface. This would support the proposal of Frost (1966, 1967, 1973) that the pathogenesis of osteomalacia is directly related to the malfunction of the osteoblast. Baylink *et al.* (1970) concluded however, that the diminished apposition was the result of hypocalcaemia and, in particular, secondary hyperparathyroidism. Frost (1973) continues to doubt that the principle bone disturbance in osteomalacia is a failure to mineralise new osteoid and argues that were this the case seams should regularly become hundreds of microns thick, or of the order of magnitude of the radius of entire osteons. He maintains that since they do not, the organic matrix must be synthesised as slowly as it is mineralised. However, Fischer *et al.* (1970) showed that in intestinal malabsorption (9 cases) and in nutritional vitamin D-deficiency (1 case) the osteoblast population (although it may be normal or increased) is always inadequate for the volume of osteoid, indicating that there is a basic deficiency in calcification which is independent of the rate of matrix apposition. Further descriptions by Baylink *et al.* (1970) confirm this (see p. 236).

There are clearly changes within the osteoblasts in osteomalacia which require careful analysis. For instance, Heller-Steinberg (1951), using the Hotchkiss procedure, demonstrated granules 0.3 to 0.6 μm in diameter inside the osteoblasts which she attributed to the presence of a polysaccharide-protein complex, similar to that in the extracellular matrix. The granules were rare in rachitic animals. At the same time, ultrastructural studies of Bonucci *et al.* (1969) imply a slower differentiation of osteoblasts from osteoprogenitor cells in patients with osteomalacia, and an accumulation of glycogen consistent with reduced activity. However, important as an understanding of the factors influencing matrix synthesis undoubtedly is to both normal and pathological conditions, the central question in osteomalacia and rickets historically, at least, concerns the calcification of bone and the translocation of mineral.

IV The Calcification of Bone and Cartilage

A THE PARADOX OF METAZOAN CALCIFICATION

Dujardin, in 1835, was the first to recognise that the elaborate shells and tests of the protozoans and diatoms were the work of a 'singular organization' of a glutinous, filamentous substance, later to be known as protoplasm. One hundred and forty years later, the central problem in calcification is still the mechanism by which the salt is laid down in relation to the protoplasm. The remarkable precision and order of the process and the variety of each arrangement despite the constancy of chemical composition in each species, is not in accord with a process of random precipitation and leaves little room for doubt that calcification in simple organisms is controlled at all stages by the cell (see Pautard, 1970 for review).

In the Protozoa the location and concentration of calcium is subject to wide variations; some free ionic calcium may be extracted from the cytoplasm, but most is associated with organelles, often as an organic complex rather than the inorganic salt. Calcium salts occur either as parts of organelles, or as crystals within vacuoles, or as structures which arise within vacuoles. In unicellular organisms (and the invertebrates in general), when mineral deposits occur, calcium carbonate is the most common, though calcium phosphate and calcium sulphate are present in some species. Towe and Cifelli (1967) in speculating on the process by which the tests of the Foraminifera mineralise suggested a system of crystal epitaxy such as Glimcher (1959) had proposed for bone. But Angell (1965) observing the construction of the test of *Rosalina floridana* described the onset of calcification with the appearance of numerous vesicles and vacuoles within pseudopodia. These formed a vacuolated sheath, the vesicles of which seemed to be the primary calcifying agent. Similarly, the unicellular coccolithophorids manufacture calcareous coccoliths, complex skeletal structures, inside membrane-bound vesicles (Wilbur and Watabe, 1963). Vesicles have been apparently associated with the development of calcium phosphate bodies in *Paramoecium caudatum* as long ago as 1894 (Schewiakoff); the same has been described more recently in *Spirostomum ambiguum* (Pautard, 1958; 1970). These simple organisms also serve to illustrate the speed with which cells can manufacture complex mineralised structures; for instance coccoliths can be made in a few minutes (Wilbur and Watabe, 1963).

Paradoxically, calcified deposits in the metazoans and particularly in the vertebrates are widely held to be the result of a nucleation and growth of crystals without direct cellular involvement, their size, shape and disposition being accounted for in terms of physical and chemical characteristics of the extracellular matrix.

B THE ULTRASTRUCTURE OF THE INORGANIC DEPOSITS OF BONE

In osteomalacic bone, according to Bonucci *et al.* (1969), although no distinct calcification front is present, clusters of apatite too small to be optically evident occur throughout the osteoid tissue. The fine structure of these crystallites is sometimes normal (see below), but sometimes abnormal consisting of amorphous or finely granular deposits which tend to sublimate under the electron beam. With mineralisation these abnormal structures grow, coalesce and become more typically crystalline in appearance.

There are many descriptions of the normal ultrastructural arrangement of bone and dentine (Robinson, 1952). The crystallites occur in clusters and sheets and are needle-shaped, or plate-like with a width or thickness of about 50 Å and a length of the order of 200 Å; according to some authors they are smallest in young bone. They may be subdivided, like a string of beads, or fused into long rods. While most authors are in agreement about the general shape, size and structure of the calcified deposits of bone, there are serious discrepancies as to the way in which these crystallites develop. Ideas vary from calcification as an extracellular event based on geometrical and chemical parameters of the matrix, to alignment by cell mediation in the matrix.

C CALCIFICATION – AN EXTRACELLULAR EVENT

1. *Collagen and Epitaxy*. Hofmeister in 1891 observed the binding of metal ions by small gelatin discs and suggested that the selective affinity of colloids for calcium ions was important in the initial phase of the calcification process. The concept was developed during the next thirty years, and interested Freudenberg and György (1924) who noted that calcium was firmly bound to the colloids of cartilage before there was any significant uptake of phosphate. Shipley (1924) found that epiphyseal cartilage calcified when immersed in serum from normal rats, whereas it would not calcify in serum from rachitic rats. He suggested that the failure was due primarily to a low concentration of inorganic phosphorus, but was unable to explain why crystal formation normally occurred only in the region of one particular zone of cells. Such considerations were superceded by the mathematical approach to the solubility of bone salt in relation to blood on the one hand, and by the development of x-ray diffraction and electron microscope techniques on the other. These verified the uniformity of the mineral particles and their orientation with the collagen, aspects which had only been suspected optically, and stimulated the theory of epitaxy. This proposes that specific sites on the collagen fibres induce the aggregation of ions to form crystal nuclei upon which the crystals grow by further deposition of calcium and phosphorus from their metastable solution in the blood.

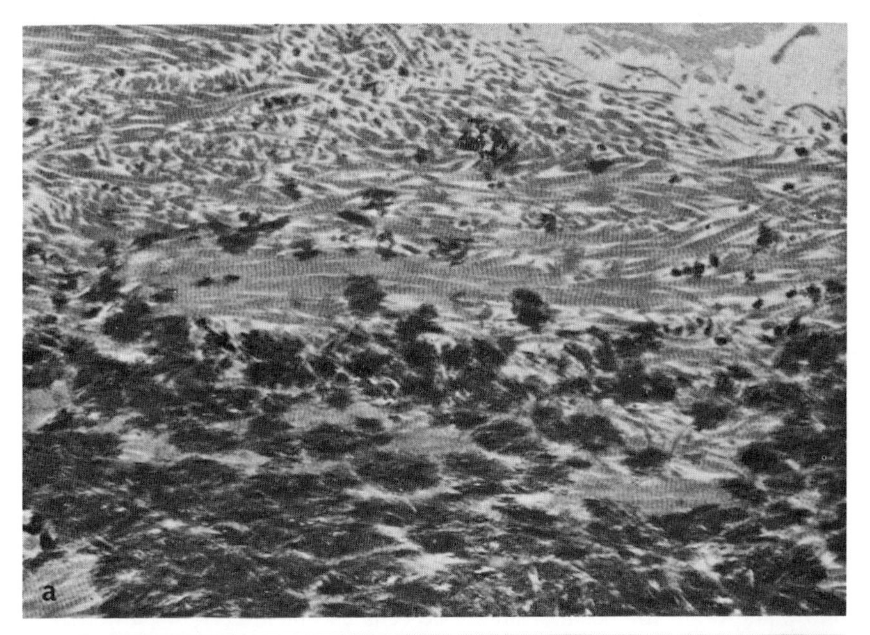

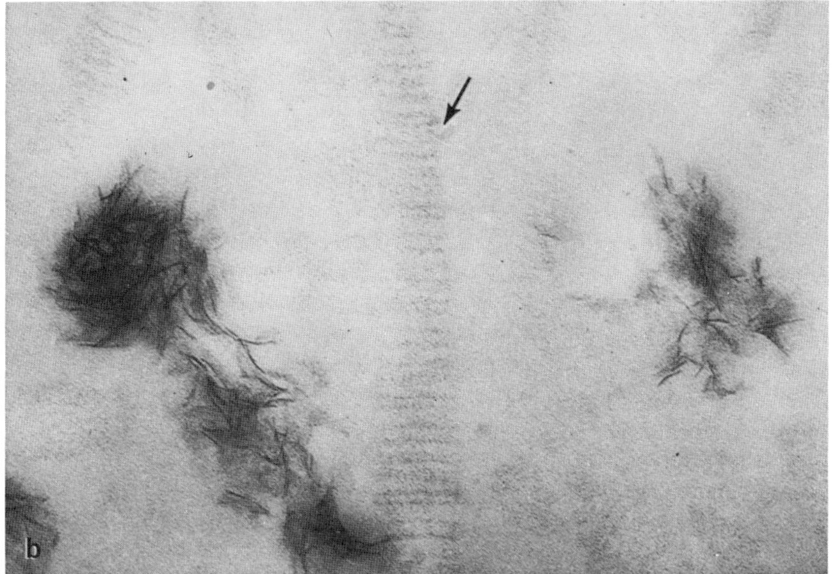

Fig. 12. Collagen and bone mineral. (a) Bone mineral appears as scattered electron-opaque areas among the collagen fibrils of the maturing matrix, becoming confluent in the deeper regions at the bottom of the figure. Embryonic avian bone, glutaraldehyde fixation, × 10 000. (b) The dense deposits are composed of clusters of crystallites 15–25Å wide, and showing no intimate association with the collagen fibrils (arrowed). × 200 000. (Photomicrographs kindly supplied by Dr B. Boothroyd)

Microcrystallites of apatite were described in the interfibrillar spaces and in the collagen fibrils where their orientation was apparently parallel with that of the fibrils (Engström and Zetterström, 1951; Robinson and Watson, 1952). Controversy arose when several authors observed random distribution and no alignment to collagen (Scott and Pease, 1956; Robinson and Cameron, 1956; Ascenzi, 1964). It was maintained, however, that whether or not the final crystallites were orientated in relation to the collagen (Fig. 12), the initial site of deposition occurred at periodic intervals along collagen fibres in embryonic chick bone (Fitton Jackson, 1957), in mouse parietal bone (Molnar, 1959), and in calcifying tendon (Nylen *et al.*, 1960). The collagen fibre came to be regarded as a chain of nucleation sites, with some characteristic of the molecular periodicity, either mechanical, or chemical, which allowed the precipitation of mineral in conditions where simple spontaneous precipitation was not thermodynamically feasible. This principle forms the basis of the various mechanisms which have been proposed by Neuman and Neuman (1958), Glimcher (1959), Sobel *et al.* (1960) and Bachra (1972), and has until recently been in accord with the electron microscope evidence that calcium phosphate does not occur inside bone cells except in certain pathological circumstances and during osteoclastic resorption. It is perhaps of some interest to note here that the osteomalacia characteristic of fibrogenesis imperfecta ossium was considered by Baker (1956) to be the consequence of a collagen abnormality and the subsequent failure of epitaxy.

Although the concept of epitaxy is consistent with the equilibrium conditions between blood and bone salt there are certain discrepancies. Pautard (1965) pointed out the exceptions to a 'unique' partnership between bone salt and collagen in the deposition of apatite in matrices lacking collagen. For example, the matrix of enamel is of the keratin-myosin-epidermin-fibrinogen group of proteins; the bone-like crystallites of baleen are deposited in a keratin matrix, and those of the Crustacea occur in association with chitin. Certain calculi not containing collagen also contain crystallites closely resembling those of bone. It may be argued that these are expressions of a mineralisation system which is mechanically orientated with respect to other proteins and polysaccharides, or that some group common to all calcifying proteins is present. But, Pautard (1966) on the basis of calcium deposits in plants found that crystal formation occurred in spaces in tissues completely independent of any of the reactive sites of the organic components. Again, Cameron (1963) described crystal-cluster formation in areas of bone distant from collagen fibres, and Bonucci (1971) was only able to find mineral granules and crystallites reinforcing collagen banding when calcification was advanced. At the same time, Dudley and Spiro (1961) have expressed uneasiness about electronmicrographs which show features described as the first mineral nuclei. Since they were able to find such particles in only one of many sections from the same specimen, they concluded that these were technical artifacts due to sublimation and reprecipitation caused by the electron beam. Finally, the accumulation of evidence for an amorphous phase (Termine and Posner, 1967), and the increasing uncertainty as to the crystalline nature of the remainder, also places the precise role of epitaxy in some doubt. Despite these anomalies the theories based on the properties of crystals and fibres continue. Long before epitaxy, however, a cellular involvement with calcification was contemplated.

2. *Alkaline Phosphatase*. Between 1923 and 1932, Robison using rachitic cartilage, proposed that an enzyme, alkaline phosphatase, entered into the localisation mechanism of calcification. He noted that alkaline phosphatase was found in the cytoplasm of hypertrophic cells in the zone of provisional calcification, and attempted to show that it produced a local supersaturation with respect to free phosphate ions, by the hydrolysis of phosphate esters. A simple precipitation of calcium phosphate would then follow. To explain the extracellular site of deposition a second mechanism was postulated, which was arrested by potassium cyanide, desiccation or fat solvents, none of which destroyed alkaline phosphatase activity.

Although the theory was accepted for many years, there were serious doubts as some authors considered the quantity of phosphate esters inadequate. Others noted the enzyme in high concentration during the first stages of bone formation, but described its disappearance as mineralisation took place (Bevelander and Johnson, 1950; Morse and Green, 1951). It was therefore suggested that the enzyme was involved in the preparation of the extracellular matrix prior to calcification, rather than in the initiation of the event itself. Thus, Fleisch and Bisaz (1962) considered that its functions may be to remove the pyrophosphate which would otherwise inhibit crystallisation. On the other hand, the optimum pH value for alkaline phosphatase activity is higher than that provided by the extracellular fluids. Others have related it to the distribution of glycogen in the hypertrophic cells and postulated its role in glycolysis (Gutman and Yu, 1950).

However, any function the enzyme might have had in calcification could not be reconciled with descriptions by Pritchard (1952) of the enzyme in soft tissues and its appearance in mesenchymal cells. The concept was subsequently neglected, and although the enzyme is always present during bone formation, any role in calcification is assumed to be indirect. But, the distribution of alkaline phosphatase, appearing first in the nucleus, then in the cytoplasm and later in the extracellular matrix is reminiscent of the distribution of calcium phosphate recently demonstrated in developing bone (see p. 243) and also in soft tissues (see p. 248), and implies that the dismissal of this enzyme from the calcification process may have been premature.

3. *Matrix 'Maturation'*. A possible role for alkaline phosphatase may be

postulated in the process loosely described as 'maturation'. Since osteoid fails to mineralise for some time after its synthesis (10 days in man), since it also differs histochemically from bone matrix, and since further histochemical changes take place in osteoid before the initiation of the mineralisation, it has been suggested that some process of 'maturation' must occur before calcification is possible. Baylink *et al.* (1970) attempted to measure the effects of vitamin D-deficiency on the rate of this process, which was found to be reduced by 50% and to the same extent as mineralisation; matrix synthesis on the other hand, was decreased by only 20%. It was concluded that 'maturation' and mineralisation are probably phases in a single event for which vitamin D is important.

A common feature of delayed mineralisation is the eventual loss by some regions of the osteoid tissue of the capacity to calcify, even when a favourable environment is restored. This results in old seams becoming buried under new calcifying tissue (Haas *et al.*, 1967; Jowsey, 1968). Such an event is generally attributed to either a defect in the organic matrix produced by the osteoblasts under the abnormal conditions (such as Steendijk *et al.*, 1965 have described in hypophosphataemic rickets), or a failure in its 'maturation'.

4. *Vesicular Structures*

(*a*) *Cartilage 'globules' and 'vesicles'*. Evidence for the ultrastructural nature of the 'maturation' process of cartilage and possibly bone has been supplied by descriptions of 'globules' and 'vesicles' in calcifying cartilage. Renaut (cited by Schuscik, 1920) put forward the view that calcification involved the release of calcium salts from small globules of a complex of calcium, fat and protein which stained densely with haematoxylin. Recently Bonucci (1967) has also reported 'globules' in calcifying cartilage and from these observations an alternative theory of calcification has developed. 'Globules' are described as membrane-bound structures which have an amorphous osmiophilic matrix and a distinct biochemistry (Figs. 13a and b). They are of cellular origin, yet are considered as separate from the cell and they apparently contain a calcium-binding glycoprotein (de Bernard *et al.*, 1977). Resembling these structures are the 'vesicles' observed by Anderson (1968) and Ali *et al.* (1970) in epiphyseal cartilage (Fig. 13c). The association of such structures with dense deposits has inevitably led to their designation as the epitactic sites previously ascribed to collagen, and to their assignment in relation to the crystallite 'ghosts' (Fig. 14), an organic phase thought to be a protein-polysaccharide (Sundström *et al.*, 1970; Appleton, 1971). The 'ghosts' occur in clusters, are 50 Å in diameter, 500–1000 Å in length and consist of strings of electron-dense spherical bodies, surrounded by an electron dense material. The 'globules' and 'vesicles' are found throughout the epiphyseal plate, even in those regions not actively calcifying; those in the resting zone are

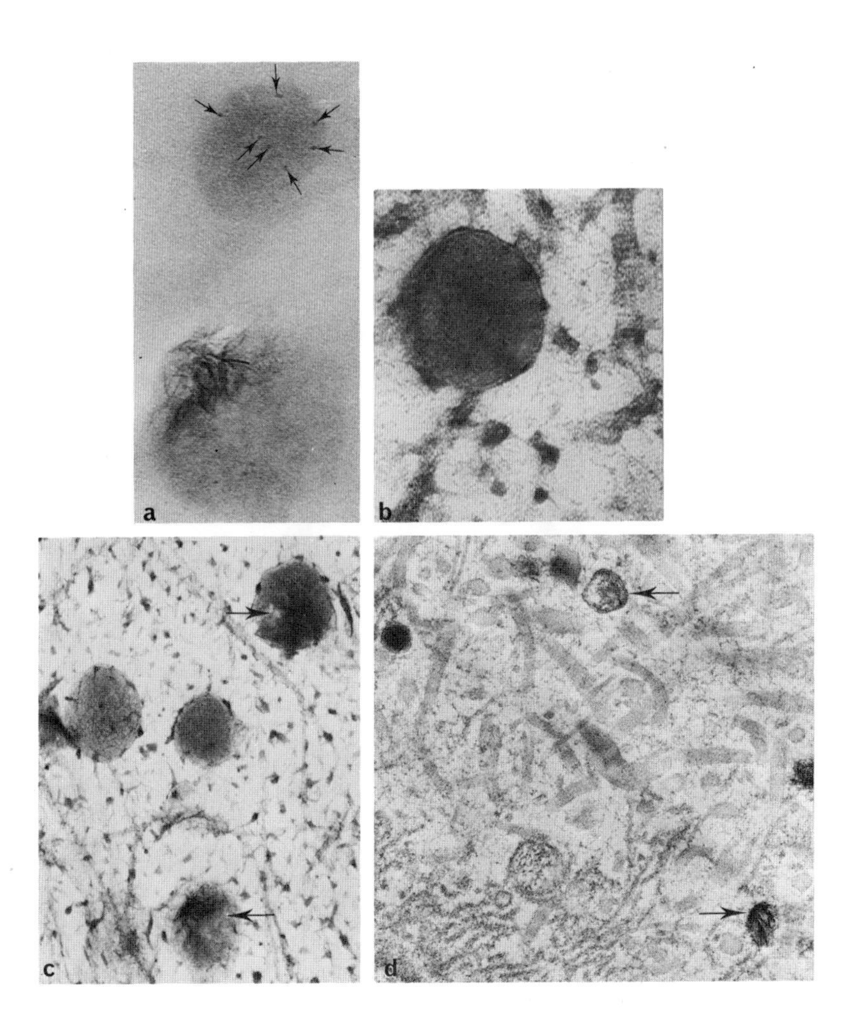

Fig. 13. 'Globules', 'vesicles' and 'buds' (a) 'Globules' in the maturing zone of the epiphyseal cartilage, one containing mineral granules (arrowed), the other a crystal cluster. Osmium post-fixation, unstained, ×100 000. (From Bonucci, 1971.) (b) Uncalcified 'globule' showing a 3-layered membrane. Osmium post-fixation, uranyl acetate and lead citrate staining ×100 000. (From Bonucci, 1971.) (c) Matrix 'vesicles' in the epiphyseal cartilage of rabbit tibia, some empty, some containing electron-dense needles of apatite (arrowed). Uranyl acetate and lead citrate staining, ×58 000. (Photomicrograph kindly supplied by Dr S. Y. Ali.) (d) 'Buds' (arrowed) in association with crystals in predentine. Osmium post-fixation, uranyl acetate and lead citrate staining, ×23 000. (From Bernard, 1972)

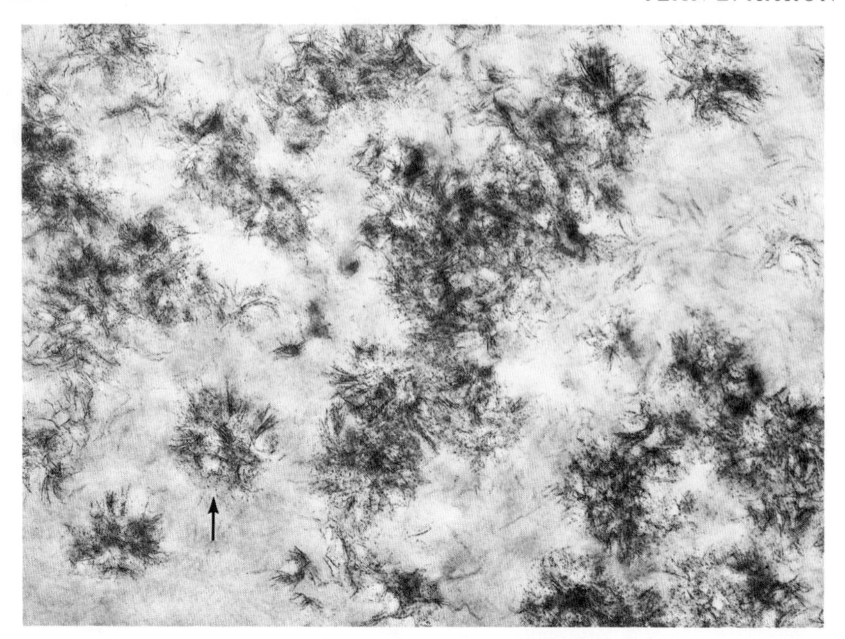

Fig. 14. Crystallite 'ghosts'. An organic phase (arrowed) closely resembles the clusters of crystallites (Fig. 12b) in shape and distribution. Mandibular condylar cartilage from newborn rats, post-fixed, decalcified, and stained with chromium sulphate, pH 4.3, papain-digested, ×46 000. (From Appleton, 1971)

free of mineral, those in the hypertrophic zone contain electron dense granules and clusters of crystals. Whether or not the 'globules' or 'vesicles' are present but in an unmineralised state in rachitic cartilage is not clear (Fig. 15). However, vesicles have been described in cartilage which normally does not calcify and it has been suggested that these may lack, among other things, alkaline phosphatase (Ali *et al.*, 1970).

Slavkin (1972) and Katchburian (1977) have described similar vesicles in dentine which have been named 'buds' by Bernard (1972, Fig. 13d). These contain not only calcium phosphate, but also alkaline phosphatase (Slavkin, 1972). Whether such features occur in bone, however, is less clear.

(b) *Membrane-bound structures and the osteoblast*

The osteoblast has always been regarded as the cell responsible for providing the localised conditions permitting calcification, an event often described as taking place in two stages. During the first stage, 50 to 70% of the mineral is deposited within the first few hours (Johnson, 1964; Harris and Heaney, 1969) or days (Frost, 1967); further mineralisation is slower, taking months (Amprino and Engström, 1952; Lacroix, 1956) or years (Frost, 1967). It is the first stage of calcification for which the activity of osteoblasts is

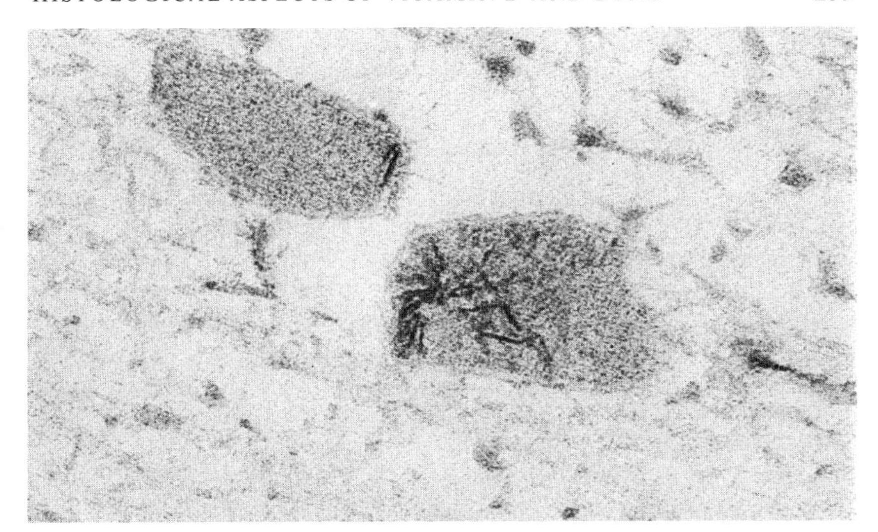

Fig. 15. Matrix 'vesicles' in the epiphyseal cartilage of the rachitic rat. Although the regions outside the vesicles have not calcified, electron-dense needles resembling apatite occur within vesicles in some areas. Osmium post-fixation, uranyl acetate and lead citrate staining, × 173 000. (From Anderson, 1972)

regarded as essential (Frost, 1967; Merz and Schenk, 1970a). As early as 1965 Hancox and Boothroyd reported isolated membrane-bound structures containing crystallites, in close proximity to osteoblasts. These were identified as sectioned cytoplasmic processes. Arnott and Pautard (1967) were unable to find evidence of such membrane-bound deposits, although they did observe a close association between 'dense ribbons of crystallites' and the filament-like processes from osteoblasts. Subsequent studies by Bernard and Pease (1969) have concerned the further description of the 'islands of crystallites' or bone 'nodules' in relation to 'extrusions' from osteoblasts. Despite the conjecture, however, structures resembling the 'globules', 'vesicles' and 'buds' are rarely reported in calcifying bone (see Anderson and Reynolds, 1973 for exception).

Since the vesicular structures are generally considered to be created in the cell and to pass through the cell wall to the extracellular matrix before they are mineralised, the mechanism differs from collagen epitaxy only in the precise nature of the initial site of calcification and both theories finally unite in the idea of an extracellular epitaxy. Both mechanisms are therefore directly subject to the vagaries of the blood biochemistry. There is, however, evidence to suggest that the process of mineralisation may be more complex than this. Also there are regular cellular processes during which large numbers of vesicles are created and extruded for a variety of purposes. Many such structures in the extracellular matrix may then be concerned with activities other than calcification.

Dr M. Parfitt (personal communication) has recently drawn attention to the fact that after labelling the calcification front (i.e. the first stage of calcification) with tetracycline, not only do some seams with cuboidal osteoblasts fail to fluoresce, but also conversely, some seams labelled with tetracycline (and therefore calcifying) frequently lack 'active' osteoblasts (see also Parfitt, 1973). This implies that it may be a mistake to regard both matrix apposition and the initiation of calcification as dependent upon the same cell. While it may be argued that the time interval between labelling and biopsy would be sufficient to allow osteoblasts originally present to regress, this possibility is eliminated when activity at the calcification front is demonstrated at the time of biopsy using tinctorial procedures as described on p. 221. Then, while 60 % or more, of the osteoid surface is actively calcifying in normal bone, the extent of osteoblasts is considerably less than this (35.6% of the osteoid surface in the young, 14.8% in the old, Merz and Schenk, 1970a). Recent evidence, to be described, suggests that it is the osteocyte (Fig. 11) and not the osteoblast which is responsible for the calcification of bone. The 'maturation' period above may then be the time during which the osteoblast modulates into an osteocyte before beginning a separate cycle of activity commencing with the calcification of its environment. It follows that when osteomalacia responds to vitamin D, the calcification of the accumulated osteoid will depend not so much upon the presence of osteoblasts, as upon the nature of the osteocytes in that region and whether or not they are stimulated to 'switch-on' for mineralisation.

D CALCIFICATION – AN INTRACELLULAR EVENT

1. *Optical Evidence*. Watt (1928) advocated that interstitial calcium and phosphate was first diffused into the osteoblasts and chondrocytes and then secreted into the matrix to initiate calcification. However, he based his hypothesis on subjective and circumstantial evidence and could not demonstrate calcium or phosphate within these cells. Consequently, his theory of mineral secretion, proposed during the years when Robison's alkaline phosphatase concept gained popularity, was not taken seriously.

But, the presence of calcium in cells of calcifying tissues other than bone has been reported by several authors using a variety of techniques. Deposits of calcium phosphate, closely resembling the mineral phase in bone have been described in certain unicellular organisms (see p. 231), and in the keratins (Pautard, 1965). The appearance of calcium deposits within cells is also a common feature of pathological conditions; thus Dahl (1952) described them in rat kidneys after parenteral administration of uranium nitrate, before any cellular damage could be demonstrated by histological examination. In skeletal tissues, mineralisation within chondrocytes has been shown micro-radiographically in the epiphyseal plate of the slider turtle (Suzuki, 1963), while Bohatirchuk (1965), in an extensive historadiographic study of mammalian cartilage showed that some cells were calcium free, while others were partly or completely mineralised (see also Gaillard *et al.*, 1975).

Recently, however, reports of a distribution of mineral inside bone cells have increased in number and the evidence which Watt lacked to support his theory is now accumulating. Mineral particles in the osteoblasts and osteocytes of bone have been reported by Kashiwa (1970), who suggested that they may be connected with the appearance of similar deposits in the extracellular matrix. At the same time Rolle (1969) showed a correlation

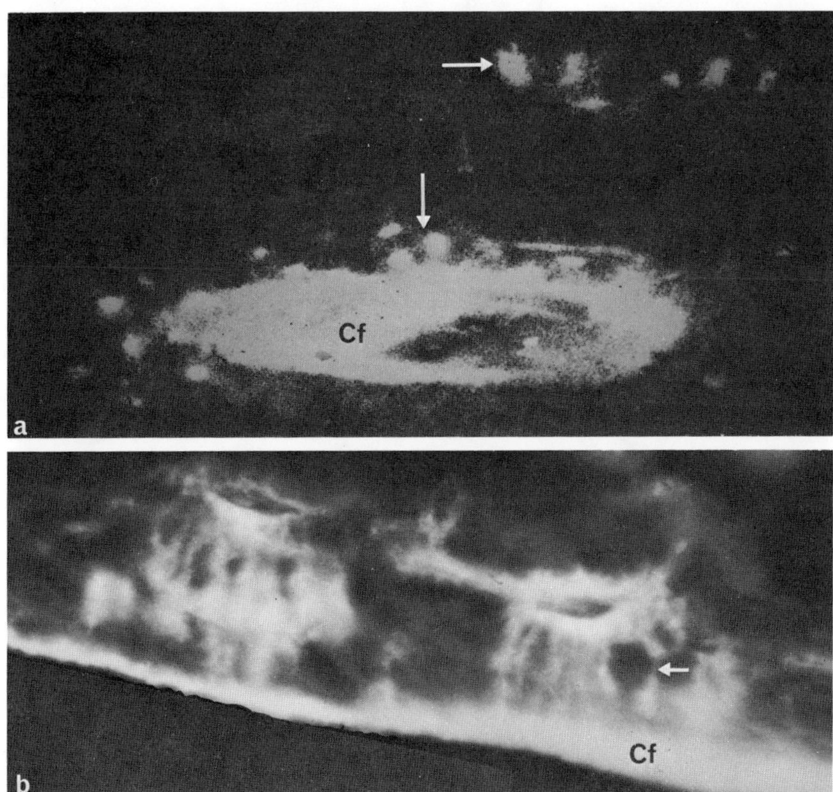

Fig. 16. Tetracycline staining of osteocytes in a region of new bone formation in the human iliac crest. (a) Osteocytes (vertical arrow) adjacent to the fluorescent calcification front (Cf) stain densely with tetracycline. Osteocytes in deeper regions of the bone are generally unstained but may switch on for mineral translocation (horizontal arrow). Undecalcified bone, UV light, ×265. (b) The canalicular processes (arrowed) leading to the calcification front (Cf) also stain densely in some instances. Undecalcified bone, UV light, ×700

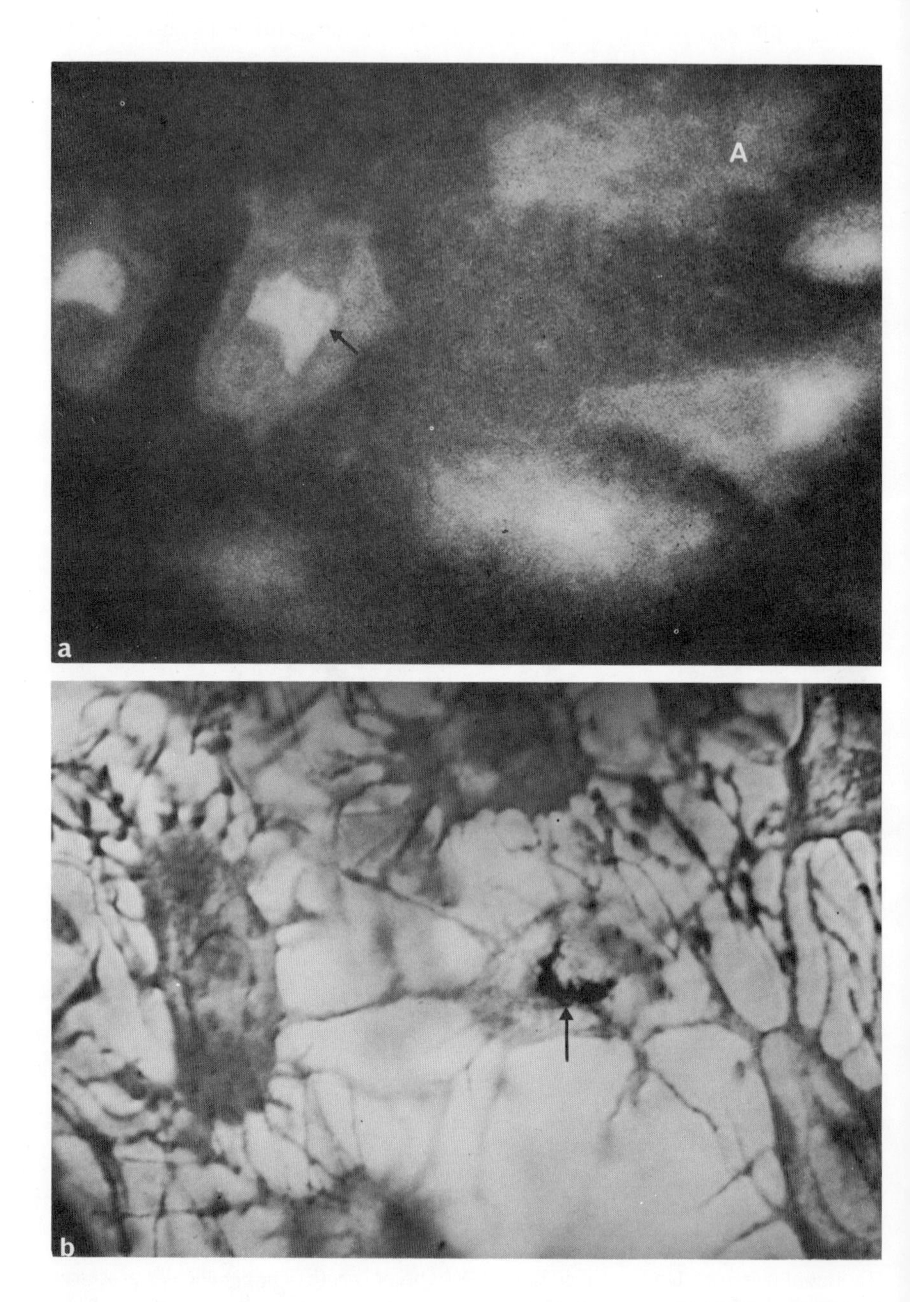
A
a
b

between the amount of calcium within the cells and the degree of mineralisation of the adjacent matrix of chick embryo bone. These histochemical observations are supported by autoradiographic studies (Johnston, 1958) and chemical analysis (Hirschman and Nichols, 1972). A systematic study of the histochemical distribution of 'calcium' and 'phosphate' (or carbonate) in developing bone (Aaron, 1973, 1974) has led to the conclusion that the mineral is more closely associated with the osteocyte than with the osteoblast and that the relationship is complex and takes place in sequence over a short period of time. In such an arrangement, the cell is first mineral-free, then goes through various phases of activity before becoming mineral-free again, and on this basis it has been proposed that osteocytes undergo a cycle of mineral 'loading' and 'unloading'. The role of the osteocyte in mineralisation may have been overlooked because of this transitory nature of the mineral in a rapidly 'packaging' cell.

Further evidence is provided by tetracycline stain (Fig. 16) when, in addition to the characteristic extracellular fluorescent zones described earlier (see p. 225), a pattern of intracellular fluorescence is apparent. The regional and discontinous nature of the intracellular fluorescence again suggests a periodic mechanism of some kind where cells 'switch on' and 'switch off' for the fabrication of the tetracycline-binding complex. In sections of developing long bone or calvarium of young mice, or regions of bone formation in the human iliac crest, the binding increases in the order osteoprogenitor cell–osteoblast–osteocyte. The concentration of tetracycline in the vicinity of the nucleus and the juxtanuclear apparatus with a more diffuse staining of the cytoplasm (Fig. 17a), is of particular significance. The dynamic evidence afforded by tetracycline, allied to previous histochemical studies (Fig. 17b), suggests that the calcium phosphate (or carbonate) is exported from the cell and that a cell cycle for bone mineralisation is present (Fig. 18). Here the osteoblast is not the primary source of mineral, but as it modulates into an osteocyte it progressively loads with calcium. While calcium is dispersed in a general manner throughout the cell, phosphate appears first in the nuclear region, before spreading into the cytoplasm (Fig. 19). During this time the

---

Fig. 17 The juxtanuclear distribution of the calcium phosphate (or carbonate) complex in osteocytes of an intact 5-day-old mouse calvarium. (a) Intracellular tetracycline stain concentrates in the juxtanuclear apparatus (arrowed) which appears as a fluorescent crescent-shaped structure containing bright granules. The cytoplasm also fluoresces, but less brightly. Not all osteocytes stain in this way and the juxtanuclear region of cell A fails to fluoresce. Undecalcified bone, tetracycline stain, UV light $\times$ 1750. (b) The juxtanuclear region (arrowed) also stains densely with silver. Undecalcified bone, von Kossa stain, followed by glyoxal-bis-(2-hydroxyanil) (now known as di-(2-hydroxyphenyl-imino)-ethane) stain (GBHA) polarisation interference contrast (Nomarski) optics for transmitted light, $\times$ 1500

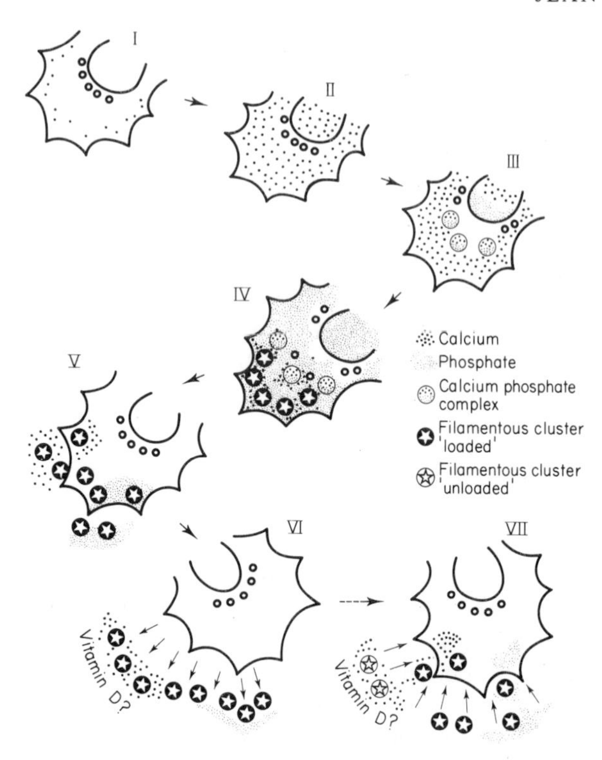

Fig. 18. Proposed cell cycle for mineralisation in the osteocyte. I. The cytoplasm begins to 'load' with calcium. The juxtanuclear apparatus is compact and intimately associated with the nucleus. II. The cytoplasm 'loads' further with calcium, which also enters the nuclear region. III. The juxtanuclear apparatus 'switches on' for mineral packaging with the proliferation and growth of vacuoles. The accumulation of phosphate (or carbonate) becomes apparent in the nuclear region. IV. The juxtanuclear apparatus extends into a network. Phosphate (or carbonate) activity spreads throughout the cytoplasm and calcium phosphate (or carbonate) complexes are formed. Some of these are discrete structures composed of filamentous clusters. V. The mineral complexes are exported from the cell to the calcification front. VI. The mature osteocyte has 'unloaded' and the juxtanuclear apparatus is again compact. VII. In response to specific stimuli the osteocyte may eventually resorb bone mineral, the filamentous clusters being engulfed intact, or 'unloading' their mineral to the cells. The precise role of vitamin D in these processes of mineral translocation is not clear

juxtanuclear apparatus (Fig. 20a) is 'switched on' for mineral packaging (Aaron and Pautard, 1973a; 1975; Aaron, 1974). Finally, the calcium and phosphorus in some complexed form appear outside the cell, and the activity of the juxtanuclear apparatus diminishes (Fig. 20b) as the osteocytes become surrounded by a calcified matrix.

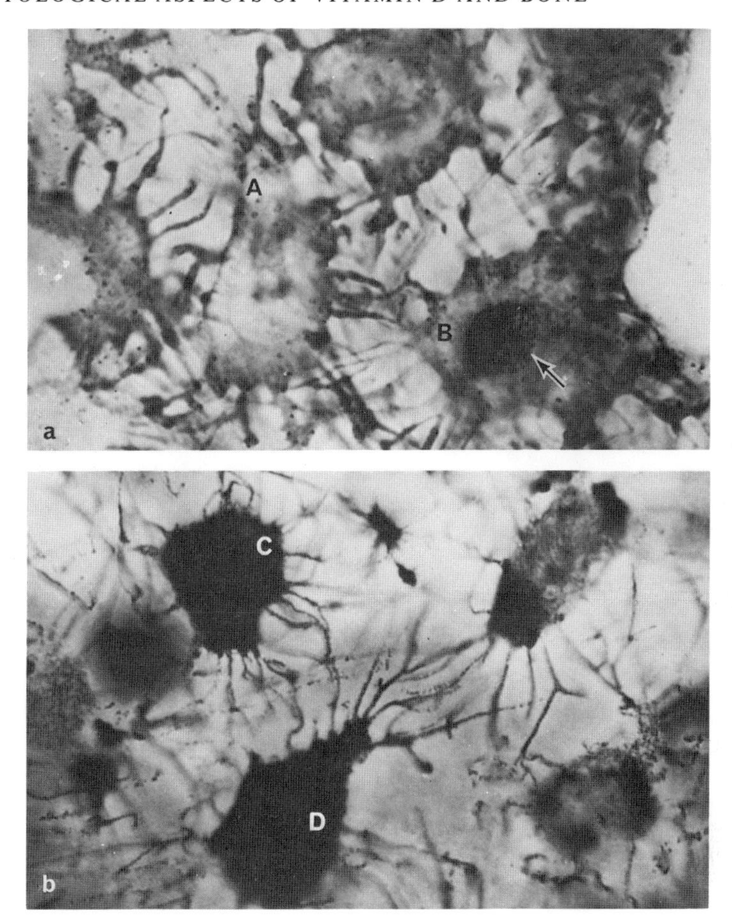

Fig. 19. The intracellular distribution of calcium and phosphate in osteocytes of an intact 5-day-old mouse calvarium. (a) Osteocytes in the 'young' peripheral regions stain predominantly for calcium. Cell A contains only calcium while cell B, in the same focal plane, also contains phosphate (or carbonate), principally localised in the juxtanuclear region (arrowed). (b) Osteocytes C and D from more mature central areas of the bone stain densely with silver and are apparently 'loaded' with (calcium) phosphate or carbonate. Undecalcified bone, von Kossa stain followed by GBHA stain, Nomarski optics for transmitted light, ×1100

Little is known of the nature of the fluorescing complex. However, if the tetracycline complex within the cell is the same as, or similar to, the tetracycline complex outside the cell it must be concluded that the mineral in the matrix commenced as such within the cell. Moreover, the association of the 'mineral particles' within the juxtanuclear apparatus tends to confirm that these, at least, are being synthesised within the cell and are not the products of

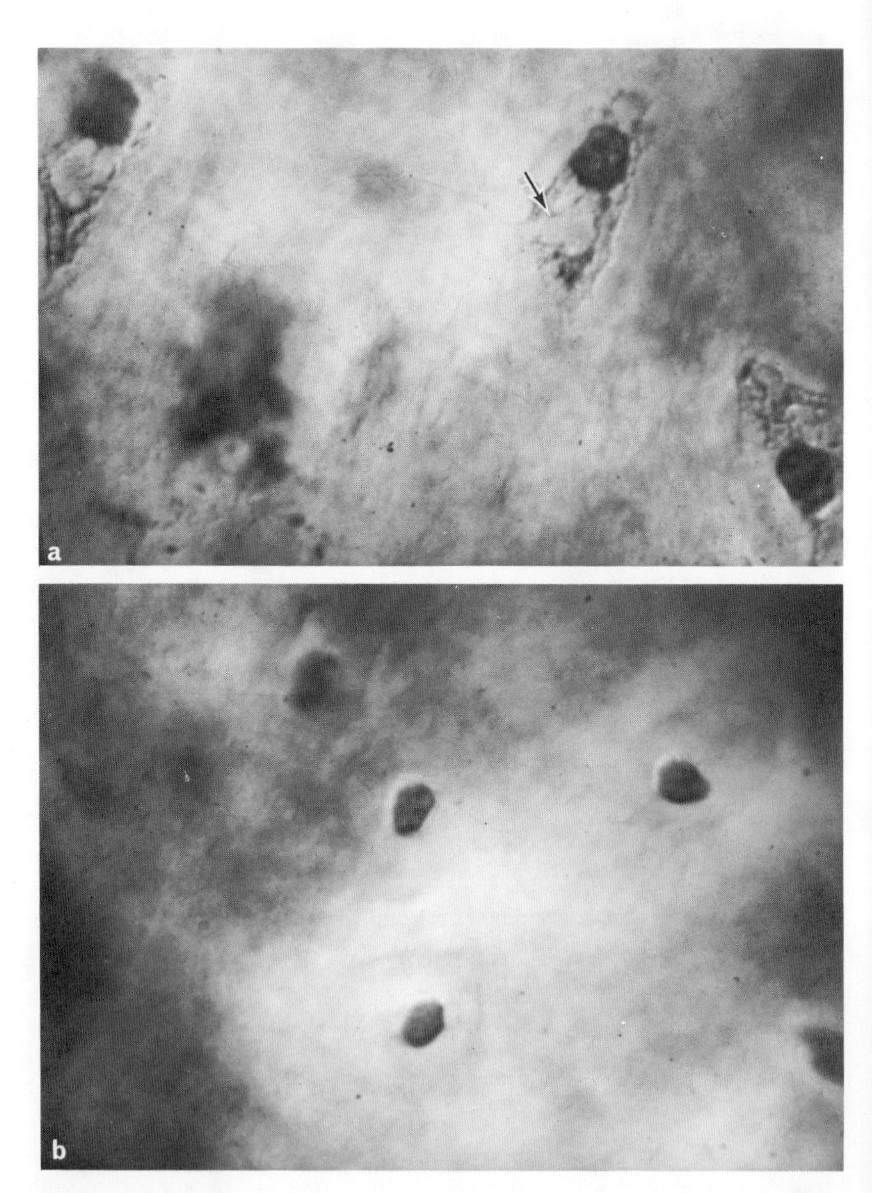

Fig. 20. The 'switch-on' 'switch-off' mechanism of juxtanuclear activity in osteocytes of an intact 5-day-old mouse calvarium. (a) Osteocytes in which the juxtanuclear apparatus has developed into a network (arrowed) which extends throughout the cytoplasm. (b) Osteocytes with a compact juxtanuclear apparatus. Undecalcified bone, neutral red stain, Nomarski optics for transmitted light, ×1500

resorption from the surrounding matrix, as Zichner (1971) has described. It also seems clear that the failure to observe cell fluorescence in specimens labelled with tetracycline, in contrast to specimens stained with tetracycline may be only a matter of concentration and time. *In vivo* the toxicity of tetracycline precludes the use of heavy doses and any fluorescence in the cells will be small in comparison to the fluorescence in the calcification zone outside the cells, where the tetracycline would be steadily accumulated during the labelling period. It seems that after periods of pulse-labelling of less than an hour, or in those pathological circumstances where tetracycline excretion is less effective than normal, (as in renal failure) bone cells do show appreciable binding of tetracycline in a manner similar to, though less intense than, the manner after staining. In addition, there is an increasing similarity of the tetracycline labelled pattern in the iliac crest to the staining pattern, when the biopsy is taken a short time after labelling.

The view that calcium and phosphate are not always present in the same place at the same time proposed by Pautard (1972) and Aaron (1973) is supported by Heeley and Irving (1973) who observed that calcium was deposited before phosphate in the mineralisation process. It is unlikely that a diffusion artifact can be the explanation, since adjacent cells in the same focal plane often differ considerably in their relative staining patterns, (Fig. 19). Moreover, the development and distribution of intracellular mineral closely resembles that described by Pritchard (1952) for alkaline phosphatase. Finally, the appearance *in situ* of the osteocyte in the living animal, using incident light interference contrast optics (Aaron and Pautard, 1973b), seems to be the result of a fortunate coincidence. It provides an opportunity to examine anatomical changes as they take place *in vivo* without the use of histological procedures, which may themselves be suspect (see for example Shida, 1970). The close resemblance of the pattern of light scattering to the mineralisation pattern determined by histology, and the presence of features morphologically similar to, though not yet chemically defined as, the calcium phosphate of stained preparations, suggests that the changing luminosity is connected with mineral transport (Fig. 21). If this is so, the 'loading' and 'unloading' activities each take approximately 15 minutes and are probably aided by the intricate nature of the cell process as seen *in situ*, together with a capacity to move these processes through the matrix.

That the etiology of metabolic bone disease might be expressed in terms of osteocyte 'types' and their capacity to build the mineral complex now seems likely. Preliminary studies, for example, suggest that there is a minimal binding of tetracycline in nutritional osteomalacia (Fig. 10b), which is increased soon after the administration of vitamin D. Present evidence (Aaron, Pautard, Robertson and Thompson, in preparation) also suggests that the mineral particles, although they become increasingly impacted in the

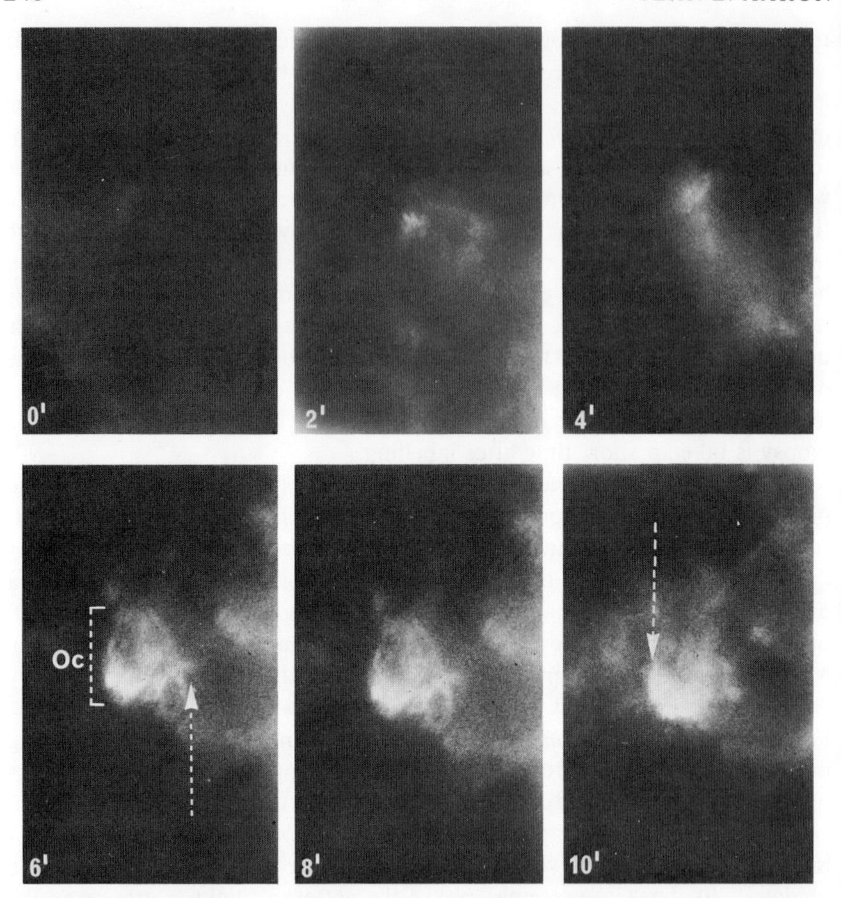

Fig. 21. A living osteocyte *in situ* in the calvarium of an anaesthetised 5-day-old mouse viewed by incident light interference contrast (Nomarski) microscopy and photographed at 2 min intervals. The osteocyte which is dimly illuminated at 0 min, becomes progressively more luminous. By 6 min the cell (Oc) is distinct. Part of the cell edge (arrowed) is poorly defined and associated with a diffuse network of fine processes. After 10 min some of these have faded or retracted and the opposite cell edge (arrowed) becomes brighter and more diffuse, ×900

maturing extracellular matrix, may retain their integrity throughout the life of the tissue (Fig. 25a). This would explain the granular nature of the bone which is apparent at the calcification front, and in the microfissured and partly mineralised 'feathered' regions (see Aaron, 1976a) common to osteomalacia.

Some soft tissues also stain with tetracycline and this may indicate no more than a separate phenomenon (Aaron, 1974; Aaron and Pautard, 1975). But it may be that the difference between bone cells and other cells is only a matter of degree. Thus liver, muscle, spleen and brain may manufacture calcium phosphate complexes in the same way as bone. The end product, however, may not be exported but instead recycled immediately for metabolic and cytoskeletal purposes. In other words, the production of bone salt by the osteocyte may be an extension of normal cell activity, the malfunction of which brings about ectopic calcification at one extreme, and perhaps myopathy at the other.

2. *Ultrastructural Evidence*. Present evidence from optical studies is not easily reconciled with reports in the literature of the same structures in the electron microscope, where there is no support for the view that normal osteocytes possess intracellular features of inorganic salt consistent with the optical picture. A typical electron micrograph of an osteocyte generally presents as a structure containing many empty vacuoles. This anomaly has to be explained before any intracellular concept of calcification is acceptable.

The procedures of electron microscopy have been developed principally for the examination of soft tissues. Their direct application to hard tissues has passed unchallenged, with the exception of some uneasiness expressed by Durning (1958) and by Boothroyd (1964), who observed the loss of mineral

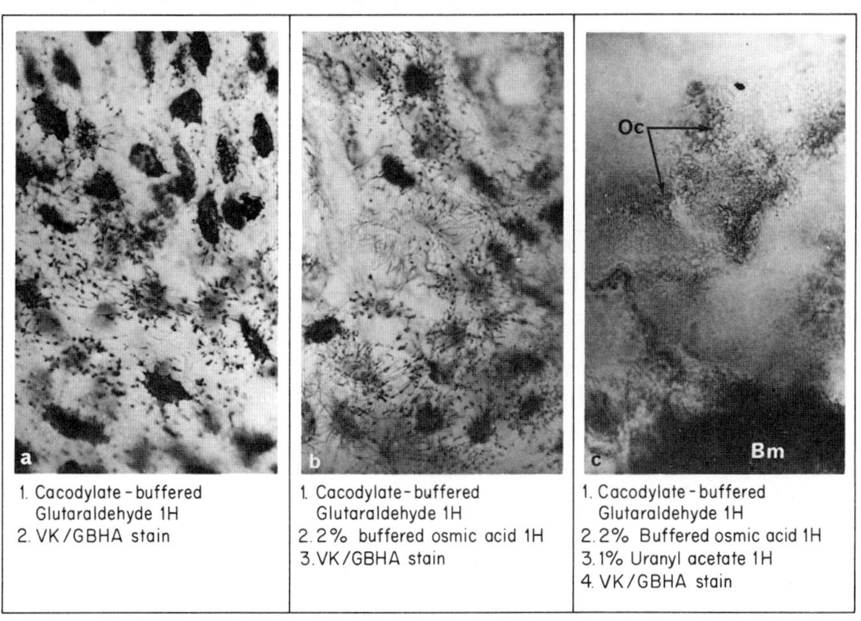

Fig. 22. Effects of electron microscope procedures on the distribution of intracellular mineral. Intact 5-day-old mouse calvarium, stained with the von Kossa stain (VK) followed by GBHA stain (a) The calcified matrix stains lightly or not at all but the osteocytes are densely stained. (b) The calcified matrix remains unstained; the cells stain, but less densely than in (a). (c) The calcified matrix (Bm) stains densely and there is a general diffuse calcium stain; the osteocytes (Oc) are pale and indistinct. $\times 350$

during sectioning when specimens are cut and floated in distilled water. The mineral was removed to the extent of showing the 'weave' of collagen fibres in some instances. He suggested the precaution of floating sections into a saturated solution of calcium phosphate, but this is doubtful cytologically because of the risk of false localisation and precipitation. Moreover, Boothroyd was concerned with the retention of the relatively stable extracellular mineral and not with the intracellular material which is particularly unstable and soluble. Any intracellular deposits remaining have to survive a sequence of fixatives and stains, which must now be considered as effective demineralising agents (Aaron and Pautard, 1972; Pautard, 1972; Aaron, 1974). Uranyl acetate is the principal agent since it effectively removes all traces of intracellular mineral even from *intact* mouse calvarium such that the optical picture becomes consistent with the accepted electron microscope picture (Fig. 22). It follows that in *ultrathin sections*, flotation and drop-staining must cause instant removal of mineral. The recent evidence from Termine (1972) confirms this. Using synthetic calcium phosphates he found that 5 to 100% of the calcium phosphate in amorphous precipitates was lost into the medium during the course of routine preparation for electron microscopy (which in his case did not include uranyl acetate). He attributed this loss principally to dissolution in water at the various stages particularly in the presence of carbon dioxide, although he suspected that osmium also might interfere with mineral morphology. Bearing in mind present doubts about crystallinity, the above evidence can only mean that the extensive literature about the distribution of mineral in bone at the ultrastructural level must now be viewed with caution. Any objections raised to interpretations of the optical image from an ultrastructural viewpoint may then be due to the application of the wrong preparative techniques, such that the first-formed mineral is lost.

The problem of retaining and visualising the fine structure of the mineral within the osteocyte has been overcome to some extent by the use of the von Kossa silver method after brief glutaraldehyde fixation (Aaron and Pautard, 1972). However, even with the right techniques, the choice of wrong cell (the osteoblast at too early a stage), at the wrong time (when the cell is not 'switched on' for calcium phosphate) and in the wrong place (a mature region instead of a developing region) will produce negative results. Unless the tissue and site for investigation are chosen with care, there is little chance of observing a particular cell in its mineralising phase, and tissue maps are essential (Aaron and Pautard, 1972; Aaron, 1973; Aaron, 1974). After the optical identification of 'loaded' osteocytes (Fig. 23a) and their subsequent preparation for the electron microscope (Fig. 23b), the resultant ultrastructural picture indicates that the distribution of intracellular mineral is more complex than is apparent from the simple particulate nature of the optical picture (Aaron and Pautard, 1972; Fig. 24). The discrete deposits 0.2 to 2 μm

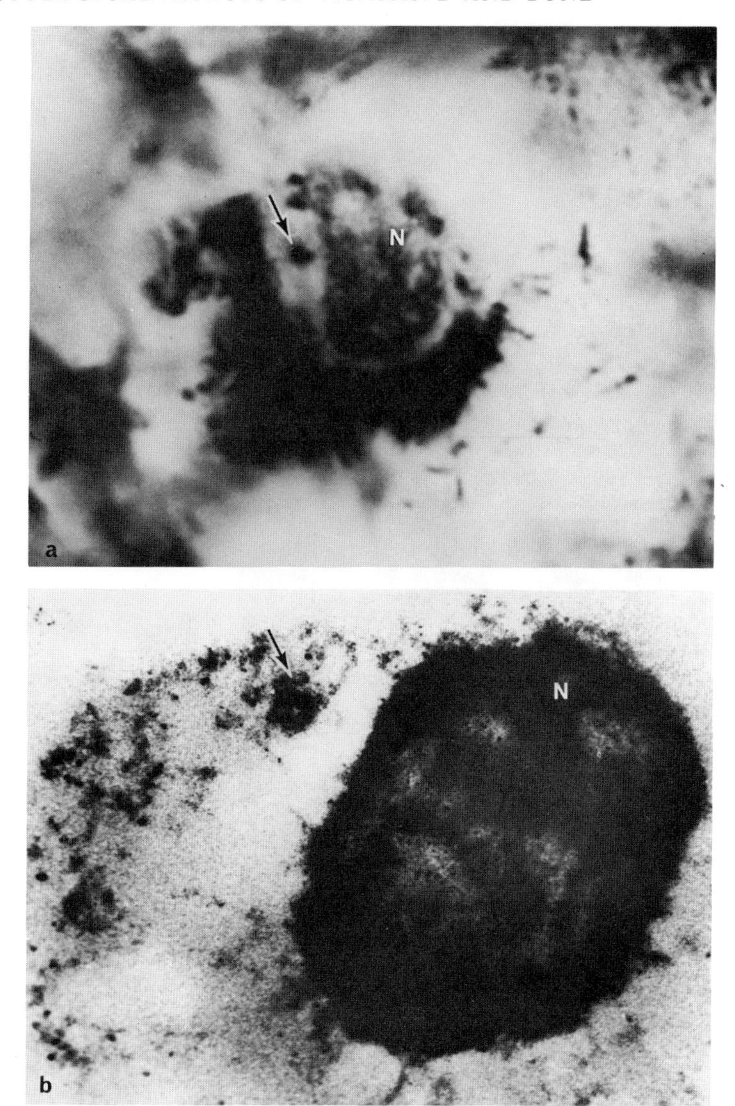

Fig. 23. Comparison of the optical (a) and ultrastructural (b) images of 'loaded' osteocytes stained with silver nitrate. The nuclear region (N) stains densely and discrete particles (arrowed) are apparent in the cytoplasm. Undecalcified bone from a 5-day-old mouse calvarium, von Kossa stain, (a) ×2100, (b) ×17 500

in diameter are composed of clusters of filaments (Fig. 24b), the important feature of which seems to be the constancy of their dimensions. These filamentous clusters closely resemble the 'islands of crystallites' described in

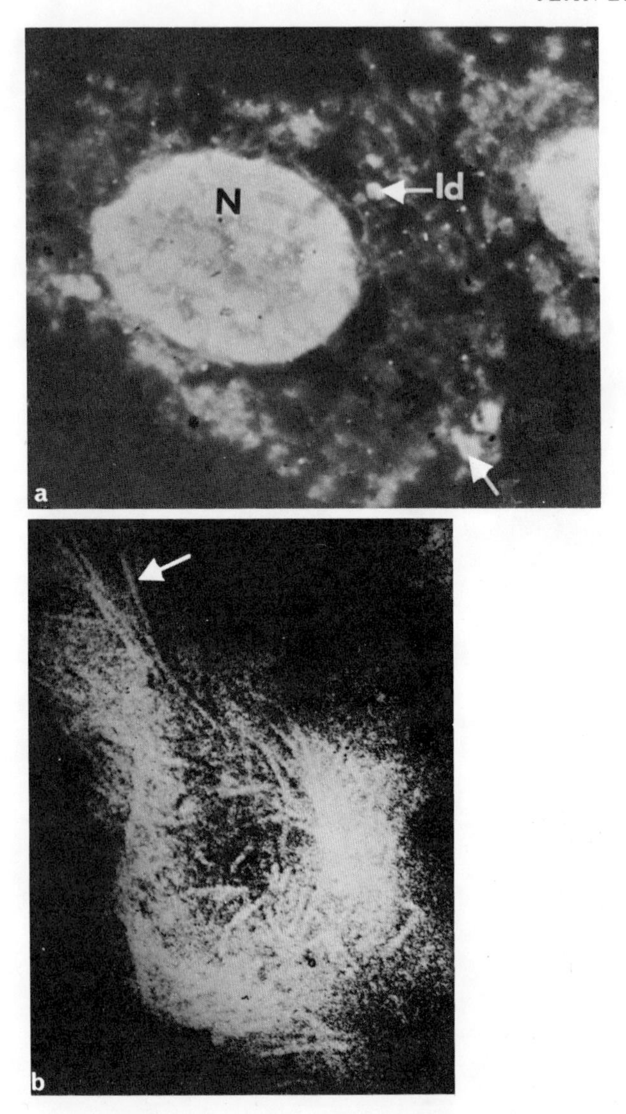

Fig. 24. Further ultrastructural features of osteocytes after staining with silver nitrate, printed as negatives for better definition. (a) The nuclear region (N) stains clearly and the cytoplasm contains both discrete intracellular deposits (Id) and diffuse areas of density, × 10 500. (b) Enlargement of the dense feature (bottom arrow in a) shows its composition. Filaments 50 Å in diameter (arrowed) are arranged into a skein with a less dense centre. Undecalcified bone from a 5-day-old mouse calvarium, von Kossa stain, × 150 000. (From Aaron and Pautard, 1972)

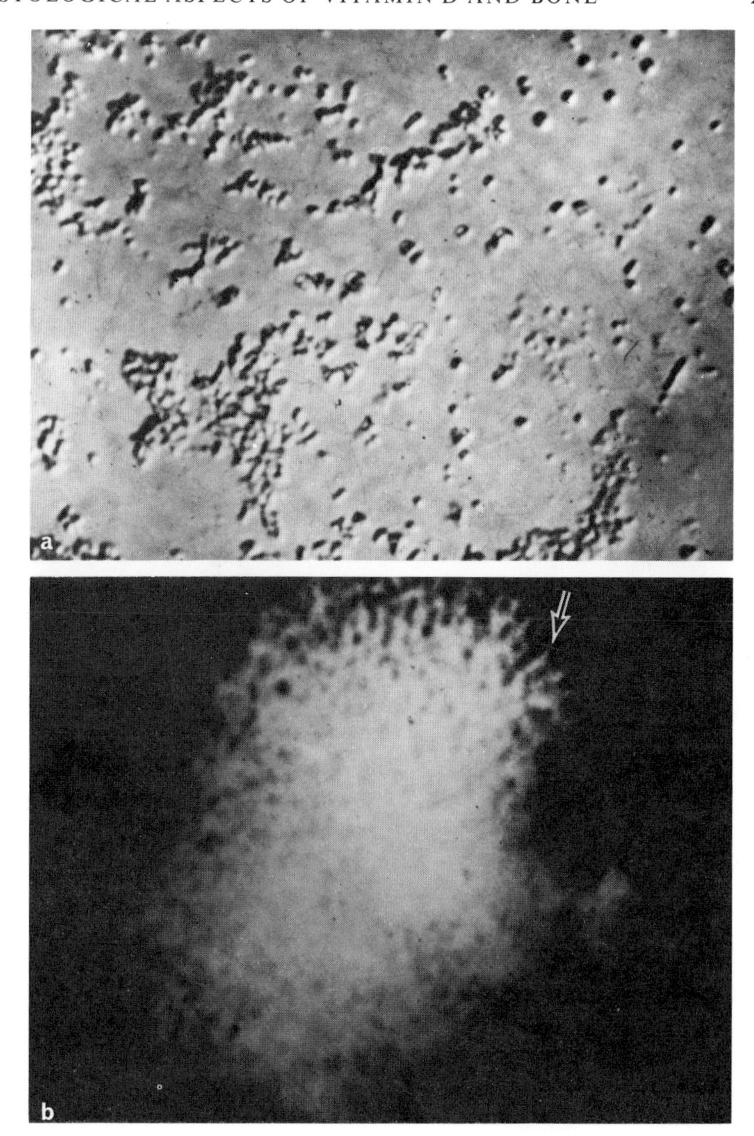

Fig. 25. After digestion with collagenase of the calvarium of the 5-day-old mouse the bones disintegrate and the mineral is released as discrete rounded structures (a) approximately 1 μm in diameter. Nomarski optics for transmitted light, × 1500. (b) When sectioned and examined in the electron microscope, these have a distinct organisation composed of filaments (arrowed), each 50 Å in diameter. Printed as the negative image for better definition, × 172 000

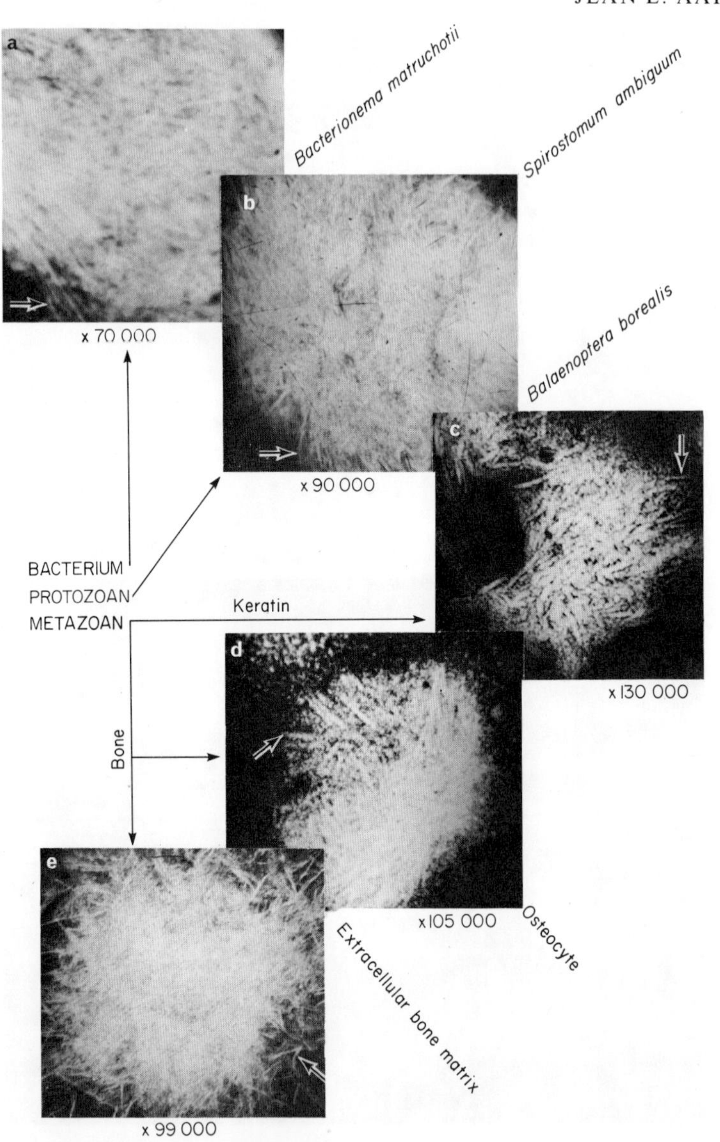

Fig. 26. Filamentous clusters (filaments arrowed) mineralised with calcium phosphate, from diverse tissues and organisms. (a) Osmic acid/potassium dichromate fixation, detail based upon Ennever and Creamer, 1967, prepared by Takazoe. (b) Osmic acid vapour fixation only, photomicrograph kindly supplied by Dr F. G. E. Pautard. (c) Unfixed, stained in uranyl acetate, photomicrograph kindly supplied by Dr F. G. E. Pautard. (d) Glutaraldehyde fixation, stained in silver, from Aaron and Pautard, 1972. (e) Glutaraldehyde/osmic acid fixation, photomicrograph kindly supplied by Dr F. G. E. Pautard

the extracellular matrix of mineralising bone (Fig. 25b) and the intracellular deposits of other calcifying forms (Fig. 26, and Pautard, 1975). Their structure suggests that the mineral matter is surrounded by an organic envelope of some kind, the nature of which is not known.

(*a*) *The role of mitochondria.* A feature which may be connected with the origin of the intracellular deposits is the mitochondrion. While intramitochondrial mineral deposits have not so far been observed in actively forming bone, their appearance in hypertrophic chondrocytes has been described by several authors (Fig. 27). Martin and Matthews (1969) studying the

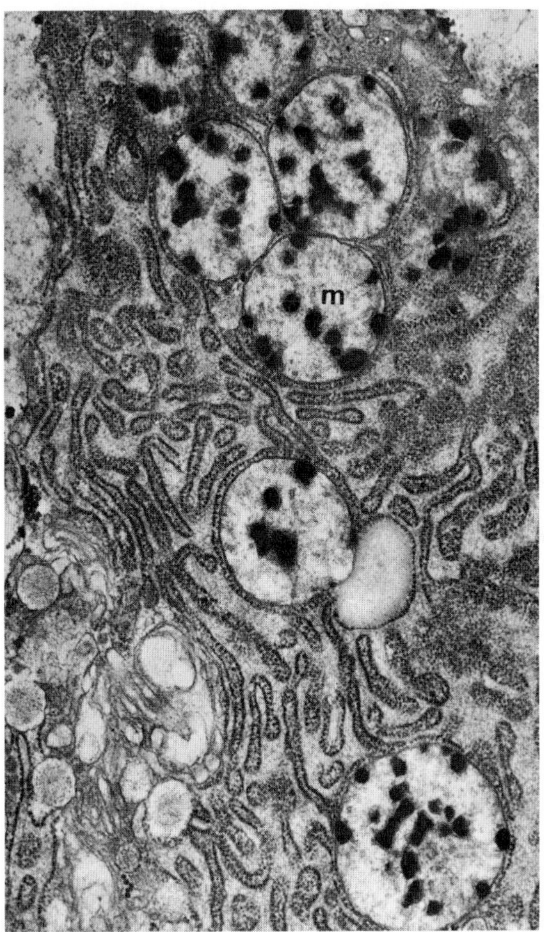

Fig. 27. Mitochondrial granules. Electron-dense granules 500–1000 Å in diameter in the mitochondria (m) of a hypertrophic chondrocyte in the zone of provisional calcification. Epiphyseal plate of mouse rib, osmic acid/glutaraldehyde fixation, uranyl acetate and lead citrate staining, ×20 000. (From Holtrop, 1972)

epiphyseal plate of the rat, described a gradient of mitochondrial granules, which increased from the proliferative zone to the zone of provisional calcification. These contained calcium phosphate, magnesium, phospholipid, ribonucleic acid and protein (Matthews and Martin, 1971). The subsequent absence of the granules from the mature cells, together with evidence that there are fewer mitochondrial granules in rachitic rats (Matthews *et al.*, 1970) has led to the suggestion that the mitochondrion is responsible for the marshalling of calcium phosphate prior to its export from the cell. Although differing in some respects from descriptions by Holtrop (1972), the concept is supported by the evidence of Brighton and Hunt (1974) and Lehninger (1970) who has proposed the production of 'micro-packets' 20–30 Å in diameter which become precursors of extracellular hydroxyapatite.

While in calcifying cartilage calcified deposits are now established as features of the mitochondria of certain chondrocytes, in bone it is the cells associated with resorptive processes which have the largest number of mitochondria (osteocytes and osteoblasts have relatively few), and paradoxically the cells containing the highest complement of intramitochondrial granules are the osteoclasts (Matthews and Martin, 1971). Any descriptions of their occurrence within mitochondria in other bone cells seems also to be associated with either resorption (Salomon and Volpin, 1970) or the administration of parathyroid hormone (Rasmussen and Ogata, 1966; Cameron *et al.*, 1967; Matthews and Martin, 1971). In addition it is well recognised that mitochondria in both animals and plants may accumulate dense deposits of calcium phosphate under abnormal and pathological conditions (Table 3).

Table 3. Some observations of electron-opaque deposits of insoluble calcium salts in mitochondria *in situ*. (Based upon Lehninger, 1970)

Observation	Reference
Osteoclasts in healing bone fractures	Gonzales and Karnovsky (1961)
Shell-gland epithelium of fowl	Hohman and Schraer (1966)
Chondrocytes in calcifying cartilage	Martin and Matthews (1969)
Kidney after calcification induced by PTH and excess of Ca^{2+}	Caulfield and Schrag (1964)
Kidney after administration of excess vitamin D	Scarpelli (1965)
Liver after carbon tetrachloride poisoning	Reynolds (1965)
Heart after isoproterenol administration	Bloom and Cancilla (1969)
Skeletal muscle after tetanus toxin	Zacks and Sheff (1964)
Hypoxic myocardium	Lin (1972)
Hypertrophic osteocytes	Salomon and Volpin (1970)
Stressed skin fibrocytes	Matthews (1972)

In contrast to the extracellular mineralisation of 'globules' and 'vesicles', the proposal that calcification begins in the mitochondrion is at least in accord with the optical evidence for intracellular calcium phosphate. But, the size and morphology of the particles is generally clearly different from the intracellular filamentous clusters described above. For instance, Holtrop (1972) observed electron-dense granules, 500 to 1000 Å in diameter and composed of a fine granular material with a less dense core (Fig. 27). Also, these granules are able to survive the preparative procedures (which usually include uranyl acetate), implying a stability in the nature of the mineral, inconsistent with the nascent material of the intracellular filaments. On the other hand, with recent descriptions by Matthews (1972) and Brighton and Hunt (1974) that the disappearance of mitochondrial granules in cartilage is associated with an increased density in the extracellular vesicles, the possibility arises that two hitherto separate ideas of calcification may now be united. However, without a more clearly defined relationship, opinion will inevitably vary as to the precise significance of the intramitochondrial event.

(*b*) *The role of the golgi apparatus.* The most prominent feature of bone cells at certain stages of their development is a complex arrangement of saccules and cisternae close to the nucleus (see for example Cameron, 1968) known as the golgi network (or juxtanuclear apparatus). The function of the golgi apparatus has always been considered as one of secretion of diverse structures. Passing reference was made to it in relation to bone by Taves (1965) who proposed its role in concentrating calcium. Matthews *et al.* (1968) observed pronounced labelling with ^{45}Ca of the golgi apparatus of hypertrophic chondrocytes, and a recent report by Park and Kashiwa (1975) describes calcium localized in juxtanuclear granules of epiphyseal chondrocytes. With these exceptions the golgi apparatus has received little attention in calcification in the vertebrates, other than as a site of enzyme activity. However, the general optical evidence for the distribution of the intracellular bone salt described above suggests coincidence with the nucleus and the adjacent network of vacuoles and vesicles in the juxtanuclear apparatus. The development of the golgi apparatus in the osteoblast is in accord with its role in the synthesis of the organic matrix, but as the cell modulates into an osteocyte, so the synthetic activity of this region changes, and is 'switched on' for the packaging of bone salt. On completion of its complement of filamentous clusters the golgi 'switches off'. Further ultrastructural details relating mineral with cell features are now being sought (Aaron and Pautard, in preparation), but until a suitable staining procedure is forthcoming there is no clear evidence that vacuoles are involved.

The presence of filamentous clusters within the osteocytes dissociates the calcification of bone from present concepts of calcification in cartilage and dentine and implies differences in the manner in which the two tissues calcify.

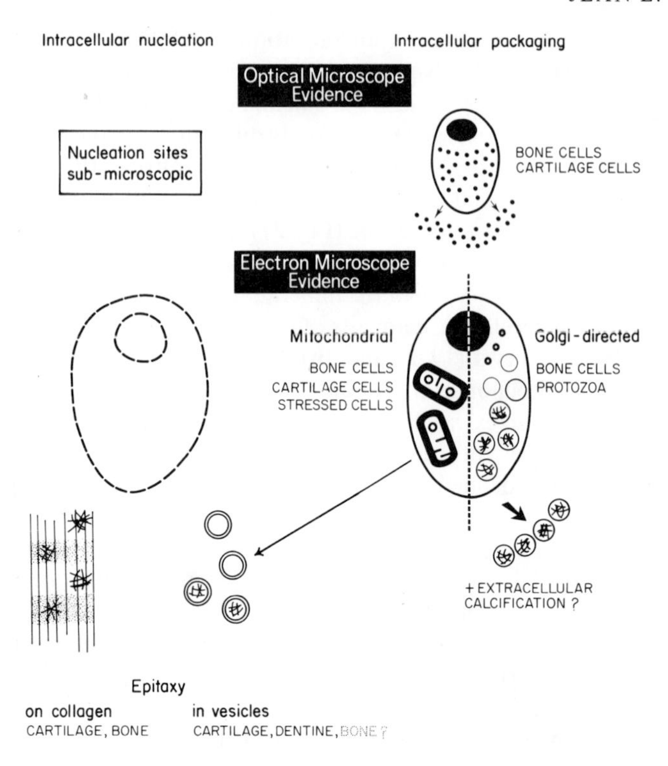

Fig. 28. Mechanism of mineralisation. Theories can be divided into those proposing extracellular nucleation based upon the ultrastructural relationship of the mineral to either collagen or membrane bound vesicles, and those proposing an initial intracellular packaging before export to the extracellular matrix based upon optical evidence of mineral granules within cells and their ultrastructure in relation to mitochondria (as dense deposits) or to the golgi apparatus (as filamentous clusters). That the intracellular mineral is in some manner transferred to the extracellular vesicles (large arrow) has also been suggested. [::::], bone mineral; [ooo], intramitochondrial mineral deposits; [✲✲✲], bone crystallites or calcified filamentous clusters

It is tempting though to describe the 'globules' of Bonucci and the 'vesicles' of Anderson and Slavkin as products of the golgi apparatus, from which the filamentous clusters have been removed or disturbed by processing. Lest the sequence of events in golgi synthesis described here seem extraordinary, such a cell differentiation process is entirely in accord with the known behaviour of calcifying cells and tissues in the invertebrates (Pautard, 1970; Abolinŝ-Krogis, 1970; Outka and Williams, 1971). Such a mechanism not only puts the calcification of bone inside the cell, but places the synthesis of the calcifying structures in the proximity of the nucleus, that most crucial of all cell organelles. In the labyrinthine intracellular environment, extracellular ion products become less significant and any direct effect vitamin D (or other factors influencing bone mineral) might have, may now need to be considered in terms of its affect on the golgi apparatus. It is too early to say how much of the extracellular mineral has been transported by the osteocyte, how much mineral is present in the intracellular filamentous clusters, and how much is added after leaving the cell. In the absence of quantitative data, the possibility remains that all the mechanisms proposed in Fig. 28 are in operation at some time.

Acknowledgements

I am indebted to Professor B. E. C. Nordin for advice and useful criticism.

References

Aaron, J. E. (1973). *Calcif. Tiss. Res.* **12**, 259.
Aaron, J. E. (1974). PhD Thesis, University of Leeds.
Aaron, J. E. (1976a). *In* 'Calcium, Phosphate and Magnesium Metabolism: Clinical Physiology and Diagnostic Procedures' (Ed. B. E. C. Nordin) p. 298. Churchill Livingstone, Edinburgh and London.
Aaron, J. E. (1976b). *In* 'XIIth European Symposium on Calcified Tissues', p. 54. University Printing Service, Leeds.
Aaron, J. E. (1977). *Calcif. Tiss. Res.* **22** (Suppl.). 247.
Aaron, J. E. and Pautard, F. G. E. (1972). *Israel J. Med. Sci.* **8**, 625.
Aaron, J. E. and Pautard, F. G. E. (1973a). *In* 'The Cell Cycle in Development and Differentiation' (Ed. M. Balls and F. S. Billett) p. 325. University Press, Cambridge.
Aaron, J. E. and Pautard, F. G. E. (1973b). *In* 'Calcified Tissue 1972', Proceedings of the IXth European Symposium on Calcified Tissues (Ed. H. Czitober and J. Eschberger) p. 197. Facta-Publication, Vienna.
Aaron, J. E. and Pautard, F. G. E. (1975). *In* 'Calcium Metabolism, Bone and Metabolic Bone Diseases' (Ed. F. Kuhlencordt and H. P. Kruse) p. 211. Springer-Verlag, Berlin, Heidelberg and New York.
Aaron, J. E., Gallagher, J. C., Anderson, J., Stasiak, L., Longton, E. B., Nordin, B. E. C. and Nicholson, M. (1974a). *Lancet* **I**, 229.
Aaron, J. E., Gallagher, J. C. and Nordin, B. E. C. (1974b). *Lancet* **II**, 84.
Aaron, J. E., Gallagher, J. C. and Nordin, B. E. C. (1974c). *Lancet* **I**, 572.
Abolinš-Krogis, A. (1970). *L. Z. Zellforsch* **108**, 501.
Ackerknecht, E. H. (1953). 'Rudolf Virchow, Doctor, Statesman, Anthropologist.' University of Wisconsin Press, Madison, U.S.A.
Albright, F., Burnett, C. H., Parson, W., Reifenstein, E. C. and Roos, A. (1946). *Medicine* **25**, 399.
Ali, S. Y., Sajdera, S. W. and Anderson, H. C. (1970). *Proc. Natl. Acad. Sci. USA* **67**, 1513.
Amprino, R. and Engström, A. (1952). *Acta. anat.* (Basel) **15**, 1.

Amprino, R. and Marotti, G. (1964). *In* 'Bone and Tooth' (Ed. H. J. J. Blackwood) p. 21. Pergamon Press, Oxford, New York and Paris.
Anderson, H. C. (1968). *In* 'Electron Microscopy' (Ed. D. S. Bocciarelli) Vol. 2, p. 437. Tipografia Poliglotta Vaticana, Rome.
Anderson, H. C. (1972). *In* 'The Comparative Molecular Biology of Extracellular Matrices' (Ed. H. C. Slavkin) p. 201. Academic Press, New York and London.
Anderson, H. C. and Reynolds, J. J. (1973). *Dev. Biol.* **34**, 211.
Angell, R. W. (1965). PhD Thesis, University of Chicago.
Appleton, J. (1971). *Calcif. Tiss. Res.* **7**, 307.
Arnott, H. J. and Pautard, F. G. E. (1967). *Israel J. Med. Sci.* **3**, 657.
Ascenzi, A. (1964). *In* 'Bone and Tooth' (Ed. H. J. J. Blackwood) p. 231. Pergamon Press, Oxford.
Atkins, D. and Peacock, M. (1974). *J. Endocr.* **61**, lxxix.
Bachra, B. N. (1972). *Calcif. Tiss. Res.* **8**, 287.
Baker, S. L. (1956). *J. Bone Jt. Surg.* **38B**, 378.
Barnicot, N. A. (1951). *J. Anat.* (London) **85**, 120.
Bast, T. H. (1921). *Amer. J. Anat.* **29**, 139.
Baylink, D., Stauffer, M., Wergedal, J. and Rich, C. (1970). *J. clin. Invest.* **49**, 1122.
Bernard, G. W. (1972). *J. Ultrastruct. Res.* **41**, 1.
Bernard, G. W. and Pease, D. C. (1969). *Amer. J. Anat.* **125**, 271.
Bevelander, G. and Johnson, P. L. (1950). *Anat. Rec.* **108**, 1.
Bloom, S. and Cancilla, P. A. (1969). *Amer. J. Path.* **54**, 373.
Bohatirchuk, F. (1965). *Amer. J. Anat.* **117**, 287.
Bohatirchuk, F. and Jeletzky, T. (1971). *Invest. Radiol.* **6**, 122.
Bonucci, E. (1967). *J. Ultrastruct. Res.* **20**, 33.
Bonucci, E. (1971). *Clin. Orthop.* **78**, 108.
Bonucci, E., Matrajt, H. D., Tun Chot, S. and Hioco, D. J. (1969). *J. Bone Jt. Surg.* **51B**, 511.
Boothroyd, B. (1964). *J. Cell Biol.* **20**, 165.
Bordier, P. J., Hioco, D., Rouquier, M., Hepner, G. W. and Thompson, G. R. (1969). *Calcif. Tiss. Res.* **4**, 78.
Bordier, P. J. and Tun Chot, S. (1972). *Clin. Endocr. Metabol.* **1**, 197.
Bordier, P. J., Woodhouse, N. J. Y., Sigurdsson, G. and Joplin, G. F. (1973). *Clin. Endocr.* **2**, 377.
Brighton, C. T. and Hunt, R. M. (1974). *Clin. Orthop.* **100**, 406.
Burkhardt, J. M. and Jowsey, J. (1966). *Mayo Clin. Proc.* **41**, 663.
Burland, C. (1918). *Practitioner* **100**, 391.
Byers, P. D. (1962). *J. Bone Jt. Surg.* **44B**, 226.
Cameron, D. A. (1963). *Clin. Orthop.* **26**, 199.
Cameron, D. A. (1968). *Clin. Orthop.* **58**, 191.
Cameron, D. A., Paschall, H. A. and Robinson, R. A. (1967). *J. Cell Biol.* **33**, 1.
Canas, F., Brand, J. S., Neuman, W. F. and Terepka, A. R. (1969). *Amer. J. Physiol.* **216**, 1092.
Caulfield, T. B. and Schrag, P. E. (1964). *Amer. J. Path.* **44**, 365.
Chalmers, J., Conacher, W. D. H., Gardner, D. L. and Scott, P. J. (1967). *J. Bone Jt. Surg.* **49B**, 403.
Clarke, E. (1962). *Bull. Hist. Med.* **36**, 45.
Cohnheim, J. (1889). 'Lectures on General Pathology' **2**. Adlard and Son, London.
Collins, D. H. (1966). *In* 'Pathology of Bone'. Butterworths, London.
Dahl, L. D. (1952). *J. exp. Med.* **97**, 681.

DeBernard, B., Furlan, G., Stagni, N., Vittur, F. and Zanetti, M. (1977) *Calcif. Tiss. Res.* **22** (Suppl.), 191.
Delesse, M. A. (1848). *Annales De Mines* **13**, 379.
Dewhurst, K. (1962). *Brit. med. J.* **ii**, 1466.
Dudley, R. H. and Spiro, D. (1961). *J. biophys. biochem. Cytol.* **11**, 627.
Dujardin, F. (1835). *C. R. Acad. Sci.* (Paris) **1**, 338.
Durning, W. C. (1958). *J. Ultrastruct. Res.* **2**, 245.
Eastwood, J. B., Bordier, P. J. and De Wardener, H. E. (1975). *In* 'Calcium Metabolism, Bone and Metabolic Bone Diseases' (Ed. F. Kuhlencordt and H.-P. Kruse) p. 82. Springer-Verlag, Berlin, Heidelberg and New York.
Ell, B. (1972). *Lancet* **I**, 1113.
Ellis, H. A. and Peart, K. M. (1972). *J. clin. Path.* **25**, 277.
Engström, A. and Zetterström, R. (1951). *Exp. Cell. Res.* **2**, 268.
Ennever, J. and Creamer, H. (1967). *Calcif. Tiss. Res.* **1**, 87.
Exton-Smith, A. N. (1971). *Brit. J. Hosp. Med.* **5**, 639.
Faccini, J. M., Exton-Smith, A. N. and Boyde, A. (1976). *Lancet* **I**, 1089.
Fischer, J. A., Binswanger, U., Schenk, R. K. and Merz, W. (1970). *Horm. Metabol. Res.* **2**, 110.
Fitton Jackson, S. (1957). *Proc. Roy. Soc. B* **146**, 270.
Fleisch, H. and Bisaz, S. (1962). *Nature* (London) **195**, 911.
Fraser, D. (1957). *Amer. J. Med.* **22**, 730.
Fraser, R., Harrison, M. and Jones, E. (1960). *In* 'Radioaktive Isotope in Klinik und Forschung' (Ed. K. Fellinger and R. Höfer) p. 45. Munich.
Freudenberg, E. and György, P. (1924). *Med. Kinderheilkunde* **24**, 17.
Frost, H. M. (1960). *Henry Ford Hospital med. Bull.* **8**, 220.
Frost, H. M. (1962). *Clin. Orthop.* **25**, 175.
Frost, H. M. (1963). *In* 'Bone Remodeling Dynamics'. Charles C. Thomas, Springfield (Illinois).
Frost, H. M. (1966). *In* 'The Bone Dynamics in Osteoporosis and Osteomalacia', Charles C. Thomas, Springfield (Illinois).
Frost, H. M. (1967). *In* 'L'Osteomalacie' (Ed. D. J. Hioco) p. 3. Masson et Cie, Paris.
Frost, H. M. (1969). *Calcif. Tiss. Res.* **3**, 211.
Frost, H. M. (1973). *In* 'Bone Remodeling and its Relationship to Metabolic Bone Diseases'. Charles C. Thomas, Springfield (Illinois).
Frost, H. M., Villanueva, A. R. and Roth, H. (1960). *Stain Technol.* **35**, 135.
Gaillard, P. J., Herrmann-Erlee, M. P. M. and Hekkelman, J. W. (1975). *In* 'Calcified Tissues 1975'. Proceedings of the XIth European Symposium on Calcified Tissues (Ed. S. Pors Nielson and E. Hjørting-Hansen) p. 70. Fadl's Forlag, Copenhagen.
Gallagher, J. C. (1976). M.D. Thesis, University of Manchester.
Garner, A. and Ball, J. (1966). *J. Path. Bact.* **91**, 545.
Garrick, R., Ireland, A. W. and Posen, S. (1971). *Ann. Internal Med.* **75**, 221.
Gee, S. (1868). *St. Bart. Hosp. Rep.* **4**, 69.
Gerlach, J. von (1858). *In* 'Carleton's Histological Technique' p. 99. Oxford University Press, New York, Toronto, 1967.
Glimcher, M. J. (1959). *Rev. mod. Phys.* **31**, 359.
Gonzales, C. H. and Karnovsky, M. J. (1961). *J. biophys. biochem. Cytol.* **9**, 299.
Gutman, A. B. and Yu, T. F. (1950). *In* 'Metabolic Interrelations' p. 167. Josiah Macy Jr. Foundation, New York.
Haas, H. G., Müller, J. and Schenk, R. K. (1967). *Clin. Orthop.* **53**, 213.
Hancox, N. M. and Boothroyd, B. (1965). *Clin. Orthop.* **40**, 153.

Harris, W. H. and Heaney, R. P. (1969). *New Engl. J. Med.* **280**, 193, 253 and 303.
Harris, W. H., Jackson, R. H. and Jowsey, J. (1962). *J. Bone Jt. Surg.* **44A**, 1308.
Heeley, J. D. and Irving, J. T. (1973). *Calcif. Tiss. Res.* **12**, 169.
Heller-Steinberg, M. (1951). *Amer. J. Anat.* **89**, 347.
Hennig, A. (1958). *Zeiss Werkzschr.* **30**, 78
Hirschman, P. N. and Nichols, G. (1972). *Calcif. Tiss. Res.* **9**, 67.
Hofmeister, F. (1891). *Naunyn-Schmiedeberg's Arch. exp. Path. Pharmak.* **28**, 211.
Hohman, W. and Schraer, H. (1966). *J. Cell Biol.* **30**, 317.
Holtrop, M. E. (1972). *Calcif. Tiss. Res.* **9**, 140.
Hoyte, D. A. N. (1968). *Amer. J. Physical Anthropol.* **29**, 157.
Irving, J. T. (1960). *Clin. Orthop.* **17**, 92.
Irving, J. T. and Wuthier, R. E. (1968). *Clin. Orthop.* **56**, 237.
Johnson, L. C. (1964). *In* 'Bone Biodynamics' Henry Ford Hospital International Symposium (Ed. H. M. Frost) p. 543. Little, Brown and Co., Massachusetts.
Johnston, P. M. (1958). *J. biophys. biochem. Cytol.* **4**, 163.
Jowsey, J. (1963). *In* 'Mechanisms of Hard Tissue Destruction' (Ed. R. F. Sognnaes) p. 447. American Association for the Advancement of Science, Washington.
Jowsey, J. (1968). *In* 'Parathyroid Hormone and Thyrocalcitonin (Calcitonin)' (Ed. R. V. Talmage and L. F. Bélanger) p. 137. Exerpta Medica, New York.
Jowsey, J., Kelly, P. J., Riggs, B. L., Bianco, A. J., Scholz, D. A. and Gershon-Cohen, J. (1965). *J. Bone Jt. Surg.* **47A**, 785.
Juster, M., Oligo, N. and Laval-Jeantet, M. (1967). *In* 'L'Ostéomalacie' (Ed. D. J. Hioco) p. 39. Masson et Cie, Paris.
Kaitila, I. (1971). *Calcif. Tiss. Res.* **7**, 46.
Kashiwa, H. K. (1970). *Clin. Orthop.* **70**, 200.
Katchburian, E. (1977). *Calcif. Tiss. Res.* **22** (Suppl.), 179.
Keevil, J. J. (1954). *J. Hist. Med. allied Sci.* **9**, 407.
Kember, N. F. (1971). *Clin. Orthop.* **76**, 213.
Kent, P. W., Jowsey, J., Steddon, L. M., Oliver, R. and Vaughan, J. (1956). *Biochem. J.* **62**, 470.
Kilian, H. F. (1857). *In* 'Das Halisteresische Becken'. Bonn.
Klebs, A. (1869). *Arch. Mikrosk. Anat. Entw. Mech.* **5**, 164.
Lacroix, P. (1954). *In* 'Proceedings of the Radioisotope Conference', p. 134. Butterworth, London.
Lacroix, P. (1956). *In* 'Bone Structure and Metabolism'. Ciba Foundation Symposium (Ed. G. E. W. Wolstenholme and C. M. O'Connor) p. 36. Churchill, London.
Lacroix, P. (1970). *Arch. Biol.* (Liège) **81**, 275.
Lehninger, A. L. (1970). *Biochem. J.* **119**, 129.
Lin, J. J. (1972). *Arch. Path.* **94**, 366.
Little, K. (1973). *In* 'Bone Behaviour'. Academic Press, New York and London.
Looser, E. (1908). *Mitt. Grenzgeb. Med. Chir.* **18**, 678.
Looser, E. (1920). *Dtsch. Z. Chir.* **152**, 210.
Martin, J. H. and Matthews, J. L. (1969). *Calcif. Tiss. Res.* **3**, 184.
Matrajt, H. and Hioco, D. (1966). *Stain Technol.* **41**, 97.
Matrajt, H., Bordier, P. and Hioco, D. (1967). *In* 'L'Osteomalacie' (Ed. D. J. Hioco) p. 101. Masson et Cie, Paris.
Matthews, J. L. (1972). *In* 'The Comparative Molecular Biology of Extracellular Matrices' (Ed. H. C. Slavkin) p. 218. Academic Press, New York and London.
Matthews, J. L. and Martin, J. H. (1971). *Amer. J. Med.* **50**, 589.

Matthews, J. L., Martin, J. H. and Collins, E. J. (1968). *Clin. Orthop.* **58**, 213.
Matthews, J. L., Martin, J. H., Sampson, H. W., Kunin, A. S. and Roan, J. H. (1970). *Calcif. Tiss. Res.* **5**, 91.
McLean, F. C. and Bloom, W. (1940). *Anat. Rec.* **78**, 333.
Melvin, K. E. W., Hepner, G. W., Bordier, P., Neale, G. and Joplin, G. F. (1970). *Quart. J. Med.* **39**, 83.
Merz, W. A. and Schenk, R. K. (1970a). *Acta Anat.* **76**, 1.
Merz, W. A. and Schenk, R. K. (1970b). *Acta Anat.* **75**, 54.
Meunier, P., Courpron, P., Edouard, C., Bernard, J., Bringuier, J. and Vignon, G. (1973). *Clin. Endocr. Metabol.* **2**, 239.
Milch, R. A., Rall, D. P. and Tobie, J. E. (1957). *J. Nat. Cancer. Inst.* **19**, 87.
Milkman, L. A. (1930). *Amer. J. Roentgenol.* **24**, 29.
Molnar, Z. (1959). *J. Ultrastruct. Res.* **3**, 39.
Morgan, D. B., Lever, J. V., Paterson, C. R., Woods, C. G., Pulvertaft, C. N. and Fourman, P. (1967). *In* 'L'Ostéomalacie' (Ed. D. J. Hioco) p. 321. Masson et Cie, Paris.
Morgan, D. B., Stanley, J. and Fourman, P. (1968). *Clin. Sci.* **35**, 337.
Morse, A. and Green, R. O. (1951). *Anat. Rec.* **111**, 193.
Neuman, W. F. and Neuman, M. (1958). *In* 'The Chemical Dynamics of Bone Mineral'. University of Chicago Press.
Nordin, B. E. C., Smith, D. A., MacGregor, J. and Anderson, J. (1965). *In* 'Proceedings of a Conference on Bone Densitometry, International Aeronautics and Space Administration'. Washington.
Nordin, B. E. C. and Smith, D. A. (1967). *In* 'L'Ostéomalacie' (Ed. D. J. Hioco) p. 379. Masson et Cie, Paris.
Nordin, B. E. C., Gallagher, J. C., Aaron, J. E. and Horsman, A. (1975). *Front. Hormone Res.* **3**, 131.
Nylen, M. U., Scott, D. B. and Mosley, V. M. (1960). *In* 'Calcification in Biological Systems' (Ed. R. F. Soggnaes) p. 129. American Association for the Advancement of Science, Washington.
Olah, A. J., Reutter, F. W. and Schenk, R. K. (1975). *In* 'Calcium Metabolism, Bone and Metabolic Bone Diseases' (Ed. F. Kuhlencordt and H.-P. Kruse) p. 146. Springer-Verlag, Berlin, Heidelberg and New York.
Outka, D. E. and Williams, D. C. (1971). *J. Protozool.* **18**, 285.
Parfitt, A. M. (1973). *In* 'Clinical Aspects of Metabolic Bone Disease' (Ed. B. Frame, A. M. Parfitt, H. Duncan) Exerpta Medica, Amsterdam.
Park, H. Z. and Kashiwa, H. K. (1975). *Calcif. Tiss. Res.* **19**, 189.
Paterson, C. R., Woods, C. G. and Morgan, D. B. (1968). *J. Path. Bact.* **95**, 449.
Pautard, F. G. E. (1958). *Biochim. Biophys. Acta* **28**, 514.
Pautard, F. G. E. (1965). *In* 'Les Congrès et Colloques de L'Université de Liège', Vol. 31, p. 347.
Pautard, F. G. E. (1966). *In* 'Third European Symposium on Calcified Tissues' (Ed. H. Fleisch, H. J. J. Blackwood and M. Owen) p. 108. Springer-Verlag, Berlin, Heidelberg and New York.
Pautard, F. G. E. (1970). *In* 'Biological Calcification, Cellular and Molecular Aspects' (Ed. H. Schraer) p. 105. Appleton-Century-Crofts, New York Educational Division, Meredith Corporation.
Pautard, F. G. E. (1972). *In* 'The Comparative Molecular Biology of Extracellular Matrices' (Ed. H. C. Slavkin) p. 231. Academic Press, New York and London.

Pautard, F. G. E. (1975). *In* 'Physico-Chimie et Cristallographie Des Apatites D'Intérêt Biologique', p. 93. Colloques Internationaux C.N.R.S. No. 230 Éditions C.N.R.S., Paris.
Pommer, G. A. (1885). *In* 'Osteomalacie und Rachitis'. Vogel, Leipzig.
Pritchard, J. J. (1952). *J. Anat.* **86**, 259.
Raina, V. (1972). *J. clin. Path.* **25**, 229.
Rambourg, A. and Leblond, C. P. (1967). *J. Cell. Biol.* **32**, 27.
Rasmussen, H. and Ogata, E. (1966). *Biochemistry* **5**, 733.
Reynolds, E. S. (1965). *J. Cell Biol.* **25**, 53.
Reynolds, J. J., Holick, M. F. and DeLuca, H. F. (1973). *Calcif. Tis Res.* **12**, 295.
Robinson, R. A. (1952). *J. Bone Jt. Surg.* **34A**, 389.
Robinson, R. A. and Watson, M. L. (1952). *Anat. Rec.* **114**, 383.
Robinson, R. A. and Cameron, D. A. (1956). *J. biophys. biochem. Cytol.* **2**, (Suppl. 4), 253.
Robison, R. (1923). *Biochem. J.* **17**, 286.
Robison, R. (1932). 'The Significance of Phosphoric Esters in Metabolism'. New York University Press.
Rolle, G. K. (1969). *Calcif. Tiss. Res.* **3**, 142.
Salomon, C. D. and Volpin, G. (1970). *Calcif. Tiss. Res.* **4** (Suppl.), 80.
Scarpelli, D. G. (1965). *Lab. Invest.* **14**, 123.
Schenk, R. K., Merz, W. A. and Müller, J. (1969). *Acta Anat.* **74**, 44.
Schewiakoff, W. (1894). *Z. wiss. Zool.* **58**, 32.
Schmorl, G. (1909). *Ergebn. Inn. Med. Kinderheilk.* **4**, 403.
Schneider, B. J. (1968). *Amer. J. Physical Anthropology* **29**, 197.
Schuscik, O. (1920). *Z. wiss. Mikr.* **37**, 215.
Scott, B. L. and Pease, D. C. (1956). *Anat. Record* **126**, 465.
Shida, H. (1970). *Exp. Cell Res.* **63**, 385.
Shipley, P. G. (1924). *Johns Hopk. Hosp. Bull.* **35**, 304.
Sissons, H. A., Holley, K. J. and Heighway, J. (1967). *In* 'L'Ostéomalacie' (Ed. D. J. Hioco) p. 19. Masson et Cie, Paris.
Slavkin, H. C. (1972). *In* 'The Comparative Molecular Biology of Extracellular Matrices' (Ed. H. C. Slavkin) p. 47. Academic Press, New York and London.
Smerdon, G. T. (1950). *J. Hist. Med.* **5**, 397.
Sobel, A. E., Burger, M. and Nobel, S. (1960). *Clin. Orthop.* **18**, 103.
Stanbury, S. W. (1972). *Clin. Endocr. Metabol.* **1**, 239.
Stanbury, S. W. and Lumb, G. A. (1967). *In* 'L'Ostéomalacie' (Ed. D. J. Hioco) p. 367. Masson et Cie, Paris.
Steendijk, R., Van Den Hooff, A. and Nielsen, H. R. (1965). *Nature* (London) **207**, 426.
Stein, I., Stein, R. O. and Beller, M. L. (1955). *In* 'Living Bone'. Pitman Medical Publishing Co. Ltd., London.
Sundström, B., Takuma, S. and Nagai, N. (1970). *Calcif. Tiss. Res.* **4**, 305.
Suzuki, H. K. (1963). *Ann. N.Y. Acad. Sci.* **109**, 351.
Taves, D. R. (1965). *Clin. Orthop.* **42**, 207.
Termine, J. D. (1972). *In* 'The Comparative Molecular Biology of Extracellular Matrices' (Ed. H. C. Slavkin) p. 443. Academic Press, New York and London.
Termine, J. D. and Posner, A. S. (1967). *Calcif. Tiss. Res.* **1**, 8.
Thomas, W. C. (1961). *J. Bone Jt Surg.* **43A**, 419.
Towe, K. M. and Cifelli, R. (1967). *J. Paleontol.* **41**, 442.

Trummel, C. L., Raisz, L. G., Blunt, J. W. and DeLuca, H. F. (1969). *Science* **163**, 1450.
Van Nguyen, V. and Jowsey, J. (1970). *Acta orthop. scand.* **40**, 708.
Villanueva, A. R. (1967). *Amer. J. clin. Path.* **47**, 78.
Villanueva, A. R., Sedlin, E. D. and Frost, H. M. (1963). *Anat. Rec.* **146**, 209.
Vincent, J. (1963). *Clin. Orthop.* **26**, 161.
Wakamatsu, E. and Sissons, H. A. (1969). *Calcif. Tiss. Res.* **4**, 147.
Watt, J. C. (1928). *Arch. Surg.* **17**, 1017.
Weibel, E. R. (1963). *Lab. Invest.* **12**, 131.
Wilbur, K. M. and Watabe, N. (1963). *Ann. N.Y. Acad. Sci.* **109**, 82.
Wilson, R. V., Ramser, J. R. and Frost, H. M. (1966). *Clin. Orthop.* **49**, 119.
Woodhouse, N. J. Y., Doyle, F. H. and Joplin, G. F. (1971). *Lancet* **II**, 283.
Woods, C. G. (1976). *In* 'Bone Morphometry' (Ed. Z. F. G. Jaworski) p. 201. University of Ottawa Press, Ottawa.
Woods, C. G., Morgan, D. B., Paterson, C. R. and Gossmann, H. H. (1968). *J. Path. Bact.* **95**, 441.
Zacks, S. I. and Sheff, M. F. (1964). *J. Neuropath. exp. Neurol.* **23**, 306.
Zichner, L. (1971). *Israel J. Med. Sci.* **7**, 359.

7 Biochemistry of Bone in Relation to the Function of Vitamin D

M. J. BARNES and D. E. M. LAWSON

I Introduction

It is the purpose of this chapter to consider bone in the context of the function of vitamin D and to what extent the known role of the vitamin in mobilisation (resorption) can account in entirety for its role in bone formation and growth. To this end, we shall briefly review present knowledge of the constituents of the organic matrix, including their possible role in the mineralisation process and then describe what is known of the influence of vitamin D status on the synthesis or structure of such constituents. Mineralisation of bone is unquestionably impaired in the absence of vitamin D giving rise to the classical nutritional deficiency known as rickets. However, it is not clear whether the lack of mineralisation is solely attributable to the lack of constituent elements arising through the impaired intestinal absorption occuring in vitamin D-deficiency or whether some metabolite(s) of the vitamin may play a vital role in this process, either in the synthesis of a matrix of precise structure suitable for calcification or the synthesis of a specific protein(s) that may be involved in the transport (as occurs in the intestine, chapter 5), or the fixation of the mineralising elements.

II Constituents of the Organic Matrix of Bone and Epiphyseal Cartilage

Since the epiphyseal cartilage is intimately involved in bone growth through the process of endochondral ossification, this review will consider constituents of the organic matrix of both bone as such and epiphyseal cartilage.

A COLLAGEN IN BONE AND EPIPHYSEAL CARTILAGE

The basic collagen molecule, rod-shaped, of dimensions approximately 300 $\times$ 1.5 nm, contains three polypeptide chains, designated α-chains, each containing around 1000 amino acid residues. For most of its length, each chain, in helical conformation, is entwined about the other two in a further super-helix so forming a rigid triple-super-helical structure. At each end of the molecule, however, the terminal portion of each constituent chain is not

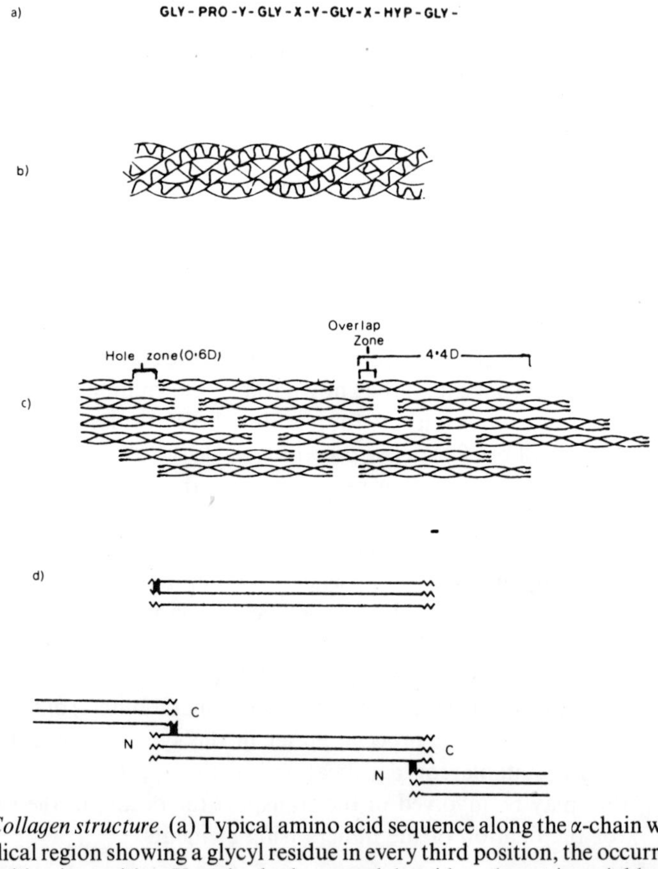

a) GLY - PRO - Y - GLY - X - Y - GLY - X - HYP - GLY -

b)

c) Hole zone (0·6D) Overlap Zone 4·4 D

d) C N N C

Fig. 1. *Collagen structure.* (a) Typical amino acid sequence along the α-chain within the triple helical region showing a glycyl residue in every third position, the occurrence of a prolyl residue in position X and a hydroxyprolyl residue almost invariably in the Y position; (b) Diagrammatic representation of the helical structure of tropocollagen; (c) The two-dimensional aggregation of tropocollagen molecules, illustrating the quarter stagger (by a length D where the collagen molecule is 4.4 D in length) and the end overlap (by an amount 0.4 D) creating a hole zone, 0.6 D in length; (d) Diagrammatic representation of intra- and inter-molecular cross-links showing the involvement of the *N*- and *C*-terminal telopeptides. The symbol, ~~ represents the telopeptide regions. (Reproduced by permission from Bailey and Robins, 1976)

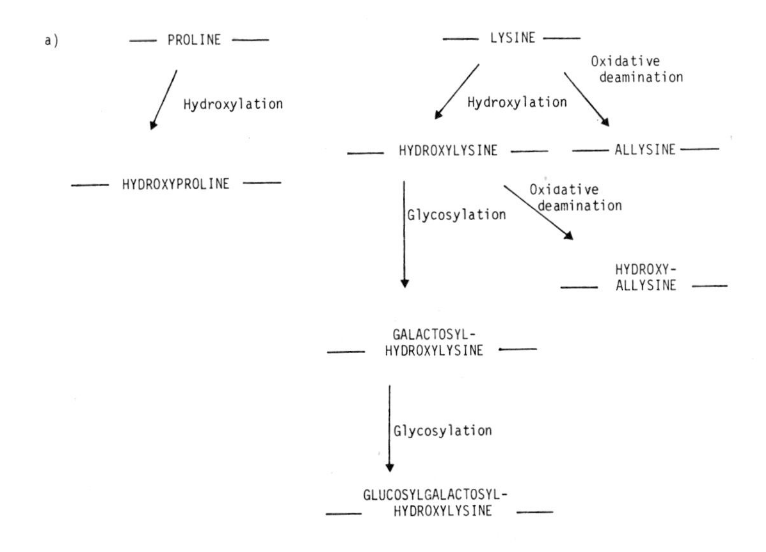

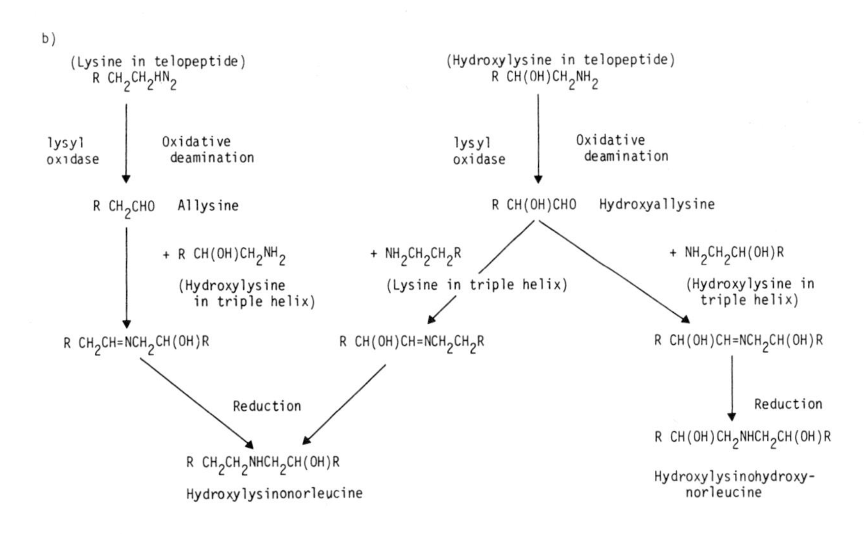

Fig. 2 (a) Post-translational modifications in collagen synthesis; (b) Derivation of the main intermolecular cross-links in collagen as isolated after reduction with borohydride. Hydroxylysinohydroxynorleucine is derived from two residues of hydroxylysine, one located in the telopeptide as hydroxyallysine following oxidation. Hydroxylysinonorleucine may be derived from allysine in the telopeptide and hydroxylysine in the main body of the adjacent molecule or from hydroxyallysine in the telopeptidyl site and a lysyl residue within the triple helical structure of a neighbouring molecule, R,-$CH_2CH_2CH(NH_2)COOH$.

bound in the triple-helical configuration. This relatively short extra-helical region, referred to as either the *N*- or *C*-terminal telopeptide, depending upon its location, is important in regard to the formation of interchain cross-links. Within the triple-helical region, every third residue in each chain is a glycyl residue. Approximately one sixth of the total residues in the molecule is an imino acid residue derived from either proline or hydroxyproline which are present in roughly equal proportions. Hydroxyproline which plays a vital role in the stability of the triple-helical structure, is derived by hydroxylation of specific prolyl residues after their incorporation within the polypeptide chain. Similarly a certain proportion of the lysyl residues are converted to hydroxylysine, an amino acid which is, like hydroxyproline, highly singular to collagen, and some of which can participate directly in cross-link formation.

Collagen molecules aggregate extracellularly in a highly-ordered manner to form fibrils which then assemble into fibres. Covalent cross-links between molecules impart tensile strength to the fibres. These essential features of collagen structure are illustrated diagrammatically in Figs. 1 and 2. (For

Table 1. Characteristics of collagens I, II and III

Type	Chain composition	Tissue distribution	% Hydroxylation		% Glycosylation
			proline	lysine	
I	$[\alpha1(I)]_2\alpha2$	Skin, bone, dentin, tendon blood vessel wall, gastrointestinal tract	45 (95–105)	20 (7)	35 (2)
II	$[\alpha1(II)]_3$	Cartilage	45 (95–105)	60 (23)	40 (9)
III	$[\alpha1(III)]_3$	Skin, blood vessel wall, gastrointestinal tract, dentin	55 (115–125)	15 (5)	—

The various α-chains differ in amino acid composition to a degree that clearly indicates their genetically distinct origin (see Miller, 1973; Chung and Miller, 1974). They also differ in the level of post-translational modifications. In this respect the data presented above are not precise since there can be considerable variation even within the single collagen type but the figures do serve to indicate the sort of level normally seen within a particular type and more especially serve to emphasize the very much higher level of hydroxylysine and glycosylated residues in Type II relative to Types I and III. The figures in parenthesis refer to numbers of residues per 1000 total.

The tissue distribution as shown should not be regarded as a complete list of tissues containing one or other of the collagen types in question. The amount of Type III relative to Type I varies considerably from a roughly equal proportion in the vascular wall to virtually none at all in bone and tendon (Epstein and Munderloh, 1975). Dentin from unerupted bovine teeth has been shown to contain a proportion of Type III (Volpin and Veis, 1973).

Other collagen types are also known, as for example the collagen occurring in basement membranes (Kefalides, 1973).

general basic reviews on collagen the reader is referred to Bailey 1968, and Grant and Prockop, 1972.)

Bone collagen, which comprises some 90% of the total organic matrix of bone, is identified as Type I collagen with a chain composition described by the formula $[\alpha 1(I)]_2\ \alpha 2$ (Table 1). The rather more basic α2-chain differs slightly in amino acid composition from the α1(I)-chain and can be separated from the latter chromatographically. Type I collagen is the most abundant collagen in the body and is found in 'soft' tissues such as skin and tendon as well as other 'hard' tissues such as dentin. It appears to be the sole collagen in bone matrix (Epstein and Munderloh, 1975) and indeed, appearance of any other type of collagen here may have deleterious effects. Thus it is considered that in some cases of osteogenesis imperfecta the skeletal defect may conceivably be attributable to the appearance of the genetically-distinct Type III collagen in bone, alongside the normal Type I (Penttinen *et al.*, 1975; Müller *et al.*, 1975).

In contrast epiphyseal cartilage contains a different collagen, defined as Type II, genetically-distinct from Type I (and Type III) and mostly confined to cartilagenous tissues (Table 1). Type II collagen has a chain composition given by the formula $[\alpha 1(II)]_3$. The α1(II)-chain differs from the α1(I)- and α2-chains of Type I collagen in primary structure and in the extent of certain post-translational modifications, particularly the (in general) relatively higher proportion of hydroxylysine and the greater number of hydroxylysyl residues undergoing glycosylation (see Miller, 1973). Collagen in epiphyseal cartilage constitutes approximately 60% of the total organic matrix. Type II collagen appears to represent, as in most other cartilages, the principal species. A proportion of Type I has however been detected in bovine epiphyseal cartilage for instance (Seyer *et al.*, 1974) and also in human rib cartilage (Eyre and Glimcher, 1972).

Collagen is clearly essential for the formation of a properly-functioning bone as evidenced by the skeletal defects that occur when its synthesis is impaired or altered as for example in certain nutritional disorders e.g. scurvy, copper deficiency (see Barnes, 1973) or in those cases of osteogenesis imperfecta already alluded to where the defect is considered to be either the partial replacement of Type I collagen by Type III or more simply a reduction in the level of Type I. For reasons outlined below, it is considered that bone collagen (or for that matter any collagen located in a calcifying matrix) may contain within its structure some particular feature(s) that distinguishes it from other collagens (in non-calcifying tissues) and that is essential for the fulfilment of its particular role(s) in the formation and functioning of the mineralised tissue. It is not unreasonable to further consider that the appearance of such a feature could be vitamin D-dependent and that its absence, for example, in rickets could contribute to the impaired skeletal formation in that disease.

Thus collagen is important in bone structure (as in other collagenous tissues) partly for its intrinsic tensile strength, dependent upon the presence of intermolecular covalent cross-links. Each tissue collagen including Type I of bone appears to exhibit a distinctive pattern of cross-links (see below) thereby imparting to the tissue of origin a characteristic cross-link structure which may conceivably relate to the precise function of that tissue. Secondly, bone collagen is important in providing a suitable framework for the deposition of the mineral phase. There is a very definite spatial relationship between the crystals of hydroxyapatite and the collagen fibrils within which they are located (Glimcher and Krane, 1968; Cameron, 1972; Engström, 1972). Evidence has been presented by Katz and Li (1973) that collagen fibrillar architecture, defined by the way collagen molecules pack together in a three-dimensional array, differs in mineralised tissues to that in 'soft' tissues. The intermolecular space (within the fibril) is greater, the molecules being spaced further apart, and this is considered important in rendering this space accessible to mineral ions. It seems likely that such specific molecular packing could depend upon some particular structural feature of the collagen molecule. Thirdly, important interactions may exist between collagen and other constituents in the matrix, e.g. phosphoproteins (Section II, B2) or alternatively 'bone morphogenetic substances' (Urist *et al.*, 1974; Reddi, 1976) that may be critical in the formation of bone. Such interactions may be governed by particular structural features of the collagen molecule. Finally, bone collagen may serve as an actual nucleator of hydroxyapatite. Although with the advent of the extracellular vesicle as the site of *initial* nucleation (Anderson, 1976a) the role of collagen as a nucleating agent in bone mineralisation is less clear, there is no doubt that the molecule in the native state (even when derived from soft tissues) can act in this capacity *in vitro* (Glimcher and Krane, 1968) and it seems likely still that this property must be of importance in mineralisation *in vivo*, (see Howell, 1976; Howell and Pita, 1976; Katz and Li, 1973; Höhling *et al.*, 1974) albeit that such nucleation may be subsequent to and perhaps in some as yet undefined way even dependent upon initial nucleation within the vesicle. Much attention has been paid to those aspects of collagen structure that may be essential for nucleation. In particular carboxylic acid and carbonyl groups have been implicated (see Glimcher and Krane, 1968; Urry, 1971; Davis and Walker, 1972). These groups are not specific to bone (or cartilage) collagen alone, however. Indeed since the primary structure of Type I collagen in the chick, for example, is identical in both bone and a 'soft' tissue such as skin (Miller *et al.*, 1969; Lane and Miller, 1969; Kang *et al.*, 1969a, b) then any consideration of essential specific structural features of calcifying collagens, whether this be in regard to the tensile strength of the molecule, to fibrillar architecture, to specific interactions with other molecules or to the nucleation process, ought perhaps to be concerned more with the post-translational modifications imposed upon the molecule rather than the primary structure itself.

During collagen synthesis, the molecule undergoes a number of post-translational alterations (see Fig. 2), including the hydroxylation of certain prolyl and lysyl residues, the glycosylation of a proportion of the hydroxylysyl residues and the oxidative deamination of specific lysyl and hydroxylysyl residues which precedes cross-link formation (for reviews see Grant and Prockop, 1972; Barnes and Kodicek, 1972; Tanzer, 1973, 1976; Bailey *et al.*, 1974; Bornstein, 1974; Cardinale and Udenfried, 1974; Gallop and Paz, 1975; Prockop *et al.*, 1976).

Hydroxylation of collagen proline seems to show relatively little variation overall at least within a single collagen type. Hydroxylation of collagen lysine, however, can show wide variation not only from one type of collagen to another (Miller, 1973; Kefalides, 1973; Chung and Miller, 1974), but from one tissue to another in respect of a single collagen type, or from one species to another in respect of a single tissue (Piez and Likins, 1960; Barnes, 1973; Stolz *et al.*, 1973; Barnes *et al.*, 1974). It has been suggested that the level of lysine hydroxylation may be controlled by the rate of triple helix formation (see Kivirikko and Risteli, 1976), since once the α-chains are incorporated within this structure hydroxylation of further lysyl residues appears to cease. The significance of the variation is obscure, but it is tempting to suggest it is related to the function of collagen within its particular tissue and that in bone it may be related to the mineralisation process, a critical state of hydroxylation being necessary for calcification. In fact it has been shown that mineralisation of turkey leg tendon collagen is associated with a decrease in the extent of hydroxylation of lysine in the mineralising collagen in comparison to that found in the uncalcified collagen (Likins *et al.*, 1960). There is also evidence that in certain instances of osteogenesis imperfecta, the defect may be attributable to an increased hydroxylysine content in bone collagen (Eastoe *et al.*, 1973; Trelstad *et al.*, 1977). However, there is no obvious straightforward correlation between the extent of collagen-lysine hydroxylation and the ability of the tissue in which the collagen is located to calcify. Thus dentin collagen appears invariably to have a relatively high level of hydroxylysine whilst bone collagen generally reveals a low level. In rat bone collagen on the other hand a relatively high proportion of the lysyl residues are hydroxylated (Piez and Likins, 1960; Butler, 1972a; Volpin and Veis, 1973; Stolz *et al.*, 1973; Barnes *et al.*, 1973a, 1974). Further the state of lysine hydroxylation within a particular collagen may not be constant (Miller *et al.*, 1967; Barnes *et al.*, 1971b). Thus in the chick embryo both skin and bone collagen are enriched in hydroxylysine. Shortly after hatching, however, the hydroxylation level falls from approximately 40% in the embryo to a constant value post-embryonically of around 20% for skin and 15% for bone (Barnes *et al.*, 1974).

Yet bone collagen would appear to calcify over the whole hydroxylation range whilst skin collagen does not calcify at any stage.

Glycosylation of hydroxylysyl residues, the function of which remains undefined, but which may be important in defining fibre architecture (Morgan *et al.*, 1970), in cross-link structure (Bailey *et al.*, 1974) or in the binding of phosphopeptides in mineralising tissues (see Section II B2), also shows variation from one collagen to another in the same sort of way that the hydroxylysine content can vary. It is reasonable to conjecture again that such variations may be related to function. There is variation not only in the extent i.e. the number of residues glycosylated, but also in the precise nature of the glycosylation, with variation in the relative proportion of residues linked either to a single galactose molecule or to the disaccharide glucosylgalactose (Spiro, 1969, 1970; Grant *et al.*, 1969; Schofield *et al.*, 1971; Segrest and Cunningham, 1970; Kefalides, 1973; Miller, 1973). In the human, for example, bone collagen has a different pattern of glycosylation, in the adult, to collagen from skin. The extent of glycosylation is similar in the two instances but in the case of bone, the major glycosylated derivative is galactosylhydroxylysine whereas in skin glucosylgalactosylhydroxylysine predominates (Pinnell *et al.*, 1971; Segrest and Cunningham, 1970). However, in the chick (Royce and Barnes, 1977) glycosylation in skin and bone appears similar in the embryo (with a ratio of glucosylgalactosylhydroxylysine: galactosylhydroxylysine of about 2) whilst post-embryonically, the proportion of galactosylhydroxylysine increases in skin, remaining essentially unaltered in bone. Further, Stolz *et al.* (1973) found little difference in the type of glycosylation between rat skin and bone collagen in the young rat. There would thus appear to be no simple correlation discernible between the overall state of glycosylation of collagen and ability of the tissue of origin to calcify.

A more meaningful comparison could perhaps be achieved if post-translational modifications at specific sites were to be compared. Thus hydroxylation of the single lysyl residue occurring in each of the non-helical telopeptide regions of the collagen molecule located at each end of the collagen α-chain, is important in determining the type of cross-link found in a particular collagen. Variations in hydroxylation at this site can be correlated with differences in the pattern of cross-links (Barnes *et al.*, 1971a, b, 1974; Bailey and Robins, 1972). The major cross-links in bone collagen (see Fig. 2) are dehydrohydroxylysinohydroxynorleucine, derived from two residues of hydroxylysine, one located in the non-helical region and the other within the helical body of the molecule, and to a lesser extent, dehydrohydroxylysinonorleucine, derived from one residue each of hydroxylysine, located mostly in the non-helical region, and lysine, from the helical part of the molecule (Tanzer, 1973, 1976; Bailey *et al.*, 1974; Robins and Bailey, 1975). This pattern of cross-linking is quite distinct from that in soft tissue collagens such as skin or tendon and appears to be basically attributable to the relatively high state of hydroxylation of lysine in the telopeptide regions in the case of bone collagen, despite the generally rather low overall level of hydroxylation (Miller *et al.*, 1967; Barnes *et al.*, 1971a, 1974). Hydroxylation at this site may conceivably be under the control of a specific enzyme (Barnes *et al.*, 1974). However, a high level of hydroxylation in the non-helical regions with a resultant high proportion of cross-links occurring as dehydrohydroxylysino-hydroxynorleucine does not inevitably mean calcification. Thus sternal and articular cartilage and embryonic skin collagens are examples which display a high level of hydroxylation in non-helical regions and in which dehydro-hydroxylysinohydroxynorleucine represents a very high proportion of the total reducible cross-links without any calcification occurring in the parent tissue (Barnes *et al.*, 1971b; Bailey and Robins, 1972; Miller, 1971; Miller and Robertson, 1973; Miller *et al.*, 1973; Balian and Bailey, 1975). Indeed cross-links may not be required at all for calcification as lathyritic bone contains the normal proportion of mineral (Miller *et al.*, 1967). Nevertheless one cannot exclude the possibility that a relatively high state of hydroxylation at the telopeptidyl site may through its consequent influence upon the cross-link pattern be an essential requisite for the proper functioning of bone. Mechanic and his colleagues maintain that bone as other tissue collagens has a very specific and readily-identifiable pattern of cross-links which in this case may be directly under the control of vitamin D (Mechanic *et al.*, 1975; Section III C1).

B NON-COLLAGENOUS COMPONENTS

1 *Glycoproteins*

(*a*) *Bone*. All connective tissues contain plasma glycoproteins (for a recent review on glycoproteins in connective tissues see Anderson, 1976b). Their presence in bone has been reported by several authors (Burckard *et al.*, 1966; Triffitt and Owen, 1973; Ashton *et al.*, 1974; Dickson, 1974; Dickson *et al.*, 1975a; Owen and Triffitt, 1976) and Owen and her colleagues have demonstrated that at least some of them occur mostly in the extravascular space. One component in particular appears to be concentrated specifically in bone and thus may well be of particular relevance to mineralisation and/or bone resorption. Triffitt and Owen (1973) identified the presence of this glycoprotein in rabbit bone by labelling the constituents of the matrix with ^{14}C derived either from [^{14}C] glucosamine or plasma [^{14}C] glycoprotein. The same protein was not detected in skin, kidney, muscle, intestine or aorta. Its extraction only after demineralisation again suggests its possible involvement in the mineralisation process. The protein was identified as of α-mobility and would appear to be equivalent to the plasma α-glycoprotein isolated from

EDTA extracts of bovine cortical bone (Ashton *et al.*, 1974). This latter protein was found to be at a concentration in the bone (expressed relative to that of albumin) some 250-fold higher than in plasma. In humans, the equivalent protein has since been identified as plasma α2 HS-glycoprotein (Dickson *et al.*, 1975a; Ashton *et al.*, 1976).

Perhaps the best characterised bone glycoprotein is the calcium-binding, sialic acid-rich, acidic glycoprotein isolated by Herring and his colleagues from bovine cortical bone (Andrews *et al.*, 1967, 1969). This protein is extracted along with a number of other less-acidic glycoproteins, including the bovine analogue of α2 HS-glycoprotein referred to above, by EDTA solutions during demineralisation. The protein is characterised by, in addition to a high sialic acid content, high levels of glutamic and aspartic acids, occurring mostly as the free acid rather than in amide form, and relatively high serine, threonine and glycine levels. Some organically bound phosphate (1.4%) was detected. Ion-binding properties, including calcium binding, have been reported by Williams and Peacocke (1967), Chipperfield and Taylor (1968, 1970) and Chipperfield (1970). The sialoprotein occurs in part associated with chondroitin sulphate as a proteoglycan (Herring, 1968; Section I B3). A comparable bone sialoprotein appears to occur in rabbit cortical bone (Burckard *et al.*, 1966), human bone (Shetlar *et al.*, 1972) and possibly sheep cortical bone bound entirely to chondroitin sulphate in the latter case (Dickson, 1974). No equivalent protein was detected in tendon (Herring, 1976) but a similar type of protein may occur in dentin (Zamoscianyk and Veis, 1966). The suggestion has been made therefore that this type of sialoprotein may be specific to calcified tissues (see Herring, 1972; Anderson, 1976b).

Leaver and his colleagues (see Leaver *et al.*, 1975) have reported the isolation of three anionic proteins from human dentin that may be comparable to the bone sialoprotein in the extent of their acid nature but which differ substantially in amino acid composition. Two contain some organically bound phosphate and one of these also contained sialic acid (2.5%).

Apart from the plasma proteins which are normally readily removed, glycoproteins in connective tissues generally may be in intimate relationship with the fibrous elements, namely collagen and elastin, and drastic procedures including high pH, strongly dissociative conditions and disulphide bond-breaking agents are required for their removal. These glycoproteins have been implicated in interfibrillar interactions and in defining the precise mode of deposition of collagen and elastin fibres (Anderson, 1976b). The so-called structural glycoproteins speculatively involved in the latter function have a microfibrillar structure (Ross and Bornstein, 1969; Robert *et al.*, 1971). These glycoproteins would appear to have some particular affinity for calcium. Thus glycoproteins attached to collagen and believed to be involved in polymerisation can be removed by EDTA extraction and the collagen, previously insoluble, can then be dispersed in acetic acid. Addition of Ca^{++} ions following EDTA extraction prevents this (Steven, 1967). Also, microfibrillar glycoprotein constituents of the major blood vessels appear to be associated with calcification in this tissue (Barnes and Partridge, 1968; McCullagh *et al.*, 1973). Demineralisation with EDTA permits their extraction with hot alkali and thereby allows the preparation of a pure elastin (Keeley and Partridge, 1974).

There is evidence for the occurrence of glycoproteins of this nature existing in intimate relationship with the fibres in bone. Thus demineralisation with EDTA permits the solubilisation of approximately two-thirds of the total non-collagenous material. Subsequent disruption of the insoluble collagenous matrix by treatment with collagenase renders most of the remaining one-third soluble. Leaver *et al.* (1975) have reported the isolation of two proteins from bovine bone by these means that are not found in EDTA extracts. One was a glycoprotein, the other essentially all protein with little if any carbohydrate. Both contained low levels of phosphate. Leaver and his associates comment on the similarity between the latter component and the phosphoprotein isolated from bone by Shuttleworth and Veis (1972) (see Section II B2).

Herring has also reported on the presence of at least one component in bovine cortical bone that is solubilised only by disruption of the collagen network with collagenase (Herring, 1977). The material remaining insoluble after collagenase digestion Herring (1977) regarded as akin to the structural glycoproteins referred to above.

(*b*) *Epiphyseal cartilage*. Although glycoproteins are undoubtedly present in the cartilage, studies of this type of constituent have not been so extensive as in bone. It has been demonstrated that sialic acid-containing constituents are more abundant in ossifying than in the resting region of calf scapular cartilage (Jibril and Lindenbaum, 1965; Vittur *et al.*, 1971).

Shipp and Bowness (1975) have reported the isolation from dog rib cartilage of two glycoproteins which were obtained after extraction of proteoglycans and subsequent removal of collagen by collagenase digestion. They were solubilised by treatment with disulphide bond-breaking agents under denaturing conditions. One of them exhibited a microfibrillar form when viewed by electron microscopy and is considered comparable to similar microfibrillar structural glycoproteins associated with elastic fibres (Barnes and Partridge, 1968; Ross and Bornstein, 1969; Robert *et al.*, 1971). The presence of small amounts of hydroxyproline and uronic acid in these proteins indicated a strong association with collagen and proteoglycan. The authors suggest the glycoprotein may anchor to the collagenous framework a proteoglycan possibly involved in calcification (see Section II B6).

2 *Phosphoproteins*. A phosphoprotein containing around 0.15–0.3% phos-

phorus, organically bound to serine, has been isolated from EDTA extracts of embryonic bovine jaw and femur bone and chicken metatarsal bone (Spector and Glimcher, 1972). The protein contained high levels of aspartic and glutamic acids. The serine content was relatively low and over one half of serine residues was phosphorylated. The authors consider that anionic, phosphorus-containing proteins of this type may play a vital role in the mineralisation process.

Shuttleworth and Veis (1972) isolated from bovine bone matrix, by periodate degradation, after decalcification with EDTA, an anionic phosphoprotein with relatively high aspartic and glutamic acid, glycine and serine levels and also containing hydroxylysine. It was proposed that the phosphoprotein was covalently bound to collagen via the phosphoserine residue through a glycosylated hydroxylysl residue in collagen and released from collagen by the periodate treatment. Similar periodate treatment of insoluble dentin collagen releases a phosphoprotein appreciably richer in phosphorus (5.9%) and rich particularly in serine and aspartic acid. This protein is also believed to be covalently bound to collagen in the same manner as above (Veis and Perry, 1967; Carmichael *et al.*, 1971). Comparison of peptides derived from bovine skin and dentin collagen (Volpin and Veis, 1973) has revealed that specific peptides, from dentin only, contain organically-bound phosphate in an amount equivalent to the hexose present. This is thought to reflect the presence in dentin of the bound phosphoproteins described above. Comparable soluble phosphoproteins have been detected in dentin (Veis *et al.*, 1972; Butler *et al.*, 1972; Butler, 1972b; Carmichael and Dodd, 1973; Dickson *et al.*, 1975b). It has been suggested (Veis *et al.*, 1972) that bound phosphoprotein may serve to locate the deposition of mineral on collagen fibres and the soluble moiety to inhibit calcification of predentin by preventing nucleation of hydroxyapatite. Interestingly predentin in bovine teeth appears not to contain bound phosphoprotein (in this respect similar to rat incisor dentin; Butler *et al.*, 1972b); further the soluble phosphoprotein contained appreciably less phosphorous than the corresponding protein in dentin (Carmichael *et al.*, 1975).

3 *Proteoglycans.* Proteoglycans are a major component of the organic matrix of cartilage. Chondroitin sulphate (4- and 6-isomers) is the major glycosaminoglycan component of proteoglycans in epiphyseal cartilage but some keratan sulphate and a small amount of hyaluronate also seem to be present (see Herring, 1973).

Several studies indicate an increase in the concentration of glycosaminoglycans towards the mineralisation front from resting zone to hypertrophic zone and then a fall in concentration in the zone of provisional calcification. The glycosaminoglycans in the calcifying region are less readily extracted and appear to be of lower molecular weight and/or charge density (Lindenbaum and Kuettner, 1967; Campo and Tourtelotte, 1967; Wuthier, 1969; Vittur *et al.*, 1971; Larsson *et al.*, 1973; Lohmander and Hjerpe, 1975).

In cartilage in general, the proteoglycan subunit or monomer is comprised of glycoaminoglycan chains linked to a central protein core. Several such proteoglycan units are then attached through the mediation of a glycoprotein – the link glycoprotein – to hyaluronate to yield a very high molecular weight complex (Fig. 3; Hardingham and Muir, 1972; Gregory, 1975; Heinegard and Hascall, 1975). Aggregated proteoglycans of this nature have been considered to play an important role in the calcification of cartilage and this will be discussed later (Section II B6).

Of particular interest to the subject of this chapter are the studies by Vittur and associates (Vittur *et al.*, 1972a, b; Vittur and de Bernard, 1973) of the proteoglycan aggregate in calf scapula cartilage. These authors reported that the complex was more abundant where calcification was occurring. This may appear contrary to the findings of a decreased concentration of glycosaminoglycans associated with mineralisation already mentioned. However, the ossifying region of calf scapular cartilage as isolated by Vittur and his colleagues may not be completely equivalent in an anatomical sense wholly to the epiphyseal zone of provisional calcification. The link-glycoprotein isolated from the proteoglycan complex exhibited calcium-binding properties and alkaline phosphatase activity. This was considered of particular pertinence to calcification in view of the histochemical identification of glycoprotein in extracellular vesicles (Bonucci, 1967) and the presence of alkaline phosphatase activity (Ali *et al.*, 1970) in these structures.

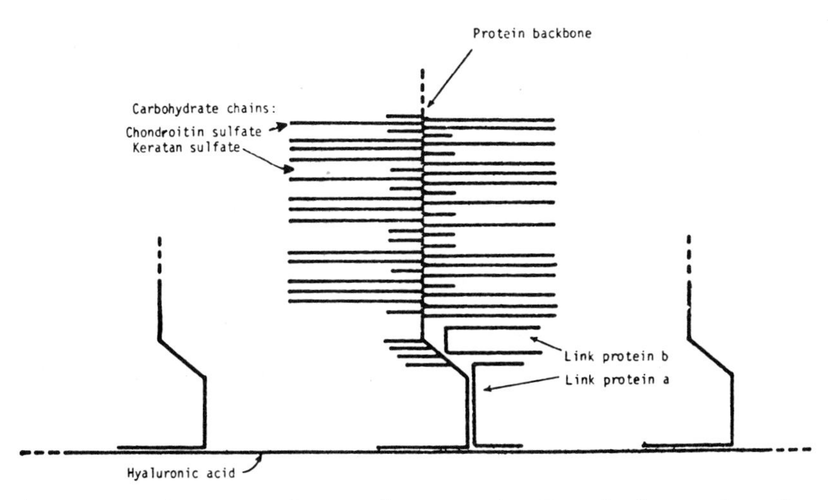

Fig. 3. Proposed structure of proteoglycan complex (from bovine nasal cartilage; taken from Gregory, 1975)

The proteoglycan fraction in bone represents a very much smaller proportion of the total organic matrix than in cartilage (see Herring, 1973). The glycosaminoglycan present appears to be mostly chondroitin-4-sulphate. The chondroitin sulphate is partly attached to the bone sialoprotein described by Herring and his colleagues referred to previously (Herring, 1968). The proteoglycan of bone differs from that in cartilage in that it does not appear to represent such a complex structure. Chondroitin sulphate chains are attached to bone sialoprotein only at the level of one or two chains per molecule of protein (Herring, 1973). It would not appear to form complex aggregates with hyaluronate.

4 *Lipids.* Irving first provided convincing evidence for the possible involvement of lipid in calcification by the histochemical demonstration of the presence of sudanophilic material at the mineralisation front (reviewed by Irving, 1976). This material is only extracted upon demineralisation and appears to be mainly acidic phospholipids, particularly phosphatidyl serine and phosphatidyl inositol (Wuthier, 1968). It is now believed that the phospholipids located at the mineralisation front reflect the presence of a high concentration of matrix vesicles in this region (Wuthier, 1976). The turnover studies of Eisenberg *et al.* (1970) and Cruess and Hong (1973) imply a probable role for these lipids in endochondral ossification. Phosphatidyl serine is known to bind Ca^{++} and this binding is enhanced in the presence of phosphate through the formation of a phospholipid-calcium phosphate complex (Cotmore *et al.*, 1971). Such a complex has been isolated from rabbit bone (Boskey and Posner, 1975).

5 *Peptides.* The matrix of bone contains a series of peptides, many dialysable, extractable by acid or EDTA. The amino acid composition varies widely, the peptides ranging from very basic to very acidic. Some at least of these peptides appear to contain organically bound phosphate. (Leaver and Shuttleworth, 1968; Leaver, 1969; Leaver *et al.*, 1975).

6 *Role of Non-collagenous Constituents in Calcification.* It is not our purpose here to describe in detail theories concerning calcification mechanisms (see for example Bowness, 1968; Glimcher and Krane, 1968; Bachra, 1970; Anderson, 1976a; Howell, 1976; Howell *et al.*, 1976; Howell and Pita, 1976; Vogel and Boyan-Salyers, 1976) but simply to consider the evidence for the involvement of the non-collagenous constituents of the matrix in this process. If so involved, then clearly alteration in the amount of such a constituent or its structure, under the influence of calciferol or one of its metabolites, could directly effect the mineralisation process.

The presence of proteins specifically associated with mineralising tissue as indicated in the preceding pages and particularly their solubilisation during demineralisation has led of course to the thought that they may be involved in the mineralisation process. They could for instance play a role in vesicle function or alternatively in facilitating the intra-fibrillar deposition of mineral in collagen or in the movement of the mineralising elements in the extracellular space. The precise mechanism of their involvement however remains obscure and the evidence on the whole is still rather circumstantial. The studies of Pugliarello *et al.* (1970) and Nusgens *et al.* (1972) indicating a reduction in the amount of non-collagenous protein as the degree of mineralisation increases whilst the amount of collagen per unit volume remains essentially constant, has pointed to a possible involvement of these proteins in the initiation or control of mineralisation. A similar loss of proteinaceous material with mineralisation is known to occur in enamel. The radioautographic studies of Weinstock *et al.* (1972) using labelled fucose and Weinstock and Leblond (1973) using ^{32}P and ^{3}H-serine has indicated the accumulation of glycoprotein and phosphoprotein at the predentin–dentin junction in the rat incisor. The authors consider that this protein(s) may be responsible for the predentin–dentin transformation. Histological techniques (see Irving, 1976) have demonstrated the presence of a sudanophilic component(s) at the mineralisation front possibly implicating, when considered in conjunction with the above radioautographic studies, the involvement of lipoproteins in the onset of mineralisation. It has been suggested that the sudanophilic material may be associated with the membranes of matrix vesicles occurring in high concentration at the mineralisation front, and considered the site of initial nucleation of hydroxyapatite. The lipid components may be directly involved in sequestering calcium ions (Howell and Pita, 1976; Irving, 1976; Vogel and Boyan-Salyers, 1976; Wuthier, 1976).

As already mentioned, Veis and his colleagues suggest that phosphoprotein, covalently bound to collagen may serve to direct the deposition of mineral within the collagen fibre whilst unbound phosphoprotein might inhibit calcification in predentin or osteoid by binding Ca^{++} and rendering it unavailable for hydroxyapatite formation (II B2). A similar inhibitory role has been suggested for calcium-binding glycoproteins (see Herring, 1972, 1973).

A large number of studies all indicate loss of proteoglycans associated with the onset and the increasing intensity of mineralisation in ossifying cartilage, bone and dentin. Further the proteoglycan remaining appears to be less highly aggregated and the constituent glycosaminoglycans to be of lower molecular weight (Lindenbaum and Kuettner, 1967; Campo and Tourtelotte, 1967; Wuthier, 1969; Pugliarello *et al.*, 1970; Vittur *et al.*, 1971, 1972; Baylink *et al.*, 1972; Engfeldt and Hjerpe, 1972; Larrsson *et al.*, 1973; Lohmander and Hjerpe, 1975; Nicholson *et al.*, 1975; Engfeldt and Hjerpe, 1976). The studies of Howell and his colleagues indicate that proteoglycan aggregates inhibit the growth of mineral crystals (see Howell and Pita, 1976; Howell *et al.*, 1976). It has been considered that depolymerisation of proteoglycans could reduce their calcium binding ability and in effect increase the concentration of Ca^{++} in solution (see reviews quoted above) perhaps thereby permitting nucleation of hydroxyapatite. The calcium-binding link-glycoprotein described by Vittur *et al.* (1972a, b) may be relevant here. Howell and his colleagues however feel that proteoglycan aggregates inhibit mineral growth more directly by binding with the mineral forming agent (Cuervo *et al.*, 1973). It is not entirely clear whether the latter represents an early mineral phase formed in the extracellular vesicles or the matrix vesicles themselves or both (Howell *et al.*, 1976). Specific enzymes have been implicated in the depolymerisation or degradation of cartilage proteoglycan aggregates, particularly lysozyme (Kuettner *et al.*, 1975) but direct proof for the involvement of any one specific enzyme is still lacking (Howell and Pita, 1976).

The identification in mineralised tissue of the calcium-binding amino acid, γ-carboxyglutamic acid, known to be responsible for the calcium-binding activity of prothrombin, has been reported (Hauschka *et al.*, 1975; Price *et al.*, 1976). The γ-carboxyglutamic acid residues appear to be located in a single protein, extracted during demineralisation with EDTA, of low molecular weight and low isoelectric point. Clearly this protein could be of primary importance in the mineralisation process. It has been detected in bone and dentin but appears to be absent from epiphyseal cartilage (and enamel). It binds to hydroxyapatite, but strongly inhibits crystallisation of the latter, a property which Price *et al.* (1976) consider may be relevant to its function *in vivo*. It is considered that this protein may be one of the strongly anionic phosphoproteins isolated by a number of workers from EDTA extracts of bone and dentin (Section II B2).

III Effects of Calciferol

This section deals with the metabolism of calciferol in bone and the role of the active metabolites in the physiological and biochemical processes of this tissue. Evidence will be presented in favour of 1,25-dihydroxycholecalciferol as the form of calciferol active in stimulating resorption and the information available on the interrelationship of this hormone with parathyroid hormone in bone metabolism will be reviewed.

A METABOLITES OF CALCIFEROL IN BONE

Since about 15% of the body weight of animals is accounted for by bone and as this tissue is a target organ of calciferol it is not surprising to find that of all the tissues of animals bone contains the highest proportion of an administered dose of the vitamin (Neville and DeLuca, 1966). In a series of experiments on the turnover of radioactive cholecalciferol in rachitic rats it was found that four hours after a dose of radioactive cholecalciferol the skeleton of rachitic rats contained as much as 27% of the dose. The half-life of this radioactive material was relatively slow in that 16% of the dose was still present at 48 h. On the reasonable assumption that this radioactivity is mainly located within the cells of bone, Neville and DeLuca (1966) concluded that only intestinal mucosal tissue and bone cells had a higher concentration of this steroid and its metabolites than plasma. The pattern of cholecalciferol metabolites in bone differs from that found in the intestine (chapter 5). Whereas in the intestine 1,25-dihydroxycholecalciferol accounts for the majority of the calciferol derived steroids, in bone, 25-hydroxycalciferol is the major metabolite accounting for over 50% of the total and the hormone itself accounting for less than 35% (Weber *et al.*, 1971; Lawson *et al.*, 1969, 1971; Wong *et al.*, 1972; Tanaka and DeLuca, 1971; Edelstein *et al.*, 1975). The relative proportions of these two metabolites varies according to the time that the analysis is made after the dose of cholecalciferol. At very early time intervals of course, the vitamin itself accounts for most of the bone radioactivity but its level falls rapidly as it is metabolised (probably by the liver). The level of 25-hydroxycholecalciferol rises steadily for between 6–8 h falling slowly thereafter. The changes in the content of these two steroids in bone appears to reflect the changes occurring in their plasma levels rather than metabolism of calciferol by bone. It was reported that bone cells have a higher concentration of cholecalciferol metabolites relative to plasma (Neville and DeLuca, 1966) and since 25-hydroxycholecalciferol represented the major fraction it would seem that bone is able to accumulate this metabolite against a concentration gradient. If this inference can be established by direct investigation it would imply a role for this substance not previously recognised. In addition bone contains two proteins which appear to be able to specifically bind 25-hydroxycholecalciferol but similar proteins for 1,25-dihydroxycholecalciferol have not so far been described (Lawson *et al.*, 1976).

The complexity of bone anatomy (chapter 6 and chapter 7, section II) makes it essential to know the location of the metabolites as between the diaphyseal, metaphyseal and epiphyseal areas and the various cell types and the intracellular matrix occurring within these areas. The autoradiographic localisation within rat bone of radioactive 25-hydroxycholecalciferol and the metabolites formed from it showed them to be present only in areas of active mineralisation (Wezeman, 1976). The radioactivity was incorporated into epiphyseal hypertrophic cells, metaphyseal osteoblasts and osteocytes and into the surrounding matrix. Radioactivity was not present in osteoclasts nor in the resting and proliferative zones of the cartilage. There has been only one attempt to establish the pattern of metabolites in the bone compartments by more biochemical means. Weber *et al.* (1971) divided bone of rachitic chicks

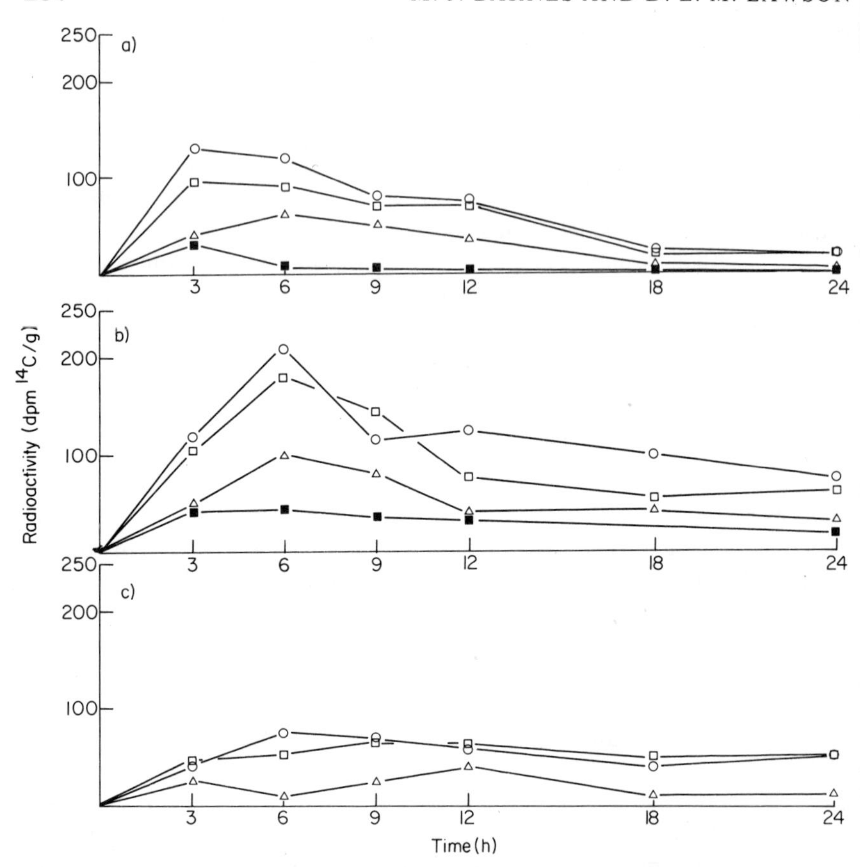

Fig. 4. Time course of appearance of cholecalciferol and metabolites in compartments of chick bone. Vitamin D-deficient chicks were dosed with 0.5 μg [4-^{14}C,1,2-^{3}H]cholecalciferol. (a) cholecalciferol; (b) 25-hydroxycholecalciferol; (c) 1,25- dihydroxycholecalciferol. ○, metaphysis; △, epiphysis; □, diaphysis; ■, plasma. Steroid concentration expressed as dpm/mg DNA or dpm/ml of plasma (Weber *et al.*, 1971)

dosed with labelled cholecalciferol into epiphyseal, metaphyseal and diaphyseal fractions. The changes in 25-hydroxycholecalciferol levels in these compartments were consistent with the changes described above for the whole bone. On the other hand there were small differences in the time after the dose at which maximum levels of 1,25-dihydroxycholecalciferol were reached in these three fractions (Fig. 4). The significance of these differences is not apparent at present. These authors were also able to show that, as in the intestine, the major calciferol-derived steroid in the bone cell nuclei was 1,25-dihydroxycholecalciferol and that the 25-hydroxy-metabolite was located in the 100 000 g fraction (cytoplasm). However, because of the different roles played by several cell types found in bone it would be most valuable to establish the pattern of cholecalciferol metabolites located specifically within them.

The metabolism of an administered dose of radioactive 1,25-dihydroxycholecalciferol has also been followed in both rachitic rats and chicks (Frolik and DeLuca, 1972; Wong *et al.*, 1972). These two investigations showed that the active form of calciferol in bone as regards calcium mobilisation is 1,25-dihydroxycholecalciferol. At time intervals at which calcium mobilisation was maximum, as measured by raised plasma calcium under conditions of dietary calcium restriction, the hormone represented over 80% of the total calciferol derived metabolites in the tissue. At later time intervals other metabolites were present which are currently unidentified. Following an intravenous dose of the hormone, maximum accumulation in bone occurs within 1 h but in contrast to the intestine the level falls slowly for the first few hours (4 h in chicks and 7 h in rats) before appearing to decline more rapidly. A good correlation has been found between changes in bone 1,25-dihydroxycholecalciferol levels and calcium mobilisation. Other evidence in favour of 1,25-dihydroxycholecalciferol being the active form of calciferol as regards bone mobilisation is discussed in the following sections.

B BONE RESORPTION

Resorption of bone, involving the dissolution of both bone mineral and matrix, is a normal part of bone growth and maintenance. Histological evidence indicates that this process can take place through the action of both osteoclasts and osteocytes. Most of the information available on resorption and its relationship to bone formation has been provided by histological investigations, but these studies have not been able to resolve whether it is the matrix or the bone mineral which is removed first. The current view considers that the process is partly extracellular and partly intracellular. There is some evidence that osteoclasts can take up the incompletely degraded bone mineral and matrix for more complete dissolution and hydrolysis (Hancox and Boothroyd, 1965). Possible roles in this process have been suggested for mitochondria and lysosomes for instance.

There is very little biochemical information on the metabolic processes involved in resorption. Most studies have concentrated on the stimulatory effect of parathyroid hormone and calciferol on this process. The effect of these two substances can be studied *in vivo* in parathyroidectomised or vitamin D-deficient animals on a low calcium diet, in which case changes in plasma calcium and phosphate levels are held to be due to bone mineral resorption. Alternatively resorption can be studied *in vitro* in embryonic bone incubated in a suitable culture medium; in this case the bone mineral is pre-labelled with ^{45}Ca or ^{32}P either *in vivo* or *in vitro*.

1 *1,25-Dihydroxycholecalciferol and Bone Mobilisation.* Calciferol can only cause resorption *in vivo*, being completely inert if added to the bone culture system. Although a number of the analogues and metabolites of calciferol can stimulate bone resorption *in vitro* the information presently available strongly suggests that 1,25-dihydroxycholecalciferol is the active form of cholecalciferol regulating the rate at which this process occurs *in vivo*. Among the evidence in favour of this view is the finding that calciferol is inactive in anephric rats whereas the hormone is fully active in such animals (Wong *et al.*, 1972). In addition 1,25-dihydroxycholecalciferol is the most potent substance known with calcium mobilising activity whether measured *in vivo* (Wong *et* al., 1972b) or *in vitro* (Reynolds, 1974; Stern *et al.*, 1975).

Studies on the metabolism of the hormone (Section IIIA) in both rat and chick support the view that this substance is the active form of calciferol in bone. It should be appreciated that histological data by Baylink *et al.* (1970) show that bone mobilisation is 80% higher in vitamin D-deficient rats than in pair-fed controls so that factors other than the calciferol metabolites can stimulate this process. Rachitic rats on a low calcium diet, however, are unable to respond to factors which normally cause increased bone mobilisation whilst the calciferol replete animals can do so.

The features of the 1,25-dihydroxycholecalciferol molecule conferring biological activity as measured *in vitro* in the bone resorption system have been assessed (Stern *et al.*, 1975; DeLuca and Schnoes, 1976). The relative contribution of the different groups in the hormone is indicated by the relative activity of the following compounds: $1\alpha,25\text{-}(OH)_2D_3 > 3\text{-deoxy-}1\alpha,25\text{-}(OH)_2D_3 > 1\alpha\text{-OH-}D_3 \simeq 25\text{-OH-}D_3 > 3\text{-deoxy-}1\alpha\text{-OH-}D_3 \gtrsim 3\text{-deoxy-}25\text{-OH-}D^3 > D_3 \simeq 5,6\text{-}trans\text{-}25\text{-OH-}D_3$. 24,25-Dihydroxycholecalciferol and its 1-hydroxy-metabolite also stimulate bone resorption with an activity a little less than that shown by 25-hydroxycholecalciferol (Peacock *et al.*, 1976). It is only the 24R and not the 24S form which shows this activity. There is almost no information on the mechanism by which these steroids stimulate bone resorption. The studies with actinomycin D (Eisenstein and Passavoy, 1964) imply that the effect requires continuing protein synthesis and by analogy with the intestinal events suggests that the synthesis of one or more proteins involved in resorption is controlled at the transcriptional stage by 1,25-dihydroxycholecalciferol. In contrast to events observed in the intestine, no one has yet detected calcium-binding protein in bone cells, even under conditions in which bone resorption should be maximal (i.e. low calcium diet).

2 *Parathyroid Hormone and Bone Mobilisation.* Much evidence indicates that parathyroid hormone stimulates adenyl cyclase activity leading to an accumulation of cyclic AMP in bone cells before mobilisation of bone mineral

occurs (Chase and Aurbach, 1970; Wells and Lloyd, 1969; Rasmussen *et al.*, 1968). It appears that this hormone never enters its target cells but acts at the plasma membrane to increase cAMP levels which in turn activates the processes involved in resorption.

Parathyroid hormone has a number of other effects on bone, of course, but in connection with its relationship to calciferol it is perhaps worth referring to the rapid increase in RNA and protein synthesis in osteoclasts caused by this hormone. Puromycin and actinomycin D inhibit the calcium mobilising response to parathyroid hormone (Rasmussen *et al.*, 1964; Tashjian *et al.*, 1964; Kunin and Krane, 1965). In addition an increased incorporation of ^{3}H-uridine into RNA and of ^{3}H-leucine into proteins in response to parathyroid hormone has been observed in osteoclasts (Bingham *et al.*, 1969).

3 *1,25-Dihydroxycholecalciferol and Parathyroid Hormone Interrelationships in Bone Mobilisation.* Since the resorption activity of calciferol is due to 1,25-dihydroxycholecalciferol it follows that the same activity shown by parathyroid hormone may be either as a result of a direct action or due to its regulation of 1,25-dihydroxycholecalciferol synthesis. The degree to which these two hormones are dependent on each other to affect bone mobilisation is a continuing problem, the complexities of which are only now beginning to be appreciated. With regard to a possible direct action of parathyroid hormone, bone mobilisation is not stimulated *in vivo* by this substance given to vitamin D-deficient rats (Harrison *et al.*, 1958), but in kidney in contrast, parathyroid hormone activity was unaffected by the vitamin D-status of the animal (Rasmussen *et al.*, 1963). That parathyroid hormone has a direct action on bone is shown by stimulation of adenyl cyclase activity in bone cell fractions from vitamin D-deficient rats effected *in vitro* by parathyroid hormone (Kakuta *et al.*, 1975). As shown by others the hormone had no effect on calcium mobilisation from bones of such animals. It could be envisaged therefore that mobilisation of calcium involves a number of biochemical steps one of which is stimulated by cAMP (and through which the effect of parathyroid hormone is mediated), and that subsequent steps involve a protein(s) the synthesis of which is 1,25-dihydroxycholecalciferol dependent. Vitamin D-deficiency results in the failure of the bone cells to produce this protein(s) and consequently the mobilisation activity of parathyroid hormone would be inhibited. In parathyroidectomised animals the level of cAMP in the cells should be limiting so that the effect of 1,25-dihydroxycholecalciferol is either severely impaired in extent or even completely inhibited. The results of Garabedian *et al.* (1974) showing that 1,25-dihydroxycholecalciferol had only partial mobilising activity in parathyroidectomised rats is consistent with this view. Other interpretations of these findings are possible however. There may be a parathyroid hormone-sensitive, calciferol-independent mechanism for stimulating calcium mobilisation which is maximally activated in the vitamin

D-deficient state (there is always a marked hyperparathyroidism in such animals). Consequently the administration of parathyroid hormone to rachitic animals may increase cAMP levels but not mobilisation if some later step was rate limiting. Furthermore experimental evidence indicating the presence of additional mechanisms of bone mobilisation has been obtained by Reynolds *et al.* (1976) who found that cultures of bone from thyroparathyroidectomised mice responded to 1,25-dihydroxycholecalciferol. In addition the pattern of phosphate resorption in response to 1,25-dihydroxycholecalciferol and other stimuli suggests that other mechanisms of mineral resorption are present in bone cells additional to those that have been revealed by the studies of calcium mobilisation alone.

4 *Phosphate Resorption and 1,25-Dihydroxycholecalciferol.* Since the discovery of an activation of calcium translocation by calciferol at the vitamin's target tissues there have been many attempts to show that phosphate is similarly affected. Most studies have found that phosphate transport across the intestinal cell occurred as a consequence of calcium transport and only relatively recently has it become clear that the effect of 1,25-dihydroxycholecalciferol on phosphate absorption occurs somewhat later than that on calcium absorption (Wasserman and Taylor, 1973; Chen *et al.*, 1974). The effect of calciferol on phosphate metabolism assumed a new dimension with the finding that the hormonal form also increased phosphate mobilisation from bone of parathyroidectomised rats (Castillo *et al.*, 1975). This latter finding corroborated the previous histological observations that resorption of bone mineral was increased in hypophosphataemic animals and that the effect could be observed in thyroparathyroidectomised animals (Baylink *et al.*, 1971; Thompson *et al.*, 1975).

This effect of 1,25-dihydroxycholecalciferol on phosphate transport is further complicated by the changes in calciferol metabolism in response to variations in plasma phosphate levels. Hypophosphataemia results in an accumulation of 1,25-dihydrocholecalciferol in its target tissues and some evidence has been presented that it is due to an increase in the kidney 1-hydroxylase by a process not requiring the presence of parathyroid hormone (Tanaka and DeLuca, 1973). However, mobilisation of embryonic bone in culture is also increased if the incubation is carried out in low phosphate medium (Raisz and Niemann, 1969) so that hypophosphataemia may cause phosphate mobilisation from bone by either directly affecting the bone or maintaining high tissue levels of the steroid hormone over a prolonged period. The parathyroid hormone-independent bone mobilising action of 1,25-dihydroxycholecalciferol mainly affects bone phosphate but some mobilisation of calcium also occurs.

C SYNTHESIS OF BONE CONSTITUENTS AND CALCIFICATION

Probably the major outstanding problem at present as regards the role of calciferol in bone metabolism is to understand how a deficiency of the vitamin leads to a failure of calcification in bone. The available information suggests that at least one metabolite, 1,25-dihydroxycholecalciferol has a direct action on bone in stimulating bone mineral mobilisation. It is the purpose of this section to consider whether there is in addition an involvement of calciferol metabolites directly in the processes that lead to the deposition of mineral.

Lack of calcification in rickets may perhaps be due wholly to reduced plasma Ca levels consequent to reduced bone mobilisation and reduced intestinal absorption together with increased renal excretion (DeLuca, 1967).

Some experimental evidence for this view has been provided; for example calcification can apparently be observed in isolated bones from rachitic rats placed in normal serum but not in serum from rachitic rats (Shipley *et al.*, 1926; Neuman, 1958). In addition Fraser *et al.* (1958) have infused inorganic phosphate into patients with nutritional rickets and observed radiographically new bone mineral formation. Similar observations have been made by others (Gran, 1960; Yoshiki *et al.*, 1974).

On the other hand, it has been considered entirely reasonable that the uptake of mineral ions by bone and their utilisation during calcification may be controlled directly by a metabolite of calciferol. Wuthier (1971a) for example observed that the concentration of mineral ions in the proliferative and hypertrophic zones of epiphyseal cartilage was affected in rickets more severely than the serum levels of these constituents and concluded that there might be a direct effect of vitamin D-deficiency on the ability of bone to produce mineral. Baylink *et al.* (1970) have concluded from histological observations that the onset of mineralisation is delayed in rickets and have proposed that this arises from a reduced rate of 'maturation' of osteoid. They maintain that the osteoid matrix in some as yet unidentified way is altered to a state suitable for mineralisation and that this alteration occurs more slowly in rickets. Furthermore in contrast to the studies of Fraser *et al.* (1958) and others referred to above, Eastwood *et al.* (1974) found that in patients with chronic renal failure the associated osteomalacia did not respond to large intakes of calcium sufficient to maintain near normal plasma levels.

Techniques for the quantitative assessment of the extent of osteomalacia in bone are still not in widespread use and furthermore their utilisation requires some degree of expertise. Only one comparison has been made with these techniques of the healing produced by calciferol as against phosphate. Using the per cent of osteoid with a calcification front as the criterion of the extent of osteomalacia, Rasmussen and Bordier (1974) reported that osteomalacic patients only showed an increase in the calcification front after vitamin D therapy and not after treatment with phosphate. Treatment with the latter ions induces only a diffuse mineralisation. This is a most important observation which has not received the attention it deserves since it appears to show for the first time an unequivocal effect of calciferol on bone mineralisation. It furthermore means that future studies that require an assessment of changes in mineralisation in rachitic bone should involve this type of histological examination.

There are of course numerous reports of the anti-rachitic effect of calciferol, and of its analogues and metabolites. Until relatively recently most of the available information on the features of this molecule necessary for biological activity had come from assessments of the curative power of these substances as anti-rachitic agents *in vivo*. As with other responses such as intestinal absorption and bone mobilisation, the maximum anti-rachitic response of calciferol in animals requires the three double-bonds, a 25-hydroxyl group and an intact side chain of the cholesterol type (25-OHD$_3$ has 40% greater anti-rachitic activity than D$_3$; Blunt *et al.*, 1968). Intriguingly the introduction of a hydroxyl group at C-1 of 25-hydroxycholecalciferol does not always produce a significantly greater response and recently it has been reported that 1,25-dihydroxycholecalciferol treatment of patients with osteodystrophy as a result of chronic renal failure does not restore in all cases a normal histological appearance to the bone (Coburn *et al.*, 1977).

It will be clear from the above that there are some grounds for belief that calcification may be influenced directly by a derivative of calciferol. This article has briefly considered the organic constituents of the matrix undergoing calcification that may play some part in this process and whose synthesis may conceivably be controlled by calciferol whether the function of such constituents is in the carriage or supply of mineral ions to the site of mineralisation, in the formation of hydroxyapatite itself or in the provision of a precisely-defined matrix required for a properly functioning mineralised tissue. As will be appreciated from what is described below studies on the effect of calciferol, or its lack, on the biosynthetic activity of bone cells, which may give rise to changes either in the quantity or the precise composition of the matrix, are not extensive and evidence for a direct and vital role for calciferol in bone formation remains inconclusive as yet.

1 *Collagen*. The precise effect of calciferol on the matrix as a whole and on collagen, its major constituent, is not entirely clear. Two aspects need to be taken into consideration: namely the effect of the deficiency itself which may be indirect, and any direct action of the calciferol metabolites. There are reports of a reduced level of organic matrix in rachitic bone (Canas *et al.*, 1969; Baylink *et al.*, 1970; Hjertquist *et al.*, 1970); but this presumably could be due to an increased turnover or decreased synthesis of matrix. The direct

investigation of collagen synthesis in the deficient state has produced conflicting data (Canas *et al.*, 1969; Barnes *et al.*, 1973a; Paterson and Fourman, 1968), although the most carefully controlled studies have shown that the changes in synthesis in this condition are minimal. Consequently the reduced collagen levels in rachitic animals is probably due to an increased degradation of this protein (Hjertquist *et al.*, 1970). The increased excretion of hydroxproline in patients with rickets or osteomalacia and in rachitic rats also points to increased degradation of bone collagen in this condition (Kivirikko, 1970; Parsons *et al.*, 1973).

The effect of calciferol on bone of rachitic rats is to cause an increased incorporation of radioactive precursor amino acids into collagen. This effect is only observed with collagen of bone and not of skin (Canas *et al.*, 1969; Barnes *et al.*, 1973a). It is considered to be a direct effect of a metabolite of the vitamin and not consequent upon a raising of the plasma calcium levels (Canas *et al.*, 1969). It is not clear as to which of the calciferol metabolites is responsible for this effect since 25-hydroxycholecalciferol appears active in parathyroidectomised rats in as much as an increase in bone hydroxyproline occurs (Russell and Avioli, 1975). The increased excretion of hydroxyproline following administration of calciferol to patients with osteomalacia may reflect increased resorption associated with remodelling during healing, but may also reflect increased collagen synthesis since invariably a significant proportion of newly-synthesised collagen is degraded rather than retained within the tissue as insoluble fibre and increased collagen synthesis is therefore accompanied by increased excretion of hydroxyproline. In summary a lack of calciferol results primarily in reduced retention of both new collagen and previously mineralised collagen and therefore osteoid accumulates primarily because of the reduction in mineralisation rather than because of any increase in the rate of synthesis of organic matrix. The action of calciferol (or a metabolite) is to effect a temporary increase in collagen synthesis during the repletion period. Likewise studies of Morava *et al.* (1973) on bones in culture and Parsons *et al.* (1973) on hydroxyproline excretion in healing rickets in rats support the concept of increased collagen synthesis in response to calciferol metabolites.

The nature of bone collagen in rickets has also been studied (Toole *et al.*, 1972; Barnes *et al.*, 1973a). Both groups concluded that the collagen synthesised in richitic bone was Type I as in normal bone, but that it differed from normal by a marked increase in the extent of collagen lysine hydroxylation. Collagen in the epiphyseal plate was normal Type II collagen with no change in composition. Similarly no change in lysine hydroxylation was observed in skin collagen (Toole *et al.*, 1972). Gross and his colleagues proposed that the increased hydroxylation of collagen lysine in bone collagen might be accompanied by increased glycosylation (either in absolute terms or as an increase in the proportion of glucosylgalactosyl- to galactosylhydroxylysine) and that the latter increase, if occurring in the region of the 'holes' of the collagen fibre, might, by steric hindrance, prevent the deposition of hydroxyapatite within the 'hole' regions, thus impeding mineralisation. They further proposed that the 'hole' regions in osteoid collagen might normally be 'closed' by glycosylated residues and that the maturation of osteoid as visualised by Baylink *et al.* (1970) might involve the enzymic modification of such glycosylated residues so that the 'holes' became available for the deposition of mineral. However, glycosylation of chick bone collagen was found to be only marginally increased in rickets and there was no increase in disaccharide relative to monosaccharide substitution (Royce and Barnes, 1977). Further glycosylation in the vicinity of the 'hole' region, at least in some bone collagens, is normally likely to be complete or nearly so and mostly in the form of the disaccharide-substituted derivative without any apparent impairment in calcification (see Royce and Barnes, 1977).

In accord with the hydroxylation changes there are alterations in the pattern of bone collagen cross-links in rickets with an increase in the proportion of dehydrohydroxylysinohydroxynorleucine relative to dehydrohydroxylysinonorleucine (Mechanic *et al.*, 1972, 1975). These changes in hydroxylation and in the cross-links of bone collagen may reflect a direct effect of calciferol on bone metabolism (as advanced by Mechanic and his colleagues; Mechanic *et al.*, 1975; Gonnerman *et al.*, 1976) but similar changes have been observed in response to dietary calcium deficiency and following parathyroidectomy (Barnes *et al.*, 1973b). It was noted that tendon collagen was not similarly affected by these factors. As the change in hydroxylation was also observed in vitamin D-deficient, phosphate-deficient rickets where serum calcium levels were normal, it was proposed that the size of the $Ca \times PO_4$ ionic product may be the critical factor. Incubation *in vitro* in the presence of labelled lysine of either periosteal membrane from the tibiae of rachitic chicks or metaphyseal tissue taken from the tibiae of calcium-deficient birds, confirmed the elevation in collagen lysine hydroxylation in either situation. Further a short preincubation in the presence of calcium caused a marked reduction in the hydroxylation value towards normal levels. This appeared to confirm the more direct effect of calcium level rather than vitamin D status as such (M. J. Barnes and L. F. Morton, unpublished).

The change in hydroxylation presumably reflects an increase in bone lysyl hydroxylase activity in the vitamin D-deficient and calcium-deficient animal. This could reflect increased amounts of enzyme as such or, as we believe, that bone lysyl hydroxylase activity, is normally controlled by calcium, resulting in increased enzymic activity when calcium is low. In this regard the finding by Ryhanen (1976) that partially purified lysyl hydroxylase from chick embryo is inhibited by calcium (50% inhibition by 15 mM Ca^{++}) is particularly interesting. The absence of significant changes in hydroxylation in rickets and dietary calcium deficiency in tissues other than bone may arise if calcium levels are normally such that inhibition of hydroxylase activity occurs only in bone. Other enzymes involved in post-translational modifications of bone collagen may be increased in rachitic tissues such as lysyl oxidase (Gonnerman *et al.*, 1976).

An increase in lysyl oxidase activity has also been reported in healing rickets (Siegel *et al.*, 1975), perhaps indicative of the stimulation of collagen synthesis under these conditions. Against this, there was however, no change in prolyl hydroxylase activity. The activity of other enzymes was not reported.

The significance of the increased hydroxylation and attendant changes in cross-links in relation to the impaired bone formation in rickets is unclear but as already indicated some evidence exists that the precise state of hydroxylation might be important as regards mineralisation (Section IIA).

2 *Proteoglycans.* As in the case of collagen, it is difficult to conclude from the available data that there is any consistent change in the rate of synthesis of proteoglycans in vitamin D-deficiency. Reports have been made of an increase in glycosaminoglycans in rat diaphyseal bone and in epiphyseal cartilage of puppies (Hjerquist, 1964; Hjerquist *et al.*, 1970) but the opposite finding has been made by others (Howell, 1965). The explanation for these contrasting conclusions may be found in the studies of Simmons and Kunin (1971) who showed that changes in glycosaminoglycan synthesis in rickets varies according to the area of the tissue analysed. Synthesis is unaffected in the cells of the proliferative zone of the cartilage and is decreased in the hypertrophic zone. There are, however, a number of studies which imply an increase in synthesis in response to calciferol and support the idea therefore of increased matrix formation in healing rickets. Thus an increase both in concentration of glycosaminoglycan constituents and in their rate of incorporation in healing rachitic cartilage has been observed (Dziewiatkowski, 1954; Cipera *et al.*, 1960; Howell and Carlson, 1965; Hjerquist, 1964).

3 *Phospholipids.* Wuthier has reported an increase in rickets of acidic phospholipids, particularly phosphotidyl serine and inositol, in proliferative and hypertrophic cartilage and cancellous bone i.e. at sites where calcification is initiated (Wuthier, 1971b). It was noted that these phospholipids were less extractable despite the reduced mineral content (usually the acidic phospholipids are least extractable when mineralisation is greatest). It is thought this may reflect the accumulation in rickets of a complex between acidic phospholipid and amorphous calcium phosphate. It is postulated such a complex may be involved in the mineralisation process. Degradation of this complex would normally occur as mineralisation proceeded and crystalline hydroxyapatite formed. As previously noted, it is considered that the phospholipids associated with mineralisation are derived from the matrix

vesicles (Wuthier, 1976). Since these structures appear to be present in normal number in rachitic cartilage and since initiation of crystal formation can be induced at these sites either *in vivo* by the intraperitoneal administration of phosphate to vitamin D- and phosphate-deficient rats or *in vitro* by incubation of rachitic cartilage in the presence of adequate calcium and phosphorus (Anderson and Sajdera, 1976), it might be concluded that synthesis and functioning in calcification of phospholipids associated with matrix vesicle membranes is not affected by calciferol.

These findings of Anderson and Sajdera imply not only that the function of the extracellular vesicle itself is intrinsically unimpaired by rickets, but also that the supply of mineral ions to these structures possibly involving chondrocyte mitochondria (see Davis *et al.*, 1976; Ali, 1976; Brighton and Hunt, 1976), does not require the direct participation of calciferol. Of course, the possibility remains as already under discussion, that mineralisation of the matrix following primary vesicular nucleation may be under the influence of the vitamin.

4 *Other Constituents.* Owen and her colleagues have investigated the influence of rickets in the context of albumin and the 'α2 HS-glycoprotein' component in rabbit bone. Both these proteins are synthesised outside the skeletal system and subsequently located in bone extravascularly. A decreased amount in rachitic bone has been observed. Uptake by bone is not impaired apparently but retention is reduced due to the decreased formation of hydroxyapatite to which these proteins strongly adsorb (Owen and Triffitt, 1974; M. E. Owen, private communication).

The influence of calciferol on the synthesis in bone of other specific constituents such as the sialo-protein described by Herring and his colleagues or the phosphoprotein described in Section II B2 is so far unknown. The effect on the post-translational introduction of γ-carboxy groups into glutamic acid residues in the protein described by Hauschka *et al.*, 1975, and Price *et al.*, 1976, would clearly be of interest. Up to now the presence of a vitamin D-dependent calcium-binding protein analogous to that involved in intestinal transport of calcium has not been detected in bone and yet its presence may seem a very reasonable proposition. It should be borne in mind perhaps that the intestinal protein is intracellular whilst the bone proteins referred to here appear to be extracellular.

IV Summary

The complexity of the structure of bone is probably the main reason why our understanding of the growth and maintenance of this tissue and of the factors controlling these two processes has developed relatively slowly. Two aspects of bone mark it out from most other tissues. Firstly, like many other 'connective tissues' it consists of a high proportion of extracellular matrix and in the case of bone of course this is a calcified matrix. Secondly bone as such is really, at least during development, a mixture of two tissues, cartilage and true bone. Both bone and cartilage contain a variety of different cells some of which reflect the presence of different cell types, others representing different stages of development within the single cell type. In addition to the differences in cell types between these two tissues (chapter 6) there are important differences in the nature of the components of the matrix as indicated in this chapter.

The nature of bone is severely affected by the absence of calciferol in a manner dependent essentially upon the age of the bone. The end result of the deficiency of the vitamin is manifested in a defective mineralisation. Such is the complexity of bone structure and of the process of mineralisation that the action of the vitamin may be on one or more of several metabolic steps in a long and complicated mechanism (chapter 6).

In this chapter we have reviewed the evidence in favour of 1,25-dihydroxycholecalciferol as the active form of calciferol responsible for bone mobilisation. However, 25-hydroxycholecalciferol also displays some mobilisation activity *in vitro* and its concentration in bone is such that consideration should be given to the possibility that it has a role in bone metabolism supplementary to that of 1,25-dihydroxycholecalciferol. Only a small number of studies have considered calciferol metabolism in relation to bone and none have so far taken into account the variety of cells present. An answer to the problem of which cell types in bone and in cartilage are affected by these two metabolites may be found through the autoradiographic approach even despite the well recognised problems of this technique. Perhaps the failure to find calciferol metabolites in osteoclasts (traditionally thought to be the site of calciferol stimulated mobilisation) in the most recent report utilising this technique underlines the need to appreciate the limitations of the data on which our current views are based.

Because of the relative technical ease with which mobilisation can be studied, more is known about the role of calciferol on this process than on mineralisation. The interrelationship of parathyroid hormone and the calciferol metabolites in bone calcium mobilisation has been the subject of several investigations but, as indicated in this chapter, doubts about the exact degree of dependence of one upon the other remain. In biochemical terms further progress in this area and in understanding the mechanisms by which calciferol metabolites control bone resorption would be greatly aided by studies with preparations of isolated cells. In this connection the recent reports by Binderman *et al.*, 1974 and Luben *et al.*, 1976 hold out some promise of progress in this direction.

Although it is held that mobilisation is a necessary prerequisite for mineralisation and consequently that the effect of calciferol metabolites on this latter process is explicable on the basis of an action through the control of mobilisation there is now some indication that calciferol metabolites have an additional affect in bone which is one directly upon the mineralisation process itself.

This chapter has therefore considered those components of bone that may be involved in this process and has examined the available evidence that may signify some influence of calciferol metabolism upon their synthesis, structure or function. Since extracellular vesicles considered to be involved in the onset of mineralisation, appear to be present in normal number in rachitic cartilage and since upon return of serum calcium and phosphate levels to normal these structures are able to induce crystal formation without the intervention of calciferol metabolites, it may be thought that both the supply of mineral ions to the vesicles and the ability of the latter to initiate mineralisation are normally calciferol independent processes. The possibility must be considered, however, that structural features of the matrix or aspects of its metabolism may be important in the control of mineralisation beyond its initiation at the vesicular site and that it may be here that calciferol metabolites may exert some influence on the overall mineralisation process. Matrix formation undoubtedly appears to be stimulated in healing rickets. Furthermore, the structure of bone collagen is affected by calciferol status in as much as hydroxylysine, the level of which in collagen may be important in permitting the precise type of mineralisation required for bone to function properly, is increased in rachitic bone. The effects, however, may be related more directly to changes in the concentration of the mineralising elements rather than reflecting a genuine control by calciferol derived substances. As reviewed in this chapter, bone contains a number of components that appear to be specific to mineralising tissues but so far any direct dependence on calciferol either in terms of their synthesis or structure has yet to be established. No calciferol-dependent protein equivalent to the intestinal calcium-binding protein has yet been found in bone. The impression gained is that the fundamental action of the vitamin in this regard has yet to be discovered. The nature of the involvement of calciferol in mineralisation may only be satisfactorily established by a study of the action of the vitamin's metabolites on isolated bone cells, a point already stressed. Such action may conceivably influence the rate of division or maturation of a particular cell type or its biosynthetic activity as expressed in specific enzyme levels. It is of interest here that Bisaz *et al.* (1975) have concluded from histological studies that there is an accumulation of cells of the proliferative zone in rachitic cartilage suggesting that calciferol affects the maturation of these cells.

References

Ali, S. Y. (1976). *Fed. Proc.* **35**, 135.
Ali, S. Y., Sajdera, S. W. and Anderson, H. C. (1970). *Proc. Natl. Acad. Sci. USA* **67**, 1513.
Anderson, H. C. (1976a). *Fed. Proc.* **35**, 105.
Anderson, H. C. and Sajdera, S. W. (1976). *Fed. Proc.* **35**, 148.
Anderson, J. C. (1976b). *Inter. Rev. Connec. Tiss. Res.* **7**, 251.
Andrews, A. T. de B., Herring, G. M. and Kent, P. W. (1967). *Biochem. J.* **104**, 705.
Andrews, A. T. de B., Herring, G. M. and Kent, P. W. (1969). *Biochem. J.* **111**, 621.
Ashton, B. A., Triffitt, J. T. and Herring, G. M. (1974). *Europ. J. Biochem.* **45**, 525.
Ashton, B. A., Hohling, H. J. and Triffitt, J. T. (1976). *Calc. Tiss. Res.* **22**, 27.
Bachra, B. N. (1970). *Inter, Rev. Connec. Tiss. Res.* **5**, 165.
Bailey, A. J. (1968). *Comprehensive Biochemistry* **26B**, 297.
Bailey, A. J. and Robins, S. P. (1972). *FEBS Lett.* **21**, 330.
Bailey, A. J. and Robins, S. P. (1976). *Sci. Prog. Oxf.* **63**, 419.
Bailey, A. J., Robins, S. P. and Balian, G. (1974). *Nature* (London) **251**, 105.
Balian, G. and Bailey, A. J. (1975). *Annals Rheum. Dis.* **34**, (Suppl. 2) 41.
Barnes, M. J. (1973). *In* 'Hard Tissue Growth, Repair and Remineralisation'. Ciba Foundation Symposium II, p. 247. Elsevier, Excerpta Medica, North Holland, Amsterdam.
Barnes, M. J. and Partridge, S. M. (1968). *Biochem. J.* **109**, 883.
Barnes, M. J. and Kodicek, E. (1972). *Vitam. Horm.* **30**, 1.
Barnes, M. J., Constable, B. J., Morton, L. F. and Kodicek, E. (1971a). *Biochem. J.* **125**, 433.
Barnes, M. J., Constable, B. J., Morton, L. F. and Kodicek, E. (1971b). *Biochem. J.* **125**, 925.
Barnes, M. J., Constable, B. L., Morton, L. F. and Kodicek, E. (1973a). *Biochem. J.* **132**, 113.
Barnes, M. J., Constable, B. J., Morton, L. F. and Kodicek, E. (1973b). *Biochem. Biophys. Acta* **328**, 373.
Barnes, M. J., Constable, B. J., Morton, L. F. and Royce, P. M. (1974). *Biochem. J.* **139**, 461.
Baylink, D., Stauffer, M., Wergedal, J. and Rich, C. (1970). *J. Clin. Invest.* **49**, 1122.
Baylink, D., Wergedal, J. and Stauffer, M. (1971). *J. Clin. Invest.* **50**, 2519.
Baylink, D., Wergedal, J. and Thompson, E. (1972). *J. Histochem. Cytochem.* **20**, 279.
Binderman, I., Duskin, D., Harell, A., Katzir, E. and Sachs, L. (1974). *J. Cell Biol.* **61**, 427.
Bingham, P., Brazell, I. and Owen, M. (1969). *J. Endocrinol.* **45**, 387.
Bisaz, S,., Schenk, R., Kunin, A. S., Russell, R. G. G., Muhlbauer, R., Fleisch, H. (1975). *Calc. Tiss. Res.* **19**, 139.
Blunt, J. W., Tanaka, Y. and DeLuca, H. F. (1968). *Proc. Natl. Acad. Sci. USA* **61**, 1503.
Bonucci, E. (1967). *J. Ultrastruc. Res.* **20**, 33.
Bornstein, P. (1974). *Ann. Rev. Biochem.* **43**, 567.
Boskey, A. L. and Posner, A. S. (1975). *Calc. Tiss. Res.* **19**, 273.
Bowness, J. M. (1968). *Clin. Orthop. Rel. Res.* **59**, 233.
Brighton, C. T. and Hunt, R. M. (1976). *Fed. Proc.* **35**, 143.
Burckard, J., Havez, R. and Dantrevaux, M. (1966). *Bull. Soc. Chim. Biol.* **48**, 851.
Butler, W. T. (1972a). *Biochem. Biophys. Res. Commun.* **48**, 1540.

Butler, W. T. (1972b). *In* 'The Comparative Molecular Biology of Extracellular Matrix' (Ed. Skavein, H. C.) p. 255. Academic Press, New York and London.
Butler, W. T., Finch, J. E. and Desteno, C. V. (1972). *Biochem. Biophys. Acta* **257**, 167.
Cameron, D. A. (1972). *In* 'The Biochemistry and Physiology of Bone' (Ed. Bourne, G. H.) p. 191. Academic Press, New York and London.
Campo, R. D. and Tourtelotte, C. D. (1967). *Biochem. Biophys. Acta* **141**, 614.
Canas, F., Brand, J. S., Neuman, W. F. and Terepka, A. R. (1969). *Amer. J. Physiol.* **216**, 1092.
Cardinale, G. and Udenfried, S. (1974). *Adv. Enzymol.* **41**, 245.
Carmichael, D. J. and Dodd, C. M. (1973). *Biochem. Biophys. Acta* **317**, 187.
Carmichael, D. J., Veis, A. and Wang, E. T. (1971). *Calc. Tiss. Res.* **7**, 331.
Carmichael, D. J., Chovelon, A. and Pearson, C. H. (1975). *Calc. Tiss. Res.* **17**, 263.
Castillo, L., Tanaka, Y. and DeLuca, H. F. (1975). *Endocrinol.* **97**, 995.
Chase, L. R. and Aurback, G. D. (1970). *J. Biol. Chem.* **245**, 1520.
Chen, T. C., Castillo, L., Korycka-Dahl, M. and DeLuca, H. F. (1974). *J. Nutr.* **104**, 1056.
Chipperfield, A. R. (1970). *Biochem. J.* **118**, 36P.
Chipperfield, A. R. and Taylor, D. M. (1968). *Nature* (London) **219**, 609.
Chipperfield, A. R. and Taylor, D. M. (1970). *Europ. J. Biochem.* **17**, 581.
Chung, E. and Miller, E. J. (1974). *Science* **183**, 1200.
Cipera, J. D., Migicovsky, B. B. and Belanger, L. F. (1960). *Can. J. Biochem. Physiol.* **38**, 807.
Coburn, J. W., Brickman, A. S., Sherrard, D. J., Singer, F. R., Baylink, D. J., Massry, S. G. and Norman, A. W. (1977). *In* '3rd Workshop on Vitamin D' (Ed. Norman, A. W.) p. 657. Walter de Gruyter, Berlin and New York.
Cotmore, J. M., Nichols, G. and Wuthier, R. E. (1971). *Science* **172**, 1339.
Cruess, R. L. and Hong, K. C. (1973). *Calc. Tiss. Res.* **13**, 305.
Cuervo, L. A., Pita, J. C. and Howell, D. S. (1973). *Calc. Tiss. Res.* **13**, 1.
Davis, N. R. and Walker, T. E. (1972). *Biochem. Biophys. Res. Commun.* **48**, 1656.
Davis, W. L., Matthews, J. L., Talmage, R. E. and Martin, J. H. (1976). *Calc. Tiss. Res.* **21** (Suppl.), 59.
DeLuca, H. F. (1967). *Vitam. and Horm.* **25**, 315.
DeLuca, H. F. and Schnoes, H. K. (1976). *Ann. Rev. Biochem.* **45**, 631.
Dickson, I. R. (1974). *Calc. Tiss. Res.* **16**, 321.
Dickson, I. R., Poole, A. R. and Veis, A. (1975a). *Nature* (London) **256**, 430.
Dickson, I. R., Dimizio, M. T., Volpin, D., Anathanarayanan, S. and Veis, A. (1975b). *Calc. Tiss. Res.* **19**, 51.
Dziewiatkowski, D. D. (1954). *J. Exp. Med.* **100**, 25.
Eastoe, J. E., Martens, P. and Thomas, N. R. (1973). *Calc. Tiss. Res.* **12**, 91.
Eastwood, J. B., Bordier, P. J., Clarkson, E. M., Tun Chot, S. and De Wardener, H. E. (1974). *Clin. Sci. Mol. Med.* **47**, 23.
Edelstein, S., Harrell, A., Bar, A. and Hurwitz, S. (1975). *Biochim. Biophys. Acta* **385**, 438.
Eisenberg, E., Wuthier, R. E., Frank, R. B. and Irving, J. T. (1970). *Calc. Tiss. Res.* **6**, 32.
Eisenstein, R. and Passavoy, M. (1964). *Proc. Soc. Exptle. Biol. and Med.* **117**, 77.
Engfeldt, B. and Hjerpe, A. (1972). *Calc. Tiss. Res.* **10**, 152.
Engfeldt, B. and Hjerpe, A. (1976). *Acta. pat. microbiol. scand. Sect A* **84**, 95.
Engström, A. (1972). *In* 'The Biochemistry and Physiology of Bone' (Ed. Bourne, G. H.) p. 237. Academic Press, New York and London.

Epstein, E. H. and Munderloh, N. H. (1975). *J. Biol. Chem.* **250**, 9304.
Eyre, D. R. and Glimcher, M. J. (1972). *Proc. Natl. Acad. Sci. USA* **69**, 2594.
Fraser, D., Geiger, D. W., Munn, J. D., Slater, P. E., Jahn, R. and Liu, E. (1958). *Amer. J. Dis. Child.* **96**, 460.
Frolik, C. A. and DeLuca, H. F. (1972). *J. Clin. Invest.* **51**, 2900.
Gallop, P. M. and Paz, M. A. (1975). *Physiol. Rev.* **55**, 418.
Garabedian, M., Tanaka, Y., Holick, M. F. and DeLuca, H. F. (1974). *Endocrinol.* **94**, 1022.
Glimcher, M. J. and Krane, S. M. (1968). *In* 'Treatise on Collagen' (Ed. Gould, B. S.) Vol. 2B, p. 67. Academic Press, London and New York.
Gonnerman, W. A., Toverud, S. V., Ramp, W. K. and Mechanic, G. L. (1976). *Proc. Soc. exp. Biol. Med.* **151**, 453.
Gran, F. C. (1960). *Acta Physiol. Scand.* **50**, 132.
Grant, M. E. and Prockop, D. J. (1972). *N. Eng. J. Med.* **286**, 194–199, 242–249, 291–300.
Grant, M. E., Freeman, I. L., Schofield, J. D. and Jackson, D. S. (1969). *Biochim. Biophys. Acta* **177**, 682.
Gregory, J. D. (1975). *Protides of the Biological Fluids* **22**, 171.
Hardingham, T. E. and Muir, H. (1972). *Biochim. Biophys. Acta* **279**, 401.
Hancox, N. M. and Boothroyd, B. (1965). *Clin. Orthopaed. Related Res.* **40**, 153.
Harrison, H. E., Harrison, H. C. and Park, E. A. (1958). *Amer. J. Physiol.* **192**, 432.
Hauschka, P. V., Lian, J. B. and Gallop, P. M. (1975). *Proc. Natl. Acad. Sci. USA* **72**, 3925.
Heinegard, D. and Hascall, V. C. (1975). *Protides of the Biological Fluids* **22**, 177.
Herring, G. M. (1968). *Biochem. J.* **107**, 41.
Herring, G. M. (1972). *In* 'The Biochemistry and Physiology of Bone' (Ed. Bourne, G. H.) p. 127. Academic Press, New York and London.
Herring, G. M. (1973). *In* 'Biological Mineralization' (Ed. Zipkin, I.) p. 75. John Wiley and Sons Inc., New York.
Herring, G. M. (1976). *Biochem. J.* **159**, 749.
Herring, G. M. (1977). *Calc. Tiss. Res.* **24**, 29.
Hjertquist, S. O. (1964). *Acta. Soc. Med. Upsal.* **69**, 83.
Hjertquist, S. O., Bergquist, E. and Sevastikoglou, J. A. (1970). *Acta. orthop. Scand. Suppl.* **136**, 53.
Höhling, H. J., Ashton, B. A. and Koster, H. D. (1974). *Calc. Tiss. Res.* **148**, 11.
Howell, D. S. (1965). *Arth. Rheum.* **8**, 337.
Howell, D. S. (1976). *Is. J. Med. Sci.* **12**, 3.
Howell, D. S. and Carlson, L. (1965). *Exp. Cell. Res.* **37**, 582.
Howell, D. S. and Pita, J. C. (1976). *Clin. Orth. Rel. Res.* **118**, 208.
Howell, D. S., Pita, J. C. and Alvarez, J. (1976). *Fed. Proc.* **35**, 122.
Irving, J. T. (1976). *Fed. Proc.* **35**, 109.
Jibril, A. O. and Lindenbaum, A. (1965). *Biochim. Biophys. Acta* **101**, 236.
Kakuta, S., Suda, T., Sasaki, S., Kimura, N. and Nagata, N. (1975). *Endocrinol.* **97**, 1288.
Kang, A. H., Igarashi, S. and Gross, J. (1969a). *Biochemistry* **8**, 3200.
Kang, A. H., Piez, K. A. and Gross, J. (1969b). *Biochemistry* **8**, 1506.
Katz, E. P. and Li, S. T. (1973). *J. Mol. Biol.* **80**, 1.
Keeley, F. W. and Partridge, S. M. (1974). *Athero* **19**, 287.
Kefalides, N. A. (1973). *Inter. Rev. Connec. Tiss. Res.* **6**, 63.
Kivirikko, K. I. (1970). *Inter. Rev. Connec. Tiss. Res.* **5**, 93.

Kivirikko, K. I. and Risteli, L. (1976). *Medical Biology* **54**, 159.
Kuettner, K. E., Sorgente, N., Eisenstein, R., Pita, J. C. and Howell, D. S. (1975). *Protides of the Biological Fluids* **22**, 437.
Kunin, A. S. and Krane, S. M. (1965). *Endocrinol.* **76**, 343.
Lane, J. M. and Miller, E. J. (1969). *Biochemistry* **8**, 2134.
Larsson, S. E., Ray, R. D. and Kuettner, K. E. (1973). *Calc. Tiss. Res.* **13**, 271.
Lawson, D. E. M., Wilson, P. W., Kodicek, E. (1969). *Biochem. J.* **115**, 269.
Lawson, D. E. M., Pelc, B., Bell, P. A., Wilson, P. W. and Kodicek, E. (1971). *Biochem. J.* **121**, 673.
Lawson, D. E. M., Charman, M., Wilson, P. W. and Edelstein, S. (1976). *Biochim. Biophys. Acta* **437**, 403.
Leaver, A. G. (1969). *Arch. Oral Biol.* **14**, 503.
Leaver, A. G. and Shuttleworth, A. (1968). *Arch. Oral. Biol.* **13**, 509.
Leaver, A. G., Triffitt, J. T. and Holbrook, I. B. (1975). *Clin. Orth. Rel. Res.* **110**, 269.
Likins, R. C., Piez, K. A. and Kunde, M. L. (1960). *In* 'Calcification in Biological Systems' (Ed. Sognnaes, R. F.) p. 143. Amer. Assn. Adv. Science, Washington.
Lindenbaum, A. and Kuettner, K. E. (1967). *Calc. Tiss. Res.* **1**, 153.
Lohmander, S. and Hjerpe, A. (1975). *Biochim. Biophys. Acta* **404**, 93.
Luben, R. A., Wong, G. L. and Chon, D. J. (1976). *Endocrinol.* **99**, 526.
McCullagh, K. G., Derouette, S. and Robert, L. (1973). *Exp. Mol. Path.* **18**, 202.
Mechanic, G. L., Toverud, S. U. and Ramp, W. K. (1972). *Biochem. Biophys. Res. Commun.* **47**, 760.
Mechanic, G. H., Toverud, S. U., Ramp, W. K. and Gonnerman, W. A. (1975). *Biochim. Biophys. Acta* **393**, 419.
Miller, E. J. (1971). *Biochem. Biophys. Res. Commun.* **45**, 444.
Miller, E. J. (1973). *Clin. Orth. Rel. Res.* **92**, 260.
Miller, E. J. and Robertson, P. B. (1973). *Biochem. Biophys. Res. Commun.* **54**, 432.
Miller, E. J., Martin, G. R., Piez, K. A. and Powers, M. J. (1967). *J. Biol. Chem.* **242**, 5481.
Miller, E. J., Lane, J, M. and Piez, K. A. (1969). *Biochemistry* **8**, 30.
Miller, E. J., Woodall, D. L. and Vail, M. S. (1973). *J. Biol. Chem.* **248**, 1666.
Morava, E., Tarjan, R. and Winter, M. (1973). *Experientia* **29**, 1225.
Morgan, P. H., Jacobs, H. G., Segrest, J. P. and Cunningham, L. W. (1970). *J. Biol. Chem.* **245**, 5042.
Müller, P. K., Lemmen, C., Gay, S. and Meigel, W. N. (1975). *Europ. J. Biochem.* **59**, 97.
Neville, P. F. and DeLuca, H. F. (1966). *Biochemistry* **5**, 2201.
Neuman, W. F. (1958). *Arch. Pathol.* **66**, 204.
Nicholson, W. A. P., Ashton, B. A., Höhling, H. J. and Boyde, A. (1975). *In* 'Calcium Metabolism, Bone and Metabolic Bone Diseases' (Ed. Kuhlencordt, F. and Kruse, H. P.) p. 181. Springer-Verlag, New York.
Nusgens, B., Chantraine, A. and Lapiere, C. M. (1972). *Clin. Orth. Rel. Res.* **88**, 252.
Owen, M. E. and Triffitt, J. T. (1974). *Is. J. Med. Sci.* **10**, 3.
Owen, M. E. and Triffitt, J. T. (1976). *J. Physiol.* **257**, 293.
Parsons, V., Davies, C. and Self, M. (1973). *Calc. Tiss. Res.* **12**, 47.
Paterson, C. R. and Fourman, P. (1968). *Biochem. J.* **109**, 101.
Peacock, M., Taylor, G. A. and Redel, J. (1976). *FEBS Lett.* 62, 248.
Penttinen, R. P., Lichtenstein, J. R., Martin, G. R. and McCusick, V. A. (1975). *Proc. Natl. Acad. Sci. USA* **72**, 586.

Piez, K. A. and Likins, R. C. (1960). *In* 'Calcification in Biological Systems' (Ed. Sognnaes, R. F.) p. 411. Amer. Assn. Adv. Science, Washington.
Pinnell, S. R., Fox, R. and Krane, S. M. (1971). *Biochim. Biophys. Acta* **229**, 119.
Price, P. A., Otsuka, A. S., Poser, J. W., Kristaponis, J. and Raman, N. (1976). *Proc. Natl. Acad. Sci. USA* **73**, 1447.
Prockop, D. J., Berg, R. A., Kivirikko, K. I. and Uitto, J. (1976). *In* 'Biochemistry of Collagen' (Ed. G. N. Ramachandran and A. H. Reddi) p. 163. Plenum Press, New York and London.
Pugliarello, M. C., Vittur, F., de Bernard, B., Bonucci, E. and Ascenzi, A. (1970). *Calc. Tiss. Res.* **5**, 108.
Raisz, L. and Niemann, I. (1969). *Endocrinol.* **85**, 446.
Rasmussen, H. and Bordier, P. (1974). *In* 'The Physiological and Cellular Basis of Metabolic Bone Disease', p. 243. Williams and Wilkins Co., Baltimore.
Rasmussen, H., DeLuca, H. F., Arnaud, C., Hawker, C. and von Stedingk, M. (1963). *J. Clin. Invest.* **42**, 1940.
Rasmussen, H., Arnaud, C. and Hawker, C. (1964). *Science* **144**, 1019.
Rasmussen, H., Pechet, M. and Fast, D. (1968). *J. Clin. Invest.* **47**, 1843.
Reddi, A. H. (1976). *In* 'Biochemistry of Collagen' (Ed. G. N. Ramachandran and A. H. Reddi) p. 449. Plenum Press, New York and London.
Reynolds, J. J. (1974). *Biochem. Soc. Spec. Publ.* **3**, 91.
Reynolds, J. J., Pavlovitch, H. and Balson, S. (1976). *Calc. Tiss. Res.* **21**, 207.
Robert, B., Szigeti, M., Derouette, J. C., Robert, L., Bouisson, H. and Fabre, M. T. (1971). *Europ. J. Biochem.* **21**, 507.
Robins, S. P. and Bailey, A. J. (1975). *Biochem. J.* **149**, 381.
Ross, R. and Bornstein, P. (1969). *J. Cell. Biol.* **40**, 366.
Royce, P. M. and Barnes, M. J. (1977). *Biochim. Biophys. Acta* **498**, 132.
Russell, J. E. and Avioli, L. V. (1975). *J. Clin. Invest.* **56**, 792.
Ryhanen, L. (1976). *Biochim. Biophys. Acta* **438**, 71.
Schofield, J. D., Freeman, I. L. and Jackson, D. S. (1971). *Biochem. J.* **124**, 467.
Segrest, J. P. and Cunningham, L. W. (1970). *J. Clin. Invest.* **49**, 1497.
Seyer, J. M., Brickley, D. M. and Glimcher, M. J. (1974). *Calc. Tiss. Res.* **17**, 25.
Shetlar, M. R., Hern, D. and Chien, S. F. (1972). *Texas, Rep. Biol. Med.* **30**, 339.
Shipley, P. G., Kramer, B. and Howland, J. (1926). *Biochem. J.* **35**, 304.
Shipp, D. W. and Bowness, J. M. (1975). *Biochim. Biophys. Acta* **379**, 282.
Shuttleworth, A. and Veis, A. (1972). *Biochim. Biophys. Acta* **257**, 414.
Siegel, R. C., Tsai, H. C. and Morris, R. C. (1975). *Clin. Res.* **23**, 136.
Simmons, D. J. and Kunin, A.S. (1971). *Is. J. Med. Sci.* **7**, 412.
Spector, A. R. and Glimcher, M. J. (1972). *Biochem. Biophys. Acta* **263**, 593.
Spiro, R. G. (1969). *J. Biol. Chem.* **244**, 602.
Spiro, R. G. (1970). *In* 'Chemistry and Molecular Biology of the Intercellular Matrix' (Ed. E. A. Balazs) p. 195. Academic Press, London and New York.
Steven, F. S. (1967). *Biochim. Biophys. Acta* **140**, 522.
Stern, P. H., Trummel, C. L., Schnoes, H. K. and DeLuca, H. F. (1975). *Endocrinol.* **97**, 1552.
Stoltz, M., Furthmayr, H. and Timpl, R. (1973). *Biochim. Biophys. Acta* **310**, 461.
Tanaka, Y. and DeLuca, H. F. (1971). *Arch. Biochem. Biophys.* **146**, 574.
Tanaka, Y. and DeLuca, H. F. (1973). *Arch. Biochem. Biophys.* **154**, 566.
Tanzer, M. L. (1973). *Science* **180**, 561.
Tanzer, M. L. (1976). *In* 'Biochemistry of Collagen' (Ed. G. N. Ramachandran and A. H. Reddi) p. 137. Plenum Press, New York and London.

Tashjian, A. H., Ontjes, D. A., Goodfriend, T. L. (1964). *Biochem. Biophys. Res. Commun.* **16**, 209.
Thompson, E. R., Baylink, D. J. and Wergedal, J. E. (1975). *Endocrinol.* **97**, 283.
Toole, B. P., Kang, A. H., Trelstad, R. L. and Gross, J. (1972). *Biochem. J.* **127**, 715.
Trelstad, R. L., Rubin, D. F. and Gross, J. (1977). *Lab. Invest.* **36**, 501.
Triffit, J. T. and Owen, M. E. (1973). *Biochem. J.* **136**, 125.
Urist, M. R., Earnest, F., Kimball, K. M., DiJulio, T. P. and Iwata, H. (1974). *Calc. Tiss. Res.* **15**, 269.
Urry, D. W. (1971). *Proc. Natl. Acad. Sci. USA* **68**, 810.
Veis, A. and Perry, A. (1967). *Biochemistry* **6**, 2409.
Veis, A., Spector, A. R. and Zamoscianyk, H. (1972). *Biochim. Biophys. Acta* **257**, 404.
Vittur, F., Pugliarello, M. C. and de Bernard, B. (1971). *Experientia* **27**, 126.
Vittur, F., Pugliarello, M. C. and de Bernard, B. (1972a). *Biochim. Biophys. Acta* **257**, 389.
Vittur, F., Pugliarello, M. C. and de Bernard, B. (1972b). *Biochem. Biophys. Res. Commun.* **48**, 143.
Vittur, F. and de Bernard, B. (1973). *FEBS Lett.* **38**, 87.
Vogel, J. J. and Boyan-Salyers, B. D. (1976). *Clin. Orth. Rel. Res.* **118**, 230.
Volpin, D. and Veis, A. (1973). *Biochemistry* **12**, 1452.
Wasserman, R. H. and Taylor, A. N. (1973). *J. Nutr.* **103**, 586.
Weber, J. C., Pons, V. and Kodicek, E. (1971). *Biochem. J.* **125**, 147.
Weinstock, A., Weinstock, M. and Leblond, C. P. (1972). *Calc. Tiss. Res.* **8**, 181.
Weinstock, M. and Leblond, C. P. (1973). *J. Cell. Biol.* **56**, 838.
Wells, H. and Lloyd, W. (1969). *Endocrinol.* **84**, 861.
Wezeman, F. H. (1976). *Science* **194**, 1069.
Williams, P. A. and Peacocke, A. R. (1967) *Biochem. J.* **105**, 1177.
Wong, R. G., Myrtle, J. F., Tsai, H. C. and Norman, A. W. (1972). *J. Biol. Chem.* **247**, 5728.
Wuthier, R. E. (1968). *J. Lipid. Res.* **9**, 68.
Wuthier, R. E. (1969). *Calc. Tiss. Res.* **4**, 20.
Wuthier, R. E. (1971a). *Calc. Tiss. Res.* **8**, 24.
Wuthier, R. E. (1971b). *Calc. Tiss. Res.* **8**, 36.
Wuthier, R. E. (1976). *Fed. Proc.* **35**, 117.
Yoshiki, S., Yanagisawa, T., Suda, T. and Sasaki, S. (1974). *Calc. Tiss. Res.* **15**, 295.
Zamoscianyk, H. and Veis, A. (1966). *Fed. Proc.* **25**, 409.

8 Physiological Aspects of Vitamin D Metabolism in Man

S. W. STANBURY AND E. B. MAWER

I Introduction

A VITAMIN D-DEFICIENCY AND VITAMIN D REQUIREMENT IN MAN

There is still no objective means of measuring, or even of defining precisely, what is meant by 'vitamin D-deficiency' in man. Its effects, in terms of the development of defective skeletal mineralisation, occur late after withdrawal of the sources of the native vitamin; and its clinical consequences in children, the development of rickets, may be critically dependent on the rate of growth of the individual. The accompanying biochemical effects of vitamin D deficiency may be detectable before clinical consequences are obvious; but the changes in serum calcium, orthophosphate and alkaline phosphatase characteristic of vitamin D-deficiency; changes in the urinary output of hydroxyproline; and even the characteristic intestinal malabsorption of calcium can all result from the operation of factors quite independent of vitamin D.

One encounters a similar difficulty with respect to the human 'requirement' for vitamin D, both in its definition in physiological terms and also in its objective measurement. It has been stated in general terms that 'the amount of vitamin D required by any human being is the amount needed to permit normal growth and mineralisation of the bones and teeth during infancy and childhood and to maintain these structures during later life, as well as to meet the increased demands of infection, pregnancy and lactation' (Kramer and Gribetz, 1971). When this generalisation is applied to a specific situation, such as the needs of the infant, it is to be appreciated that the estimated daily requirement of 10 μg is derived indirectly, as the amount of orally administered ergocalciferol adequate to prevent the development of rickets among children living in urban communities at northern latitudes; and also as a generous estimate of the daily oral dose effective in curing privational rickets. In all animal species, the degree of exposure to sunlight is the most important single factor determining the need for vitamin D in the diet (Jones, 1971); and as in animals, the human infant can obtain his total requirement from adequate exposure to sun or even to sky-shine. The estimated lesser requirement of the adult of 2.5 μg/day (Dent and Smith, 1969) may represent a true physiological difference from the infant but this cannot be regarded as established. It may simply mean that the adult meets most of his requirements from casual exposure to sunlight. In vitamin D-deficiency developing in adults as a complication of gastric surgery, a parenteral dose no greater than 2.5 μg per day is probably sufficient to cure the resulting osteomalacia (Morgan *et al.*, 1965); it is not known if privational rickets in infants would respond to the same parental dosage. It is not yet possible to measure the rate of production of cholecalciferol in the skin nor to estimate the fraction of the daily requirement derived from this endogenous source under different conditions of living or at different ages of life. From separate measurements of 25-hydroxyergocalciferol and 25-hydroxycholecalciferol in the serum, it appears that cutaneous synthesis is a quantitatively more important source in the adult than is the diet (Haddad and Hahn, 1973). The same conclusion is indicated by observations made on nuclear submariners excluded from sunlight (Preece *et al.*, 1974, 1975). As yet, there appear to have been no measurements of the two forms of 25-hydroxycalciferol in the serum of infants. Since infant feeds are supplemented with ergocalciferol, it might well prove possible to demonstrate that the artificially fed infant is principally dependent on this dietary source unless he is deliberately exposed to sunlight. Until it becomes possible to measure the total mass of cholecalciferol produced endogenously in the skin, and delivered into the circulating blood, it will remain impossible to define the human requirement with confidence; and equally difficult to assess the significance of the supposed increase of requirement caused by prematurity, infancy and rapid growth, possible genetical factors including sex (Childs *et al.*, 1962), pregnancy and advancing age.

A more direct assessment of the state of vitamin D nutrition should be provided by accurate measurement of one or other vitamin D sterol in some accessible body fluid or tissue. If a limiting lower concentration of that sterol could be equated with physiological deficiency of vitamin D, 'requirement' might be defined alternatively as the total amount of calciferol derived from all sources sufficient to sustain that concentration. It has been established that the bioassayed total antiricketic activity in the serum (Lumb *et al.*, 1971) and also the serum concentration of 25-hydroxycalciferol (Haddad and Stamp, 1974) increase in proportion to the oral intake of calciferol but such undoubtedly valid relationships were established by the inclusion of data from subjects receiving massive therapeutic dosage. The methods at present available are probably insufficiently sensitive to detect small differences in serum concentration such as might be produced by intakes between 2.5 and 10 μg per day – that is, in the range of the estimates of daily requirement. It is also evident that the total amount of 'vitamin D' in body fat and muscle may greatly exceed the total in the circulation, whether this is assayed as total antiricketic activity or as calciferol and 25-hydroxycalciferol separately (Mawer *et al.*, 1971b, 1972), and the factors determining equilibrium between the circulating pool and tissue pools or stores are unknown. None the less, measurement of serum 25-hydroxycalciferol is currently the best available index of the state of vitamin D nutrition in man. Sufficient data have been accumulated by different groups of investigators to define levels of serum 25-hydroxycalciferol at which it is reasonable to consider an individual 'insufficient' of vitamin D, and it has also been clearly demonstrated that the serum 25-hydroxycalciferol is exquisitively sensitive to variation of solar exposure (Stamp and Round, 1974; Preece *et al.*, 1973, 1974; P. de Silva and C. M. Taylor, private communication). It is, however, premature to assume that any absolute level of 25-hydroxycalciferol represents physiological deficiency in a particular individual or a particular population. Among a group of individuals acknowledged to be poorly nourished with respect to vitamin D, such as the immigrant Asian population in Britain (Holmes *et al.*, 1973), the presence of the clinical effects of physiological deficiency cannot be related predictably to the prevailing level of serum 25-hydroxycalciferol (Stanbury *et al.*, 1975b). Thus the serum 25-hydroxycalciferol provides a measure of the plane of vitamin D nutrition under ordinary conditions of life but it is unreliable as an index of relative deficiency. There are also clinical circumstances, such as massive therapeutic dosage with calciferol in the remote past, in which the serum 25-hydroxycalciferol will provide a completely erroneous reflection of the total body content of 'vitamin D' (Mawer *et al.*, 1972).

The promotion of vitamin D from the status of 'bastard nutrient born of social and economic conditions' (Stanbury, 1973) to its present accepted function as steroid hormone (Kodicek, 1974) promises the prospect of a rational resolution of these difficulties. Deficiency of 'vitamin D' can now be considered in physiological rather than nutritional terms, in relation to the availability of the hormonal effector, 1,25-dihydroxycholecalciferol; and the regulated renal synthesis of this metabolite implies that a physiological deficiency of the hormone could co-exist with a surplus of the pro-hormonal forms, cholecalciferol and 25-hydroxycholecalciferol. Similarly, deficiency at pro-hormonal level would imply an insufficiency of substrate from which to produce the currently required quantity of 1,25-dihydroxycholecalciferol. Such pro-hormonal deficiency may ultimately prove to be measurable in terms of the concentration of 25-hydroxycalciferol in the serum; but the larger extravascular pools of calciferol (Mawer *et al.*, 1972) may be capable of sustaining serum levels of 25-hydroxycalciferol which, even if very low, might still prove adequate for the synthesis of the requisite picomolar quantities of 1,25-dihydroxycalciferol. Methods are becoming available for the measurement of 1,25-dihydroxycalciferol in human serum (Section IIB) although they are, as yet, relatively insensitive. The future accurate measurement of 1,25-dihydroxycalciferol in the serum may provide a closer approach to the clinical delineation of physiological deficiency but there are reasons why even this may prove inadequate. In the first place, the relevant measure of a sufficiency of 1,25-dihydroxycalciferol will be its concentration in the target organs – intestinal mucosa, bone and perhaps kidney – rather than in the blood. As is discussed in chapter 9, Section IA, there is already evidence to suggest that the hormone is selectively concentrated from the circulating plasma into its target sites. Unless there were some proportionate relationship between the concentrations of 1,25-dihydroxycalciferol in target cells and plasma in the steady state, a single measurement of this hormone in serum might prove no more informative than the serum 25-hydroxycalciferol. However, the few measurements made to date, the results of radioiotopic studies of 25-hydroxycholecalciferol metabolism and, above all, the accumulated experience with other steroid hormones suggest that *clinically* useful information should be provided by such measurements. Whether a single measurement of 1,25-dihydroxycalciferol in serum (or even in the intestinal mucosa, if this were readily feasible) would provide physiologically significant information might well depend on whether the hormone is ultimately proved to have a permissive or direct regulatory role in the control of calcium transport. If its function is permissive, 'repletion' with vitamin D might simply imply saturation with 1,25-dihydroxycholecalciferol of the specific nuclear receptors in the target organs; and the concentration of this hormone could simultaneously indicate the degree of saturation and the degree of 'physiological deficiency'. If 1,25-dihydroxycholecalciferol has a direct regulatory control of calcium absorption, as is currently widely assumed on what we consider totally inadequate evidence, the situation will be much more difficult of interpretation. This view implies that 1,25-dihydroxycholecalciferol is produced in regulated amounts, according to prevailing requirements for calcium, and that this renal hormone determines *directly* the quantitative amount of calcium absorbed. In such circumstances, a single measurement of the concentration of the hormone – even if this were made in the target tissue – could be interpreted only in the light of prevailing physiological conditions; and, if those conditions were as imponderable as 'the prevailing requirements for calcium', precise interpretation might be impossible. This situation would necessitate application of the dynamic approach to assessment of hormonal function, as has been extensively exploited in conventional endocrinology. It is shown subsequently (Section IVA) that the quantitative production in man of labelled 1,25-dihydroxycholecalciferol from a pulse dose of radioactive cholecalciferol is related inversely to the prevailing 'state of vitamin D nutrition' as measured by the serum 25-hydroxycalciferol. This phenomenon, with the suggested implication of a closed loop system and negative feedback control, exemplifies the potential applicability of the dynamic approach. It will doubtless be possible and indeed necessary to devise other means of exploring these control systems.

Thus, although its ultimate effects are reasonably fully understood, there is still room for debate as to how vitamin D-deficiency should be defined. In attempting to ascertain the quantitative amounts of the pro-hormonal sterols needed to ensure adequate functioning of the endocrine system ('the requirement'), the nutritionist is frustrated by his inability to measure the contribution of the cutaneous endocrine gland. The endocrinological approach is at an embryonic stage; requisite methods for the simple and accurate measurement of the two pro-hormones and the effector hormone are not yet available; nor is it known how such measurements should best be exploited when methods do become available. In human studies of vitamin D metabolism in Manchester, an attempt has been made to utilise the techniques of both the nutritionist and the experimentalist. Applying the approach of the experimental physiologist and biochemist, radioisotopic studies have been restricted mainly to subjects 'relatively deficient of vitamin D'. Since the latter state can be defined only in crude and approximate terms (*vide supra*), it is impossible to ensure the degree of vitamin D-depletion attainable in the rat or chick. There is, however, no alternative method currently available to study the endocrinology of vitamin D in man. It is considered that significant and valid results have been obtained but the conclusions tentatively reached will require confirmatory studies as alternative techniques evolve. It has also been conclusively demonstrated that radioisotopic studies in individuals replete or surfeited with vitamin D provide little more than a demonstration of the existence of extensive body pools of the vitamin D sterols (Mawer *et al.*, 1971b, 1972; Stanbury *et al.*, 1972).

II Methods for the Study of Calciferol Metabolism in Man

A BIOLOGICAL ASSAY

Prior to the introduction of radioactive preparations of cholecalciferol in the 1960s, estimation of vitamin D activity in biological fluids and tissues was dependent on biological assay (Bills, 1947). In man, almost all such measurements were made on samples of serum or plasma (Warkany, 1936; Warkany and Mabon, 1940; Thomas *et al.*, 1959; Illig *et al.* 1961; Haddock and Vasquez, 1966) but estimations were also made directly on tissues or lipid extracts of tissues (Windorfer, 1938; Lumb *et al.*, 1971). The error of all available bioassays is wide and they measure the combined biological activity attributable to the native vitamins (cholecalciferol and ergocalciferol) and their 25-hydroxylated derivatives. None the less, when coupled with a prior chromatographic separation, the biological assay can yield useful information on the relative concentrations of calciferol and its 25-hydroxy-metabolite (Lumb *et al.*, 1971; Mawer *et al.*, 1971b, 1972). As a means of assessing the plane of vitamin D nutrition, the biological assay has been largely superceded by the competitive protein-binding assay for 25-hydroxycalciferol (Section IIB, 1) but no alternative satisfactory method for the measurement of unchanged calciferol has yet been described.

The technique of chromatographic separation has been extended to develop a biological assay for 1,25-dihydroxycalciferol (Hill *et al.*, 1974, 1975). Lipid extracts of serum (or intestinal mucosa) are chromatographed on columns of Sephadex LH20 to separate the fraction containing 1,25-dihydroxycalciferol, which is administered orally to vitamin D-deficient rats. Response is measured in terms of intestinal calcium transport using sacs of everted duodenum *in vitro*. The equivalent of 10–20 ml of serum is required for each assay rat, which limits the application of the method in clinical practice. It is to be noted that the chromatographic fraction used for the assay also includes 25,26-

dihydroxycalciferol but this is believed to make a negligible contribution to the activity measured.

The lack of any well-defined physiological functions for 24,25- and 25,26-dihydroxycholecalciferol makes it unlikely that these metabolites will prove amenable to biological assay.

B COMPETITIVE PROTEIN BINDING ASSAYS

1. *25-Hydroxycalciferol.* Several laboratories have published methods for estimating 25-hydroxycalciferol in human plasma or serum (Haddad and Chyu, 1971; Belsey *et al.*, 1971; Bayard *et al.*, 1972; Edelstein *et al.*, 1974); these methods all rely on preparative chromatography to separate 25-hydroxycalciferol from calciferol by means of columns of silicic acid or lipophilic Sephadex or by thin layer plates. The source of the 25-hydroxycalciferol binding protein has usually been the plasma or kidney cytosol of vitamin D-deficient rats although Bayard *et al.* (1972) used human plasma. These proteins bind 25-hydroxycholecalciferol and 25-hydroxyergocalciferol to approximately the same extent and distinction between the two forms can be made only by using a system of preparative chromatography that separates them (Haddad and Hahn, 1973). It is possible that the reported difference in affinity of the 25-hydroxylated derivatives of ergo- and cholecalciferol for receptors in the chick might form the basis of an alternative differential assay. Approximately 15 times more 25-hydroxyergocalciferol than 25-hydroxycholecalciferol is required to cause 50% displacement of ^{3}H 25-hydroxycholecalciferol from chick plasma (Belsey *et al.*, 1974a); results showing the same order of difference have been obtained for chick kidney cytosol (Greenberg *et al.*, 1974). Most values so far reported refer to the total 25-hydroxycalciferol in plasma or serum.

An assay for plasma 25-hydroxycalciferol without preparative chromatography has recently been described (Belsey *et al.*, 1974b). The mean value for normal volunteers (35.2 ± 31.1 (SD) ng/ml) was higher than those reported from the U.S.A. by Haddad and Chyu (1971) and Haddad *et al.*, (1973). Repeated assay of the same samples after conventional chromatography reduced the mean value only slightly (33.3 ± 13.9 ng/ml) but a direct comparison of individual values obtained by the two methods was not provided. It is claimed that under the rapid conditions of the assay even large amounts of calciferol do not interfere but this claim must be treated with reserve. In patients receiving 1.25 to 2.5 mg/day of calciferol, Belsey *et al.*, (1974b) obtained values for serum 25-hydroxycalciferol (500–3200 ng/ml) that were much higher than those (120–300 ng/ml) obtained by Haddad and Chyu (1971) in patients on similar dosage. Using the line test to assay the total antiricketic activity in serum, Lumb *et al.* (1971) obtained a mean value of approximately 10 i.u./ml and an upper limit of 70 i.u./ml ($\simeq$250–1750 ng/ml) for patients taking 2.5 mg/day of ergocalciferol – it is probable that at least half this assayed activity was attributable to unchanged calciferol (Mawer *et al.*, 1971b). It thus seems possible that the method of Belsey *et al.* (1974b) may measure both calciferol and its 25-hydroxy-metabolite when the intake of calciferol is high. It is particularly desirable that this simple method should not be taken into widespread use without its further validation.

2. *Calciferol.* When reporting their technique for the determination of 25-hydroxycalciferol Belsey *et al.* (1971) claimed that the method could be adapted to the separate measurement of calciferol in plasma. The load of other lipids, notably cholesterol, that appears in the same chromatographic position as the calciferols caused problems with solubility and phase separation which necessitated an incubation period of 10 days to achieve equilibration. This method does not appear to have received any significant practical exploitation and, in our hands, has failed to provide reproducible results.

3. *1,25-Dihydroxycalciferol.* A binding assay has been described for 1,25-dihydroxycalciferol using a cytosol-chromatin receptor preparation isolated from chick intestinal mucosa (Brumbaugh *et al.*, 1974a, b); 20 ml of plasma is required for a single determination but this volume could probably be reduced with the availability of radio-isotopically labelled reagents of higher specific activity. The preparation of samples by repeated chromatography is laborious and difficult but the Tucson workers have demonstrated that the method is applicable to clinical studies.

4. *24,25-Dihydroxycalciferol.* An assay for this metabolite has also been developed using the binding protein for calciferol metabolites in ricketic rat kidneys (Taylor *et al.*, 1976). Since this protein also binds all 25-hydroxylated metabolites of calciferol it is necessary to isolate the 24,25-dihydroxycalciferol from the other metabolites in the plasma lipids by a chromatographic step. The plasma concentration of 24,25-dihydroxycalciferol in seven normal subjects was 1.68 ± 0.82 ng/ml with a range of 0.92–3.28. The plasma 25-hydroxycalciferol levels in these subjects ranged from 8.8–35.7 ng/ml.

C RADIOISOTOPIC METHODS FOR THE METABOLISM OF VITAMIN D

Because of the many difficulties involved in measuring unlabelled calciferol and its metabolites, most investigations of vitamin D metabolism in man have involved the use of radioisotopic preparations (Avioli *et al.*, 1967; Gray *et al.*, 1974; Mawer *et al.*, 1969, 1971a, b, 1972, 1973, 1975; Thompson *et al.*, 1966). This is likely to continue as the technique of choice until sensitive and specific methods for individual sterols, probably involving radioim-

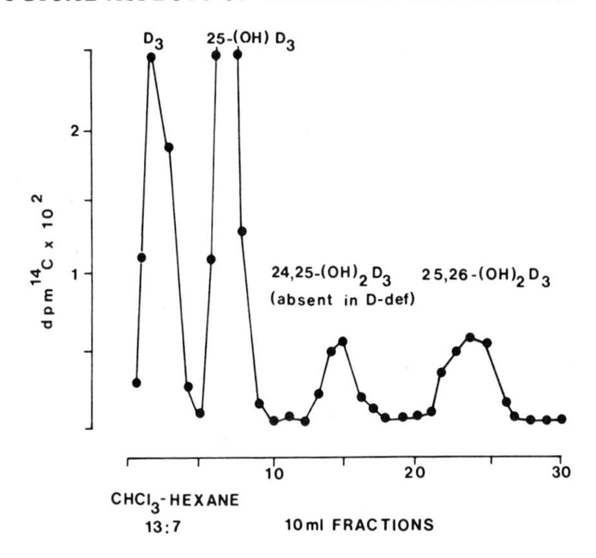

Fig. 1. Sephadex LH 20 chromatographic profile of a lipid extract of serum from a normal subject 24 h after injection of 25 μg (10 μCi) [^{3}H-^{14}C]vitamin D. The ordinate represents the dpm ^{14}C in each 10 ml fraction. (The profile obtained in a vitamin D-deficient subject would show no peak for 24,25-$(OH)_2D_3$, and any 1,25-$(OH)_2D_3$ present would co-chromatograph with 25,26-$(OH)_2D_3$)

munoassay, become available. A single pulse dose of labelled cholecalciferol is given orally or intravenously; in our laboratory the pulse is given intravenously after dispersion in a synthetic stabilised lipid emulsion. Timed serial samples of blood are taken and the concentrations of labelled cholecalciferol and its metabolites are determined after chromatography of lipid extracts of serum on columns of silicic acid (Mawer and Backhouse, 1969; Mawer *et al.*, 1971b) or Sephadex LH20 (Taylor *et al.*, 1973; Fig. 1). This permits monitoring of the rate of disappearance of cholecalciferol from the circulation, as well as the appearance in plasma and subsequent decay of individual metabolites. This technique has been used in attempts to define metabolic abnormalities in a variety of pathological conditions (chapter 9).

The combination of the protein binding assay for 25-hydroxycalciferol and pulse labelling studies has made possible calculation of the specific activity of serum 25-hydroxycalciferol and hence the derivation of an estimate of the molar concentrations of the dihydroxylated metabolites in the serum (Gray *et al.*, 1974; Mawer *et al.*, 1975; Stanbury *et al.*, 1975a; Norman and Henry, 1974).

There are disadvantages in the labelled pulse technique in man and a failure to appreciate its limitations effectively invalidated most early clinical studies with its use. In the first place, it provides no direct information concerning the size of body pools of unlabelled calciferol and its metabolites. The more important effect of pre-existing unlabelled pools on the actual interpretation of the radioisotopic data is discussed in greater detail subsequently (Section VA). Secondly, because of the mass of the labelled dose is relatively large and in excess of the estimates of daily requirements for calciferol (Section IA), metabolism is not necessarily studied in a steady state; that is, conditions do not meet the ideal requirements of a tracer study. The large size of the pulse dose is determined by the need to incorporate ^{14}C-labelled material when [1,2-^{3}H,4-^{14}C]-cholecalciferol is used to permit detection of 1,25-dihydroxy-cholecalciferol formation (Lawson *et al.*, 1969; Mawer *et al.*, 1971a). The alternative use of tritiated 25-hydroxycholecalciferol (Figs. 2, 3) is not suitable for the latter purpose since 1,25- and 25,26-dihydroxycholecalciferol have the same elution volume and cannot be separated by the usual Sephadex LH20 column system. The implications of this are not always fully appreciated and some workers, assigning a particular chromatographic peak to 1,25-dihydroxycholecalciferol are in fact recording the combined radioactivity attributable to this metabolite and the 25,26-dihydroxy-metabolite. This

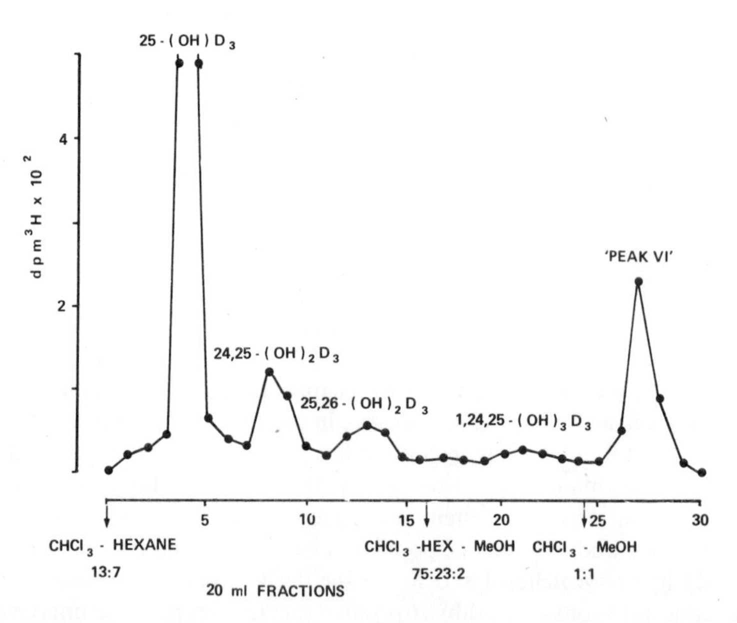

Fig. 2. Chromatographic profile (Sephadex LH 20) of a lipid extract of serum obtained 20 days after i.v. administration of 83 ng (1.5 μCi) [26-^{3}H]-25-hydroxycholecalciferol to a healthy volunteer replete with vitamin D. The ordinate represents the dpm ^{3}H in each 20 ml fraction. Since no detectable amount of radioactive 1,25-dihydroxycholecalciferol is produced in the vitamin D-replete individual (Mawer *et al.*, 1975), the peak labelled 25,26-$(OH)_2D_3$ is uncontaminated with the former metabolite (see also Fig. 3)

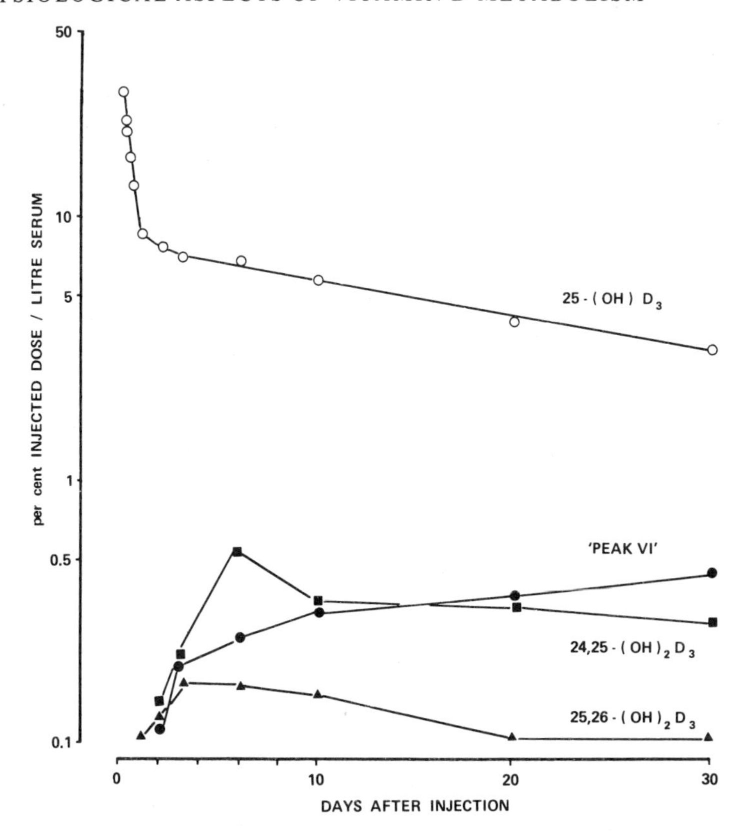

Fig. 3. The sequential changes in concentration of radioactive metabolites in the serum following i.v. administration of labelled 25-hydroxycholecalciferol (see Fig. 2)

disadvantage is most unfortunate since the high specific activity in available preparations of [26,27-^{3}H]-25-hydroxycholecalciferol makes this an otherwise attractive metabolic tracer (Schaefer *et al.*, 1971; Gray *et al.*, 1974).

III Serum (or Plasma) Concentrations of Antiricketic Activity, 25-Hydroxycalciferol and 1,25-Dihydroxycalciferol in Man

A ANTIRICKETIC ACTIVITY AND SERUM 25-HYDROXYCALCIFEROL; CONTROL DATA AND SEASONAL VARIATIONS

A mean serum antiricketic activity of 0.77 ± 0.40 i.u./ml (SD) ($\equiv 19.3 \pm 10$ ng/ml as cholecalciferol) from 26 assays in members of the staff of this department has been reported by Lumb *et al.* (1971); the mean value was higher in summer months (≡21.8 ng/ml) than in winter (≡16.5 ng/ml). It was also shown that there could be a six-fold variation of mean serum antiricketic activity in geographically different populations depending on the available sunlight and regional policies concerning vitamin D fortification of foodstuffs. From the results of radioisotopic studies and a few separate assays, it appears that most serum antiricketic activity is attributable to 25-hydroxycalciferol when the intake of vitamin D is low and that calciferol constitutes an increasing proportion of the total activity under conditions of pharmacologically high dosage (Mawer *et al.*, 1971b; and unpublished observations).

The binding assay for 25-hydroxycalciferol has been widely exploited and ranges of normal values have been reported from many sources (Table 1). Unfortunately, many of these ranges have been established using hospital or laboratory personnel and such subjects are not necessarily representative of the range of age, race and socioeconomic factors found in the population at large (chapter 9, Section IVC). Such possibly weighted normal values have been described for Americans; 27.3 ± 11.8[1] mean $\pm$SD. range 11–55 (Haddad and Chyu, 1971); 18.7, range 11–35 (Haddad *et al.*, 1973); 23.6 ± 6.4 (children aged 4–14 years, Hahn *et al.*, 1975); and for Europeans, 15.2 ± 5.6 (Edelstein *et al.*, 1974); 15.4 ± 6.1 (Stamp *et al.*, 1972); 28.8 ± 15.2 range 9–60 in summer and autumn, 16.2 ± 6, range 6–28 in spring (Mawer *et al.*, 1975); 16.5 ± 3.6 range 5–38 in school children (Goel *et al.*, 1976).

When deliberately sought, seasonal variations in serum 25-hydroxycalciferol have always been found, the values obtained in the late summer and autumn being higher than those samples taken during the winter and spring months (Stamp and Round, 1974; McLaughlin *et al.*, 1974; Gupta *et al.*, 1974; Mawer *et al.*, 1975).

B SERUM 1,25-DIHYDROXYCHOLECALCIFEROL

In the first report on the application of a binding assay for 1,25-dihydroxycholecalciferol, Brumbaugh *et al.* (1974a, b) found a mean of 62 ± 9 pg/ml for the serum concentration in 20 normal control subjects; the mean in 5 patients with renal disease was 25 ± 5 pg/ml. Almost identical results (52 ± 30 pg/ml) have been obtained in 8 healthy subjects in our laboratory using the biological assay (Hill *et al.*, 1974). The similarity of the results obtained in the two laboratories is striking in view of the fundamental difference in the assay methods used. Further confirmation of the assayed range of the hormone concentration has been obtained by calculation of the specific activity of the

[1] In accord with current clinical practice, 25-hydroxycalciferol levels are expressed as ng/ml of plasma (or serum).

Table 1. Serum 25-hydroxycalciferol levels in various clinical states

	Stamp *et al.* (1972) (London, UK)	Hahn *et al.* (1972) (Missouri, USA)	de Silva and Taylor (1975) (Manchester, UK)	Hahn *et al.* (1975) (Missouri, USA)	Hepner *et al.* (1975) (Pennsylvania, USA)
Controls	15.3 ± 6.1 (19) staff 16.3 ± 5.5 (12) schoolboys	20.5 ± 6.2 (38)	28.8 ± 15.2 (17) staff, summer 16.2 ± 6.2 (17) staff, winter 8.6 ± 4.7 (18) antenatal patients	23.6 ± 6.4 (51) pediatric outpatients	29.9 ± 9.9 (?) 'controls'
Treated epileptics	4.8 ± 2.7 (11) multiple drugs	12.8 ± 5.5 (48) phenobarbitone and phenytoin 15.2 ± 4.0 (13) phenobarbitone or phenytoin	5.8 ± 1.9 (6) overt osteomalacia	13.1 ± 4.7 (22) phenobarbitone and phenytoin	—
Asian osteomalacia	—	—	3.4 ± 0.7 (12)	—	—
D-deficiency osteomalacia	—	—	3.6 ± 1.3 (10)	—	—
Alcoholics	—	—	—	—	31.1 ± 11.7 (12)
Cirrhotics	—	—	—	—	18.2 ± 11.2 (26)

All values are given as mean ± SD. Figures in parenthesis are the numbers of individuals examined.

precursor 25-hydroxycalciferol in experiments involving the use of radioactive cholecalciferol. In subjects sufficiently vitamin D-deficient to permit detection of labelled 1,25-dihydroxycholecalciferol formation, its estimated concentration in serum was in the range 18–74 pg/ml (Stanbury *et al.*, 1975a; Mawer *et al.*, 1975). Recently 1,25-dihydroxycholecalciferol levels as measured by the binding assay have been reported as 33 pg/ml (range 21–45) in 78 normal subjects in whom 25-hydroxycalciferol levels were assayed as 25–40 ng/ml. The binding assay distinguishes between 1,25-dihydroxy- ergo-and cholecalciferol. In normal American subjects the ergocalciferol derived form was undetectable. Only in patients receiving large doses of ergocalciferol could the dihydroxylated metabolite be found (Hughes *et al.*, 1976).

C EFFECTS OF VITAMIN D INTAKE AND OF EXPOSURE TO ULTRAVIOLET IRRADIATION ON SERUM LEVELS OF 25-HYDROXYCALCIFEROL

Since man can utilise both cholecalciferol and ergocalciferol, the circulating pool of 25-hydroxycalciferol will consist of a mixture of 25-hydroxychole- and 25-hydroxyergo-calciferol reflecting the availability of the two native vitamins. Ergocalciferol is derived solely from the diet, cholecalciferol principally from the results of cutaneous irradiation and partly from the diet.

Low values of 25-hydroxycalciferol have been reported for patients with rickets or osteomalacia of privational or malabsorptive origin. Bayard *et al.* (1972) in France record values of 2–7 ng/ml and P. de Silva and C. M. Taylor (private communication) in England values of 1–6 ng/ml in such patients. In patients with biliary obstruction in the USA, Haddad and Chyu (1971) observed a range of 3–9 ng/ml. Although it can be assumed *a priori* that inadequate diet or intestinal malabsorption was of primary importance in determining these values, the very low concentration of 25-hydroxycalciferol in some of these patients implies that their illness or social conditions must also have precluded their significant exposure to sunlight.

Edelstein *et al.* (1974) observed an increase of mean serum 25-hydroxycalciferol from 15 to 36 ng/ml in four volunteers who had taken 10 μg per day of cholecalciferol for two months. Avioli and Haddad (1973) raised the serum level in a single individual from 15 to 90 ng/ml by a month's treatment with 1 mg per day of cholecalciferol. Hahn *et al.* (1972) demonstrated a significant positive linear correlation between the serum 25-hydroxycalciferol (10–36 ng/ml) and calculated intake levels of vitamin D between 0.75 and 15 μg per day; but the intake was estimated by the unreliable method of dietary recall and the scatter of data was wide. The St Louis workers have also shown a similar positive correlation in patients with hypoparathyroidism treated with doses of vitamin D between 1.25 and 2.5 mg per day; this therapy resulted in concentrations of serum 25-hydroxycalciferol between 120 and 300 ng/ml (Haddad *et al.*, 1973). Lumb *et al.* (1971) found the bioassayed total antiricketic activity of serum to be a power function of the daily vitamin D intake.

Haddad and Hahn (1973) have attempted to estimate the contribution of cutaneously synthesised cholecalciferol to the total circulating pool of 25-hydroxycalciferol by separating and assaying separately both 25-hydroxycholecalciferol and 25-hydroxyergocalciferol. In the population of their relatively sunny area of the USA (latitude 38°N) they found that 80–90 % of the total was 25-hydroxycholecalciferol. The normal ratio of the two 25-hydroxylated forms could be reversed only by treatment with relatively massive doses of ergocalciferol. In Britain, 25-hydroxyergocalciferol was undetectable in the plasma of adults but accounted for 58% of the total 25-hydroxycalciferol levels in a group of children aged 10–16 years (Preece *et al.*, 1975). In addition the seasonal variations in total 25-hydroxycalciferol already discussed are certainly a reflection of varying solar exposure; it has also been shown that a short summer vacation can produce a two- or three-fold increase in serum 25-hydroxycalciferol (P. de Silva and C. M. Taylor, private communication). Dent *et al.* (1973) have shown that the healing of rickets produced by a course of therapeutic ultraviolet irradiation was accompanied by a significant rise in serum 25-hydroxycalciferol; and Stamp (1975) has documented the very considerable rise in serum levels produced by total body irradiation to the limits of tolerance.

IV 25-Hydroxycholecalciferol

A THE FORMATION OF 25-HYDROXYCHOLECALCIFEROL IN MAN AND ITS REGULATION

Kinetic studies with the use of radioisotopically labelled cholecalciferol have provided most of the information available on the formation of 25-hydroxycholecalciferol in man; and the incorrect interpretation of radioisotopic data has also led to the promulgation of certain misconceptions regarding the formation and metabolism of 25-hydroxycholecalciferol in disease (Avioli *et al.*, 1967, 1968; Mawer *et al.*, 1971b, 1972; Stanbury *et al.*, 1972). Although the means for measuring stable 25-hydroxycalciferol in serum has been available for several years (Haddad and Chyu, 1971), there appears to have been no systematic study of the *acute* effects on the serum 25-hydroxycalciferol of a single dose of calciferol given orally or by other routes. It is not known how this response may vary with the size of dose administered nor whether pre-treatment with vitamin D modifies the response to a single pulse dose given subsequently. All these variables have been studied by the radioisotopic technique (Section 11C; Mawer *et al.*, 1971b, 1972; Stanbury *et al.*, 1973) but, as in any tracer study in which observations are limited to measurements of radioactivity alone, the interpretation of results is made difficult by the effects of dilution of the tracer and its derivatives into pre-existing body pools of vitamin D and 25-hydroxyvitamin D (Stanbury *et al.*, 1972). The rate of disappearance of injected radioactive cholecalciferol from the circulation, the rate of appearance of labelled 25-hydroxycholecalciferol, its maximum concentration in the serum and the subsequent rate of its decay from the serum are all dependent on the state of vitamin D nutrition in the subject studied (Mawer *et al.*, 1971b). The effects of vitamin D status on the serum concentration of labelled 25-hydroxycholecalciferol, 24 h after

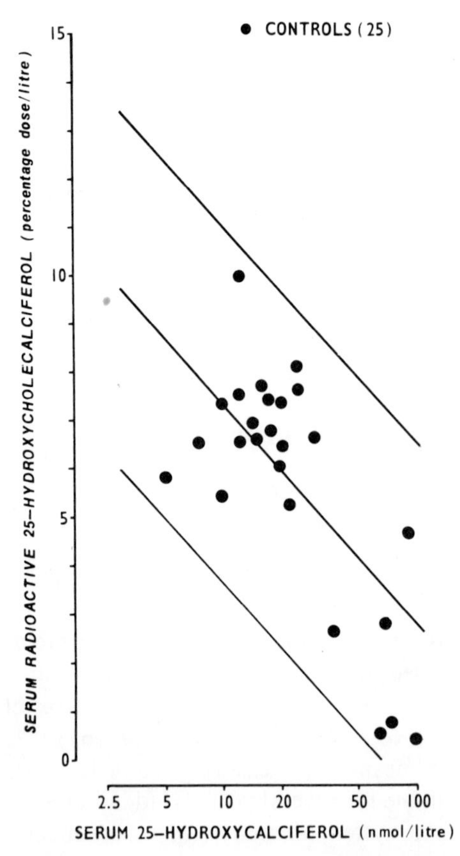

Fig. 4. The relationship between the serum concentration of unlabelled 25-hydroxycalciferol and of radioactive 25-hydroxycholecalciferol, 24 h after i.v. injection of labelled cholecalciferol

injecting radioactive cholecalciferol, are shown in Fig. 4. The highly significant negative correlation between the two variables suggests that less 25-hydroxycholecalciferol is formed the larger the body content of 25-hydroxycalciferol at the time of injection; but the relationship might represent no more than the passive consequence of pool size. Dilution of the tracer into a larger pre-existing pool of cholecalciferol would reduce the specific radioactivity of the precursor substrate and thereby determine the formation of 25-hydroxycholecalciferol of correspondingly low specific radioactivity; and dilution of the metabolically produced 25-hydroxycholecalciferol into the body pool of unlabelled metabolite would also reduce the concentration of radioactive 25-hydroxycholecalciferol in the plasma. The more rapid rate of turnover of injected cholecalciferol in vitamin D-deficient as compared with vitamin D-treated individuals (Mawer *et al.*, 1971b) suggests that the rate of formation of 25-hydroxycholecalciferol is regulated in some way by the amount of vitamin D in the body. But a complete interpretation of the relationship shown in Fig. 4 will require further observations in which serial measurements are made of the specific radioactivity of both calciferol and

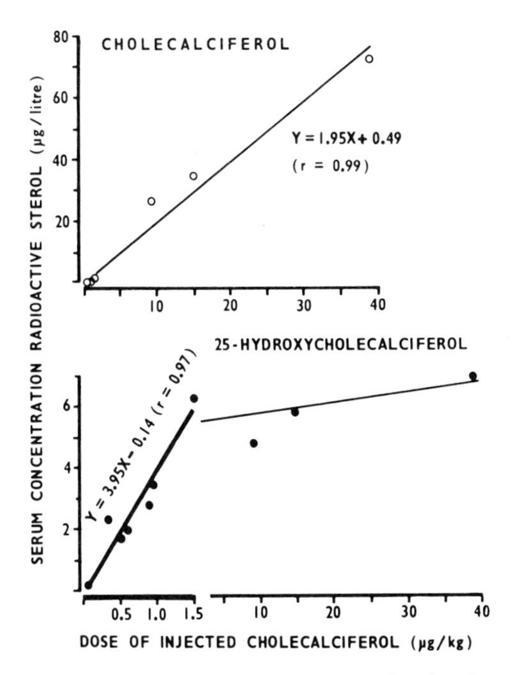

Fig. 5. The relationship between the mass of an injected pulse dose of cholecalciferol and the concentrations of cholecalciferol (above) and 25-hydroxycalciferol (below) 24 h after the injection (Mawer *et al.*, 1973). Note that each point relates to a single patient with clinically overt vitamin D-deficiency

25-hydroxycalciferol in the plasma. With present methods for measuring stable calciferol in the plasma (Section IIB, 2) this is not readily possible. In default of this, studies have been made in a group of patients with clinically overt consequences of vitamin D-deficiency, in whom it can reasonably be assumed that the body pool of vitamin D was negligible (E. B. Mawer, G. E. Mawer and S. Lucas, unpublished observations). Radioisotopically labelled cholecalciferol was injected intravenously with, in different individual patients, increasing amounts of unlabelled cholecalciferol. The relationship between the administered doses of cholecalciferol and the concentrations of radioactive cholecalciferol and radioactive 25-hydroxycholecalciferol in the serum, 24 h after the injection, are shown in Fig. 5. Throughout the whole range of dosage, the serum concentration of cholecalciferol increased in proportion to dose, to reach values approaching 80 μg/l. The serum concentration of 25-hydroxycholecalciferol also increased in a linear manner with dose but only up to a dosage of about 1.5 μg/kg (total dose 100 μg). A 20- to 25-fold increase in dose above this level produced no significant further increase in serum 25-hydroxycholecalciferol and, under these conditions of acute pulse loading, it was not possible to increase the concentration of 25-hydroxycholecalciferol above 6–8 μg/l. These observations establish that there is a finite limit to the acute production of 25-hydroxycholecalciferol by the liver and, in conjunction with the other studies already discussed (Fig. 4), they indicate that hepatic 25-hydroxylation is subject to control in some manner by the 'vitamin D' content of the body. They are analogous to the demonstration by Bhattacharyya and DeLuca (1973a) of inhibition of 25-hydroxylation in animal and *in vitro* studies; but they cannot distinguish between substrate inhibition by cholecalciferol, 'product inhibition' by 25-hydroxycholecalciferol itself and some more subtle process perhaps involving the binding capacity of the 25-hydroxylase, or of some associated carrier protein, for cholecalciferol or 25-hydroxycholecalciferol. Other observations in man make it unlikely that control of 25-hydroxylation is effected by accumulation of 25-hydroxycholecalciferol. As is discussed elsewhere (Section IVD), under conditions of high therapeutic dosage with vitamin D the concentration of 25-hydroxycalciferol in serum may reach values 100 times the limiting value encountered under conditions of acute pulse dosage (Fig. 5). The mass of 25-hydroxycalciferol produced with continued therapeutic dosage never the less represents only a minute fraction of the calciferol presented to the liver.

It is not unlikely that the relationship shown in Fig. 4 is determined partly by the influence of nutritional status on 25-hydroxylation and partly to the passive effects of dilution into body pools. The confidence limits of the regression shown are wide. This implies that any disturbance of hepatic 25-hydroxylation produced by disease would need to be gross to be detected by this technique. As shown subsequently (chapter 9, Fig. 1) data for a variety of diseases supposed to be associated with abnormal vitamin D metabolism all fall within the confidence limits.

There are a number of indications from animal experiments that the synthetic analogue, 1α-hydroxycholecalciferol must undergo 25-hydroxylation *in vivo* before acquiring its full biological potency (Reynolds *et al.*, 1974; Zerwekh *et al.*, 1974; chapter 2). A cautionary point with regard to the therapeutic use of 1α-hydroxycholecalciferol arises from the experiments of Fukushima *et al.*, (1976) on the metabolism of [2-^{3}H]1α-hydroxycholecalciferol. This group found that the only product of this analogue when perfused through rat liver was 1,25-dihydroxycholecalciferol. The hormone was produced linearly with doses of the analogue up to at least 25 μg showing that there is very little if any metabolic control of this 25-hydroxylation. Consequently much higher levels of the hormone were produced than is found after dosing with the vitamin. These observations if applicable to man may indicate the cause of the high incidence of hypercalcaemic intoxication developing in patients treated with 25 μg/day of 1α-hydroxycholecalciferol (Peacock *et al.*, 1974).

B THE FORMATION AND FATE OF 25-HYDROXYDIHYDROTACHYSTEROL$_3$ IN MAN

Dihydrotachysterol is not a naturally occurring vitamin but it is biologically active in man and is capable of reproducing most of the effects of the calciferols. It is antiricketic in man, is effective in the treatment of azotaemic rickets (Stanbury and Lumb, 1962) and has been shown to be more potent than equimolar amounts of ergocalciferol in promoting calcium absorption in dialysed uraemic patients (Kaye *et al.*, 1970). It has long been regarded as the preparation of choice for the treatment of hypoparathroidism but its principle advantage is the short duration of its therapeutic action and of its toxic effect in the case of inadvertent overdosage. Dihydrotachysterol$_3$ is biologically equally active in the intact and anephric rat and presumably does not require prior 1α-hydroxylation to produce its effects; it is assumed that 25-hydroxydihydrotachysterol$_3$ is the biologically active form. Mawer (1974) has described the chromatographic profiles of its metabolites in human serum following intravenous injection of isotopically labelled DHT$_3$. The principle metabolite in serum is 25-hydroxydihydrotachysterol$_3$; other forms include unchanged dihydrotachysterol$_3$, a less polar and presumably esterified form, and two unidentified more-polar fractions. This pattern resembles so closely the pattern of metabolites seen in the rat (Hallick and DeLuca, 1972) that one can reasonably assume that 25-hydroxydihydrotachysterol$_3$ is also the biologically active metabolite in man.

Results of kinetic studies of the metabolism of isotopically labelled dihydrotachysterol$_3$ probably explain the shorter duration of dihydrotachysterol activity. Consecutive studies with labelled cholecalciferol and labelled dihydrotachysterol$_3$ in the same vitamin D-deficient patient are shown in Fig. 6. The decay of cholecalciferol, the formation of labelled 25-hydroxycholecalciferol and its sustained high concentration in the serum are typical of the vitamin D-deficient state (Mawer *et al.*, 1971b). The decay of dihydrotachysterol$_3$ was not significantly different from that of cholecalciferol but the serum concentration of labelled 25-hydroxydihydrotachysterol$_3$ was lower than that of 25-hydroxycholecalciferol and it had virtually disappeared from the serum by the fourth day of observation. The reasons of the differences in the hepatic metabolism of cholecalciferol and dihydrotachysterol$_3$ in man are not explained; nor are the qualitatively similar differences in the rat (Bhattacharyya and DeLuca, 1973b). Possible responsible mechanisms are discussed elsewhere (Stanbury *et al.*, 1973; Mawer, 1974).

C THE RELATION BETWEEN SERUM 25-HYDROXYCHOLECALCIFEROL AND SERUM CALCIUM

25-Hydroxycholecalciferol induces resorption of bone cultured *in vitro* (Trummel *et al.*, 1969) and promotes absorption of calcium by the isolated

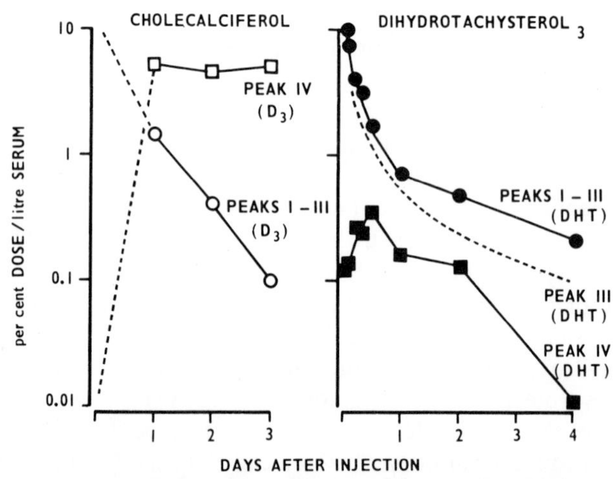

Fig. 6. A comparison of the turnover of radioactive cholecalciferol and radioactive DHT$_3$ in the same patient with chronic renal failure and relative vitamin D-deficiency. A period of 9 weeks elapsed between the two observations. Note that 'peaks 1–111' includes both the originally injected sterol (peak 111) and its esters (peak 1). Cholecalciferyl esters accounted for a constant fraction (circa 5%) of 'peaks 1–111'. From day 2 onwards, about 50% of the serum DHT$_3$ was in the ester form; the concentration of unesterified DHT$_3$ is shown as a curved interrupted line

perfused intestine (Olson and DeLuca, 1969) and by the renal tubules (Puschett *et al.*, 1972). These represent actions on each of the tissues capable of influencing the concentration of serum calcium and, although they were demonstrated originally with the use of pharmacological dosage, they suggested that 25-hydroxycholecalciferol may have a direct role in the

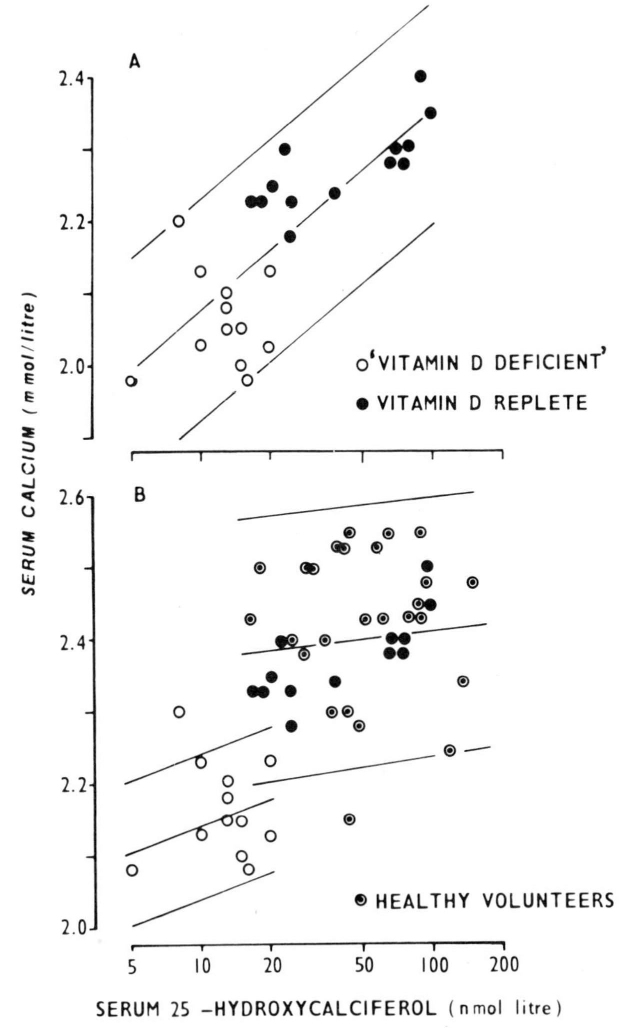

Fig. 7. The relationship between the serum concentrations of 25-hydroxycholecalciferol and calcium. A, in a mixed group of vitamin D-deficient and replete subjects; the regression and 95% confidence limits are shown. B, separately calculated regressions for vitamin D-deficient subjects and an augmented group of healthy replete subjects (see text)

regulation of the serum calcium. Apparent support for this proposition was provided by the finding of a significant direct correlation between serum 25-hydroxycalciferol and the serum calcium in a large group of epileptic patients treated with phenobarbitone and other anti-epileptic drugs (Hahn *et al.*, 1972, 1975). *A priori*, it was unlikely that this correlation represented a causal relationship: there may be a ten-fold variation of the serum 25-hydroxy-calciferol among a population of healthy normocalcaemic individuals; and a short holiday in the sun can double or treble the serum 25- hydroxycalciferol without influencing the serum calcium (P. de Silva and C. M. Taylor, private communication). Subsequently, Hahn and his collaborators have revised their views on the relation between serum 25-hydroxycalciferol and the serum calcium (Haddad *et al.*, 1973; Haddad and Stamp, 1974) but the idea of a causal relationship persists. A highly significant correlation between the two variables in a population of Asian immigrants in Britain has been found but no such relationship was found in a group of Caucasians studied simultaneously (Gupta *et al.*, 1974).

The probable reason for this paradox is best illustrated by a specific example. In Fig. 7A is shown the relationship between the serum 25-hydroxycalciferol and serum calcium in a group of 25 individuals (data extended from the study of Mawer *et al.*, 1975); there is a highly significant correlation between the two variables ($r=0.78$, $P<0.001$). This group included 13 perfectly healthy individuals, some of whom had received cholecalciferol or solar exposure, and 12 patients with clinical effects of vitamin D-deficiency or reasons for developing potential vitamin D-deficiency. In Fig. 7B, 26 additional measurements from healthy individuals have been added to the original thirteen, and the relationship between serum 25-hydroxycalciferol and serum calcium has been re-examined separately in this augmented ‘normal’ group ($r=0.17$,NS) and in the 12 patients with vitamin D-insufficiency ($r=0.36$, NS). There was thus no significant relationship between the two variables in either group and it is notable that there was a 9-fold variation in serum 25-hydroxycalciferol among the healthy subjects without change in the mean serum calcium of 9.6 mg/100 ml. Yet, if all the data in Fig. 7B are considered as a single population there is still a highly significant correlation ($r=0.64$, $P<0.001$) between serum 25-hydroxycalciferol and serum calcium. This and the correlation in Fig. 7A are thus spurious and determined by the inclusion of two functionally distinct populations, a normocalcaemic vitamin D replete group and a vitamin D insufficient group with varying degrees of hypocalcaemia. A similar spurious correlation will be found in any similar mixed population; it is known that a random group of treated epileptics (Richens and Rowe, 1970) or of Asians in Britain (Holmes *et al.*, 1973) will include unpredictable proportions of vitamin D-deficient and replete individuals. Analogous spurious correlations between serum 25-

hydroxycalciferol and the serum phosphate and serum calcium × phosphate product can also be demonstrated (Mawer *et al.*, 1975; Stanbury *et al.*, 1975a).

This analysis does not preclude the possibility that there may be a valid correlation between serum 25-hydroxycalciferol and serum calcium among subjects with varying degrees of vitamin D-insufficiency. But, even if established, such a correlation need not indicate a direct causal relationship. It would reflect the requirement of 'vitamin D' for the action of parathyroid hormone in regulating the serum calcium; and it is not yet established whether this requirement is met by 25-hydroxy- or 1,25-dihydroxy-cholecalciferol (Mahgoub and Sheppard, 1975).

D HYPERCALCAEMIC INTOXICATION WITH CALCIFEROL; MECHANISMS OF PROTECTION

Although the evidence reviewed suggests that 25-hydroxycalciferol does not have a direct role in regulating the serum calcium, excessive therapeutic dosage with vitamin D can produce potentially lethal hypercalcaemia. Individual susceptibility varies widely and unpredictably; a daily dose of 50 μg/kg of ergocalciferol is dangerous and intoxication can result from smaller doses, while some individuals can tolerate a larger amount (Fourman and Royer, 1968). The degree of induced hypercalcaemia may vary with the dietary intake of calcium, indicating that intestinal absorption contributes to

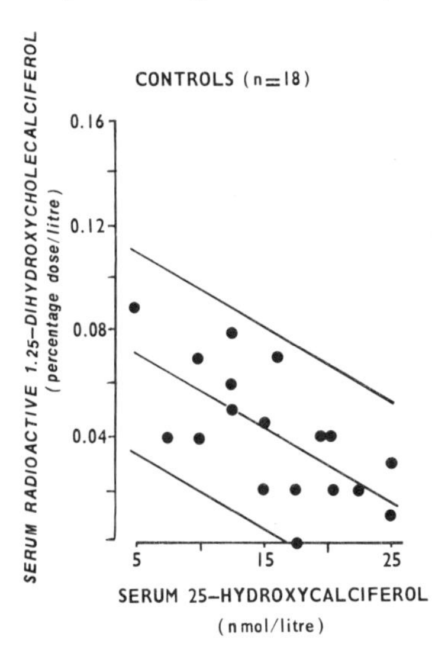

Fig. 8. The relationship between the serum concentration of 25-hydroxycalciferol and the concentration of labelled 1,25-dihydroxycholecalciferol in serum 48 h after injecting radioactive cholecalciferol

its production; but the serum calcium may remain elevated when calcium is withdrawn from the diet and, in animals, hypercalcaemia has been produced when the diet is virtually free of calcium. This implies that mobilisation of calcium from bone and possibly also an effect on the renal handling of calcium may be as important in causing hypercalcaemia as in an action on the gut. Since the formation of 1,25-dihydroxycholecalciferol from a pulse dose of cholecalciferol is apparently inhibited with moderate elevation of the serum 25-hydroxycalciferol (Fig. 8) and with any tendency to elevation of the serum calcium (Fig. 9), it is unlikely that the effects of excess vitamin D are attributable to an increased accumulation of 1,25-dihydroxycalciferol. This has now been proved by the demonstration of normal serum concentrations of 1,25-dihydroxycholecalciferol in patients with clinical intoxication (Hughes *et al.*, 1976). Serum 25-hydroxycalciferol, however, increases in proportion to the intake of vitamin D (Haddad and Stamp, 1974) and this metabolite is the most likely candidate responsible for the production of hypercalcaemic intoxication. Large doses of 25-hydroxycholecalciferol are capable of promoting calcium absorption in the anephric rat (Hill *et al.*, 1971); and similar doses (50–250 μg) will elevate the serum calcium in the anephric rat fed a negligible calcium intake (0.02% Ca), in the presence or absence of the parathyroid glands (Pavlovitch *et al.*, 1973). Thus the pharmacological effects of 25-hydroxycalciferol alone may be sufficient to account for vitamin D

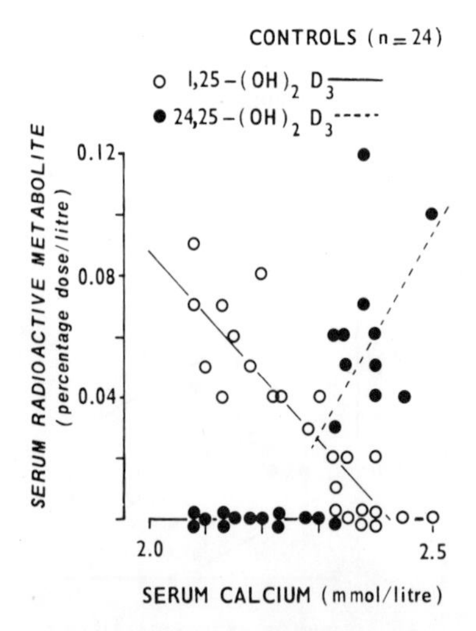

Fig. 9. The relationships between the serum calcium and the serum concentrations of labelled 1,25- and 24,25-dihydroxycholecalciferol 48 h after injecting radioactive cholecalciferol. The regression of serum 24,25-dihydroxycholecalciferol on serum calcium in control subjects (interrupted line) was calculated only for individuals with serum calcium >2.3 mmol/l

intoxication. Values of serum 25-hydroxycalciferol as high as 200–400 ng/ml have been measured in patients receiving daily doses of ergocalciferol (Mawer *et al.*, 1971b; Haddad and Chyu, 1971). Values for serum 25-hydroxycalciferol of 206, 400 and 690 ng/ml have been recorded in three intoxicated adults (Haddad and Stamp, 1974) (cf. values for healthy individuals in Table 1 and Fig. 7); but finding a value no higher than 129 ng/ml in an intoxicated infant, they caution that factors other than the serum level of this metabolite may be operating to influence the hypercalcaemic response to vitamin D. This comment is obviously valid, and one such factor could be greater reactivity of the juvenile skeleton, but two observations may be relevant to this problem. Firstly, when treatment with high doses of ergocalciferol is stopped the subsequent decay of serum antiricketic activity with time follows a series of exponential functions, the earliest component of which series is relatively rapid (Lumb *et al.*, 1971). Thus, if the blood sample for assay is taken even a relatively few days after stopping treatment with vitamin D, the result may underestimate the activity prevailing during the course of treatment. The pattern of decay of serum 25-hydroxycalciferol immediately following cessation of vitamin D treatment has not been established. If it is similar to that of serum total antiricketic activity, any delay in blood sampling could again produce an inappropriately low estimate of the serum 25-hydroxycalciferol associated with intoxication. Secondly, the tissue content of this metabolite may remain relatively high after treatment with vitamin D has stopped, and even when the serum level has returned to the 'normal range'. In a patient previously treated with enormous doses of ergocalciferol but who had received no treatment for two years, Mawer *et al.* (1972) found the 25-hydroxycalciferol content of bone to be 52 μg/kg of wet tissue when the level in serum 25-hydroxycalciferol did not exceed 23.6 μg/l. Thus 25-hydroxycalciferol may disappear more slowly from certain target tissues than from the blood. It is conceivable that its concentration in the bone cell is more relevant to the development of hypercalcaemia than its concentration in the serum.

From the high levels of serum 25-hydroxycalciferol encountered during treatment with daily pharmacological doses of vitamin D, it is evident that the inhibition of hepatic 25-hydroxylation is not complete when excess vitamin D is continually entering the blood from the intestine. The same appears to be the case when increased amounts of cholecalciferol are delivered into the circulation consequent upon increased cutaneous exposure to sunshine. Moreover, the total amount in the plasma provides an underestimate of the 25-hydroxycalciferol actually formed. Variable amounts of this metabolite also accumulate in the extravascular tissues and, although its concentration may not be high, the large bulk of tissues such as voluntary muscle may accommodate a greater mass of 25-hydroxycalciferol than is present in the circulation (Mawer *et al.*, 1972). In the patient of Mawer *et al.*, cited above, there was probably 10–20 times as much 25-hydroxycalciferol in the extravascular tissues as in the blood. Since 25-hydroxycalciferol will be capable of influencing the serum calcium only when present in the target organs – intestine, bone and kidney – its sequestration in indifferent tissues such as muscle will tend to limit its biological effects and thereby reduce its liability to produce hypercalcaemic intoxication. This mechanism may possibly be quantitatively more important in protecting against vitamin D intoxication than the mechanisms limiting the formation of 25-hydroxycalciferol in the liver. The formation of both 24,25- and 25,26-dihydroxycholecalciferols (Sections VC and VD) appears to increase in proportion to the body pool of 25-hydroxycalciferol. Since each of these triols is biologically less potent than 25-hydroxycalciferol especially in its action on bone resorption (Raisz and Trummel, 1972), their formation may also serve to limit the deleterious effects of an excess of vitamin D. But probably the most important single factor protecting against the immediate effects of excess vitamin D is the partition of unmetabolised vitamin into body fat and its binding to protein in other tissues. These passive physicochemical processes rapidly remove the greater fraction of a pulse dose of cholecalciferol from the circulating blood and thereby limit the amount available for conversion to biologically more potent metabolites (Mawer *et al.*, 1972). However, if hypercalcaemic intoxication should occur, this sequestered pool of native vitamin D may perpetuate its effect as material is returned to the circulating blood and thus into the metabolic pool. The subcutaneous fat of the cited patient of Mawer *et al.* (see above) had an assayed content of vitamin D (96 i.u/g) approaching that of cod liver oil, even although she had received no vitamin D therapy for almost two years!

V The Metabolism of 25-Hydroxycalciferol and its Regulation

A THE FALLACIES OF THE INDIRECT APPROACH

Since there is no simple means available for measuring 1,25-, 24,25- and 25,26-dihydroxycalciferols, it has not yet been possible to undertake systematic studies of the metabolism of 25-hydroxycalciferol in man. In default of such direct measurement, several attempts have been made to infer changes in the metabolism of 25-hydroxycalciferol in disease from measurements of its serum concentration in relation to arbitrary 'normal levels'. Thus a 'low' serum 25-hydroxycalciferol in drug-treated epileptic patients has been taken to imply an abnormal hepatic degradation of cholecalciferol; an 'increased' serum 25-hydroxycalciferol in 'vitamin D-dependent' rickets has been regarded as supporting the postulated defect of the renal 1-hydroxylase in this disease; and somewhat similar inferences have been made regarding the metabolism of 25-hydroxycalciferol in renal failure. In view of the sensitivity of the serum 25-hydroxycalciferol to changes of exposure to sunshine (Section IIIA) and the literal impossibility of ensuring identity of solar exposure and of cutaneous response in 'experimental' and 'control' subjects, such indirect attempts to assess 25-hydroxycalciferol metabolism are doomed to failure or, at best, to great uncertainty. Similarly, in any individual who has received large therapeutic amounts of calciferol for a prolonged period (such as is likely to be the case, for example, in all but virgin patients with 'vitamin D-dependency'), it will not be possible to assess the significance of serum 25-hydroxycalciferol levels measured even many months after stopping such treatment. After an initial rapid fall when treatment is stopped (Section IVD), the high serum levels of total antiricketic activity induced by such therapy decay very slowly (Lumb *et al.*, 1971). The therapeutically induced high serum antiricketic activity is about equally attributable to calciferol and its 25-hydroxylated metabolite (Mawer *et al.*, 1971b) and the differential decay of the two sterols after withdrawing therapy has not yet been documented. We have measured high serum concentrations of 25-hydroxycalciferol as long as 8 years after terminating a course of treatment with pharmacological doses of ergocalciferol (unpublished observations).

B THE FORMATION OF 1,25-DIHYDROXYCHOLECALCIFEROL: POSSIBLE CONTROL MECHANISMS

The formation of radioactive 1,25- and 24,25-dihydroxycholecalciferol from a pulse dose of 10 μg [1,2-^{3}H,4-^{14}C] cholecalciferol has been observed in a group of individuals with widely differing states of vitamin D nutrition (Mawer *et al.*, 1975). From these studies, it appears that the pattern of the renal metabolism of 25-hydroxycholecalciferol is chiefly dependent on the prevailing nutritional state. Subjects relatively deficient of vitamin D (serum 25-(OH)D $<$ 10 ng/ml), produced only radioactive 1,25-dihydroxycholecalciferol, whereas vitamin D replete individuals (serum 25-(OH)D $>$ 15 ng/ml) formed only radioactive 24,25-dihydroxycholecalciferol and no single individual produced significant amounts of both triols simultaneously. The maximum concentration of labelled hormone in the serum was reached 48–72 h after administration of the tracer and, whether expressed simply as dpm/1 (Mawer *et al.*, 1975) or as a derived picomolar value (Stanbury *et al.*, 1975a), it was related inversely to the prevailing serum concentration of non-radioactive 25-hydroxycalciferol (Fig. 8). This relationship suggests that the formation of the hormone from a single pulse of cholecalciferol is regulated in proportion to the prevailing degree of physiological vitamin D-deficiency, more new metabolite being produced the greater the deficiency. If confirmed by further studies, this relationship has two important potential implications. Firstly, the quantitative production of 1,25-dihydroxycholecalciferol from a standard dose of cholecalciferol might provide a means of defining and measuring 'vitamin D-deficiency' in man in physiological terms (Stanbury *et al.*, 1975b). Secondly, if physiological repletion with vitamin D implies the failure to produce additional hormone from such a pulse dose of cholecalciferol, the regression in Fig. 8 suggests that 'repletion' is represented by a *mean* serum 25-hydroxycalciferol of about 15 ng/ml. But it must be emphasised that this mean limiting value of serum 25-hydroxycalciferol is likely to have a wide standard error. The confidence limits of the regression are wide and the number of observations is small. There are no other published data bearing on this relationship.

The mechanisms by which the nutritional state modulates the renal metabolism of 25-hydroxycholecalciferol in man are unknown. In the studies of Mawer *et al.* (1975), the serum concentration of radioactive 1,25-dihydroxycholecalciferol 48 h after injecting cholecalciferol was related

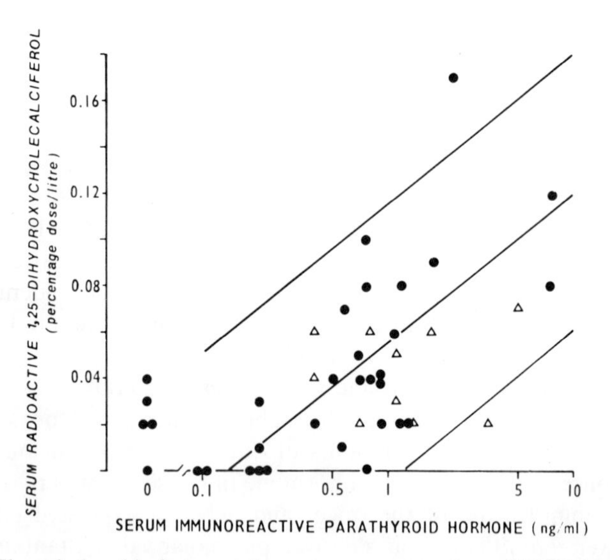

Fig. 10. The relationship between the serum concentration of iPTH (antiserum 367) and the concentration of labelled 1,25-dihydroxycholecalciferol in serum 48 h after injecting radioactive cholecalciferol. The regression and confidence limits were calculated for the 29 control subjects with measurable serum iPTH. ●, control subjects; △, primary hyperparathyroid subjects

inversely to the prevailing serum calcium (Fig. 9) and directly with the serum immunoassayable parathyroid hormone (Fig. 10), both relationships being at a high level of significance. It was thus not possible to determine whether one of these variables or some other function of the state of vitamin D nutrition (Fig. 8) was the primary determinant of the renal 1α-hydroxylation of 25-hydroxycholecalciferol. Parallel studies in primary hyperparathyroidism (chapter 9, Section IIB) by Mawer *et al.* (1975) indicated that the parathyroid hormone was probably the trophic factor determining this process.

C METABOLISM OF 1,25-DIHYDROXYCHOLECALCIFEROL

The disappearance of [26-^{3}H]1,25-dihydroxycholecalciferol from plasma of normal subjects is biphasic with a rapid-phase half-time of about 14 h (Mawer *et al.*, 1976). The half-life of the slow phase was about 18 h. After an oral dose of the labelled hormone the highest concentration in plasma was reached after 4 h. The majority of the radioactivity in plasma is due to the hormone itself with small quantities of three other substances, one of which has the polarity of 25-hydroxycholecalciferol and another co-chromatographs with 1,24,25-trihydroxycholecalciferol. In the first 24 h after an intravenous dose of the labelled hormone about 7% of the radioactivity appears in the urine in a water soluble form. Since the hormone is labelled at C-26 the original side chain is still intact in these metabolites. In the 14 days after either an oral or an intravenous dose of the hormone over 33% was excreted in the urine and faeces. Interestingly the major peak of faecal radioactivity was 1,25-dihydroxycholecalciferol even when the hormone was given intravenously. In a hypoparathyroid patient the orally administered labelled hormone caused a rapid increase in serum calcium without concomitantly increasing the plasma level of the hormone to the normal range. This may indicate that an effective concentration of hormone in the intestine can be achieved although plasma levels were low. Presumably the 1,25-dihydroxycholecalciferol reaches its active sites during the process of absorption.

D FACTORS INFLUENCING THE FORMATION OF 24,25-DIHYDROXYCHOLECALCIFEROL

There have been relatively few observations on the formation of 24,25-dihydroxycholecalciferol in man. Parathyroid hormone is not required for its production; as in animals (Garabedian *et al.*, 1972; chapter 2), the parathyroidectomised individual produces this triol in amounts appropriate to his nutritional state (Mawer *et al.*, 1975). No more than trace amounts of labelled 24,25-dihydroxycholecalciferol were detectable in the serum following administration of radioactive cholecalciferol to patients with advanced renal failure (Mawer *et al.*, 1973). Under similar conditions of study, patients with clinical vitamin D-deficiency and normal renal function also produced no labelled 24,25-dihydroxycholecalciferol but detectable amounts appeared in the serum of some clinically normal individuals with serum 25-hydroxycalciferol as low as 7–9 ng/ml (Mawer *et al.*, 1975). Thus, as in animal studies

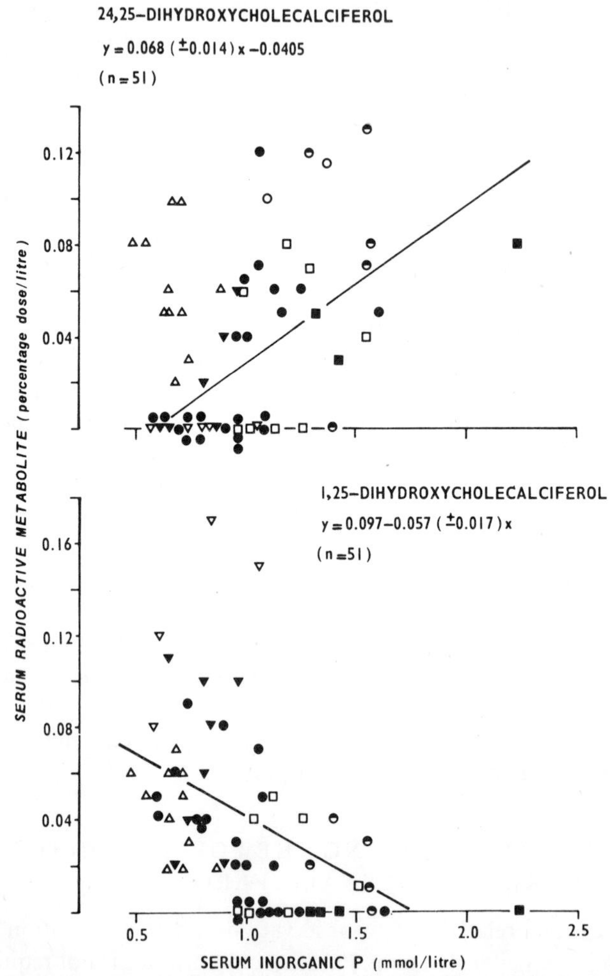

Fig. 11. The relationship between the serum concentration of orthophosphate and the serum concentration of labelled 24,25-dihydroxycholecalciferol (above) and labelled 1,25-dihydroxycholecalciferol (below) 48 h after injecting radioactive cholecalciferol ●, control subjects; △, primary hyperparathyroidism; ■, hypoparathyroidism; □, Mg deficiency; ◓, diphosphonate treated; ○, renal failure; ▽, Asian osteomalacia; ▼, epileptic osteomalacia

(Galante *et al.*, 1973), 24,25-dihydroxycholecalciferol appears to be formed preferentially by the vitamin D-replete individual and 1,25- dihydroxycholecalciferol in states of physiological deficiency. In terms of the previously discussed concept of 'physiological repletion', the production of labelled 24,25-dihydroxycholecalciferol in some individuals with relatively low values of serum 25-hydroxycalciferol would simply imply that these particular subjects were replete at such levels of 25-hydroxycalciferol. At serum levels of 25-hydroxycalciferol greater than 10–15 ng/ml, the serum concentration of labelled 24,25-dihydroxycholecalciferol was positively correlated with the serum 25-hydroxycalciferol, serum calcium and serum phosphate, (Fig. 11); no labelled 24,25-dihydroxycholecalciferol was detected in subjects with serum calcium <9.2 mg/dl and serum phosphate <3.0 mg/100 ml (Mawer *et al.*, 1975).

These various correlations of the formation of 24,25-dihydroxycholecalciferol were not statistically significant and it will be difficult to assess their meaning until the molar concentrations of 24,25-dihydroxycholecalciferol have been measured directly. The little information presently available shows that 24,25-dihydroxycholecalciferol is not present in plasma of individuals with <2 ng/ml of 25-hydroxycalciferol rising to between 2.39–4.41 ng/ml at

Table 2. Calculated concentrations of dihydroxylated derivatives of vitamin D in human serum

Subject[a] number	Assayed 25-(OH)D (μg/ml)	Calculated concentrations (ng/ml)		
		$1,25\text{-}(OH)_2D$	$24,25\text{-}(OH)_2D$	$25,26\text{-}(OH)_2D$
7	2	0.03	0	0.02
9	3.2	0.02	0	0.05
2	4.0	0.04	0	0.11
5	5.2	0.05	0	0.13
4	6.0	0.04	0	0.16
6	8.0	0.04	0	0.08
16	9.2	0.04	0.07	0.19
10	10.0	0.04	0	0.17
14[b]	28.0	n.d.	0.60	0.30
11[b]	30.0	n.d.	0.54	0.86
15[b]	38.0	n.d.	0.83	0.50
20[b,c]	27.2	n.d.	3.48	2.0
19[b,c]	40.0	n.d.	3.33	4.15

[a] Subjects taken from Table 1 of Mawer *et al.* (1975).
[b] Labelled $1,25\text{-}(OH)_2D_3$ could not be detected in these subjects.
[c] These subjects had previously received a large dose of cholecalciferol.

plasma 25-hydroxycalciferol levels of 52–186 ng/ml (Taylor *et al.*, 1976). The indirectly calculated molar concentrations of serum 24,25-dihydroxycholecalciferol in the subjects studied by Mawer *et al.* (1975) varied enormously between 0.07 and 3.48 ng/ml (see Table 2). This implies correspondingly large differences in the total pool of 24,25-dihydroxycalciferol within the circulation; previous studies of the distribution of polar metabolites in human tissue (Mawer *et al.*, 1972) make it highly likely that there is an even greater extravascular pool of this metabolite. In such circumstances observations limited to measurement of radioactivity alone are open to considerable error in interpretation (Stanbury *et al.*, 1972). The effects of dilution of metabolically produced, labelled 24,25-dihydroxycholecalciferol into pre-existing pools of this metabolite may contribute to the low order of significance in the correlation discussed.

The same factor of pre-existing pools must also potentially influence observations on the formation of labelled 1,25-dihydroxycholecalciferol; but the narrow range of the serum concentrations of 1,25-dihydroxycalciferol (Section IIIB) and the fact that its formation can be detected only in subjects deficient of 1,25-dihydroxycholecalciferol (see above) suggest that the dilutional factor is likely to be of less significance in this situation. In any event, the physiological factors regulating the formation of the hormone clearly dominate over any effect of pool size.

This may also be true of observations on the formation of labelled 24,25-dihydroxycholecalciferol in patients with primary hyperparathyroidism (chapter 9, IIIB) and low values of serum 25-hydroxycalciferol. As compared with controls having a similar range of serum 25-hydroxycalciferol (6–14 ng/ml), patients with hypercalcaemic primary hyperparathyroidism produced inappropriately large amounts of labelled 24,25-dihydroxycholecalciferol from injected radioactive cholecalciferol (Mawer *et al.*, 1975 and the concentration of this radioactive metabolite in the serum was positively correlated with the concentration of serum calcium (chapter 9, Fig. 3: $r=0.61$, $0.05<p<0.1$, $n=9$). This observation, and the positive correlation between serum concentrations of calcium and labelled 24,25-dihydroxycholecalciferol in control subjects (Fig. 9), suggests that elevation of the serum calcium may be one of the factors increasing the activity of the renal 24-hydroxylase, as in the rat (Boyle *et al.*, 1972). The positive correlation between the serum 25-hydroxycalciferol and serum radioactive 24,25-dihydroxycholecalciferol in all groups of subjects studied (Mawer *et al.*, 1975), and the very high calculated molar concentrations of serum 24,25-dihydroxycalciferol in subjects with high levels of serum 25-hydroxycalciferol (Table 2) suggest that the formation of 24,25-dihydroxycholecalciferol may increase in proportion to the size of the body pool of 25-hydroxycalciferol. This possibility will require further investigation but it is compatible with the more direct observations on the formation of 24,25-dihydroxycholecalciferol in the toad recently reported by Fraser (1975). The demonstration in man of a greater formation of labelled 24,25-dihydroxycholecalciferol from injected radioactive 25-hydroxy cholecalciferol than from radioactive cholecalciferol may also be an effect of substrate concentration (Gray *et al.*, 1974).

E 25,26-DIHYDROXYCHOLECALCIFEROL

Labelled 25,26-dihydroxycholecalciferol was detected in all subjects we have studied with radioactive cholecalciferol, irrespective of their vitamin D status or the state of their renal function. Its function and site of formation are unknown. This metabolite co-chromatographs with 1,25-dihydroxycholecalciferol in most systems (Haussler and Rasmussen, 1972) but methods are available for calculating the relative proportions of the two metabolites (Bell and Kodicek, 1970; Mawer *et al.*, 1971a). Detection of 1,25-dihydroxycholecalciferol depends upon measurement of the loss of ^{3}H from position 1 of the molecule relative to ^{14}C at position 4, and this is only possible when a double isotope labelled preparation of cholecalciferol is used as tracer. If the tracer dose given is [26,27^{3}H]25-hydroxycholecalciferol, detection of 1,25-dihydroxycholecalciferol in human serum is not possible by currently available techniques; in any event, 25,26-dihydroxycholecalciferol is normally the major component of the mixed chromatographic peak (Mawer *et al.*, 1973). Gray *et al.* (1974) claim to have detected the formation of labelled 1,25-dihydroxycholecalciferol from injected [1,2-^{3}H,4-^{14}C]-cholecalciferol in healthy subjects with a mean serum 25-hydroxycalciferol of 27 ± 3 (SEM) ng/ml. We ourselves have never detected the formation of labelled 1,25-dihydroxy-cholecalciferol from a pulse dose of cholecalciferol in normal individuals with serum 25-hydroxycalciferol levels as high as this and we suspect that the metabolite measured by these authors was 25-26-hydroxy-cholecalciferol. This suspicion is supported by the failure of Gray *et al.* to detect loss of tritium in the chromatographic fraction (Sephadex LH20) identified as 1,25-dihydroxycholecalciferol.

The indirectly calculated molar concentration of 25,26-dihydroxycalciferol in human serum (Table 2) increases with the serum 25-hydroxycalciferol. This suggests that this metabolite may be produced in proportion to the prevailing body pool of 25-hydroxycalciferol.

F METABOLITES MORE POLAR THAN THE DIHYDROXY-CHOLECALCIFEROLS

1 *1,24,25-Trihydroxycholecalciferol.* This metabolite has been detected experimentally after administration of 24,25-dihydroxycholecalciferol to vitamin D-deficient animals (Boyle *et al.*, 1973; chapter 2, Section IC) or on

incubating 24,25-dihydroxycholecalciferol in a kidney homogenate from vitamin D-deficient chicks (Holick *et al.*, 1973). 1,24,25- Dihydroxycholecalciferol can also be made by incubating the 1,25-dihydroxy-metabolite with kidney homogenates from chicks treated with EHDP (E. B. Mawer and C. M. Taylor, unpublished observations; Taylor *et al.*, 1975). The tetrol metabolite can be detected on Sephadex LH20 columns eluted with $CHCl_3$-hexane-methanol (Boyle *et al.*, 1973). We have been unable to detect significant amounts of material with this chromatographic mobility in serum from human subjects given either labelled cholecalciferol or 25-hydroxycholecalciferol (Fig. 2). It seems likely that this metabolite does not have any physiological significance in man.

2 '*Peak VI*'. A metabolite which has been designated 'peak VI' (Fig. 1) from its mobility on silicic acid columns (Mawer *et al.*, 1969; Ponchon and DeLuca, 1969) is more polar than either the tri- or tetrahydroxycalciferols, and is eluted from Sephadex LH20 with chloroform-methanol (Fig. 2). A similar peak of radioactivity was found in rat bile by Bell and Kodicek (1969) and identified as a glucuronide but the aglycone moiety produced on hydrolysis could not be characterised. Material of similar chromatographic mobility was shown to be the main vitamin D metabolite in human bile (Mawer *et al.*, 1972). A water soluble vitamin D metabolite was found in human bile, which became lipid soluble on treatment with glucuronidase (Avioli *et al.*, 1967). In the same study small amounts of water-soluble radioactivity not susceptible to glucuronidase or acid hydrolysis were found in bile and also in urine.

G SUMMARY

It is not yet possible to determine what fraction of administered cholecalciferol or 25-hydroxycholecalciferol is converted into 24,25-, 25,26-dihydroxycholecalciferol and more polar metabolites. It is possible that all are degradation products of little biological importance; but the relatively high concentrations of 24,25-dihydroxycholecalciferol in the serum of normal man (Taylor *et al.*, 1976) and its relatively long half-life in the circulation (Fig. 3) suggest that this metabolite may yet be found to have some physiological function.

An attempt has been made to estimate the circulating mass concentrations of the dihydroxylated metabolites from the radioactive concentrations by using the specific activity of their precursor 25-hydroxycalciferol (Stanbury *et al.*, 1975; Mawer *et al.*, 1975). The estimated concentration ranges are shown in Table 2. In vitamin D-replete subjects the 24,25- and 25,26-dihydroxy-metabolites each measured about 10% of the 25-hydroxycalciferol concentration although the two metabolites appear to have different half-lives in serum (Fig. 3). Recently competitive protein binding assays for 24,25-dihydroxycholecalciferol have confirmed this finding.

It is evident that not all the 25-hydroxycalciferol produced metabolically or administered extraneously remains immediately available, within the metabolic pool, for further conversion. Gray *et al.* (1974) estimate the total body pool of 25-hydroxycalciferol to be about four times the amount in the circulating blood. This size of the extravascular pool of 25-hydroxycalciferol must, however, depend on the previous intake of vitamin D sterols. In a patient previously treated with massive amounts of ergocalciferol, there was at least 20 times as much 25-hydroxycalciferol in the tissues as in the circulating blood (Mawer *et al.*, 1972). This sequestration of 25-hydroxycalciferol, by binding to the receptor proteins present in most tissues, must limit its immediate further metabolism.

From the 25-hydroxycalciferol remaining within the circulating pool, the formation of 1,25-dihydroxycalciferol appears to be quantitatively regulated; the formation of 24,25- and 25,26-dihydroxycalciferol may be a function of the concentration of circulating 25-hydroxylated metabolite, and 24-hydroxylation of the latter may also increase with the serum calcium (Fig. 9). While the scanty evidence so far available from studies in man suggests that the level of parathyroid activity may be the most important physiological determinant of 1,25-dihydroxycholecalciferol formation from a pulse of cholecalciferol, a direct influence of the serum calcium or of one or more metabolites of cholecalciferol cannot be excluded. Studies of isolated renal tubules and renal mitochondria suggest that the synthesis of 1,25-dihydroxycholecalciferol may be determined by complexly interrelated changes of ionic concentration (Ca^{2+}, HPO_4^{2-} and H^+) both outside and within the cell (Bikle and Rasmussen, 1975; Bikle *et al.*, 1975) and perhaps also by the renal cellular content of the hormone itself (Larkins *et al.*, 1974). No studies have yet been reported on the effects of changes in acid-base balance on the formation of 1,25-dihydroxycholecalciferol in man, although systemic acidosis of renal origin may be associated with the development of rickets and osteomalacia (see chapter 9, Section IC). In normal and vitamin D-deficient individuals and patients with primary hyperparathyroidism, no correlation was found between the serum phosphate and the formation of the hormone from a pulse of cholecalciferol in the original study of Mawer *et al.* (1975) but an accelerated turnover of injected [1,2-^{3}H]25-hydroxycholecalciferol was found by Gray *et al.* (1975) in subjects with experimental phosphorus depletion (chapter 9, Section IA). When the results of our studies of radioactive vitamin D metabolism in miscellaneous clinical states are aggregated with the original data of Mawer *et al.* (1975), the resulting 51 data show a significant negative correlation between serum phosphate and serum labelled 1,25-dihydroxycholecalciferol, and a positive correlation between serum phosphate and labelled 24,25-dihydroxycholecalciferol (Fig. 11).

Acknowledgements

Departmental studies of vitamin D metabolism reported in the text of this chapter and chapter 9 were supported by a grant from the Medical Research Council and the Department of Health and Social Security. We are grateful to our various colleagues, especially Dr G. A. Lumb, Dr C. M. Taylor and Mrs P. de Silva, who have allowed us to cite unpublished results from their personal researches.

References

Avioli, L. V. and Haddad, J. G. (1973). *Metabolism* **22**, 507.

Avioli, L. V., Lee, S. W., McDonald, J. E., Lund, J. and DeLuca, H. F. (1967). *J. Clin. Invest.* **46**, 983.

Avioli, L. V., Birge, S., Lee, S. W. and Slatopolsky, E. (1968). *J. Clin. Invest.* **47**, 2229.

Bayard, F., Bec, P. and Louvet, J. P. (1972). *Europ. J. Clin. Invest.* **2**, 195.

Bell, P. A. and Kodicek, E. (1969). *Biochem. J.* **115**, 663.

Bell, P. A. and Kodicek, E. (1970). *Biochem. J.* **116**, 755.

Belsey, R. E., DeLuca, H. F. and Potts, J. T. (1971). *J. Clin. Endocrinol.* **83**, 554.

Belsey, R. E., DeLuca, H. F. and Potts, J. T. (1974a). *Nature* (London) **247**, 208.

Belsey, R. E., DeLuca, H. F. and Potts, J. T. (1974b). *J. Clin. Endocr. Metab.* **38**, 1046.

Bhattacharyya, M. H. and DeLuca, H. F. (1973a). *J. Biol. Chem.* **218**, 2969.

Bhattacharyya, M. H. and DeLuca, H. F. (1973b). *J. Biol. Chem.* **248**, 2974.

Bikle, D. D. and Rasmussen, H. (1975). *J. Clin. Invest.* **55**, 292.

Bikle, D. D., Murphy, E. W. and Rasmussen, H. (1975). *J. Clin. Invest.* **55**, 299.

Bills, C. E. (1947). *Biol. Symp.* **12**, 409.

Boyle, I. T., Gray, R. W., Omdahl, J. L. and DeLuca, H. F. (1972). *In* 'Endocrinology 1971: Proceedings of 3rd International Symposium of Endocrinology' (Ed. Taylor, S.) p. 468. Heinemann, London.

Boyle, I. T., Omdahl, J. L., Gray, R. W. and DeLuca, H. F. (1973). *J. Biol. Chem.* **248**, 4174.

Brumbaugh, P. F., Haussler, D. H., Bressler, R. and Haussler, M. R. (1974a). *Science* **183**, 1089.

Brumbaugh, P. F., Haussler, D. H., Bursac, K. M. and Haussler, M. R. (1974b). *Biochemistry* **13**, 4091.

Childs, B., Cantolino, S. and Dyke, M. K. (1962). *Bull. Johns Hopkins Hosp.* **110**, 134.

Dent, C. E. and Smith, R. (1969). *Quart. J. Med.* **38**, 195.

Dent, C. E., Round, J. M., Rowe, D. J. F. and Stamp, T. C. B. (1973). *Lancet* **I**, 1282.

Edelstein, S., Charman, M., Lawson, D. E. M. and Kodicek, E. (1974). *Clin. Sci. Molec. Med.* **46**, 231.

Fourman, P. and Royer, P. (1968). *In* 'Calcium Metabolism and the Bone' (Ed. Fourman, P. and Royer, P.) p. 104. Blackwell, Oxford.

Fraser, D. R. (1975). *Proc. Nutr. Soc.* **34**, 139.

Fukushima, M., Suzuki, Y., Tohira, Y., Nishii, Y., Suzuki, M., Sasaki, S. and Suda, T. (1976). *FEBS Letters* **65**, 211.

Galante, L., Colston, K. W., Evans, I. M. A., Byfield, P. G. H., Matthews, E. W. and MacIntyre, I. (1973). *Nature* (London) **244**, 438.
Garabedian, M., Holick, M. F., DeLuca, H. F. and Boyle, I. T. (1972). *Proc. Nat. Acad. Sci.* (Washington) **69**, 1673.
Goel, K. M., Sweet, E. M., Logan, R. W., Warren, J. M., Arneil, G. C. and Shanks, R. A. (1976). *Lancet* **I**, 1141.
Gray, R. W., Weber, H. P., Dominguez, J. H. and Lehman, J. (1974). *J. Clin. Endocr. Metab.* **39**, 1045.
Gray, R. W., Dominguez, J. H. and Lehmann, J. (1975). *In* 'Vitamin D and Problems Related to Uremic Bone Disease' (Ed. Norman, A. W., Schaefer, K., Grigoleit, H. G., v. Herrath, D. and Ritz, E.) p. 331. de Gruyter, Berlin and New York.
Greenberg, P. B., Hillyard, C. J., Galanate, L. S., Colston, A. W., Evans, I. M. A. and MacIntyre, I. (1974). *Clin. Sci. Molec. Med.* **46**, 143.
Gupta, M. M., Round, J. M. and Stamp, T. C. B. (1974). *Lancet* **I**, 586.
Haddad, J. G. and Chyu, K. J. (1971). *J. Clin. Endocr.* **33**, 992.
Haddad, J. G. and Hahn, T. J. (1973). *Nature* (London) **244**, 515.
Haddad, J. G. and Stamp, T. C. B. (1974). *Amer. J. Med.* **57**, 57.
Haddad, J. G., Chyu, K. J., Hahn, T. J. and Stamp, T. C. B. (1973). *J. Lab. Clin. Med.* **81**, 22.
Haddock, L. and Vazquez, M. del C. (1966). *J. Clin. Endocr.* **26**, 859.
Hahn, T. J., Hendin, B. A., Scharp, C. R. and Haddad, J. G. (1972). *New Engl. J. Med.* **287**, 900.
Hahn, T. J., Hendin, B. A., Scharp, C. R., Boisseau, V. C. and Haddad, J. G. (1975). *New Engl. J. Med.* **292**, 550.
Hallick, R. B. and DeLuca, H. F. (1972). *J. Biol. Chem.* **247**, 91.
Haussler, M. R. and Rasmussen, H. (1972). *J. Biol. Chem.* **247**, 2328.
Hepner, G. W., Roginsky, M. and Moo, H. F. (1975). *In* 'Vitamin D and Problems Related to Uremic Bone Disease' (Ed. Norman, A. W., Schaefer, K., Grigoleit, H. G., v. Herrath, D. and Ritz, E.) p. 325. de Gruyter, Berlin and New York.
Hill, L. F., Van Den Berg, C. J. and Mawer, E. B. (1971). *Nature New Biol.* **232**, 189.
Hill, L. F., Taylor, C. M. and Mawer, E. B. (1974). *Clin. Sci. Molec. Med.* **47**, 14P.
Hill, L. F., Mawer, E. B. and Taylor, C. M. (1975). *In* 'Vitamin D and Problems Related to Uremic Bone Disease' (Ed. Norman, A. W., Schaefer, K., Grigoleit, H. G., v. Herrath, D. and Ritz, E.) p. 775. de Gruyter, Berlin and New York.
Holick, M. F., Kleiner-Bosaller, A., Schnoes, H. K., Kasten, P. M., Boyle, I. T. and DeLuca, H. F. (1973). *J. Biol. Chem.* **248**, 6691.
Holmes, A. M., Enoch, B. A., Taylor, J. L. and Jones, M. E. (1973). *Quart. J. Med.* **42**, 125.
Hughes, M. R., Baylink, D. J., Jones, P. G. and Haussler, M. R. (1976). *J. Clin. Invest.* **58**, 61.
Illig, R., Antener, I. and Prader, A. (1961). *Helv. Paediat. Acta* **16**, 469.
Jones, J. H. (1971). *In* 'The Vitamins: Chemistry, Physiology, Pathology, Methods' (Ed. Sebrell, W. H. Jr. and Harris, R. S.) Vol. 3, p. 285. Academic Press, London and New York.
Kaye, M., Chatterjee, G., Cohen, G. F. and Sager, S. (1970). *Ann. Int. Med.* **73**, 225.
Kodicek, E. (1974). *Lancet* **I**, 325.
Kramer, B. and Gribetz, D. (1971). *In* 'The Vitamins: Chemistry, Physiology, Pathology, Methods' (Ed. Sebrell, W. H. Jr. and Harris, R. S.) Vol. 3, p. 259. Academic Press, London and New York.

Larkins, R. G., MacAuley, S. J., Rapoport, A., Martin, T. J., Tullock, B. R., Byfield, P. G. H., Matthews, E. W. and MacIntyre, I. (1974). *Clin. Sci. Molec. Med.* **46**, 569.
Lawson, D. E. M., Wilson, P. W. and Kodicek, E. (1969). *Biochem. J.* **115**, 269.
Lumb, G. A., Mawer, E. B. and Stanbury, S. W. (1971). *Amer. J. Med.* **50**, 421.
Mahgoub, A. and Sheppard, H. (1975). *Biochem. Biophys. Res. Comm.* **62**, 901.
Mawer, E. B. (1974). *In* 'The Metabolism and Function of Vitamin D'. Biochemical Society Special Publication No. 3, p. 27.
Mawer, E. B. and Backhouse, J. (1969). *Biochem. J.* **112**, 255.
Mawer, E. B., Lumb, G. A. and Stanbury, S. W. (1969). *Nature* (London) **222**, 482.
Mawer, E. B., Backhouse, J., Lumb, G. A. and Stanbury, S. W. (1971a). *Nature New Biol.* **232**, 188.
Mawer, E. B., Lumb, G. A., Schaefer, K. and Stanbury, S. W. (1971b). *Clin. Sci.* **40**, 39.
Mawer, E. B., Backhouse, J., Holman, C. A., Lumb, G. A. and Stanbury, S. W. (1972). *Clin. Sci.* **43**, 413.
Mawer, E. B., Backhouse, J., Taylor, C. M., Lumb, G. A. and Stanbury, S. W. (1973). *Lancet* **I**, 626.
Mawer, E. B., Backhouse, J., Hill, L. F., Lumb, G. A., De Silva, P., Taylor, C. M. and Stanbury, S. W. (1975). *Clin. Sci. Molec. Med.* **48**, 349.
Mawer, E. B., Backhouse, J., Davies, M., Hill, L. F. and Taylor, C. M. (1976). *Lancet* **II**, 1203.
McLaughlin, M., Fairney, A., Lester, E., Raggatt, P. R., Brown, D. J. and Wills, M. R. (1974). *Lancet* **I**, 536.
Morgan, D. B., Paterson, C. R., Woods, C. G., Pulvertaft, C. N. and Fourman, P. (1965). *Lancet* **I**, 1089.
Norman, A. W. and Henry, H. (1974). *Rec. Progr. Horm. Res.* **30**, 431.
Olson, E. B. and DeLuca, H. F. (1969). *Science* **165**, 405.
Pavlovich, H., Garabedian, M. and Balsan, S. (1973). *J. Clin. Invest.* **52**, 2656.
Peacock, M., Gallagher, J. C. and Nordin, B. E. C. (1974). *Lancet* **I**, 1.
Ponchon, G. and DeLuca, H. F. (1969). *J. Nutr.* **99**, 157.
Preece, M. M., Ford, J. A., McIntosh, W. B., Dunnigan, M. G., Tomlinson, S. and O'Riordan, J. L. H. (1973). *Lancet* **I**, 907.
Preece, M. M., Ribot, C. A., Tomlinson, S., Kern, H. T. and O'Riordan, J. L. H. (1974). *Abstr. Europ. Soc. Clin. Invest.* VIIIth Ann. Meeting 59.
Preece, M. M., Tomlinson, S., Ribot, S., Ribot, C. A., Pietrek, J., Korn, H. T., Davies, D. M., Ford, J. A., Dunningan, M. G. and O'Riordan, J. L. H. (1975). *Quart. J. Med.* **44**, 575.
Puschett, J. B., Fernandes, P. C., Boyle, I. T., Gray, R. W., Omdahl, J. L. and DeLuca, H. F. (1972). *Proc. Soc. Exp. Biol. Med.* **141**, 379.
Raisz, L. G. and Trummel, C. L. (1972). *In* 'Endocrinology' (Ed. Taylor, S.) p. 480. Heinemann, London.
Reynolds, J. J., Holick, M. F. and DeLuca, H. F. (1974). *Calc. Tiss. Res.* **15**, 333.
Richens, A. and Rowe, D. J. F. (1970). *Brit. Med. J.* **4**, 73.
Schaefer, K., Opitz, A., Stratz, R., Koch, H. U. and v. Herrath, D. (1971). *Dtsch. Med. Wschr.* **96**, 798.
Stamp, T. C. B. (1975). *Proc. Nutr. Soc.* **34**, 119.
Stamp, T. C. B. and Round, J. M. (1974). *Nature* (London) **247**, 563.
Stamp, T. C. B., Round, J. M., Rowe, D. J. F. and Haddad, J. G. (1972). *Brit. Med. J.* **4**, 9.
Stanbury, S. W. (1973). *In* 'Therapeutic Aspects of Nutrition' (Ed. Jonxis, J. H. P., Visser, H. K. A. and Troelstra, J. A.) p. 28. Sternfert Kroese, Leiden.

Stanbury, S. W. and Lumb, G. A. (1962). *Medicine* (Baltimore) **41**, 1.
Stanbury, S. W., Mawer, E. B., Lumb, G. A., Hill, L. F., Holman, C. A., Jones, M. and Van Den Berg, C. J. (1972). *In* 'Endocrinology' (Ed. Taylor, S.) p. 487. Heinemann, London.
Stanbury, S. W., Mawer, E. B., Lumb, G. A., Hill, L. F., Holman, C. A., Taylor, C. M. and Torkington, P. (1973). *In* 'Clinical Aspects of Metabolic Bone Disease' (Ed. Frame, B., Parfitt, A. M. and Duncan, H.) p. 562. Excerpta Medica, Amsterdam.
Stanbury, S. W., Mawer, E. B., Hill, L. F., Taylor, C. N., de Silva, P. and Lumb, G. A. (1975a). *In* 'Calcium Regulating Hormones' (Ed. Talmage, R. V., Owen, M. and Parsons, J. A.) p. 431. Excerpta Medica, Amsterdam.
Stanbury, S. W., Mawer, E. B., Lumb, G. A., Hill, L. F., de Silva, P. and Taylor, C. M. (1975b). *In* 'Vitamin D and Problems Related to Uremic Bone Disease' (Ed. Norman, A. W., Schaefer, K., Grigoleit, H. G., v. Herrath, D. and Ritz, E.) p. 205. de Gruyter, Berlin and New York.
Stanbury, S. W., Torkington, P., Lumb, G. A., Adams, P. H., de Silva, P. and Taylor, C. M. (1975). *Proc. Nutr. Soc.* **34**, 111.
Taylor, C. M., Mawer, E. B. and Reeve, A. (1973). *Biochem. Soc. Trans.* **1**, 596.
Taylor, C. M., Mawer, E. B. and Reeve, A. (1975). *Clin. Sci. Molec. Med.* **49**, 391.
Taylor, C. M., Hughes, S. E. and de Silva, P. (1976). *Biochem. Biophys. Res. Commun.* **70**, 1243.
Thomas, W. C., Morgan, H. G., Connor, T. B., Haddock, L., Bills, C. E. and Howard, T. E. (1959). *J. Clin. Invest.* **38**, 1078.
Thompson, G. R., Lewis, B. and Booth, C. C. (1966). *J. Clin. Invest.* **45**, 94.
Trummel, C., Raisz, L. G., Blunt, J. W. and DeLuca, H. F. (1969). *Science* **163**, 1450.
Warkany, J. (1936). *Amer. J. Dis. Child.* **52**, 831.
Warkany, J. and Mabon, H. E. (1940). *Amer. J. Dis. Child.* **60**, 606.
Windorfer, A. (1938). *Klinische Wochenschrift* **17**, 228.
Zerwekh, J. E., Brumbaugh, P. F., Haussler, D. H., Cork, D. J. and Haussler, M. R. (1974). *Biochemistry* **13**, 4097.

9 Clinical Aspects of Vitamin D Metabolism in Man

S. W. STANBURY AND E. B. MAWER

I Vitamin D Metabolism in Renal Disease

A RENAL FAILURE

A relationship between chronic renal disease and the development of a form of rickets was recognised by Lucas (1883) and much later it was also shown that azotaemic adults might develop osteomalacia (Stanbury, 1957). This defective skeletal mineralisation in both children and adults was histologically indistinguishable from the osteopathy of simple vitamin D deficiency, and Liu and Chu (1943) suggested that uraemia might cause some interference with the action of the vitamin. Metabolic studies demonstrated intestinal malabsorption of calcium and other changes compatible with an 'apparent vitamin D-deficiency' or 'vitamin D-resistance' (Liu and Chu, 1943; Dent *et al.*, 1961; Stanbury and Lumb, 1962). To produce the biological effects of the vitamin, patients with advanced renal failure required a greater intake of vitamin D and higher levels of total antiricketic activity in the plasma than did normal individuals (Lumb *et al.*, 1971). But, so long as appropriate pharmacological doses of vitamin D were administered, it was invariably possible to correct the intestinal malabsorption of calcium and to heal this form of renal osteodystrophy (Stanbury and Lumb, 1962; Stanbury, 1962a, 1968a; Lumb *et al.*, 1971).

In spite of previous claims to the contrary (Avioli *et al.*, 1968a), it was shown that the uraemic patient had a normal capacity to 25-hydroxylate cholecalciferol and that the 25-hydroxy-metabolite formed *in vivo* survived normally in the circulation (Mawer *et al.*, 1971b, 1972; Stanbury *et al.*, 1972). It also became evident that the intestinal malabsorption of calcium was relatively unresponsive to high plasma concentrations of 25-hydroxycholecalciferol (Mawer *et al.*, 1971b); and, although this metabolite was unquestionably capable of healing azotaemic rickets, this therapeutic effect was produced only by pharmacological dosage (Witmer and Balsan, 1971). With the demonstration by Fraser and Kodicek (1970) of the indispensability of the kidneys for the synthesis of 1,25-dihydroxycholecalciferol, many previously unexplained aspects of renal osteodystrophy appeared to find a satisfactory explanation. Mawer *et al.* (1971a) found no formation of labelled hormone from a pulse of [1,2-$^{3}H_2$,4-^{14}C] cholecalciferol in an anephric patient; subsequently, among a group of 10 patients with advanced renal failure (endogenous creatinine clearance less than 23 ml/min), detectable formation of labelled 1,25-dihydroxycholecalciferol was found in only one (Mawer *et al.*, 1973). More direct measurement, both by biological assay (Hill *et al.*, 1974) and by protein binding assay (Brumbaugh *et al.*, 1974a, b), has demonstrated 1,25-dihydroxycholecalciferol in the serum of patients with advanced chronic renal failure but in significantly lower concentration than in healthy control subjects. The reasons for this discrepancy between the results obtained with the radioisotopic technique and by assay are not immediately apparent; but both suggest an impaired formation and a conditioned deficiency of this hormonal metabolite in advanced renal disease.

Experimental trials using biosynthetically and chemically prepared 1,25-dihydroxycholecalciferol in uraemic patients during the last four years have supported this proposition. Intestinal absorption of calcium is increased in uraemic and anephric patients given oral doses ranging from 0.28 μg/day to 5.4 μg/day (Brickman *et al.*, 1972, 1974, 1976). Bodily retention of calcium was found to increase with oral doses ranging from 0.68 μg to 1.0 μg (Silverberg *et al.*, 1975, Brickman *et al.*, 1974; and personal observations). 1α-Hydroxycholecalciferol (oral doses of 1–2 μg/day) has also been used in the treatment of the osteodystrophy in chronic renal failure with essentially identical results (Catto *et al.*, 1975; Davie *et al.*, 1976; Chan *et al.*, 1975). In patients with azotaemic rickets or osteomalacia, administration of comparably small doses of 1,25-dihydroxycholecalciferol has increased the extent of the calcification front in bone (Bordier *et al.*, 1975; personal observations) and, after an initial apparent stimulation of osteoclastic activity (Bordier *et al.*, 1975), continued administration has produced a reduction of bone resorption and of osteitis fibrosa (Coburn *et al.*, 1975; Bordier *et al.*, 1975). These beneficial effects on the bone were accompanied by a reduction of serum alkaline phosphatase and of serum iPTH[1], the latter change showing a crude inverse relationship to the induced increase in serum calcium (Coburn *et al.*, 1975; Chan *et al.*, 1975; Davie *et al.*, 1976).

The progressive healing of azotaemic rickets and reversal of the radiographic signs of secondary hyperparathyroidism with daily doses from 0.68 to 1.35 μg continued over many weeks has been observed (Henderson *et al.*, 1974; Chan *et al.*, 1975; Silverberg *et al.*, 1975; Davies *et al.*, 1977a and personal observations). It thus appears that minute doses of the hormone will reproduce, in advanced renal failure and in renal osteodystrophy, all the effects previously shown to result from the administration of 25-hydroxycholecalciferol, cholecalciferol or ergocalciferol at a level of dosage hundreds or even thousands of times greater; and it is reasonable to infer that the 'apparent vitamin D-deficiency' of the uraemic patient is actually a deficiency of 1,25-dihydroxycholecalciferol.

It is perhaps necessary to re-emphasise that all these recently documented effects of 1,25-dihydroxycholecalciferol in uraemic patients had been produced earlier by pharmacological doses of vitamins D_2 or D_3 and of the 25-hydroxy-metabolite and the therapeutic effectiveness of these materials in renal osteodystrophy has been established conclusively (Stanbury and Lumb, 1962; Stanbury, 1962a, 1966, 1967). It is intrinsically unlikely that their effects are produced by mass action, through increased formation of the hormone in the renal remnant, since the formation of this metabolite from cholecalciferol is normally related inversely to the serum concentration of 25-hydroxycalciferol (Mawer *et al.*, 1975a). A more probable explanation for their effectiveness is that the specificity of tissue receptors is relative and that an excess of 25-hydroxycholecalciferol or perhaps even of cholecalciferol, can substitute for the normal effector molecule and activate calcium transport. Such an effect has been demonstrated *in vitro* (Corradino and Wasserman, 1971) and in the anephric rat (Hill *et al.*, 1971). Since 25-hydroxylation appears to occur normally in the uraemic patient, and treatment with large oral doses of vitamin D_2 or D_3 sustains greatly elevated levels of 25-hydroxycalciferol in the serum of such patients (Mawer *et al.*, 1971b), it seems reasonable to attribute the beneficial effects of such therapy to the endogenously synthesised 25-hydroxy derivative.

1,25-Dihydroxycholecalciferol could well have distinct advantages over

[1] iPTH: immunoassayable parathyroid hormone.

ergocalciferol and 25-hydroxycholecalciferol in the treatment of renal osteodystrophy, since studies with [26-^{3}H]1,25-dihydroxycholecalciferol showed that it was rapidly metabolised (chapter 8, section VC) and clinical observations suggest that the duration of action of small doses in man is short (Brickman *et al.*, 1974; Henderson *et al.*, 1974; Coburn *et al.*, 1975). Although 1,25-dihydroxycholecalciferol is widely distributed to the tissues following its oral or intravenous administration to animals (Lawson and Emtage, 1974; Mawer *et al.*, 1975b), there are no reasons to expect that it will be stored significantly in the tissues as are the calciferols and the 25-hydroxy-metabolite (Mawer *et al.*, 1972). The requirement for calciferol or for 25-hydroxy-cholecalciferol is unpredictable in the individual uraemic patient (Lumb *et al.*, 1971) and it is conceivable that unidentified factors in the uraemic state modify the target organ responsiveness to these non-specific sterols; whereas evidence to date suggests that 'near physiological' doses of the normal effector, 1,25-dihydroxycholecalciferol, may always be effective in uraemia. Thus it should be possible to define a minimal dose of 1,25-dihydroxy-cholecalciferol, possibly within the narrow range of 0.35 to 1 μg/day, that is predictably effective in the treatment of established cases of renal osteo-dystrophy and conceivably also potentially useful as prophylaxis against the development of bone disease in patients maintained by chronic haemodialysis.

Comparably small doses of the less expensive analogue 1α-hydroxycholecalciferol should serve the same purpose but the potency ratio of the two sterols in uraemia is not yet firmly established.

It is critically important that a natural wish to utilise 1,25-dihydroxychole-calciferol and its 1α-hydroxy-analogue therapeutically should not ignore the lessons learned over many years from the use of calciferol in treating renal osteodystrophy. It is suggested frequently that these newly available sterols might be used with greater safety than surgery (Stanbury *et al.*, 1960) to reverse severe secondary hyperparathyroidism in renal failure. But it has been demonstrated that small amounts of the hormone will partly restore the impaired capacity of parathyroid hormone to raise the serum calcium in acute uraemia (Massry *et al.*, 1975); and the administration of 1,25-dihydroxycho-lecalciferol (2.7 μg/day) to a patient with overt azotaemic hyperpara-thyroidism produced an extreme degree of hypercalcaemia (Brickman *et al.*, 1972). These effects were entirely predictable on the basis of experience with calciferol. Conversely, an early rise in serum calcium should not necessarily be expected during effective treatment of azotaemic osteomalacia with 1,25-dihydroxycholecalciferol. In this condition, the production of a massive positive balance of calcium by ergocalciferol may sometimes cause no elevation of the serum calcium until the bone disease is healed (Stanbury and Lumb, 1962); we have made similar observations when treating azotaemic rickets with the hormone (unpublished observations). Once the osteomalacia has been healed, continued treatment with ergocalciferol can rapidly induce hypercalcaemia; it can be predicted confidently that continued treatment with the hormonal metabolite in the same circumstances would be at least equally hazardous. Thus the use of 1,25-dihydroxycholecalciferol and its 1-hydroxy-analogue will require the same careful surveillance of the individual patient as has been advocated in many publications from this laboratory describing the therapeutic use of calciferol in renal failure.

In spite of these cautionary strictures, there is considerable scope for further study of the effects of 1,25-dihydroxycholecalciferol in renal failure; but its safe and rational therapeutic use will depend on knowledge of its rate of turnover in man (Mawer *et al.*, 1976) and of the mechanisms of its transport in human plasma, as well as on the availability of a simple method for monitoring its plasma concentration. In animals it is established that the target tissues – intestinal mucosa, bone, kidney and also liver – concentrate 1,25-dihydroxycholecalciferol from the circulating plasma but the details of this process vary with the species and with the route of administration (Lawson and Emtage, 1974; Mawer *et al.*, 1975b). Thus, in the chick 1,25-dihydroxycholecalciferol accumulates equally rapidly in the intestinal mucosa from an oral as from an intravenous dose, and plasma levels fall rapidly; in the rat, intestinal 1,25-dihydroxycholecalciferol is built up rapidly from an oral dose but relatively slowly from an intravenous dose, and relatively high plasma levels are produced by both routes of administration (Mawer *et al.*, 1975b). These differences may be determined by the relative binding affinities or binding capacities of the plasma carrier proteins for the hormone in the two species. It is also to be emphasised that these results were obtained with single pulse dosage. Under conditions of daily therapeutic dosage in man, it is reasonable to expect that treatment would rapidly saturate the binding sites in target organs; and, if the dose administered exceeded the combined losses due to catabolism of 1,25-dihydroxycholecalciferol and desquamation of intestinal mucosal cells, any therapeutic surplus might accumulate in the plasma. Preliminary studies suggest that the binding capacity of human plasma for 1,25-dihydroxycholecalciferol may greatly exceed the amount of the hormone produced physiologically (Belsey *et al.*, 1974). 1,25-Dihydroxycholecalciferol has an uniquely potent osteolytic action, increasing bone resorption by stimulating existing osteoclasts and also by recruiting the formation of new osteoclasts (Reynolds, 1974). 1α-Hydroxycholecalciferol is approximately equally active *in vivo*, presumably through its conversion to 1,25-dihydroxycholecalciferol (Reynolds *et al.*, 1974). In attempting to reverse azotaemic hyperparathyroidism by the therapeutic use of 1,25-dihydroxycholecalciferol these osteolytic effects might thus increase the severity of the bone lesions being treated and, in concert with the effects of the hormone on the intestinal and renal tubular absorption of calcium will tend to produce an unpredictable degree of hypercalcaemia. Unless 1,25-dihydroxycholecalciferol has a direct inhibitory effect on the parathyroid glands (Section IIIB) the successful reversal of secondary hyperparathyroidism is likely to require the therapeutic maintenance of a minimum degree of hypercalcaemia. To achieve this will necessitate meticulous management of the individual patient and it will not be easy to avoid potentially toxic effects when treating azotaemic hyperparathyroidism with the hormone.

B SOME OUTSTANDING PROBLEMS OF VITAMIN D METABOLISM IN RENAL DISEASE

Clinically obvious renal osteodystrophy is encountered only in patients with advanced renal impairment, and it has seemed reasonable to assume that the development of 1,25-dihydroxycholecalciferol-deficiency in such patients is a simple consequence of the progressive loss of the tissue responsible for its production. Although there is now good evidence that parathyroid secretion may increase from the earliest stages of renal disease (see Stanbury, 1972b), there has been no systematic study of the histological state of the bone in patients with minimum renal impairment and no observations on the formation of 1,25-dihydroxycholecalciferol or of its plasma concentration in such subjects. Recently a deliberate attempt has been made to assess the state of the bone early in the course of primary renal disease. Somewhat surprisingly, clear histological evidence of osteomalacia (and, less remarkably, of secondary hyperparathyroidism) has been documented in patients with early renal impairment (serum creatinine <2.5 mg/100 ml; Ritz *et al.*, 1975) and even in patients with histologically proven primary renal disease but no significant impairment or renal function (serum creatinine, 0.58 to 1.25 mg/100 ml; glomerular filtration, 130 to 85 ml/min, Bonucci *et al.*, 1975). If the osteomalacic component in this bone disease is due to a deficiency of the hormone as postulated for the osteomalacia of advanced renal failure, it cannot be attributed to the loss of renal tissue; at this stage of renal disease the greater mass of renal tissue is intact. These observations may have one of two possible implications. Either the osteomalacia, which appears to be a true defect of mineralisation (Ritz *et al.*, 1975; Bonucci *et al.*, 1975), is not due to a deficiency of 1,25-dihydroxycholecalciferol or there is some factor operating to inhibit the formation of this substance in the structurally intact tubules of the diseased kidney. If the latter option should prove to be correct, it is obvious that the same factor may continue to operate throughout the course of the renal disease. Indeed, we have commented previously (Hill and Stanbury, 1975) that it is remarkable the failing kidney should apparently fail so completely in the synthesis of 1,25-dihydroxycholecalciferol despite increased secretion of the putative trophic stimulus, parathyroid hormone.

There have, however, been very few studies of 1,25-dihydroxycholecalciferol formation or of its serum concentration at any stage of renal disease. These recent observations indicate a need for detailed studies of the formation of both 1,25- and 24,25-dihydroxycholecalciferol in early renal disease; and it is equally desirable to observe the effects of deprivation of phosphorus on the formation of these metabolites in advanced renal failure. If the patient with early renal disease is found to be deficient of 1,25-dihydroxycholecalciferol we may be faced with the tendentious question as to whether he should be treated prophylactically with 'physiological' doses of the hormone or its 1-hydroxy-analogue.

Prophylaxis with 1,25-dihydroxycholecalciferol early in spontaneously evolving renal disease is probably unnecessary, since overt osteodystrophy can be treated fairly easily as it develops; but the situation is different in the chronically uraemic patient maintained by intermittent haemodialysis. Clinically severe bone disease has been frequent in dialysed patients and its prevention and treatment is of both academic and economic importance. The situation has been confused and difficult (see Stanbury, 1972b); from the lack of adequate documentation of the nature of the bony changes: from uncertainty whether the dialytic procedure itself contributes to producing the bone disease; and from difficulty in predicting the physiological effectiveness of the calciferols, dihydrotachysterol or 25-hydroxycholecalciferol used in its attempted treatment. The consensus of evidence now suggests that 'dialytic bone disease' can be regarded as qualitatively the same as azotaemic osteodystrophy (Krempien *et al.*, 1972; Ritz *et al.*, 1973); as such, it should be amenable to the same treatment as is bone disease in undialysed patients with renal failure. A considerable measure of success in the prevention and treatment of dialytic bone disease has been achieved by the use of massive oral doses of calcium salts and by dialysis against high concentrations of calcium. Use of the calciferols and the 25-hydroxy-metabolite has been generally eschewed because of their potential for inducing hypercalcaemic intoxication and the prolonged duration of their effects. Since very small doses of 1,25-dihydroxycholecalciferol are effective in the anephric patient and since the action of this sterol is apparently short-lived, its use might well provide an alternative and more physiological means of managing bone disease in dialysed patients. Catto *et al.* (1975) have demonstrated a progressive increase in skeletal calcium from the use of oral doses of 1 to 2 μg/day of 1α-hydroxycholecalciferol over a period of three months. As bone disease is probably already established in a majority of patients when dialysis is commenced, a case can be made for the use of the hormone or an analogue from the start of this treatment, as 'prophylaxis' against the potentially devastating effects of its progression. But, such therapy should still be regarded as tentative and experimental.

One other aspect of calciferol metabolism in renal failure warrants comment. Following the original observations of Avioli *et al.* (1968a), there have been several suggestions that the formation and metabolism of 25-hydroxycholecalciferol may be abnormal in renal failure. It has been proposed that hyperphosphataemia may interfere with the 25-hydroxylation of cholecalciferol; that a tendency to low levels of serum 25-hydroxy-calciferol in uraemia may reflect its accelerated catabolism; and that the pattern of prevailing osteodystrophy, whether predominantly osteomalacia or predominantly osteitis fibrosa, can be correlated with the prevailing serum concentration of 25-hydroxycholecalciferol. In radioisotopic studies of calciferol metabolism, we found no apparent difference between the formation of radioactive 25-hydroxycholecalciferol by uraemic patients and nutritionally matched healthy controls; the rate of decay of the metabolically produced 25-hydroxycholecalciferol was also apparently appropriate to the nutritional state of the individual patient (Mawer *et al.*, 1971b, 1972; Stanbury *et al.*, 1973). Offerman and Dittmar (1975) found no correlation between serum 25-hydroxycholecalciferol level and the type of osteodystrophy and considered that the serum level of this metabolite in the uraemic patient simply reflects his dietary intake and solar exposure. While we would tend to agree with the latter suggestion, it would be unwise to dismiss the alternative propositions without further study. In a careful study of experimental phosphorus deprivation in healthy adult volunteers, Gray *et al.* (1975) demonstrated a significantly accelerated disappearance of injected radioactive 25-hydroxycholecalciferol from the plasma of phosphorus deprived subjects. It was calculated that the mean turnover of this metabolite in the same subjects, was 5.0 μg/day during phosphorus depletion and 2.8 μg/day ($p < .02$) when eating a normal diet. Thus the metabolism of 25-hydroxycholecalciferol appears to be influenced by the state of phosphorus nutrition in man as in the rat (Tanaka and DeLuca, 1973). It remains to be determined whether the accelerated turnover of 25-hydroxycholecalciferol in the phosphorus deficient subject is entirely accountable in terms of increased formation of the hormonal metabolite or whether other metabolic pathways are also involved.

C RENAL TUBULAR DISORDERS (EXCLUDING X-LINKED HYPOPHOSPHATAEMIA, q.v.)

Recognition of the role of the kidney in the intermediary metabolism of vitamin D will necessitate re-examination of the various forms of rickets and osteomalacia associated with disorders of renal tubular function (Dent, 1952; Dent and Harris, 1958). In these conditions, which may be either genetically determined or acquired, there is impairment of one or more specific renal tubular functions and glomerular function is apparently normal or reduced in minor degree. In those cases developing rickets or osteomalacia there is either hypophosphataemia, due to reduced renal tubular reabsorption of phosphate ('Fanconi syndrome', cystine storage disease, etc.) or systemic acidosis due to impairment of the renal tubular function of hydrion secretion (renal tubular acidosis). In the primarily phosphaturic disorders, the bone disease is commonly regarded as a form of 'low phosphate rickets' and there is some evidence that the bony abnormalities may be healed by treatment with massive supplements of phosphate salts (Wilson and Yendt, 1963). It has been estimated that perhaps 25% of patients with renal tubular acidosis may develop defective mineralisation of bone (Richards *et al.*, 1972) and, in a few instances, the bone disease has apparently been cured by treatment with alkali alone (Richards *et al.*, 1972; Dundon *et al.*, 1966). Since renal tubular acidosis is commonly associated with hypophosphataemia, which is largely corrected when the acidaemia is controlled by alkali therapy (Stanbury, 1971), this form of bone disease is also commonly attributed to hypophosphataemia (Morgan, 1973).

All these conditions are relatively rare and, in most reported cases, the complicating rickets or osteomalacia has been treated successfully with variably large doses of vitamin D, sometimes without the use of alkali or supplements of phosphate. There have been few adequate studies of external mineral balance or of the intestinal absorption of calcium in these renal tubular forms of osteomalacia; but when appropriate investigations have been made an apparent intestinal malabsorption of calcium has been found in several of these syndromes (Stanbury, 1967). This, and the therapeutic response to large amounts of vitamin D, raises the question of whether calciferol metabolism may be disturbed in some of these cases, as in azotaemic osteomalacia. The improvement of bone disease on treatment with alkalis or phosphate supplements without vitamin D makes this unlikely unless, in the case of renal tubular acidosis, systemic acidosis interferes with the 1α-hydroxylation of 25-hydroxycholecalciferol. The lack of obvious signs of secondary hyperparathyroidism in renal tubular acidosis has also been taken as evidence against an involvement of cholecalciferol in the causation of the accompanying bone disease (Morgan, 1973); but increased levels of serum iPTH have recently been documented in cases of renal tubular acidosis with 'normal' levels of glomerular filtration (Gonick *et al.*, 1973). As has been indicated previously (Stanbury, 1967), there is a lack of adequate documentation of the relevant parameters of calcium metabolism in these syndromes and no studies of cholecalciferol metabolism in affected patients have yet been reported. In default of this information, further discussion would be unprofitable. However, recent observations on one of the rarer acquired forms of multifactorial renal tubular disorder – due to cadmium intoxication – suggest that further investigation of cholecalciferol metabolism should be undertaken in the whole field of 'renal tubular disorders'.

It is known that chronic industrial exposure to cadmium in various forms can give rise to a specific 'tubular' form of proteinuria and to abnormalities of renal tubular function including glycosuria, aminoaciduria, and an impaired renal excretion of acid with a tendency to hyperchloraemic acidosis (Kazantzis *et al.*, 1963). Nicaud *et al.* (1942) described osteomalacia as a complication of chronic cadmium poisoning and a single case was reported by Adams *et al.* (1969). More recently, a similar association of renal tubular disorder and osteomalacia (itai-itai or 'ouch-ouch' disease) has been reported from Japan in people consuming water and crops industrially contaminated with heavy metals; the evidence indicates that cadmium is most probably responsible (Tsuchiya, 1969). Larrson and Lorentzon (1975) have studied the metabolism of ^{3}H-labelled 25-hydroxycholecalciferol in rats exposed to 25 and 75 p.p.m. of cadmium in the drinking water. In animals receiving a diet containing 1.2% calcium and 0.7% phosphorus, there was an apparent inhibition of the formation of 1,25-dihydroxycholecalciferol with a corresponding increased formation of 24,25-dihydroxy-metabolite; this inhibitory effect of cadmium exposure on the renal 1α-hydroxylation of 25-hydroxycholecalciferol was prevented if animals were fed on a diet low in calcium (0.04% Ca.). The latter observation is of especial interest in suggesting that this effect of cadmium may be indirect and not due to a non-specific toxic destructive effect on the kidney. It is analogous to the effects of a low calcium diet in preventing the indirect inhibition of 1,25-dihydroxycholecalciferol formation in rats treated by ethane-1-hydroxy-1, 1- diphosphonate (Hill *et al.*, 1973). These observations on the effects of cadmium, and the attribution of 'strontium rickets' in the rat to inhibition of the renal 25-hydroxycholecalciferol-1-hydroxylase (Omdahl and DeLuca, 1971), reinforce the need for re-appraisal of the nature of some forms of 'renal tubular' osteomalacia. Multifactorial renal tubular disorders associated with osteomalacia may occur with the chronic cupric intoxication of Wilson's disease (Bearn *et al.*, 1957); exceptionally, similar abnormalities and rickets may complicate lead poisoning (Chisholm *et al.*, 1955). In these conditions, as well as in the renal tubular disorders associated with myelomatosis, glycogenosis and tyrosinosis – all of which may be associated with the development of rickets or osteomalacia – investigation of cholecalciferol metabolism could well prove profitable.

It is often assumed that the tubular disorder(s) in these various syndromes is an isolated functional lesion in an otherwise structurally and functionally intact kidney. While this appears to be true in some cases, others also have a greater or lesser degree of impaired glomerular function (Stanbury, 1967). In other words, even although the specific tubular abnormality may be the dominant feature, there is evidence of diffuse renal damage in such cases. Since osteomalacia has been demonstrated in patients with glomerulonephritis and 'normal' glomerular filtration (Bonucci *et al.*, 1975; Section 1B), attribution of the development of osteomalacia to a specific tubular lesion may be hazardous. Adequate understanding of the pathogenesis of bone disease in 'renal tubular disorders' requires further detailed studies of mineral metabolism and of vitamin D metabolism in the individually delineated syndromes.

II Some Forms of 'Vitamin D-Resistant Rickets' and Osteomalacia

A PSEUDO-VITAMIN D-DEFICIENCY OR VITAMIN D-DEPENDENT RICKETS

This is an autosomal recessive disorder, the clinical manifestations of which develop slowly during the first year of life and mimic in virtually all respects the syndrome of simple nutritional deficiency in vitamin D (Prader *et al.*, 1961). It is accompanied by hypocalcaemia, hypophosphataemia, raised serum alkaline phosphatase, hyperaminoaciduria and elevated serum levels of iPTH (Arnaud *et al.*, 1972); and it is associated with severe rickets, retardation of growth and other clinical features shared with vitamin D-deficiency. It differs from the latter syndrome in being curable by vitamin D but only in large doses approaching 10^3 the estimated normal requirement; and such pharmacological dosage is required throughout life to prevent relapse. As suggested previously (Stanbury, 1972a), this is the one form of genetically determined rickets in which it was reasonable to expect an innate disorder of cholecalciferol metabolism. In all cases so far studied, the dosage of 25-hydroxycholecalciferol required to control the disease has also been within the pharmacological range; requirement for ergocalciferol or cholecalciferol is 1 mg/day or more, and for 25-hydroxycholecalciferol 0.5–1.0 mg/day (Balsan and Garabedian, 1972; Fraser *et al.*, 1973). Such observations, and the demonstration of elevated concentrations of the 25-hydroxy-metabolite in the serum of patients treated with high dosage of vitamin D (Haddad *et al.*, 1973; Fraser *et al.*, 1973) indicate that any disorder of cholecalciferol metabolism is at a step subsequent to 25-hydroxylation.

Indirect evidence that the disease may arise on the basis of a deficiency or defect of renal 25-hydroxycholecalciferol-1α-hydroxylase has been provided by therapeutic observations using 1,25-dihydroxycholecalciferol. Fraser *et al.* (1973) have shown that the biochemical and clinical abnormalities can be corrected by daily intravenous doses of 1 μg of the hormone; in a small group of patients the ratios of effective dosage of vitamin D:25-

hydroxycholecalciferol:1,25-dihydroxycholecalciferol averaged 1700:500:1. Essentially similar results have been obtained with the same dose administered orally and with the oral administration of 2–3 μg/day of 1-hydroxycholecalciferol (Balsan *et al.*, 1976; Prader, 1976; Reade *et al.*, 1975; Scriver *et al.*, 1976).

Although these observations are compatible with an innate defect of 1α-hydroxylation this hypothesis will require confirmation by direct studies of 25-hydroxycholecalciferol-1α-hydroxylase in renal tissue. It is also conceivable that the syndrome is not homogeneous and it remains hypothetically possible, if unlikely, that the probands in some families could develop the effects of 'vitamin D-deficiency' on the basis of defective 25-hydroxylation or of unresponsiveness of the target cells. A young child with what is now appreciated to be vitamin D-dependent rickets was described briefly by Stanbury (1962a). After some 14 years of successful continued treatment with 2.5 mg/day of ergocalciferol, it has been possible to assay the serum of this patient for 1,25-dihydroxycalciferol. At a time when the serum 25-hydroxycalciferol was very high ($\sim$100 ng/ml) there was no assayable 1,25-dihydroxy-metabolite in two separately assayed blood samples (L. F. Hill, private communication). To date, this is the most direct evidence available for a deficiency of the renal 25-hydroxycholecalciferol-1-hydroxylase in this syndrome.

B X-LINKED HYPOPHOSPHATAEMIC RICKETS AND OSTEOMALACIA

This X-linked dominant disorder, which also causes a form of rickets developing during the first year of life, has no other features in common with the effects of simple vitamin D-deficiency or of vitamin D-dependency. There is no associated hypocalcaemia nor aminoaciduria, and serum iPTH is normal or low in the untreated patient (Arnaud *et al.*, 1971). Treatment with vitamin D or with 25-hydroxycholecalciferol (Balsan and Garabedian, 1972; Puschett *et al.*, 1975) in pharmacological dosage is only partially successful in healing the rickets and relapse is usual even when an initially effective dose is continued. A claim that 25-hydroxycholecalciferol is converted to water soluble and biologically inert metabolites in this disease (Avioli *et al.*, 1967b) has not been confirmed (Mawer and Stanbury, unpublished observations) and normal or elevated levels of 25-hydroxycalciferol are found in the serum of affected patients treated with vitamin D (Haddad *et al.*, 1973). There is thus little, either in its clinical or biochemical features or in its response to therapy, to suggest that this disease is associated with disordered vitamin D metabolism. A suggested hypothesis invokes a primary defect of the transepithelial transport of orthophosphate (Glorieux *et al.*, 1973). There is, indeed, evidence for a specific impairment of the parathyroid hormone-sensitive component of phosphate transport in the renal tubule (Glorieux and Scriver, 1972). This is responsible for the persistent hypophosphataemia in this syndrome and probably also for the defective skeletal mineralisation. On the other hand, studies of Hahn *et al.* (1975) have not confirmed these observations on the renal transport of phosphate and in addition there is no good evidence that the intestinal epithelium shares in this transport defect. In addition there are features of the bone disease in affected adults which are difficult to reconcile with a causation by a simple deficiency of phosphorus (Stanbury, 1976).

One factor furthering the belief that the action of vitamin D is disturbed in this disease was the demonstration of apparently impaired intestinal net absorption of calcium in affected children (Stickler, 1963). But failure of growth is a cardinal clinical feature of the disease and it is possible that the sub-normal absorption of calcium in children is a consequence of the retarded growth rate rather than a primary attribute of the disease itself. A recent examination in untreated affected adults suggests that their calcium absorption, both when taking a normal diet and when receiving large amounts of calcium salts orally, is within the range of normal (Stanbury, 1976). Also compatible with the exoneration of vitamin D in the pathogenesis of this syndrome, treatment with 'physiological' doses of 1,25-dihydroxycholecalciferol has proved no more effective than massive doses of the native vitamin or its 25-hydroxy-metabolite (Brickman *et al.*, 1973; Glorieux *et al.*, 1973). The latter authors demonstrated a transient restoration of normal renal tubular reabsorption of phosphate following the intravenous administration of the hormone but this effect was not sustained on continued treatment. Since a similar temporary correction of the tubular transport defect can be produced by infusion of calcium salts (Glorieux and Scriver, 1972), they suggest that the acute effects of 1,25-dihydroxycholecalciferol may also be due to its effects on renal cellular calcium. These observations are essentially of pharmacological interest and they do not in any way support the idea of disordered calciferol metabolism in this disorder. There are many bizarre and puzzling features of X-linked hypophosphataemia, more especially in the later life of affected individuals, for which none of the prevailing hypotheses provides adequate explanation. It is unlikely that further studies of calciferol metabolism will add materially to the problem.

C MAGNESIUM DEFICIENCY AND 'MAGNESIUM-DEPENDENT' RICKETS

Magnesium deficiency and hypomagnesaemia arise most commonly as a complication of diarrhoea and intestinal malabsorption syndromes (MacIntyre *et al.*, 1961; Heaton and Fourman, 1965); less frequently in association with alcoholism and various other diseases (Wacker and Parisi, 1968); and rarely as a disease *sui generis* ('primary hypomagnesaemia'; Paunier *et al.*, 1968; Friedman *et al.*, 1967). In a significant proportion of such patients with hypomagnesaemia the serum calcium is also reduced, to levels causing frank tetany, and this hypocalcaemia is corrected promptly on restoration of the magnesium deficit (Shils, 1969; Muldowney *et al.*, 1970). The pathogenesis of this hypocalcaemia has been the subject of debate. Observations based largely on hypomagnesaemic patients with alcoholism or intestinal malabsorption suggested that the hypocalcaemia was due to unresponsiveness of the target organs, especially the bone, to parathyroid hormone (Estep *et al.*, 1969; Muldowney *et al.*, 1970). More recent studies in primary hypomagnesaemia strongly suggest that magnesium depletion causes impaired synthesis or secretion of parathyroid hormone (Suh *et al.*, 1973; Anast *et al.*, 1972) and this conclusion is also supported by experimental studies in the puppy and monkey (Suh *et al.*, 1971; Dunn, 1971).

Hypomagnesaemia is often first detected in hypocalcaemic patients with intestinal malabsorption when treatment with calcium salts and massive doses of ergocalciferol has failed to restore the serum calcium. In this respect, and in contrast to the usual satisfactory response of patients with idiopathic hypoparathyroidism (Section IIIA) similarly treated, such patients can be regarded as relatively resistant to pharmacological doses of vitamin D. In the presence of hypomagnesaemia, the hypocalcaemia of hypoparathyroidism may also be unresponsive to treatment with vitamin D. A daily dose of 30 mg (1.2×10^6 i.u.) of ergocalciferol failed to influence the hypocalcaemia in a patient with hypoparathyroidism; after correction of the associated hypomagnesaemia, the hypocalcaemia was controlled by a dose of 2.5–5 mg/day (Rösler and Rabinowitz, 1973). Qualitatively comparable observations have been reported in other cases of hypoparathyroidism. Although these observations are concerned with the effects of pharmacological doses of vitamin D, they raise the possibility that magnesium deficiency may interfere with the conversion of calciferol to its biologically more potent hydroxylated derivatives. The situation has become further complicated with the recent reporting of apparently 'magnesium-dependent' rickets. Reddy and Sivakumar (1974) described two Indian children with what appeared to be simple vitamin D-deficiency rickets, which failed to show biochemical or radiographic response to treatment with large doses (15 mg/day) of ergocalciferol until the associated hypomagnesaemia was corrected. The time allowed to assess responsiveness to the administered vitamin D was, in our opinion, short but the recorded effects of magnesium administration were impressive none the less. These effects suggested that administration of magnesium salts increased greatly the biological effectiveness of vitamin D given. (Parenthetically, in a large personal experience of nutritional rickets and osteomalacia among Asians in this country, we have encountered no case with hypomagnesaemia comparable to the levels recorded by Reddy and Sivakumar; the cause of the low serum magnesium in their patients was not established.) A third example of apparently magnesium-dependent rickets has been reported from Spain (Rapado *et al.*, 1975) in a child with hypercalciuria and nephrocalcinosis. Treatment with cellulose phosphate and chlorothiazide, in an attempt to reduce the hypercalciuria, was followed by the development of hypomagnesaemia, hypocalcaemia and the radiographic signs of rickets. Subsequent treatment with magnesium sulphate corrected the acquired biochemical abnormalities and was followed by radiographic healing of the rickets. While these interesting cases suggest a possible effect of magnesium deficiency on vitamin D metabolism, their investigation was insufficiently detailed to establish or refute this possibility.

In patients developing hypomagnesaemia and hypocalcaemia as a consequence of intestinal resection, studies in this laboratory have shown the

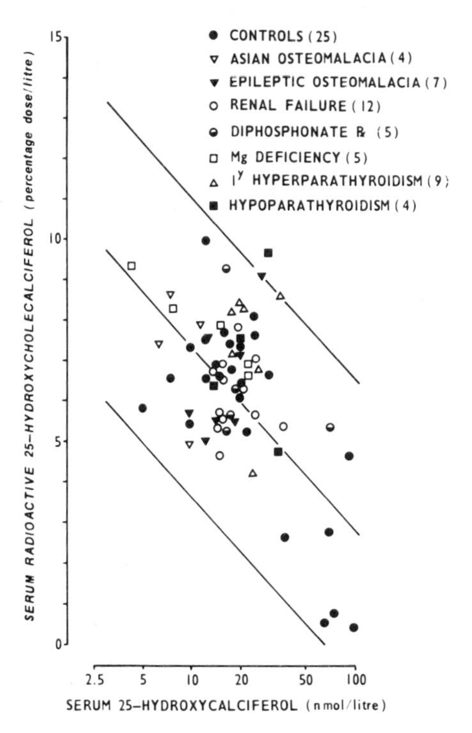

Fig. 1. The relationship between the serum concentration of unlabelled 25-hydroxycalciferol and of radioactive 25-hydroxycholecalciferol, 24 h after i.v. injection of labelled cholecalciferol. The regression and 95% confidence limits were calculated for the 25 control data only

serum iPTH to be inappropriately low or undetectable; correction of the hypomagnesaemia produced simultaneous increase in the serum concentrations of both calcium and iPTH (Dr G. A. Lumb, unpublished). These results agree with the observations in primary hypomagnesaemia (*loc. cit.*) and open the possibility that an acquired functional hypoparathyroidism in magnesium-deficiency might secondarily influence the renal metabolism of 25-hydroxycholecalciferol. Our studies of the metabolism of radioactive cholecalciferol in these patients have as yet been inconclusive. In five patients the formation of labelled 25-hydroxycholecalciferol was appropriate to their prevailing state of vitamin D nutrition, as measured by the serum 25-hydroxycalciferol (Fig. 1). There was thus no support for the suggestion of Rösler and Rabinowitz (1973) that magnesium-deficiency might impair the 25-hydroxylation of cholecalciferol. The concentration of labelled 1,25-dihydroxycholecalciferol in the serum tended to be low as compared with nutritionally matched controls (Fig. 2) but this was not a consistent finding and the formation of labelled hormone was not appreciably increased after correction of the magnesium-deficiency. Studies of cholecalciferol metabolism in experimental animals have also been difficult to interpret. Coburn *et al.* (1973) found the *in vitro* production of 1,25-dihydroxycholecalciferol from the 25-hydroxy-metabolite by homogenates of the kidneys of magnesium-deficient chicks to be 70% less than that of the kidneys of control animals. Yet, following the administration of radioactive cholecalciferol, greater amounts

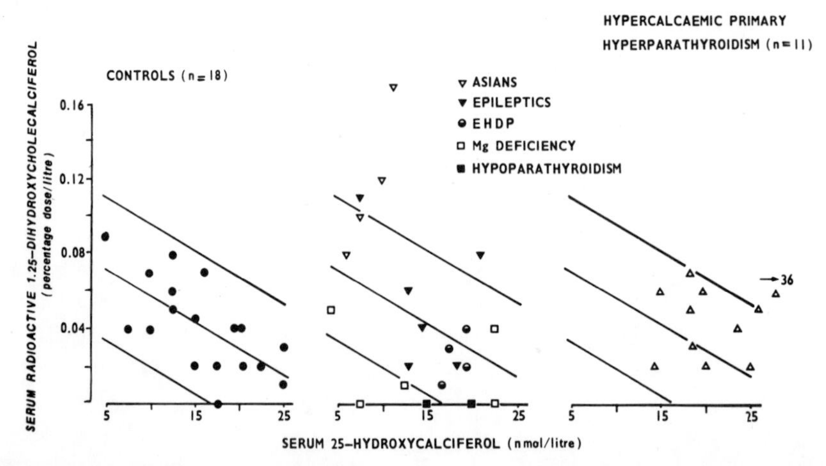

Fig. 2. The relationship between the serum concentration of 25-hydroxycalciferol and the concentration of labelled 1,25-dihydroxycholecalciferol in serum 48 h after injecting radioactive cholecalciferol. The regression and 95% confidence limits were established for the 18 control subjects with degrees of vitamin D-deficiency. Data from patients with primary hyperparathyroidism (right) and from miscellaneous clinical conditions (centre) are related to this control regression

of the hormone were found in the intestinal mucosa of magnesium-deficient chicks than in their controls. There is obvious need for further studies of the effects of magnesium deficiency on vitamin D metabolism, both in the clinical situation and in animals.

III Primary Disorders of Parathyroid Function

A HYPOPARATHYROIDISM

Vitamin D and dihydrotachysterol are conventionally used in the treatment of the hypocalcaemia of hypoparathyroidism. Very large doses are required, response in terms of elevation of the serum calcium is variable and unpredictable, and the development of hypercalcaemia with temporary or permanent impairment of renal function is common (Avioli, 1974). Recent reports suggest that small and 'apparently physiological' doses of 1,25-dihydroxycholecalciferol are effective in restoring normocalcaemia in these patients. Russell *et al.* (1974) found that oral doses of 0.68 to 2.7 μg/day of either 1,25-dihydroxycholecalciferol or the 1α-hydroxy analogue corrected the hypocalcaemia in two patients; 1 μg/day of the hormone was similarly effective in children, whereas the smaller dose of 0.25 μg/day was inadequate (Kind *et al.*, 1976). The mechanism of this effect of 1,25-dihydroxycholecalciferol has not been adequately studied. It appears to be due primarily to an increased intestinal absorption of calcium and the effectiveness of treatment is influenced by the level of calcium intake in the diet (Davies *et al.*, 1977a); but an increase in the ratio of calcium to creatinine in the urine in the fasting state, and a concomitant increase in the urinary excretion of hydroxyproline, suggest that an increase of bone resorption produced by these sterols may also contribute to raising the serum calcium (Russell *et al.*, 1974).

Although needing conformation these observations have interesting physiological implications. The effectiveness of small doses of 1,25-dihydroxycholecalciferol in hypoparathyroidism is as impressive as the effects produced by the same dosage in vitamin D-dependent rickets and in renal failure (Sections IA, IIA); and, as in the later conditions, the therapeutic response might be considered compatible with the correction of a deficiency of the hormone. Measurements made in a few patients by competitive protein binding assay suggest that the serum concentration of 1,25-dihydroxycholecalciferol may be significantly lower in hypoparathyroidism than in healthy individuals (Brumbaugh *et al.*, 1974b). Similarly, in a small number of patients with hypoparathyroidism complicating thyroidectomy, we found no detectable formation of radioactive hormone from an administered pulse of [1,2-$^{3}H_2$,4-^{14}C] cholecalciferol (Mawer *et al.*, 1975a). These observations are compatible with the results of animal experiments suggesting that either the lack of parathyroid hormone (Garabedian *et al.*, 1972) or the accompanying hyperphosphataemia (Tanaka and DeLuca, 1973) may reduce the renal capacity to synthesise 1,25-dihydroxycholecalciferol. Similar conclusions have been drawn from the studies by Kooh *et al.* (1975) on the relative effectiveness of 25-hydroxy- and 1,25-dihydroxycholecalciferol in the treatment of this disease compared to their efficacy in simple vitamin D-deficiency.

If there is a deficiency of the hormone in hypoparathyroidism, one must account for the absence of rickets and osteomalacia in this disease; and, since hypoparathyroidism may sometimes be congenital, it must be explained how affected children acquire the calcium required for mineralisation of the growing skeleton. There is no certain answer to either of these questions. It is generally considered that the hyperphosphataemia of hypoparathyroidism is sufficient to account for the absence of defective skeletal mineralisation. This accords with the long held clinical belief that secondary hyperparathyroidism and consequential hypophosphataemia is an essential factor in the development of osteomalacia in vitamin D-deficiency; and with the belief of some biochemists that vitamin D has no direct influence on the mineralisation of osteoid (Omdahl and DeLuca, 1973). On the other hand, the biochemical syndrome of hypoparathyroidism – hypocalcaemia and hyperphosphataemia – may accompany rickets or osteomalacia in simple vitamin D deficiency (Lumb and Stanbury, 1974) and in chronic azotaemic renal failure (Stanbury, 1967, 1968a). And both mineral retention (Stanbury *et al.*, 1969) and histological evidence of the mineralisation of osteoid (Eastwood *et al.*, 1974) can be detected, during the treatment of azotaemic osteomalacia with vitamin D, in the absence of change in the plasma calcium × plasma phosphate product. It is thus premature to assume that hyperphosphataemia protects against the development of defective mineralisation in hypoparathyroidism, and equally premature to assume that there is an absolute deficiency of the hormone in this disease. Hypoparathyroidism in children may be associated with retarded growth, and correction of the hypocalcaemia by treatment with vitamin D may be followed by a spurt of catch-up growth; but most untreated children continue to grow and must thus accumulate a sizeable mass of calcium in their bones. If 1,25-dihydroxycholecalciferol is essential for the intestinal absorption of this calcium, there cannot be an absolute deficiency of the hormone and the few data of Brumbaugh *et al.* (1974b) support this conclusion. It is also conceivable that the process of growth might stimulate the formation of 1,25-dihydroxycholecalciferol despite the lack of parathyroid hormone and the presence of hyperphosphataemia (see Adams *et al.*, 1975). These various problems of hypoparathyroidism should prove a fruitful field for further clinical studies of calciferol metabolism.

1,25-Dihydroxycholecalciferol increases the intestinal absorption of phosphorus as well as calcium and must mobilise both ions simultaneously from the bone; since it also apparently increases the renal tubular reabsorption of phosphorus (Puschett *et al.*, 1972), it must be explained how treatment with this hormone reduces the elevated serum phosphate in hypoparathyroidism (Russell *et al.*, 1974; Kind *et al.*, 1976). Probably of most significance in this respect is the demonstration that sustained elevation of the serum calcium, produced in hypoparathyroidism by infusion of calcium salts, will reduce the renal tubular reabsorption of phosphate and correct the hyperphosphataemia, presumably through some effect of calcium on the renal tubular cell (Eisenberg, 1965).

In a group of patients with hypoparathyroidism the serum calcium was increased from ~6 to ~9.5 mg/100 ml by massive oral dosage with calcium salts; the rise in serum calcium was accompanied by proportionate reduction of the serum phosphate and of the renal tubular reabsorption of phosphate. Indistinguishable effects on the renal tubular handling of phosphate were produced in the same patients when the serum calcium was elevated to the same extent by treatment with 1,25-dihydroxycholecalciferol (Davies *et al.*, 1977a). Thus the effect of 1,25-dihydroxycholecalciferol in raising the serum calcium, by its actions on gut, bone and perhaps on the renal tubular reabsorption of calcium (Puschett *et al.*, 1972), appears to counter its other actions that tend to raise the serum phosphate. Experience in treating hypoparathyroidism with large doses of ergocalciferol has shown that sometimes it is difficult or impossible to raise the serum calcium without simultaneously reducing the dietary availability of phosphorus or greatly increasing the intake of calcium. In such circumstances, one must assume that the direct effects of 'vitamin D' on phosphorus metabolism effectively nullify its action in raising the serum calcium. Our personal experience of the use of 1,25-dihydroxycholecalciferol in hypoparathyroidism indicates that it may be necessary to supplement the intake of calcium until the serum calcium is restored to normal and the serum phosphate has fallen; thereafter, a daily oral dose of 0.5 to 1 μg of the hormone alone may be sufficient to maintain normocalcaemia (Hill *et al.*, 1975).

B PRIMARY HYPERPARATHYROIDISM

As judged by the appearance of labelled 1,25- and 24,25-dihydroxycholecalciferol in the serum following the intravenous injection of 10 μg of [1,2^{3}H$_2$,4^{14}C-]cholecalciferol, the metabolism of cholecalciferol in primary hyperparathyroidism differs from normal in at least two respects (Mawer *et al.*, 1975a; Stanbury *et al.*, 1975a, b). All patients studied produced the labelled hormone in the same amounts as in nutritionally matched controls, although the serum calcium (mean 12.7 mg/100 ml, SD 1.1) in each of them was above the level (9.6 mg/100 ml) at which the formation of this metabolite becomes undetectable in control subjects. Within the relatively narrow nutritional range so far studied (serum 25-(OH)D 6–14 ng/ml), the formation of 1,25-dihydroxycholecalciferol also appeared to be independent of the prevailing state of vitamin D nutrition. Secondly, all patients produced labelled 24,25-dihydroxycholecalciferol in amounts inappropriately high for their nutritional state. The reasons for this are not apparent but a positive correlation between serum levels of calcium and labelled 24,25-dihydroxycholecalciferol suggests that it could be related to the hypercalcaemia of these patients. Since normal subjects in general produce *either* 1,25- or 24,25-dihydroxycholecalciferol from a single pulse dose of labelled cholecalciferol, depending on their nutritional state (Mawer *et al.*, 1975a), the simultaneous production of significant amounts of both renal metabolites in primary hyperparathyroidism implies a third difference from the normal. It further implies an increased renal turnover of 25-hydroxycholecalciferol in this disease which, if 24,25-dihydroxycholecalciferol has no specific function, could involve a net wastage of 25-hydroxycholecalciferol.

These studies will require amplification and, more especially, confirmation by alternative techniques permitting direct measurement of the molar concentrations of 1,25- and 24,25-dihydroxycholecalciferol in their serum.

Preliminary measurements by competitive binding assay indicate that the molar concentration of 24,25-dihydroxycalciferol is significantly higher in patients with primary hyperparathyroidism than in normal adults with comparable levels of serum 25-hydroxycalciferol (Taylor, 1976). Even within the limitations of the radioisotopic technique, these observations may be relevant to several aspects of the morbid physiology of primary hyperparathyroidism. They suggest that the formation of the hormone in this disease is independent of two factors, the serum calcium and the serum 25-hydroxycalciferol that normally correlate with its production (Mawer *et al.*, 1975a). This would be reasonable if the parathyroid hormone were the trophic factor determining the 1α-hydroxylation of 25-hydroxycholecalciferol. Primary hyperparathyroidism is associated with intestinal hyperabsorption of calcium (Hodgkinson, 1963; Stanbury, 1968b, 1973a, 1976); this has been attributed to a direct action of parathyroid hormone on the intestine but it is more probably an indirect consequence of parathyroid overactivity. There are no recorded measurements of serum 1,25-dihydroxycalciferol, or of the formation of labelled hormone from radioactive cholecalciferol, in patients with primary hyperparathyroidism complicated by advanced secondary renal disease. In such patients, the phenomenon of hyperabsorption is no longer evident and intestinal net absorption of calcium may be effectively nil (Stanbury, 1968b), as in patients with advanced primary renal failure. It seems reasonable to infer that 1,25-dihydroxycholecalciferol is essential for the increased absorption of calcium in primary hyperparathyroidism but it is an open question whether the hormone itself determines and regulates the quantitative amount of calcium absorbed. In the patients with primary hyperparathyroidism studied by Mawer *et al.* (1975a) the formation of labelled 1,25-dihydroxycholecalciferol was no greater than in appropriate controls; but a moderate degree of renal impairment (mean creatinine clearance 63 ml/min, SD 26; range 38 to 112 ml/min) in this sample of patients could have reduced quantitatively the renal capacity to hydroxylate 25-hydroxycholecalciferol. In a small number of observations, Brumbaugh *et al.* (1974a, b) found the assayed serum 1,25-dihydroxycalciferol in patients with primary hyperparathyroidism to be about twice the mean value in their control subjects. Such increased values might well be compatible with 1,25-dihydroxycholecalciferol directly determining the increased intestinal absorption of calcium. When studied by conventional metabolic balance techniques, a majority of patients with primary hyperparathyroidism is found to be in external equilibrium for calcium; that is, the intestinal net absorption and urinary output of calcium are closely equivalent (Stanbury, 1968b, 1973a). This suggests a causal relationship between these two variables but it is not clear whether the hypercalciuria or the increased intestinal net absorption of calcium in primary hyperparathyroidism should be regarded as the independent variable. If the high intestinal absorption of calcium is directly dependent on a sustained, inappropriate formation of 1,25-dihydroxycholecalciferol, the quantitatively equivalent urinary output of calcium would be a passive consequence of the inappropriate intestinal absorption. This option has the appeal of logical simplicity but hypercalciuria in primary hyperparathyroidism may be sustained in the fasted patient; and there are other indications that the urinary output of calcium in this disease is largely independent of intestinal absorption. The converse option, that the urinary output of calcium is the independent variable, would imply the operation of homeostatic mechanisms that regulate the intestinal absorption of calcium to offset or compensate for the urinary losses (Stanbury, 1968b, 1973a). Elucidation of the mechanisms controlling the quantitative intestinal absorption of calcium in primary hyperparathyroidism, both before and after parathyroidectomy, remains an outstanding and challenging problem. It should prove one of the most profitable fields for the study of the clinical endocrinology of vitamin D.

Vitamin D may have other important effects in primary hyperparathyroidism. A sufficient number of cases has now been reported to suggest that the occurrence of bone disease, in some patients with primary hyperparathyroidism, may be determined by the development of vitamin D-deficiency (Woodhouse *et al.*, 1971; Stanbury, 1962b, 1972a). Such bone disease shows the changes of both osteomalacia and classical osteitis fibrosa, and the evidence suggests that the latter lesion results from an increased secretion of parathyroid hormone consequent on the development of vitamin D-deficiency. In patients with osteomalacia complicating primary hyperparathyroidism, the mass of parathyroid tissue is inappropriately great for the height of the serum calcium (Stanbury, 1973b): in hypercalcaemic osteomalacia, correction of vitamin D-deficiency has been followed by a slow exponential fall in serum iPTH, compatible with structural involution of parathyroid tissue, and by concomitant healing of both components of the bone disease (Lumb and Stanbury, 1974). These observations have been taken to suggest that 'vitamin D', most probably in the form of the hormonal metabolite, may act directly on the parathyroid glands. This proposition finds some support in the demonstration that administration of cholecalciferol or the 25-hydroxy metabolite to vitamin D-deficient individuals can reduce serum iPTH without inducing detectable change of serum calcium (Rasmussen *et al.*, 1974); and similar observations have been made in vitamin D-deficient puppies (Oldham *et al.*, 1974).

Woodhouse *et al.* (1971) have further suggested that primary hyperparathyroidism may itself occasion the development of 'vitamin D-deficiency' or cause an increased 'requirement' for vitamin D in this disease. This suggestion was probably based on the reported inhibitory effect of parathyroid hormone on the production of 1,25-dihydroxycholecalciferol in the rat (Galante *et al.*, 1972) but it is evident that this effect is not operating in human primary hyperparathyroidism (*vide supra*; Mawer *et al.*, 1975a). In our own experience, the development of vitamin D-deficiency in primary hyperparathyroidism has been accounted for adequately by dietary insufficiency and inadequate solar exposure or by associated intestinal malabsorption; and in the two patients reported by Woodhouse, one a mental defective and the other an immigrant Asian, similar factors may have been operating. None the less, the demonstrated increased renal turnover of 25-hydroxycholecalciferol in primary hyperparathyroidism could hypothetically cause a conditioned deficiency of 'vitamin D'. On the basis of radioisotopic studies alone, it is difficult to judge whether this increased production of renal metabolites is quantitatively sufficient to cause depletion of the body pool of 25-hydroxycalciferol (and, secondarily, of cholecalciferol). An adequate appraisal of this and the other problems of vitamin D metabolism in primary hyperparathyroidism will require sensitive methods for the direct measurement of the dihydroxylated metabolites in the serum.

IV Miscellaneous Diseases

A OSTEOMALACIA COMPLICATING GASTRIC SURGERY AND INTESTINAL MALABSORPTION

It is widely believed that the commonest cause of osteomalacia in temperate 'developed' countries is vitamin D-deficiency arising as a consequence of gastric surgery or of intestinal malabsorption. This point is perhaps open to question in view of the frequency with which osteomalacia develops in all types of bilateral renal disease and, in this country, the frequency of privational vitamin D-deficiency in immigrant Asians and in the indigenous elderly. It is also argued that the frequency of post-gastrectomy osteomalacia has often been overestimated (Morgan, 1973). Despite this general awareness of gastrointestinal disease as a cause of osteomalacia, there has been surprisingly little application of available modern techniques to the study of the pathogenesis of vitamin D-deficiency in these conditions.

Osteomalacia develops as long as 10 years after an operation involving partial resection of the stomach (Morgan *et al.*, 1970); the reasons for this delayed development are unknown. There is no doubt that the condition is due to vitamin D-deficiency; the bioassayed antiricketic activity in the plasma is very low or undetectable (Thompson *et al.*, 1966c); it responds to very small (2.5 μg/day) parenteral doses of calciferol (Morgan *et al.*, 1965). In view of the observation that infantile rickets is more common in boys than girls (Childs *et al.*, 1962; Fraser *et al.*, 1967), it is of interest that post-gastrectomy osteomalacia is many times more frequent in women than in men (Morgan, 1973); this too is unexplained. A few studies of the absorption of a large (1 mg) oral dose of radioactive cholecalciferol have suggested that *some* gastrectomised patients may have a minor malabsorption of the vitamin (Thompson *et al.*, 1966b). Some patients may show impaired absorption of 25-hydroxycholecalciferol when tested with a comparatively large (10 μg/kg) oral dose (Stamp, 1974); but other studies have not confirmed this (von Lilienfeld-Toal and Becker, 1975). The fragmentary evidence available suggests that the trivial impairment of the intestinal absorption of calciferol sterols after gastrectomy is not predictably related to the rate of gastric emptying, to the presence of steatorrhoea, or to the presence of bone disease; but too few studies have been made to warrant any firm conclusions. There is a good deal of evidence that the dietary intake of vitamin D is low in patients with post-gastrectomy osteomalacia but not necessarily any lower than in operated patients without osteomalacia. Nothing is known of the possible contribution of inadequate exposure to sunlight but post-gastrectomy osteomalacia has been reported from Australia and from sunny areas of the United States. The problem remains unresolved and warrants further study.

The pathogenesis of vitamin D-deficiency is better understood in the osteomalacia complicating idiopathic steatorrhoea, which for all practical purposes can be regarded as synonymous with gluten enteropathy. Studies with labelled cholecalciferol have clearly demonstrated impaired intestinal absorption of the vitamin (Thompson *et al.*, 1966a; Miravet et al., 1969), there being an inverse relation between the net absorption of the oral dose and the degree of steatorrhoea. There is little doubt that this is the principal factor responsible for the vitamin D-deficiency although, in our experience, the vitamin D intake of osteomalacic patients has often been very low (Stanbury, 1972a). It has, however, been shown that the presence of osteomalacia in idiopathic steatorrhoea may be accompanied by normal levels of bioassayed antiricketic activity in the plasma (Thomas *et al.*, 1959). Also, although the bone disease may respond to parenterally administered doses of vitamin D that were ineffective orally, it has been considered that the clinical response and also the induced increase in calcium absorption are less than in simple privational vitamin D-deficiency (Badenoch and Fourman, 1954; Nassim *et al.*, 1959). These observations, and the failure of rickets in children with coeliac disease to respond to sunlight (Fanconi, 1928), might be taken to suggest an abnormality of vitamin D metabolism. However, no detectable difference has been found between the metabolism of a pulse dose of labelled cholecalciferol in osteomalacia due to privational deficiency, to gastrectomy or to coeliac disease (Mawer *et al.*, 1971b, 1972, 1975a). Nassim *et al.* (1959) showed that large parenteral doses (15 mg/day) of ergocalciferol might fail to produce an increase of calcium absorption in patients with idiopathic steatorrhoea until the institution of a gluten-free diet. Since the metabolism of cholecalciferol is apparently normal even in patients eating a normal diet, the most reasonable explanation for both the malabsorption of the vitamin and the relative unresponsiveness of calcium absorption to pharmacological parenteral doses of vitamin D is the villous atrophy and the functional abnormality of the enterocyte induced by gluten.

B OSTEOMALACIA AND RICKETS IN ASIAN IMMIGRANTS

During the past decade, clinical experience has revealed that rickets and osteomalacia are common among Asian immigrants in Britain (Dunnigan *et al.*, 1962; Dunnigan and Smith, 1965), and random surveys in this population have uncovered a high incidence of the clinical and biochemical signs of vitamin D-deficiency among apparently healthy individuals (Holmes *et al.*, 1973). The re-appearance in Britain of rickets apparently due to vitamin D-deficiency has provoked considerable interest and a remarkable amount of speculation as to its possible cause. The high phytate content of the Asian diet, the consumption of chappatis, skin pigmentation and a genetical abnormality of vitamin D metabolism have been invoked as possible causes. Based on assessment of the available epidemiological evidence and an extensive personal experience of the response to therapy, we consider that none of these hypotheses is valid and that the condition is simply one of privational deficiency due to a low dietary intake of vitamin D and minimum exposure to sunshine (Holmes *et al.*, 1973; Hodgkin *et al.*, 1973; Stanbury *et al.*, 1975b). In general support of this belief, the serum 25-hydroxycholecalciferol in the Asian immigrants is very low and it has been claimed that the levels in patients with rickets or osteomalacia are 'unmeasurable' (Preece *et al.*, 1973). The last finding is almost certainly attributable to the insensitivity of the method used to measure 25-hydroxycalciferol. In 12 Asians with overt bone disease, we found the mean serum 25-hydroxycalciferol to be 3.4 ng/ml, SD 0.7; an identical value (3.6 ng/ml), was found in a group of Caucasians with vitamin D-deficiency osteomalacia due to intestinal malabsorption and allied causes.

Several years ago, we were able to induce healing of rickets and to document the production of a positive mineral balance in dark-skinned Asian adolescents by treatment with ultraviolet irradiation (unpublished observations). Recently, this has been further documented in a patient eating chappatis and shown to be accompanied by a brisk rise in serum 25-hydroxycalciferol to levels 'above normal' (Dent *et al.*, 1973). In a deliberate study of the effects of ultraviolet irradiation, Stamp (1975) found similar increments in serum 25-hydroxycalciferol in white- and dark-skinned subjects following exposure of the whole body. There is no evidence that dark pigmentation reduces skin synthesis of cholecalciferol; and none for the seemingly plausible hypothesis of Loomis (1967) based on the converse assumption. Epidemiological studies undertaken 30 years ago by Wilson and Widdowson (1942) had virtually established the critical role of sunshine in preventing rickets in the Asian in India. The recent limited survey in the Punjab by Hodgkin *et al.* (1973) provides further evidence in confirmation; and Stamp and Round (1974) have documented the spontaneous correction of vitamin D-deficiency in Asians in Britain during the summer months.

Studies with labelled cholecalciferol show that Asians with osteomalacia have a normal capacity to produce both 25-hydroxycholecalciferol and 1,25-dihydroxycholecalciferol (Fig. 2). Because radioisotopically labelled cholecalciferol can be used only in subjects older than 40 years, it has been possible to undertake studies in only five of the many Asian patients we have encountered. In three of these patients, the concentration of labelled 1,25-dihydroxycholecalciferol at 48 h was outside the confidence limits of Fig. 2, and the mean value for the group was above that of Caucasian controls during six days of observation (Mawer, 1974). As is to be expected in vitamin D-deficiency, no patients produced labelled 24,25-dihydroxycholecalciferol but the mean serum concentration of labelled 25,26-dihydroxycholecalciferol, as well as of 1,25-dihydroxycholecalciferol was higher than in Caucasian controls. Without further study, we are unable to assess the significance of this difference between the Caucasian and Asian patients with vitamin D-deficiency.

C RICKETS AND OSTEOMALACIA DEVELOPING DURING ANTICONVULSANT THERAPY

Since the original description (Kruse, 1968) of the occurrence of rickets and osteomalacia among epileptic patients chronically treated with anticonvulsant drugs ('treated epileptics'), this problem has probably received as much attention as any clinical situation involving vitamin D. Dent *et al.* (1970) postulated that anticonvulsant drugs caused wastage of vitamin D through hepatic enzyme induction and the conversion of cholecalciferol to metabolically inactive derivatives. This plausible hypothesis has been widely accepted but never proved in man, and it is supported only indirectly by circumstantial evidence. Measurements by photon absorptiometry have shown that the estimated bone mineral mass is lower in treated epileptics than in matched controls; treatment with supplementary calciferol (50 μg/day) and calcium (390 mg/day) increased the mineral mass in the epileptics but not in the controls (Christiansen *et al.*, 1973). Caspary *et al.* (1975) found a significant reduction in the intestinal absorption of ^{47}Ca in treated epileptics as compared with controls; this malabsorption was reversed by cholecalciferol (25 μg/day) or the 25-hydroxy-metabolite (50 μg/day) but the improved absorption relapsed to its original state some months after withdrawing this treatment. These observations and the demonstration of the effectiveness of 25-hydroxycholecalciferol in treating overt cases of osteomalacia in epileptics (Stamp *et al.*, 1972) simply serve to demonstrate that epileptic patients treated with anticonvulsant drugs tend to become deficient in vitamin D. This much could be inferred from earlier surveys (Richens and Rowe, 1970; Hunter *et al.*, 1971), but none of these studies indicates how or why vitamin D deficiency should develop.

Hahn *et al.* (1972a) observed a reduction in the half-life of injected labelled cholecalciferol in plasma following two weeks' treatment with phenobarbitone in two subjects (one healthy volunteer, one child with rickets). In epileptic patients chronically treated with phenobarbitone these authors found a reduced half-life of plasma cholecalciferol, an accelerated formation and decay from plasma of 25-hydroxycholecalciferol and an increased formation of more polar metabolites, as compared with 'control subjects'; but they appreciated that this observed pattern of the metabolism of radioactive cholecalciferol in treated epileptics might simply reflect a lower pool of vitamin D in these individuals (Mawer *et al.*, 1971b). In a review of the problem of enzyme induction, Hunter (1974) claims that treatment with barbiturates reduces the half-life of radioactive cholecalciferol in plasma whereas the half-life of metabolically produced 25-hydroxycalciferol remains within the range found in 'untreated control subjects'. Since control and treated groups consisted of different individuals not necessarily matched for nutritional status, the significance of this observation is uncertain. In a group of eight epileptic patients developing overt osteomalacia in the course of treatment, we found their formation of labelled 25-hydroxy- and 1,25-dihydroxycholecalciferol (Fig. 12) from radioactive cholecalciferol to be appropriate to their nutritional state; the half-lives of both cholecalciferol and 25-hydroxy-metabolite in the serum were also appropriate to the prevailing concentration of 25-hydroxycalciferol. During a period of six days observation, the serum concentration of labelled 1,25-dihydroxycholecalciferol fell more rapidly than in a control group but the difference was not significant (Mawer, 1974). Thus the radioisotopic technique demonstrates that the treated epileptic has a normal capacity to produce the biologically active metabolites of cholecalciferol; it has not so far proved capable of detecting any abnormal hepatic degradation of cholecalciferol that might be caused by enzyme induction. This is probably also true of enzyme induction studies in animals; although claims have been made to detect abnormal degradation of both cholecalciferol and 25-hydroxycholecalciferol in phenobarbitone and phenytoin treated rats, reported results are open to differing interpretations. In this laboratory, P. Torkington, P. de Silva and Berthoud (unpublished observations) treated rats with phenobarbitone for six months and at the end of that time found only a trivial increase in the rate of turnover of cholecalciferol. This produced no detectable biological effect; was considered to be quantitatively insignificant; and had not reduced the serum 25-hydroxycalciferol below the levels in their strictly pair-fed controls.

Against the background of these generally negative or inconclusive results from radioisotopic studies, it is necessary to examine the significance of the finding of 'low values' of serum 25-hydroxycalciferol in treated epileptic patients. Some recorded values and their miscellaneous 'controls' are shown in Table 1 of the previous chapter. Each group of investigators making measurements of serum 25-hydroxycalciferol in drug treated epileptics finds their mean values to be lower than in the chosen control subjects but the proportionate lowering varies enormously between investigations. Hahn *et al.* (1972b) found the mean serum 25-hydroxycalciferol in outpatient epileptics treated with phenobarbitone and/or phenytoin to be 62–72% of the mean of controls taken from hospital general outpatients. Stamp *et al.* (1972) obtained a mean value of serum 25-hydroxycalciferol in their epileptics which was no higher than 30% of the mean of their control subjects; but their epileptics were institutionalised and receiving high dosage of several drugs, whereas their controls were hospital and academic staff or adolescent schoolboys – two groups privileged in terms of their exposure to sunshine. If the epileptics with osteomalacia studied by P. de Silva and C. M. Taylor (unpublished observations) are compared with a similarly privileged control group, their mean serum 25-hydroxycalciferol is 20% of the control values in summer and

36% of the control values taken in winter: but, if a casual group of women attending a local antenatal clinic were taken as the control group, the mean serum 25-hydroxycalciferol in the osteomalacic epileptics would be 70% of the 'control mean'. In other words, the values of serum 25-hydroxycalciferol cannot be used as indirect evidence for abnormal calciferol metabolism unless it is certainly known that experimental and control groups had an identical pattern of solar exposure and dietary intake of vitamin D. This is not possible of achievement. From the data of de Silva and Taylor (Table 1, chapter 8) it would be equally logical (or illogical) to postulate that pregnancy produces a massive disturbance of vitamin D metabolism. This is not mere pedantry; the situation appears different to those constantly managing epileptic patients than it may to investigators invading their clinical field. Livingston *et al.* (1973) have recognised no instance of 'drug induced' osteomalacia or rickets in an experience of 15 000 epileptic patients during a period of 36 years; and they found no biochemical abnormalities in the serum of a sample of this population. These authors emphasise that an 'adequate diet' is by no means the rule in institutionalised patients and it is evident that more severe epilepsy needing large doses of multiple drugs also tends to cause limited activity and sequestration from sunlight. Thus the hypothesis of hepatic enzyme induction as a cause for the vitamin D deficiency has not yet been proved by hard facts; and it is important that the attractiveness of the hypothesis should not pervert the interpretation of the inadequate information provided by measurements of serum 25-hydroxycalciferol. Some cases of osteomalacia in epileptic patients have been complicated by other metabolic abnormalities (e.g. case 2 of Stamp *et al.*, 1972). Among cases of 'epileptic osteomalacia' studied in this laboratory, some patients have been proved to have gluten enteropathy; others responded to as little as 11.3 μg of ergocalciferol per day; an exceptional case required 1.25 mg per day to produce a therapeutic response – a situation not readily explained by the enzyme induction hypothesis or by any other recognised abnormality. Livingston *et al.* (1973) question whether 'epileptic osteomalacia' might not usually be due to simple nutritional deficiency and exceptionally to some coincidental abnormality.

D LIVER DISEASE AND VITAMIN D METABOLISM

Bone disease is a not infrequent complication of primary chronic diseases of the liver but it takes the form of osteoporosis more often than of defective mineralisation (Atkinson *et al.*, 1956; Kehayoglou *et al.*, 1968). The development of rickets or osteomalacia correlates well with the degree of biliary obstruction but has occasionally been observed in the absence of jaundice, and rickets is said to be common in neonatal hepatitis (Yu *et al.*, 1971). Obstructive jaundice is associated with impaired intestinal absorption of both cholecalciferol (Thompson *et al.*, 1966a) and 25-hydroxycalciferol

(Stamp, 1974) and low values in serum of the latter metabolite have been recorded in patients with biliary cirrhosis (Haddad and Chyu, 1971). In most circumstances, therefore, the occurrence of defective skeletal mineralisation is explained adequately on a basis of simple vitamin D-deficiency resulting from intestinal malabsorption of the vitamin.

The essential role of the liver in the initial stage of vitamin D metabolism not unnaturally leads to the expectation that hepatic cellular damage might disturb this function and produce conditioned secondary deficiencies of 25-hydroxy-and 1,25-dihydroxycholecalciferol. In recording the development of osteomalacia within six months of the onset of hepatocellular jaundice, Atkinson *et al.* (1956) express doubt that this could have been caused by simple malabsorption of vitamin D; as have other authors before and since, they suggest that destruction of liver cells may interfere with the metabolism of the vitamin. There has been no systematic study of the intermediary metabolism of labelled cholecalciferol in the various forms of hepatitis or in cirrhosis. Avioli *et al.* (1967a) reported that labelled cholecalciferol disappeared more slowly from the blood in four patients with alcoholic cirrhosis than in their control subjects, but, in the absence of evidence concerning pool size in the groups compared, it is impossible to interpret these data. In six patients with primary biliary cirrhosis, the formation and survival of labelled 25-hydroxycholecalciferol were indistinguishable from the processes in matched control subjects (Krawitt *et al.*, 1977). Four of these patients showed impaired intestinal absorption of cholecalciferol and five excreted excessive amounts of polar metabolites in the urine.

The indirect approach, of measuring serum levels of 25-hydroxycalciferol, has been used by Hepner *et al.* (1975) in a study of patients with alcoholic cirrhosis. They found the serum 25-hydroxycalciferol in these patients to be about one half the mean values in their control subjects and in a group of alcoholic patients with normal liver function and histology (Table 1, chapter 8). They were also able to derive significant correlations between the serum 25-hydroxycalciferol and the serum albumin concentration and other indices of hepatocellular function. This may suggest an impairment of 25-hydroxylation in cirrhosis but there is the same difficulty in interpreting the data as has been discussed in relation to treatment with anticonvulsant drugs. The alcoholic with normal liver function may eat no more than the patient with cirrhosis; but if the cirrhosis is severe enough to reduce the serum albumin the patient is ill and thus less likely to be active and exposed to sunshine out of doors. Since sunshine rather than diet is the principal source of serum 25-hydroxycalciferol (Haddad and Hahn, 1973), lowered values could arise from lack of solar exposure independently of biochemical events in the liver.

This is a relatively neglected field in the clinical study of vitamin D metabolism and there is scope for further investigation. Two recent publications have documented the occurrence of low levels of serum 25-hydroxycalciferol in both parenchymal and cholestatic liver disease without clarifying the mechanisms responsible for this finding (Long *et al.*, 1976; Wagonfeld *et al.*, 1976). In patients with primary biliary cirrhosis the low serum 25-hydroxycalciferol increased after oral administration of 25-hydroxycholecalciferol but it was uninfluenced by oral or parenteral administration of vitamin D (Wagonfeld *et al.*, 1976). This failure of large parenteral doses (2,500–12 500 μg) of vitamin D to increase significantly the serum level of 25-hydroxycalciferol was taken to imply an impairment of hepatic 25-hydroxylation. But, the parenteral dose was given subcutaneously and thus, presumably, largely into subcutaneous fat; and it is doubtful if significant amounts of the lipophilic sterol would be absorbed into the circulation. Failure to increase serum 25-hydroxycalciferol is more reasonably explained by failure of its precursor to reach the liver. (Parenthetically, a single intramuscular dose of 7500 μg of cholecalciferol given to vitamin D-deficient patients with normal liver function may increase the serum 25-hydroxycalciferol by no more than 2–5 ng/ml) (P. de Silva, private communication). In patients with hepatocellular disease who had had recent prolonged exposure to sunshine, the serum 25-hydroxycalciferol was unequivocally normal (Long *et al.*, 1976). This and our own observations in pre-terminal biliary cirrhosis (Stanbury, 1972a) suggest that low levels of 25-hydroxycalciferol in liver disease are determined by a reduced availability of its precursor – that is, by privational deficiency of vitamin D due to inadequate diet and solar exposure or to intestinal malabsorption.

There is, however, no good reason to believe that vitamin D is involved in the pathogenesis of the more common bone disease, osteoporosis, in chronic liver disease.

E SARCOIDOSIS: IDIOPATHIC HYPERCALCAEMIA OF INFANCY

These two conditions, clinically and aetiologically distinct, may have in common a characteristic disorder of calcium metabolism that stimulates closely the syndrome of vitamin D intoxication. Each may be associated with intestinal hyperabsorption of calcium, hypercalcaemia and hypercalciuria; and, in both conditions, it has been postulated that an abnormality of vitamin D metabolism or an unexplained 'sensitivity to vitamin D' is responsible for the disordered mineral metabolism.

The frequency of the hypercalcaemic syndrome in sarcoidosis is uncertain and there is suggestive evidence that it may vary with geographic region; hypercalciuria is probably more frequent than hypercalcaemia. A seasonal incidence of hypercalcaemia, correlating with variation in the availability of natural ultraviolet irradiation (Taylor *et al.*, 1963), and the occasional relatively acute development of hypercalcaemic symptoms after exposure to sunlight (see below) suggests some close linkage with vitamin D. Hypercalcaemia may develop in patients with sarcoidosis following treatment with relatively small doses of ergocalciferol (Anderson *et al.*, 1954; Mather, 1957) and its improvement has been documented after institution of an artificial diet free of vitamin D (Hendrix, 1966). There is evidence that increased bone resorption (Henneman *et al.*, 1956; Hendrix, 1966) as well as intestinal hyperabsorption of calcium (Anderson *et al.*, 1954) contributes to its production. In spite of this highly suggestive evidence, there have been few direct studies of vitamin D metabolism in this syndrome. In a small number of determinations, the bioassayed antiricketic activity of serum has been within the range found in the healthy population (Thomas *et al.*, 1959; Bell *et al.*, 1964; Mawer *et al.*, 1971a) but there appear to be no recorded measurements of serum 25- hydroxycalciferol in this disease. Possibly related to the relatively low vitamin D status of our northern British population (Lumb *et al.*, 1971; Stanbury *et al.*, 1972), we encounter few cases of hypercalcaemic sarcoidosis but have been able to study the metabolism of isotopically labelled cholecalciferol in two patients (Mawer *et al.*, 1971a). Both patients produced labelled 25-hydroxy- and 1,25-dihydroxycholecalciferol in amounts apparently appropriate to their prevailing nutritional state, as assessed by serum antiricketic activity. (Unfortunately, we were not then able to measure the formation of labelled 24,25-dihydroxycholecalciferol.) One patient was a farmer, who first developed hypercalcaemia after taking a vitamin D preparation but in whom symptoms tended to recur annually when he sowed seed in late spring. The liability to hypercalcaemia was controlled during summer months by corticosteroid therapy. Radioisotopic studies were done in January when the patient was not receiving steroid therapy and the serum calcium was 10.4 mg/100 ml. The latter value is at the upper extreme of the laboratory range (8.9–10.4 mg/100 ml) but it is above the highest level (9.6 mg/100 ml) of serum calcium at which we have seen significant production of labelled 1,25- dihydroxycholecalciferol (Fig. 3). This, although an isolated observation, suggests the possibility that the formation of 1,25-dihydroxycholecalciferol continues inappropriately in patients with sarcoidosis when the serum calcium is elevated. Such a state of affairs might seem analogous to the findings in primary hyperparathyroidism (Section IIIB) but hypercalcaemia in sarcoidosis is apparently invariably associated with absence of iPTH from the blood (Dr Eric Reiss, personal communication). There is an exception to this generalisation, since ‘primary’ hyperparathyroidism occurs relatively frequently in association with sarcoidosis (Dent and Watson, 1966); fortuitously and unfortunately, our second patient studied with labelled cholecalciferol came into this category (Fig. 3).

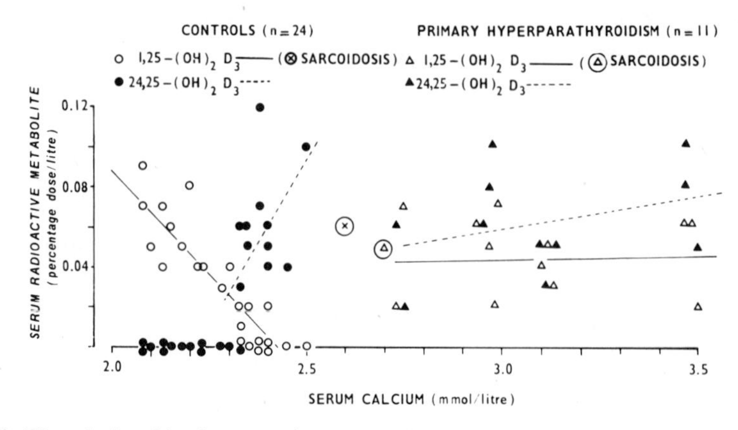

Fig. 3. The relationships between the serum calcium and the serum concentrations of labelled 1,25- and 24,25-dihydroxycholecalciferol 48 h after injecting radioactive cholecalciferol. The regression of serum 24,25-dihydroxycholecalciferol on serum calcium in control subjects (interrupted line) was calculated only for individuals with serum calcium >2.3 mmol/l. Note the continued production of labelled hormone in the hypercalcaemic patients with primary hyperparathyroidism and in two patients with sarcoidosis (see text)

This problem of hypercalcaemia in sarcoidosis warrants further detailed investigation by all available modern techniques and especially with measurements of the molar concentration of 1,25-dihydroxycholecalciferol in the serum. If it should be found that this hormone is produced in the face of two influences that normally inhibit its synthesis – hypercalcaemia and functional hypoparathyroidism – this might explain the development of the hypercalcaemic syndrome and also provide further insight into mechanisms controlling the renal metabolism of 25-hydroxycholecalciferol.

The features of infantile hypercalcaemia and the problems of its pathogenesis have been reviewed extensively elsewhere (Fraser *et al.*, 1966; Seelig, 1969). It occurs in so-called 'mild' and 'severe' forms. The cause of neither type has been established with certainty but the weight of evidence suggests that the milder form may be a manifestation of vitamin D intoxication caused by ingestion of excess vitamin D in milk feeds. The more severe type (Fanconi *et al.*, 1952; Schlesinger *et al.*, 1956) is rare, it apparently arises *in utero* and is not predictably related to the intake of vitamin D by the child or its mother. Isolated observations on individual patients have demonstrated an apparent 'sensitivity' to relatively small doses of vitamin D; elevated serum antiricketic activity in the absence of recognisable excessive intake (Fellers and Schwarz, 1958; Smith *et al.*, 1959; Garcia *et al.*, 1964); and an 'abnormal' elevation and persistence of antiricketic activity in serum after administration of small doses of cholecalciferol (Manios *et al.*, 1966). There have, however, been too few observations made in normal infants to establish a normal range of response with which these supposed 'abnormal' responses can be compared. It is notable that Cuthbertson (1963) found normal serum antiricketic activity in a group of patients with the severe type of infantile hypercalcaemia; and Lindquist (1962) has stressed the differences between infantile hypercalcaemia and vitamin D intoxication.

Evidence of hyperparathyroidism and benefit from parathyroidectomy in two children with classical features of severe idiopathic hypercalcaemia has been noted by Rasmussen (1969 and personal communication). Clayton *et al.* (1976) has measured inappropriately normal serum levels of iPTH in infants with hypercalcaemia; this is analogous to findings in many patients with primary hyperparathyroidism (Arnaud *et al.*, 1971; Lumb and Stanbury, 1974). In a classical severe case surviving to the age of 16 years, we found greatly elevated serum iPTH and apparent autonomy of parathyroid secretion (Stanbury, 1976). In spite of advanced secondary renal impairment (creatinine clearance, 16 ml/min), net intestinal absorption of calcium in this patient was relatively high (40 % of dietary intake). But, as in other patients with primary renal disease and a comparable degree of renal impairment (Mawer *et al.*, 1973), there was no detectable formation of labelled hormone from an administered pulse of radioactive cholecalciferol.

These fragmentary recent observations in infantile hypercalcaemia simply emphasise the need for a detailed re-examination of the disordered mineral metabolism in this syndrome. Because of the central role of calciferol in controlling calcium absorption by the intestine, it has seemed appropriate to seek some disorder of the action or the metabolism of calciferol in clinical states associated with intestinal hyperabsorption of calcium. Factors are known capable of simulating the action of calciferol (chapter 3) and it is not beyond the bounds of possibility that some such factor could be produced metabolically – either as an inborn error in infantile hypercalcaemia or as an acquired abnormality in a multi-system disease such as sarcoidosis.

F EFFECTS OF ADRENAL GLUCOGENIC CORTICOSTEROIDS (GLUCOCORTICOIDS)

Relatively large doses of cortisone are capable usually of reversing the hypercalcaemia induced by overdosage with calciferol (Winberg and Zetterstrom, 1956; Verner *et al.*, 1958) and this effect can occur without change in the assayable antiricketic activity in the serum of the patient treated (Thomas *et al.*, 1959). It has also been demonstrated that the hypercalcaemia and the intestinal hyperabsorption of calcium in sarcoidosis (Dent *et al.*, 1953; Anderson *et al.*, 1954; Henneman *et al.*, 1956; Jackson and Dancaster, 1959) and in infantile hypercalcaemia (Morgan *et al.*, 1956; Forfar *et al.*, 1956; Illig and Prader, 1959) can be similarly reversed by cortisone. Collectively, these observations have been taken to imply that there is an 'antagonism' between the actions of vitamin D and of the glucocorticoids. This concept has in turn tended to reinforce the belief that infantile hypercalcaemia and hypercalcaemia in sarcoidosis (Section IVE) are manifestations of the action of vitamin D.

Outside of these clinical therapeutic observations, there has been relatively little investigation of the effects of glucocorticoids on the intestinal absorption of calcium or on the metabolism of vitamin D in man. The problem has been explored almost exclusively in experimental animals and especially in the rat. In this species it has been established that steroid treatment reduces the capacity of the intestine to transport calcium both *in vivo* and *in vitro*. It must be emphasised, however, that the dose of steroid used to demonstrate this effect has greatly exceeded, on a basis of body weight, the therapeutic dosage effective in man: and the experimental design has usually involved the steroid treatment of vitamin D-deficient animals, with observations on the effects of such treatment on the responsiveness of calcium absorption to subsequent administration of vitamin D.

Avioli *et al.* (1968b) investigated the metabolism of an oral pulse dose of isotopically labelled cholecalciferol before and after treatment with prednisone (30 mg/day for 10 days). This treatment produced an accelerated disappearance of cholecalciferol from the circulation and an apparent increase in the production of biologically inactive more polar metabolites. These results have been interpreted to imply an effect of adrenal glucocorticoids on the metabolism of vitamin D and taken to support the concept of antagonism between the two steroids but they were undertaken before it was possible to monitor the formation of 1,25-dihydroxycholecalciferol in man. There appear to be no reported studies of this aspect of vitamin D metabolism in man but treatment with large doses of cortisone or prednisolone does not reduce the capacity of the vitamin D-deficient rat to produce 1,25-dihydroxycholecalciferol (Lukert *et al.*, 1973; Favus *et al.*, 1973). In both studies cited, steroid treatment was shown to inhibit active intestinal transport of calcium in spite of the presence of normal amounts of the hormone in the intestinal mucosa. Cortisone did not influence the localisation of the hormone in the nuclei of the intestinal target cell (Favus *et al.*, 1973) nor the capacity of these cells to synthesise the specific, vitamin D-dependent, calcium binding protein (Kimberg *et al.*, 1971). On this basis, there appears to be no 'antagonism' between vitamin D and adrenal glucocorticoids, the latter producing their effects on calcium transport by some independent action on the target cell.

None the less, in both the study of Lukert *et al.* (1973) and that of Favus *et al.* (1973), there was evidence that steroid treatment may have induced significant changes in vitamin D metabolism; if similar changes occur in man, they could be clinically relevant. The one group found evidence suggesting an increased formation of 1,25-dihydroxycholecalciferol after steroid treatment, the other group an increased formation of 24,25-dihydroxycholecalciferol. Both claims appear to be valid in terms of the data presented but, most unfortunately, the methods used were inadequate for the one group to confirm or refute the findings of the other. The simultaneous production of both 1,25- and 24,25-dihydroxycholecalciferol from a pulse of cholecalciferol would be aberrant in a vitamin D-deficient rat and is not usually seen in man (chapter 8, Sections VB and D); it is reminiscent of the pattern of vitamin D metabolism in primary hyperparathyroidism (Section IIIB). There is considerable evidence for the development of secondary hyperparathyroidism in rats treated with adrenal glucocorticoids; recently it has also been demonstrated that both chronic and acute treatment with such steroids in man produce a significant increase in the serum concentration of immunoassayable parathyroid hormone (Fucik *et al.*, 1975). These findings may be relevant to the development of severe osteoporosis in Cushing's syndrome and in patients treated with adrenal glucocorticoids. There is scope for further studies of parathyroid function, calciferol metabolism and their interrelations in patients under the influence of excess adrenal glucocorticoids.

G DIPHOSPHONATE TREATMENT

Treatment of rats with high dosage (40 mg/kg/day) of the synthetic diphosphonate, ethane-1-hydroxy-1, 1-diphosphonate (EHDP), produces defective mineralisation of bone (King *et al.*, 1971) and an apparently indirect inhibition of the renal synthesis of 1,25-dihydroxycholecalciferol (Hill *et al.*, 1973). Similar effects have been produced in chicks by the same high dose (Taylor *et al.*, 1975). EHDP has also been used in man in the attempted treatment of Paget's disease, myositis ossificans and various types of calcinosis. The therapeutic dose in man has been smaller (8–20 mg/kg/day) but treatment with EHDP has caused defective mineralisation not only of the dystrophic bone in myositis ossificans but also of the patient's normal bone (Jowsey *et al.*, 1971; Stanbury, 1972a). Although this treatment can thus cause the development of a form of osteomalacia, it is unlikely to have inhibited the formation of the hormone since the intestinal absorption and urinary output of calcium are not reduced in EHDP treated patients (Russell *et al.*, 1974). We have investigated the metabolism of a pulse dose of labelled cholecalciferol in five patients treated with EHDP (unpublished). In each patient the formation of labelled 25-hydroxycholecalciferol was apparently normal (Fig. 1) and the serum concentration of labelled 1,25-dihydroxycholecalciferol at 48 h was appropriate to the prevailing serum concentrations of 25-hydroxycalciferol and calcium (Figs 2 and 3). The concentrations of labelled 24,25-dihydroxycholecalciferol in the serum at the same time tended to be high; the mean value was higher than in any other group studied (including hypoparathyroidism and primary hyperparathyroidism, q.v.) and individual concentrations in two patients were the highest we have encountered in studies of this kind. Treatment of adults with EHDP causes elevation of the serum phosphate but, in the two patients cited, the concentration of labelled 24,25-dihydroxycholecalciferol appeared also to be relatively high for the prevailing level of serum phosphate. These data are quantitatively inadequate to establish statistical significance but the apparent tendency to produce increased amounts of 24,25-dihydroxycholecalciferol resembles one of the effects of EHDP in the rat and chick (Hill *et al.*, 1973; Taylor *et al.*, 1975). Further studies would be of academic interest but of doubtful relevance to the development of defective mineralisation in EHDP treated patients which is most probably caused by a direct action of the drug on the bone.

H OSTEOPOROSIS

The cause of osteoporosis in the elderly is unknown but the reduction of bone mass has been regarded as a consequence of calcium deficiency arising on the basis of intestinal malabsorption of calcium. An apparently impaired absorption has been demonstrated in some but by no means in all patients with osteoporosis; when present, it is questionable whether it should be regarded as a contributory cause or as a consequence of the bony condition. Bullamore *et al.* (1970) found a progressive fall in calcium absorption with age in both sexes after about 60 years and they suggested that this may be due to vitamin D deficiency. No direct evidence was provided in support of this suggestion but it was subsequently reported that 'quite small doses' of vitamin D will improve this malabsorption (Nordin, 1971). It is also often mooted that the 'requirement for vitamin D' is increased in the elderly but there is little or no tangible evidence for this; and similarly no evidence for the speculative suggestion that the ageing kidney may have a reduced capacity to synthesise 1,25-dihydroxycholecalciferol. Exton-Smith *et al.* (1966) produced evidence that the development of osteomalacia in the elderly may contribute to the reduced radiographic density of their bones. More recently, Aaron *et al.* (1974) have described histological changes, which they interpret to imply the presence of osteomalacia, in a large proportion of older patients with fractures of the upper end of the femur. This they attribute to vitamin D-deficiency; they further speculate that a degree of vitamin D-deficiency insufficient to cause osteomalacia might cause impaired calcium absorption and thereby contribute to development of the osteoporotic component of the bone disease. There is no evidence for or against this suggestion and we suggest that it confuses the issue to seek a common cause for two different bone diseases which have little in common. Of more importance is the danger that propagation of a 'vitamin D-deficiency hypothesis' for osteoporosis could lead to widespread use of vitamin D and synthetic analogues as 'treatment' for this 'disease'. The observations of Peacock *et al.* (1974) have demonstrated conclusively the hazards attending overdosage with 1α-hydroxycholecalciferol in patients with osteoporosis.

We have undertaken no detailed studies of vitamin D metabolism in patients with osteoporosis but one half of the control subjects in the study of Mawer *et al.* (1975a) were of reasonably advanced age (55 to 71 years); their production of labelled hormone from a pulse of radioactive cholecalciferol was not apparently different from that of younger patients of similar nutritional status. We have, however, studied the effects of 1,25-dihydroxycholecalciferol in a daily oral dose of 1 μg in a small group of elderly patients with well established osteoporosis (Davies *et al.*, 1977b). There was an immediate increase in the urinary output of calcium, which equalled and in some cases exceeded any increase of intestinal absorption of calcium produced by the treatment; the external calcium balance was thus not improved. These results were fully anticipated and the study was undertaken deliberately, to demonstrate the expected ineffectiveness of this form as therapy and to provide a warning against the indiscriminate use of 1,25-dihydroxycholecalciferol in osteoporotic patients.

References

Aaron, J. E., Gallagher, J. C., Anderson, J., Stasiak, L., Longton, E. B., Nordin, B. E. C. and Nicholson, M. (1974). *Lancet* **I**, 229.
Adams, R. G., Harrison, J. F. and Scott, P. (1969). *Quart. J. Med.* **38**, 425.
Adams, P. H., Hill, L. F., Wain, D. and Taylor, C. M. (1975). *Calcif. Tiss. Res.* **16**, 293.
Anast, C. S., Mohs, J. M., Kaplan, S. L. and Burns, T. W. (1972). *Science* **177**, 606.
Anderson, J., Dent, C. E., Harper, C. and Philpot, G. R. (1954). *Lancet* **II**, 720.
Arnaud, C. D., Tsao, H. S., Littledyke, T. (1971). *J. Clin. Invest.* **50**, 21.
Arnaud, C. D., Glorieux, F. and Scriver, C. R. (1972). *Pediatrics* **49**, 837.
Atkinson, M., Nordin, B. E. C. and Sherlock, S. (1956). *Quart. J. Med.* **25**, 299.
Avioli, L. V. (1974). *Amer. J. Med.* **57**, 34.
Avioli, L. V., Lee, S. W., McDonald, J. E., Lund, J. and DeLuca, H. F. (1967a). *J. Clin. Invest.* **46**, 983.
Avioli, L. V., Williams, T. F., Lund, J. and DeLuca, H. F. (1967b). *J. Clin. Invest.* **46**, 1907.
Avioli, L. V., Birge, S., Lee, S. W. and Slatopolsky, E. (1968a). *J. Clin. Invest.* **47**, 2229.
Avioli, L. V., Birge, S. J. and Lee, S. W. (1968b). *J. Clin. Endocr.* **28**, 1341.
Badenoch, J. and Fourman, P. (1954). *Quart. J. Med.* (N.S.) **23**, 165.
Balsan, S. and Garabedian, M. (1972). *J. Clin. Invest.* **51**, 749.

Balsan, S., Garabedian, M., Sorgniard, R., Dommergnes, J. P., Courtecuisse, V., Holick, M. F. and DeLuca, H. F. (1976). *In* 'Vitamin D and Problems Related to Uremic Bone Disease' (Ed. Norman, A. W., Schaefer, K., Grigoleit, H. G., v. Herrath, D. and Ritz, E.) p. 249. De Gruyter, Berlin and New York.

Bearn, A. G., Yu, T. F. and Gutman, A. B. (1957). *J. Clin. Invest.* **36**, 1107.

Bell, N. H., Gill, J. R. and Bartter, F. C. (1964). *Amer. J. Med.* **36**, 500.

Belsey, R. E., Clark, M. B., Bernat, M., Glowacki, J., Holick, M. F., DeLuca, H. F. and Potts, J. T. (1974). *Amer. J. Med.* **57**, 50.

Bonucci, E., Maschio, G., D'Angelo, A., Ossi, E., Lupo, A. and Valvo, E. (1975). *In* 'Vitamin D and Problems Related to Uremic Bone Disease' (Ed. Norman, A. W., Schaefer, K., Grigoleit, H. G., v. Herrath, D. and Ritz, E.) p. 523. De Gruyter, Berlin and New York.

Bordier, P. J., Marie, P., Arnaud, C. D., Gueris, J., Ferriere, C. and Norman, A. W. (1975). *In* 'Vitamin D and Problems Related to Uremic Bone Disease' (Ed. Norman, A. W., Schaefer, K., Grigoleit, H. G., v. Herrath, D. and Ritz, E.) p. 133. De Gruyter, Berlin and New York.

Brickman, A. S., Coburn, J. W. and Norman, A. W. (1972). *J. Clin. Invest.* **51**, 15a.

Brickman, A. S., Coburn, J. W., Kurokawa, K., Bethune, J. E., Harrison, H. E. and Norman, A. W. (1973). *New Eng. J. Med.* **289**, 495.

Brickman, A. S., Coburn, J. W., Massry, S. A. and Norman, A. W. (1974). *Ann. Int. Med.* **80**, 161.

Brickman, A. S., Coburn, J. W., Friedman, G. R., Okamura, H., Massry, S. G. and Norman, A. W. (1976). *J. Clin. Invest.* **57**, 1540.

Brumbaugh, P. F., Haussler, D. H., Bressler, R. and Haussler, M. R. (1974a). *Science* **183**, 1089.

Brumbaugh, P. F., Haussler, D. H., Bursac, K. M. and Haussler, M. R. (1974b). *Biochemistry* **13**, 4091.

Bullamore, J. R., Gallagher, J. C., Wilkinson, R., Nordin, B. E. C. and Marshall, D. H. (1970). *Lancet* **II**, 535.

Caspary, W. F., Hesch, R. D., Matte, R., Ritter, H., Kattermann, R. and Emrich, D. (1975). *In* 'Vitamin D and Problems Related to Uremic Bone Disease' (Ed. Norman, A. W., Schaefer, K., Grigoleit, H. G., v. Herrath, D. and Ritz, E.) p. 737. De Gruyter, Berlin and New York.

Catto, G. R. D., MacLeod, M., Pelc, B. and Kodicek, E. (1975). *Brit. Med. J.* **1**, 12.

Chan, J. C. M., Oldham, S. B., Holick, M. F. and DeLuca, H. F. (1975). *J. Amer. Med. Assoc.* **234**, 47.

Childs, B., Cantolino, S. and Dyke, M. K. (1962). *Bull. Johns Hopkins Hosp.* **110**, 134.

Chisholm, J. J., Harrison, H. F., Eberlein, W. R. and Harrison, H. E. (1955). *Amer. J. Dis. Child* **89**, 159.

Christiansen, C., Rødbro, P. and Lund, M. (1973). *Brit. Med. J.* **4**, 695.

Clayton, B. E., Fairney, A., Flynn, D. and Jackson, D. (1976). *In* 'Inborn Errors of Bone Metabolism' (Ed. Bickel, H. and Stern, J.) p. 63. Medical and Technical, Lancaster, England.

Coburn, J. W., Reddy, C. R., Brickman, A. S., Hartenbower, D. L., Friedler, R. M. and Norman, A. W. (1973). *Fed. Proc.* **32**, 918 abs.

Coburn, J. W., Brickman, A. S. and Hartenbower, D. L. (1975). *In* 'Vitamin D and Problems Related to Uremic Bone Disease' (Ed. Norman, A. W., Schaefer, K., Grigoleit, H. G., v. Herrath, D. and Ritz, E.) p. 219. De Gruyter, Berlin and New York.

Corradino, R. A. and Wasserman, R. H. (1971). *Science* **172**, 731.

Cuthbertson, W. F. J. (1963). *Proc. Nutr. Soc.* **22**, 146.
Davie, M. W. J., Chalmers, T. M., Hunter, J. O., Pelc, B. and Kodicek, E. (1976). *Ann. Int. Med.* **84**, 281.
Davies, M., Hill, L. F., Taylor, C. M. and Stanbury, S. W. (1977a). *Lancet* **I**, 55.
Davies, M., Mawes, E. B. and Adams, P. H. (1977b). *J. clin. Endocr. Metab.* **45**, 199.
Dent, C. E. (1952). *Journal of Bone and Joint Surgery* **34-B**, 266.
Dent, C. E. and Harris, H. (1958). *J. Bone J. Surg.* **38-B**, 204.
Dent, C. E. and Watson, L. (1966). *Brit. Med. J.* **1**, 646.
Dent, C. E., Flynn, F. V. and Nabarro, J. D. N. (1953). *Brit. Med. J.* **2**, 808.
Dent, C. E., Harper, C. M. and Philpot, G. R. (1961). *Quart. J. of Med.* **30**, 1.
Dent, C. E., Richens, A., Rowe, D. J. F. and Stamp, T. C. B. (1970). *Brit. Med. J.* **4**, 69.
Dent, C. E., Round, J. M., Rowe, D. J. F. and Stamp, T. C. B. (1973). *Lancet* **I**, 1282.
Dundon, S., Travis, L., Dodge, W. and Roberts, F. J. (1966). *J. Ir. Med. Ass.* **59**, 87.
Dunn, M. J. (1971). *Clin. Sci.* **41**, 333.
Dunnigan, M. G., Paton, J. P. J., Haase, S., McNicol, G. W., Gardner, M. D. and Smith, C. M. (1962). *Scot. Med. J.* **7**, 159.
Dunnigan, M. G. and Smith, C. M. (1965). *Scot. Med. J.* **10**, 1.
Eastwood, J. B., Bordier, P. J., Clarkson, E. M., Tun Chot, S. and de Wardener, H. E. (1974). *Clin. Sci. Molec. Med.* **47**, 23.
Eisenberg, E. (1965). *J. Clin. Invest.* **44**, 942.
Estep, H., Shaw, W. A., Watlington, C., Hobe, R., Holland, W. and Tocker, S. (1969). *J. Clin. Endocr.* **29**, 842.
Exton-Smith, A. N., Hodkinson, M. H. and Stanton, B. R. (1966). *Lancet* **II**, 999.
Fanconi, G., (1928). Der intestinale infantilisms (Berlin).
Fanconi, G., Girardet, P., Schlesinger, B., Butler, N. and Black, J. (1952). *Helv. Paediat. Acta* **7**, 314.
Favus, M. J., Kimberg, D. V., Miller, G. N. and Gershon, E. (1973). *J. Clin. Invest.* **52**, 1328.
Fellars, F. X. and Schwartz, R. (1958). *New Eng. J. Med.* **259**, 1050.
Forfar, J. O., Balf, C. L., Maxwell, G. M. and Tompsett, S. L. (1956). *Lancet* **I**, 981.
Fraser, D., Kidd, B. S. L., Kooh, S. W. and Paunier, L. A. (1966). *Pediat. Clin. N. Amer.* **13**, 503.
Fraser, D., Kooh, S. W. and Scriver, C. R. (1967). *Pediat. Res.* **1**, 425.
Fraser, D., Kooh, S. W., Kind, H. P., Holick, M. F., Tanaka, Y. and DeLuca, H. F. (1973). *New Eng. J. Med.* **289**, 817.
Fraser, D. R. and Kodicek, E. (1970). *Nature* (London) **228**, 764.
Friedman, M., Hatcher, G. and Watson, L. (1967). *Lancet* **I**, 703.
Fucik, R. F., Kukreja, S. C., Hargis, C. K., Bowser, E. N., Henderson, W. J. and Williams, G. A. (1975). *J. Clin. Endocr.* **40**, 152.
Galante, L., MacAuley, S., Colston, K. and MacIntyre, I. (1972). *Lancet* **I**, 985.
Garabedian, M., Holick, M. F., DeLuca, H. F. and Boyle, I. T. (1972). *Proc. Natl. Acad. Sci. USA* **69**, 1673.
Garcia, R. E., Friedman, W. F., Kaback, M. M. and Rowe, R. D. (1964). *New Eng. J. Med.* **271**, 117.
Glorieux, F. H. and Scriver, C. R. (1972). *Science* **175**, 997.
Glorieux, F. H., Scriver, C. R., Holick, M. F. and DeLuca, H. F. (1973). *Lancet* **II**, 287.
Gonick, H. C., Lee, D. B. N., Drinkard, J. P. and Coulson, W. C. (1973). *In* 'Clinical Aspects of Metabolic Bone Disease' (Ed. Frame, B., Parfitt, A. M. and Duncan, H.) p. 403. Excerpta Medica, Amsterdam.

Gray, R. W., Dominguez, J. H. and Lemann, J. (1975). *In* 'Vitamin D and Problems Related to Uremic Bone Disease' (Ed. Norman, A. W., Schaefer, K., Grigoleit, H. G., v. Herrath, D. and Ritz, E.) p. 331. De Gruyter, Berlin and New York.
Haddad, J. G. and Chyu, K. J. (1971). *J. Clin. Endocr.* **33**, 992.
Haddad, J. G. and Hahn, T. J. (1973). *Nature* (London) **244**, 515.
Haddad, J. G., Chyu, K. J., Hahn, T. J. and Stamp, T. C. B. (1973). *J. Lab. Clin. Med.* **81**, 22.
Hahn, T. J., Birge, S. J., Scharp, C. R. and Avioli, L. V. (1972a). *J. Clin. Invest.* **51**, 741.
Hahn, T. J., Hendin, B. A., Scharp, C. R. and Haddad, J. G. (1972b). *New. Eng. J. Med.* **287**, 900.
Hahn, T. J., Scharp, C. R., Halstead, L. R., Haddad, J. G., Karl, D. M. and Avioli, L. V. (1975). *J. Clin. Endocr. Metab.* **41**, 926.
Heaton, F. W. and Fourman, P. (1965). *Lancet* **II**, 50.
Henderson, R. G., Russell, R. G. G., Ledingham, J. G. G., Smith, R., Oliver, D. O., Walton, R. J., Small, D. G., Preston, C., Warner, G. T. and Norman, A. W. (1974). *Lancet* **I**, 379.
Hendrix, J. Z. (1966). *Ann. Intern. Med.* **64**, 797.
Henneman, P. H., Dempsey, E. F., Carroll, E. L. and Albright, F. (1956). *J. Clin. Invest.* **35**, 1229.
Hepner, G. W., Roginsky, M. and Moo, H. F. (1975). *In* 'Vitamin D and Problems Related to Uremic Bone Disease' (Ed. Norman, A. W., Schaefer, K., Grigoleit, H. G., v. Herrath, D. and Ritz, E.) p. 325. De Gruyter, Berlin and New York.
Hill, L. F. and Stanbury, S. W. (1975). *Nephron.* **15**, 369.
Hill, L. F., Van Den Berg, C. J. and Mawer, E. B. (1971). *Nature New Biol.* **232**, 189.
Hill, L. F., Lumb, G. A., Mawer, E. B. and Stanbury, S. W. (1973). *Clin. Sci.* **44**, 335.
Hill, L. F., Taylor, C. M. and Mawer, E. B. (1974). *Clin. Sci. and Molec. Med.* **47**, 14P.
Hill, L. F., Davies, M., Taylor, C. M. and Stanbury, S. W. (1975). *Clin. Endocr.* **5** (Suppl), 1675.
Hodgkin, P., Kay, G. H., Hine, P. M., Lumb, G. A. and Stanbury, S. W. (1973). *Lancet* **II**, 167.
Hodgkinson, A. (1963). *Clin. Sci.* **25**, 321.
Holmes, A. M., Enoch, B. A., Taylor, J. L. and Jones, M. E. (1973). *Quart. J. Med.* **42**, 125.
Hunter, J. (1974). *J. Roy. Coll. Phys.* (London) **8**, 163.
Hunter, J., Maxwell, J. D., Stewart, D. A., Parsons, V. and Williams, R. (1971). *Brit. Med. J.* **4**, 202.
Illig, R. and Prader, A. (1959). *Helv. Paediat. Acta* **14**, 618.
Jackson, W. P. U. and Dancaster, C. P. (1959). *J. Clin. Endocr.* **19**, 658.
Jowsey, J., Riggs, B. L., Kelly, P. J. and Hoffman, D. L. (1971). *J. Lab. Clin. Med.* **78**, 574.
Kazantzis, G., Flynn, F. V., Spowage, J. S. and Trott, D. J. (1963). *Quart. J. Med.* (N.S.) **32**, 165.
Kehayoglou, A. K., Agnew, J. E., Holdsworth, C. D., Whelton, M. J. and Sherlock, S. (1968). *Lancet* **I**, 715.
Kimberg, D. V., Baerg, R. D., Gershon, E. and Grandusius, R. T. (1971). *J. Clin. Invest.* **50**, 1309.
Kind, H. P., Prader, A. and DeLuca, H. F. (1976). *In* 'Inborn Errors of Bone Metabolism' (Ed. Bickel, H. and Stern, J.) p. 76. Medical and Technical, Lancaster, England.
King, W. R., Francis, M. D. and Michael, W. R. (1971). *Clin. Orthop.* **78**, 251.

Kooh, S. W., Fraser, D., DeLuca, H. F., Holick, M. F., Belsey, R. E., Clark, M. B. and Murray, T. M. (1975). *New Eng. J. Med.* **293**, 840.
Krawitt, E. L., Grundman, M. J. and Mawer, E. B. (1977). *Lancet* **II**, 1246.
Krempien, B., Ritz, E., Beck, U. and Keilbach, H. (1972). *Virchows Archs A* **357**, 257.
Kruse, R. (1968). *Mschr. Kinderheilk* **116**, 378.
Larrson, S. E. and Lorentzon, R. (1975). *In* 'Vitamin D and Problems Related to Uremic Bone Disease' (Ed. Norman, A. W., Schaefer, K., Grigoleit, H. G., v. Herrath, D. and Ritz, E.) p. 68. De Gruyter, Berlin and New York.
Lawson, D. E. M. and Emtage, J. S. (1974). *In* 'The Metabolism and Function of Vitamin D', p. 75. Biochemical Society Special Publication No. 3.
Lilienfeld-Toal, H. von and Becker, W. M. (1975). *In* 'Vitamin D and Problems Related to Uremic Bone Disease' (Ed. Norman, A. W., Schaefer, K., Grigoleit, H. G., v. Herrath, D. and Ritz, E.) p. 355. De Gruyter, Berlin and New York.
Lindquist, B. (1962). *Acta Paediat.* (Uppsala) **51,** (Suppl.) 135, 144.
Livingstone, S., Berman, W. and Pauli, L. L. (1973). *J. Amer. Med,. Assoc.* **224**, 1634.
Liu, S. H. and Chu, H. I. (1943). *Medicine* (Baltimore) **22**, 103.
Long, R. G., Skinner, R. K., Wills, M. R. and Sherlock, S. (1976). *Lancet* **II**, 650.
Loomis, W. F. (1967). *Science* **157**, 501.
Lucas, R. C. (1883). *Lancet* **I**, 993.
Lukert, B. P., Stanbury, S. W. and Mawer, E. B. (1973). *Endocrinol.* **93**, 718.
Lumb, G. A. and Stanbury, S. W. (1974). *Amer. J. Med.* **56**, 833.
Lumb, G. A., Mawer, E. B. and Stanbury, S. W. (1971). *Amer. J. Med.* **50**, 421.
MacIntyre, I., Hanna, S., Booth, C. C. and Read, A. E. (1961). *Clin. Sci.* **20**, 297.
Manois, S., Panagou, M., Tsakalidis, D. and Kovatsis, A. (1966). *Arch. Franc. Pédiat.* **23**, 63.
Massry, S. G., Stein, R., Garty, J., Arieff, A. I., Coburn, J. W. and Norman, A. W. (1975). *In* 'Vitamin D and Problems Related to Uremic Bone Disease' (Ed. Norman, A. W., Schaefer, K., Grigoleit, H. G., v. Herrath, D. and Ritz, E.) p. 619. De Gruyter, Berlin and New York.
Mather, G. (1957). *Brit. Med. J.* **1**, 248.
Mawer, E. B. (1974). *In* 'The Metabolism and Function of Vitamin D', p. 27. Biochemical Society Special Publication No. 3.
Mawer, E. B., Backhouse, J., Lumb, G. A. and Stanbury, S. W. (1971a). *Nature New Biol.* (London) **232**, 188.
Mawer, E. B., Lumb, G. A., Schaefer, K. and Stanbury, S. W. (1971b). *Clin. Sci.* **40**, 39.
Mawer, E. B., Backhouse, J., Holman, C. A., Lumb, G. A. and Stanbury, S. W. (1972). *Clin. Sci.* **43**, 413.
Mawer, E. B., Backhouse, J., Taylor, C. M., Lumb, G. A. and Stanbury, S. W. (1973). *Lancet* **I**, 626.
Mawer, E. B., Backhouse, J., Hill, L. F., Lumb, G. A., De Silva, P., Taylor, C. M. and Stanbury, S. W. (1975a). *Clin. Sci. Molec. Med.* **48**, 349.
Mawer, E. B., Backhouse, J., Hill, L. F. and Taylor, C. M. (1975b). *In* 'Vitamin D and Problems Related to Uremic Bone Disease' (Ed. Norman, A. W., Schaefer, K., Grigoleit, H. G., v. Herrath, D. and Ritz, E.) p. 603. De Gruyter, Berlin and New York.
Miravet, L., Rambaud, J. C., Lousi, C. and Hioco, D. (1969). *Sem Hôp. Paris* **45**, 531.
Morgan, B. (1973). Osteomalacia, Renal Osteodystrophy and Osteoporosis. Charles C. Thomas, Springfield, Illinois.
Morgan, D. B., Paterson, C. R., Woods, C. G., Pulvertaft, C. N. and Fourman, P. (1965). *Lancet* **I**, 1089.

Morgan, D. B., Hunt, G. and Paterson, C. R. (1970). *Quart. J. Med.* **39**, 395.
Morgan, H. G., Mitchell, R. G., Stowers, J. M. and Thomson, J. (1956). *Lancet* **I**, 925.
Muldowney, F. P., McKenna, T. J., Kyle, L. H., Greaney, R. and Swan, M. (1970). *New Eng. J. Med.* **282**, 61.
Nassim, J. R., Saville, P. D., Cook, P. B. and Mulligan, L. (1959). *Quart. J. Med.* (n.s.) **28**, 141.
Nicaud, P., Lafitte, A. and Gros, A. (1942). *Arch. Mal. Prof.* **4**, 192.
Nordin, B. E. C. (1971). *Brit. Med. J.* **1**, 571.
Offermann, G. and Dittmar, F. (1975). *In* 'Vitamin D and Problems Related to Uremic Bone Disease' (Ed. Norman, A. W., Schaefer, K., Grigoleit, H. G., v. Herrath, D. and Ritz, E.) p. 295. De Gruyter, Berlin and New York.
Oldham, S. B., Arnaud, C. D. and Jowsey, J. (1974). *In* 'Endocrinology 1973' (Ed. Taylor, S.). Heinemann, London.
Omdahl, J. L. and DeLuca, H. F. (1971). *Science* **174**, 949.
Omdahl, J. L. and DeLuca, H. F. (1973). *Physiol. Rev.* **53**, 327.
Paunier, L., Radde, I. C., Kooh, S. W., Coven, P. E. and Fraser, D. (1968). *Pediatrics* **41**, 385.
Peacock, M., Gallagher, J. C. and Nordin, B. E. C. (1974). *Lancet* **I**, 385.
Prader, A. (1976). *In* 'Inborn Errors of Bone Metabolism' (Ed. Bickel, H. and Stern, J.) p. 115. Medical and Technical, Lancaster, England.
Prader, A., Illig, R. and Heierli, E. (1961). *Helv. Paediat. Acta* **16**, 452.
Preece, M. M., Ford, J. A., McIntosh, W. B., Dunnigan, M. G., Tomlinson, S. and O'Riordan, J. L. H. (1973). *Lancet* **I**, 907.
Puschett, J. B., Fernandez, P. C., Boyle, I. T., Gray, R. W., Omdahl, J. L. and DeLuca, H. F. (1972). *Proc. Soc. Exp. Biol. Med.* **141**, 379.
Puschett, J. B., Genel, M., Rasteger, A., Anast, C., DeLuca, H. F. and Friedman, A. (1975). *Clin. Pharm. Therap.* **17**, 202.
Rapado, A., Castrillo, J. M., Arrayo, M., Traba, M. L. and Calle, H. (1975). *In* 'Vitamin D and Problems Related to Uremic Bone Disease' (Ed. Norman, A. W., Schaefer, K., Grigoleit, H. G., v. Herrath, D. and Ritz, E.) p. 453. De Gruyter, Berlin and New York.
Rasmussen, H. (1969). *New Engl. J. Med.* **280**, 1416.
Rasmussen, H., Bordier, P., Kurokawa, K., Nagata, N. and Ogata, E. (1974). *Amer. J. Med.* **56**, 751.
Reade, T. M., Scriver, C. R., Glorieux, F. H., Nogrady, B., Devlin, E., Poirier, R., Holick, M. F. and DeLuca, H. F. (1975). *Pediat. Res.* **9**, 593.
Reddy, V. and Sivakumar, B. (1974). *Lancet* **I**, 963.
Reynolds, J. J. (1974). *In* 'Metabolism and Function of Vitamin D', p. 91. Biochemical Society Special Publication No. 3.
Reynolds, J. J., Holick, M. F. and DeLuca, H. F. (1974). *Calc. Tiss. Res.* **15**, 333.
Richards, P., Chamberlain, M. J. and Wrong, O. M. (1972). *Lancet* **II**, 994.
Richens, A. and Rowe, D. J. F. (1970). *Brit. Med. J.* **4**, 73.
Ritz, E., Krempien, B., Mehls, O. and Malluche, H. (1973). *Kidney International* **4**, 116.
Ritz, E., Mehls, O., Malluche, H., Krempien, B., Schmidt-Gay, K. H. and Heimberg, H. (1975). *In* 'Vitamin D and Problems Related to Uremic Bone Disease' (Ed. Norman, A. W., Schaefer, K., Grigoleit, H. G., v. Herrath, D. and Ritz, E.) p. 497. De Gruyter, Berlin and New York.
Rösler, A. and Rabinowitz, D. (1973). *Lancet* **I**, 803.
Russell, R. G. G., Smith, R., Walton, R. J., Preston, C., Basson, R., Henderson, R. G. and Norman, A. W. (1974). *Lancet* **II**, 14.

Scriver, C. R., Glorieux, F. H., Reade, S., Terenhouse, S. and Delvin, E. (1976). *In* 'Inborn Errors of Bone Metabolism' (Ed. Bickel, H. and Stern, J.) p. 150. Medical and Technical, Lancaster, England. In press.
Schlesinger, B. E., Butler, N. R. and Black, J. A. (1956). *Brit. Med. J.* **1**, 127.
Seelig, M. S. (1969). *Ann. N.Y. Acad. Sci.* **147**, 537.
Shils, M. E. (1969). *Medicine* (Baltimore) **48**, 61.
Silverberg, D. S., Bettcher, K. B., Dossetor, J. B., Overton, T. R., Holick, M. F. and DeLuca, H. F. (1975). *Canad. Med. Assoc. J.* **112**, 192.
Smith, D. W., Blizzard, R. M. and Harrison, H. E. (1959). *Pediatrics* **24**, 258.
Stamp, T. C. B. (1974). *Lancet* **II**, 121.
Stamp, T. C. B. (1975). *Proc. Nutr. Soc.* **34**, 119.
Stamp, T. C. B. and Round, J. M. (1974). *Nature* (London) **247**, 563.
Stamp, T. C. B., Round, J. M., Rowe, D. J. F. and Haddad, J. G. (1972). *Brit. Med. J.* **4**, 9.
Stanbury, S. W. (1957). *Brit. Med. Bull.* **13**, 57.
Stanbury, S. W. (1962a). *In* 'Renal Disease' (Ed. Black, D. A. K.) first edition, p. 508. Blackwell, Oxford.
Stanbury, S. W. (1962b). *Swiss Med. J.* **92**, 883.
Stanbury, S. W. (1966). *Ann. Int. Med.* **65**, 1133.
Stanbury, S. W. (1967). *In* 'Renal Disease' (Ed. Black, D. A. K.) second edition, p. 665. Blackwell, Oxford.
Stanbury, S. W. (1968a). *Amer. J. Med.* **44**, 714.
Stanbury, S. W. (1968b). *In* 'Nutrition in Renal Disease' (Ed. Berlyne, G. M.) p. 118. Livingstone, Edinburgh.
Stanbury, S. W. (1971). *In* 'Phosphate et Métabolisme Phospho-calcique' (Ed. Hioco, D. J.) p. 187. Expansion Scientifique Francaise, Paris.
Stanbury, S. W. (1972a). *Clin. Endocr. Metab.* **1**, 239.
Stanbury, S. W. (1972b). *Clin. Endocr. Metab.* **1**, 267.
Stanbury, S. W. (1973a). *In* 'Atti Simposi Internazzionali sul Metabolismo Dell Acqua e Degli Elettroliti', p. 241. Sclavo, Siena, Italy.
Stanbury, S. W. (1973b). Proceedings IVth International Congress Endocrinology, Washington, 1972.
Stanbury, S. W. (1976). *In* 'Inborn Errors of Bone Metabolism' (Ed. Bickel, H. and Stern, J.) p. 21. Medical and Technical, Lancaster, England.
Stanbury, S. W. and Lumb, G. A. (1962). *Medicine* (Baltimore) **41**, 1.
Stanbury, S. W., Lumb, G. A. and Nicholson, W. F. (1960). *Lancet* **I**, 793.
Stanbury, S. W., Lumb, G. A. and Mawer, E. B. (1969). *Arch. Intern. Med.* (Chicago) **124**, 274.
Stanbury, S. W., Mawer, E. B., Lumb, G. A., Hill, L. F., Holman, C. A., Jones, M. and Van Den Berg, C. J. (1972). *In* 'Endocrinology 1971' (Ed. Taylor, S.) p. 487. Heinemann, London.
Stanbury, S. W., Mawer, E. B., Lumb, G. A., Hill, L. F., Holman, C. A., Taylor, C. M. and Torkington, P. (1973). *In* 'Cllnical Aspects of Metabolic Bone Disease' (Ed. Frame, B., Parfitt, A. M. and Duncan, H.) p. 562. Excerpta Medica, Amsterdam.
Stanbury, S. W., Mawer, E. B., Hill, L. F., Taylor, C. M., de Silva, P. and Lumb, G. A. (1975a). *In* 'Calcium Regulating Hormones' (Ed. Talmage, R. V., Owen, M and Pasons, J. A.) p. 431. Excerpta Medica, Amsterdam.
Stanbury, S. W., Mawer, E. B., Lumb, G. A., Hill, L. F., de Silva, P. and Taylor, C. M. (1975b). *In* 'Vitamin D and Problems Related to Uremic Bone Disease' (Ed. Norman, A. W., Schaefer, K., Grigoleit, H. G., v. Herrath, D. and Ritz, E.) p. 205. De Gruyter, Berlin and New York.

Stickler, G. B. (1963). *J. Pediat.* **63**, 942.
Suh, S. M., Csima, A. and Fraser, D. (1971). *J. Clin. Invest.* **50**, 2668.
Suh, S. M., Tashjian, A. H., Parkinson, D. K. and Fraser, D. (1973). *In* 'Clinical Aspects of Metabolic Bone Disease' (Ed. Frame, B., Parfitt, A. M. and Duncan, H.) p. 667. Excerpta Medica, Amsterdam.
Tanaka, Y. and DeLuca, H. F. (1973). *Arch. Biochem. Biophys.* **154**, 566.
Taylor, C. M. (1976). *Clin. Sci. Molec. Med.* **51**, 76P.
Taylor, C. M., Mawer, E. B. and Reeve, A. (1975). *Clin. Sci. Molec. Med.* **49**, 391.
Taylor, R. L., Lynch, H. J. and Wysor, W. G. (1963). *Amer. J. Med.* **34**, 221.
Thomas, W. C., Morgan, H. G., Connor, T. B., Haddock, L., Bills, C. E. and Howard, T. E. (1959). *J. Clin. Invest.* **38**, 1078.
Thompson, G. R., Lewis, B. and Booth, C. C. (1966a). *J. Clin. Invest.* **45**, 94.
Thompson, G. R., Lewis, B. and Booth, C. C. (1966b). *Lancet* **I**, 457.
Thompson, G. R., Neale, G., Watts, J. M. and Booth, C. C. (1966c). *Lancet* **I**, 623.
Tsuchiya, K. (1969). *Keio J. Med.* **18**, 181.
Verner, J. V., Engel, F. L. and McPherson, H. T. (1958). *Ann. Intern. Med.* **48**, 765.
Wacker, W. E. C. and Parisi, A. F. (1968). *New Engl. J. Med.* **278**, 658, 712–717, 772.
Wagonfeld, J. B., Nemchausky, B. A., Bolt, M., Horst, J. V., Boyer, J. L. and Rosenberg, I. H. (1976). *Lancet* **II**, 391.
Wilson, D. C. and Widdowson, E. M. (1942). Indian Medical Research Memoirs, No. 34.
Wilson, D. R. and Yendt, E. R. (1963). *Amer. J. Med.* **35**, 487.
Winberg, J. and Zetterström, R. (1956). *Acta Paediat.* (Uppsala) **45**, 96.
Witmer, G. and Balsan, S. (1971). European Society for Pediatric Research: Working Party on Mineral Metabolism (abstract).
Woodhouse, N. J. Y., Doyle, F. H. and Joplin, G. F. (1971). *Lancet* **II**, 283.
Yu, J. S., Walker-Smith, J. A. and Burnard, E. D. (1971). *Med. J. Aust.* **1**, 790.

10 Functional Interactions between Vitamin D Metabolism and other Calcium-Regulating Hormones

J. A. PARSONS

I Introduction

The total quantity of calcium in the body and its concentration in extracellular fluid are variables of such biological importance that they have led to the evolution of two major endocrine regulating systems, based respectively on the differential biological activity of the vitamin D secosteroids and of the straight-chain parathyroid peptide or peptides. A third endocrine system based on 32-residue peptides with amidated carboxyl terminals and a strongly conserved amino-terminal sulphur-containing ring, the calcitonins, undoubtedly contribute to the regulation of extracellular fluid calcium in mammalia, especially during development, specifically by temporarily inhibiting the osteolytic component of bone turnover (for reviews see Hirsch and Munson, 1969; Copp, 1969, 1970; Munson, 1976).

Although in mammals the calcitonins have been shown to play an important part in protecting against the risks of transient hypercalcaemia during intestinal absorption of large calcium loads (e.g. in breast feeding), it seems to the present reviewer highly unlikely that they originally evolved as calcium regulators. The calcitonins have at most a minor and inconstant hypocalcaemic action in non-mammalian vertebrates (Copp, 1976), and their main physiological role outside the mammalia probably remains to be established.

A MULTIPLE LEVELS OF INTERACTION

As in the case of other equally well regulated variables such as the fluid volume and blood pressure, either of the two major calcium-regulating systems can ensure survival when the other is disabled. The complex interactions between these duplicate systems at the secretory and target-organ levels have presented investigators with extremely difficult problems, many of which still remain to be solved.

In the twelve years since bioactive metabolites of calciferol were first shown to exist (Norman *et al.*, 1964), it has become accepted that the most active compound 1,25-dihydroxycholecalciferol plays the biological role of a hormone. (For reviews see Kodicek, 1972; DeLuca, 1974, Norman and Henry, 1974.)

This role of 1,25-dihydroxycholecalciferol was established by evidence that its synthesis is markedly accelerated by calcium deprivation and that it acts to increase the calcium content of extra-cellular fluid both by enhancing intestinal absorption and causing bone breakdown. As will be further discussed below, DeLuca and his colleagues, and most recently MacIntyre *et al.* (1976), have emphasised that the synthesis of the steroid hormone is also stimulated by hypophosphataemia and that its actions on calcium intake and mobilisation are paralleled by effects on phosphate. It is thus a matter for continuing debate whether the need for calcium or phosphate homeostasis represented the original stimulus to evolution of the secosteroid control system.

There is little doubt that the parathyroid control system evolved in relation to calcium homeostasis (for discussion see Parsons, 1976a). Its effects on phosphate and acid-base balance are best accounted for as an adaptation to the function of bone as an emergency calcium reservoir (Froeling and Bijvoet, 1974), both phosphate and bicarbonate being liberated as counterions during osteolysis. It is well established that the secretion of parathyroid hormone (PTH) is accelerated by hypocalcaemia and that it acts on the kidney to enhance tubular calcium reabsorption. PTH has both anabolic and catabolic actions on bone, but the latter predominate during acute parathyroid hyperactivity, which mobilises calcium by an effect on existing cells as well as stimulating proliferation of osteoclasts and temporarily arresting bone formation. (For further details, see recent reviews of parathyroid physiology by Parsons and Potts, 1972; Aurbach and Phang, 1974; Talmage, 1975; Parfitt, 1976; Parsons, 1976a.)

The functional relationship between the parathyroid and secosteroid calcium-regulating systems is of such importance in clinical medicine as well as theoretical biology that it has been intensively investigated, in spite of the remarkable technical difficulty of studying the circulating levels of such potent agents, which are active at picomolar concentrations. The evidence will first be examined that in addition to the long-established interaction between calciferol and parathyroid hormone on calcium transport in the bone and kidney, the steroid and peptide systems interact at the level of the tissues in which the humoral mediators themselves are formed.

B EFFECTS OF CALCIFEROL ON THE PARATHYROIDS

A study by Oldham *et al.* (1974) in dogs chronically deprived of cholecalciferol provided the first experimental indication of a direct effect of the vitamin and its 25-hydroxy metabolite on parathyroid secretion. Within 72 h of vitamin repletion with either compound, the calcium-binding activity in the parathyroid glands had almost doubled in all animals (measured as a percentage of ^{45}Ca bound/mg protein). As expected, levels of circulating immunoreactive PTH (iPTH) were restored almost to normal by the vitamin repletion. However a study of the time course of the effect strongly indicated that it was a direct one, and not due to relief of the hypocalcaemia. The iPTH fell 50 per cent within 12 h of intravenous injection of 25-hydroxycholecalciferol although at this time the serum calcium concentration had risen only 0.2 mg/100 ml in one animal and decreased in the other three, while the serum phosphate showed a 20 per cent rise, which would presumably have *reduced* the intracellular level of free calcium.

Oldham *et al.* (1974) concluded that their results probably pointed to the existence of a cholecalciferol-dependent mechanism for transport of calcium into the parathyroid cell, which would decrease the concentration of extracellular calcium required for effective suppression of PTH secretion. Cholecalciferol-dependence of the ‘set-point’ at which parathyroid secretion is cut off by rising plasma calcium was independently proposed (though without direct evidence) by Lumb and Stanbury (1974) as the most probable explanation for the progressive involution of signs of hyperparathyroidism and of measured levels of circulating iPTH, which occurred (without an accompanying rise in plasma calcium concentration) during calciferol repletion of several of their patients with severe simple vitamin D-deficiency.

The existence of this postulated direct effect of calciferol or its metabolites on the parathyroid gland is a question of major physiological importance, both because it would represent a refinement of the feedback control mechanism and because it might explain many otherwise paradoxical observations, for example the well-documented occasional occurrence of hypercalcaemia in azotaemic osteodystrophy as well as in simple vitamin D-deficiency (Stanbury and Lumb, 1966; Lumb and Stanbury, 1974). However evidence is still being published both for and against the hypothesis. In its favour are:

(1) The finding of Henry and Norman (1975) that chick parathyroid glands contain a calciferol acceptor system capable of binding exogenous or endogenous 1,25-dihydroxycholecalciferol to a weight-for-weight concentration at least 4-fold higher than the level in circulating blood. Within a few hours of administration of labelled cholecalciferol metabolite the parathyroids came to contain nearly as high a concentration as did the intestine (known to contain specific binding proteins for 1,25-dihydroxycholecalciferol) and a higher level than bone, which is the other established target tissue for the 1,25-dihydroxy-compound.

(2) The study by Chertow *et al.* (1975) of the effects of 1,25-dihydroxycholecalciferol on plasma calcium and iPTH in rats, both alone and during the stimulation of PTH secretion by injected phosphate. The iPTH measured by the particular antiserum used (which was said to be principally carboxy-terminal in specificity and would thus have responded only slowly to changes in parathyroid secretion) fell 43 per cent during 4 h after injection of the cholecalciferol metabolite, in a dose of only 130 pmol (54 ng). There was no accompanying change in measurements of total plasma calcium and the possibility that the effect might still have been mediated by a small rise in ionic calcium was much reduced by the finding that the 1,25-dihydroxycholecalciferol also greatly inhibited the rise in iPTH elicited by phosphate injection. *In vitro* evidence was also obtained that release of iPTH was inhibited by adding the steroid hormone to the culture medium at a concentration of 1 nM. Although the interpretation of *in vitro* experiments in terms of *in vivo* control function must be largely speculative, at least the effect was statistically significant and in the right direction to support *in vivo* findings.

(3) In preliminary experiments reported by Care *et al.* (1975), 1,25-dihydroxycholecalciferol added at a concentration of 125 pg/ml (0.3 pmol) to the medium perfusing goat parathyroid glands isolated in situ caused a significant reduction in PTH secretion, though 200-fold higher doses were without effect.

However, evidence of some significance against the postulated 'negative feedback' effect of 1,25-dihydroxycholecalciferol on parathyroid secretion was obtained by Canterbury *et al.* (1976), who gave bolus injections of 0.25 μg (650 pmol) into the thyroid arteries of dogs and observed an immediate doubling of the concentration of PTH in the thyroid venous effluent. This would represent a small *positive* feedback effect, but no change occurred in peripheral levels of iPTH or plasma calcium. On the other hand a similar bolus of the alternative metabolite 24,25-dihydroxycholecalciferol caused a remarkable decrease in PTH secretion (268 → 10 arbitrary units), followed by an equally striking fall in peripheral levels. This inhibition of PTH secretion by the 24,25-dihydroxy metabolite confirms findings originally described by Care *et al.* (1975), whereas the small rise caused by the bolus of 1,25-dihydroxycholecalciferol at what must have been an unphysiological concentration recalls the zero response which Care *et al.* (1975) reported at high doses.

On balance, the reviewer believes the evidence is in favour of the concept that calciferol is somehow involved in the secretory responses of the parathyroid glands to circulating levels of plasma calcium. However it is not yet clear whether this is a calciferol-dependent or metabolite-regulated system (a distinction discussed in greater detail below). The dose-response relationships are still obscure, and much remains to be learned about the physiological and pathological consequences of such steroid-peptide interaction at the secretory level.

If one of the calciferol metabolites *does* normally exert a depressor influence on parathyroid secretion, a recent careful clinical study provides further evidence that it is unlikely to be 1,25-dihydroxycholecalciferol. Small oral doses of the latter given to normal volunteers affected serum levels of iPTH only in the direction and to the extent expected from concomitant changes in plasma calcium (Llach *et al.*, 1977). However the intriguing reports from two laboratories on depression of parathyroid secretion by the 24,25-dihydroxy-derivative, whose possible biological significance is further discussed below, still keeps open the possibility of this extra functional sophistication in what is already known to be a highly refined control mechanism.

II Biological Significance of the Calciferol Metabolites

Intensive study in several laboratories during the past decade has shown the existence of hydroxylated metabolites of calciferol which have far more potent biological activity *in vivo* and *in vitro* than the parent secosteroid. It now seems clear that under all normal physiological circumstances the activities formerly attributed to the vitamin itself are entirely mediated by formation of these metabolites. Thus identification of the organs in which the specific hydroxylations occur and investigation of the mechanisms by which they are controlled has provided one of the most exciting areas of advance in the understanding of calcium metabolism.

The stages by which present understanding was reached and the main characteristics of the control system revealed have been well reviewed by three of the chief protagonists (Kodicek, 1972, 1974; DeLuca, 1974, 1976; Norman and Henry, 1974). The present discussion will be limited to more recent functional evidence regarding the influence of other hormones on this calciferol system, with particular reference to some of the physiological questions which still remain unanswered.

The three metabolites which appear at present to be of major regulatory significance are 25-hydroxycholecalciferol; 1,25-dihydroxycholecalciferol and 24,25-dihydroxycholecalciferol.

A 25-HYDROXYCHOLECALCIFEROL

This compound was the first metabolite shown to be more potent and faster-acting than cholecalciferol, and was for a short time thought to be the final active form of the vitamin (Blunt *et al.*, 1968a; Blunt and DeLuca, 1969; Ponchon *et al.* 1969).

Under all normal physiological circumstances, 25-hydroxycholecalciferol is the most abundant circulating compound of the cholecalciferol group. Once formed, it has a circulating half-life of the order of 2–3 weeks, many times longer than that of ingested cholecalciferol (Smith and Goodman, 1971; Mawer *et al.*, 1972; Haddad and Rojanasathit, 1976). (These figures for the final rate of metabolic disappearance must of course be carefully distinguished from the faster rates of plasma fall seen during the redistribution phase, which may last for several days after administration of exogenous 25-hydroxycholecalciferol or tracers. They also ignore extensive fat storage of calciferol itself.)

Individual plasma levels of 25-hydroxycholecalciferol vary so widely with exposure to sunlight and the dietary content of cholecalciferol that only extreme values have much diagnostic significance. Levels up to 80 ng/ml were found in healthy lifeguards after prolonged exposure to sun (Haddad and Chyu, 1971), whereas the concentration must fall below about 4 ng/ml before significant disturbances of calcium metabolism can be demonstrated (based on an informative study of 21 Indian subjects living in Britain by Gupta *et al.*, 1974).

In the normal physiological range, no correlation was found between individual levels of the 25-hydroxy metabolite and simultaneous measurements of plasma calcium, phosphate or iPTH (Haddad and Stamp, 1974). Neither has it been established that the mean plasma concentration or the circulating half-life of 25-hydroxycholecalciferol is significantly altered in physiological stress, such as that involved in pregnancy. However the severe consequences of vitamin D-deficiency in pregnancy have been known for centuries and it has recently been pointed out that earlier statistical studies failed to take account of the normal two-fold seasonal variation in levels of 25-hydroxycholecalciferol (Turton *et al.*, 1977), so that the last word has not yet been said on this question.

These measurements of circulating levels of 25-hydroxycholecalciferol indicate that up to 20-fold variation is tolerated, but this is much less than the range of total vitamin D intakes compatible with normal health. This probably extends from as little as 50 to as much as 10 000 i.u. per day, calculated by summing the contributions from the diet and skin under various conditions (Lumb *et al.*, 1971; Haddad and Stamp, 1974; Stamp *et al.*, 1977). Partially regulated formation of the 25-hydroxy metabolite is thus presumably the first stage of vitamin D regulation, but the detailed mechanism of this control is not well understood.

In vitro and *in vivo* experiments in rats were originally thought to indicate that the activity of the 25-hydroxylase was simply product-inhibited by the circulating level of the metabolite itself (for reviews, see DeLuca, 1974). However the data obtained from acute *in vivo* experiments show only a superficial similarity to the *in vitro* phenomenon of product inhibition familiar to organic chemists, and the analogy breaks down when more chronic experiments are considered. There is also a possibility of significant species differences, because Tucker *et al.* (1973), who found little evidence of product inhibition, detected the occurrence of significant amounts of 25-hydroxylation in the intestine and kidney as well as the liver of chicks, whereas in the rat it seems clear that the liver is the major, if not the exclusive site of this reaction (DeLuca, 1974).

Experiments depending on the *in vitro* study of hydroxylation in tissues or homogenates removed after *in vivo* administration of various forms of vitamin D are always open to the fundamental criticism that loss of anatomical integrity itself affects the enzymic activity of cells or sub-cellular organelles and might destroy evidence of a regulatory process important in the intact organism. *In vivo* measurements of circulating metabolite levels are thus indispensable for the investigation of control mechanisms.

Experiments in man with isotopically labelled vitamin D agree in showing that the rate of formation of 25-hydroxycholecalciferol is high in vitamin D deficiency and relatively low in subjects adequately supplied with the vitamin and with pre-existing high plasma levels of the metabolite (Mawer *et al.*, 1971, 1972). The possible influence of changes in pool size in the latter observations did not allow firm conclusions on the role of product-inhibition in human vitamin D metabolism, but more recent experiments of the Manchester group using a calciferol tracer in the presence of varying additions of the unlabelled vitamin indicate that the lowering in rates of 25-hydroxylation may more closely reflect levels of calciferol itself rather than those of its metabolite (Mawer, 1977).

A practical impression of the way in which circulating levels of 25-hydroxycholecalciferol vary with the total vitamin D intake can be obtained from the extensive data reported by Stamp *et al.* (1977), see Fig. 1. On a log-log

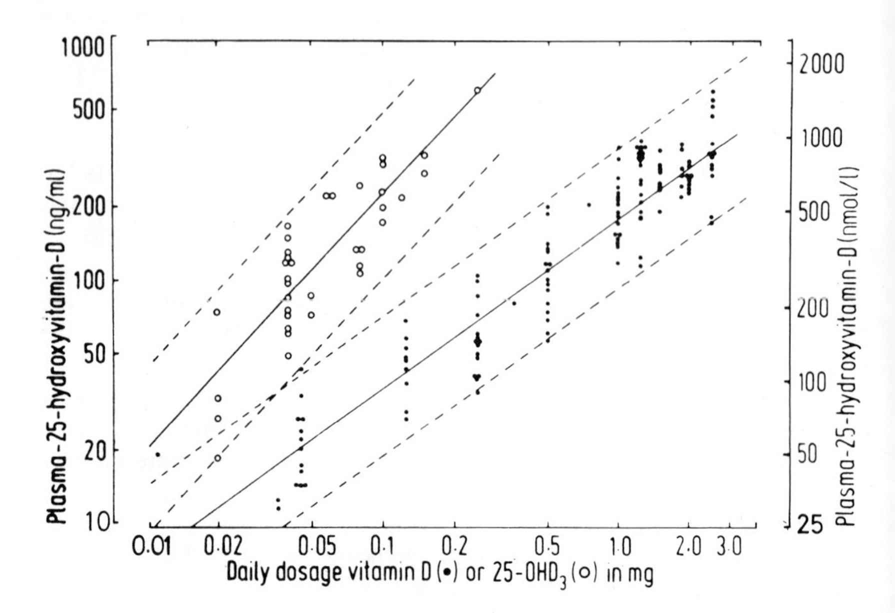

Fig. 1. Plasma concentrations of 25-hydroxycholecalciferol in 164 subjects receiving daily long-term treatment with various doses of ergocalciferol or cholecalciferol (●) or receiving 25-hydroxycholecalciferol itself (○). Regression lines calculated for each form of treatment are shown with 95 per cent confidence limits. (Reproduced by permission from Stamp *et al.*, 1977.)

scale, this shows a clear linear relationship over a very wide range, and a closely similar relationship was seen in rats given graded intakes of vitamin D by Clark and Potts (1977).

The implication of these important studies is that under conditions of chronic exposure to high vitamin D intake, levels of 25-hydroxycholecalciferol are not in fact very closely controlled but continue to rise slowly, as might be expected from the very long half-life of this metabolite already referred to. This suggests that the relatively restricted range of circulating concentrations of the metabolite encountered in clinical practice is more likely to be a consequence of deliberate avoidance of continuous excessive intake, at least by those whose skin does not darken enough to afford much protection.

Whatever down-regulation of the rate of 25-hydroxylation does occur must, however, give considerable protection against transient high vitamin D intake. This is consistent with the finding of Stamp *et al.* (1977) that circulating levels of the metabolite rose much more steeply in response to graded oral doses of 25-hydroxycholecalciferol itself than it did to the parent vitamin.

It has been shown in animal studies that even without further metabolic transformation, 25-hydroxycholecalciferol can stimulate intestinal calcium transport (Olson and DeLuca, 1969) and bone resorption (Raisz *et al.*, 1972a, b; Reynolds *et al.*, 1973). Similar evidence is available in man from the fact that the 25-hydroxy-metabolite can cause hypercalcaemia in anephric patients (Blondin and Rutherford, 1975). The quantitative *in vitro* comparisons of Reynolds *et al.* (1973) indicate that 25-hydroxycholecalcerol is about 100-fold less potent than the dihydroxycholecalciferol shortly to be discussed, at least so far as stimulation of bone resorption is concerned. However the plasma levels of this first metabolite are often so high in relation to those of other circulating forms of the vitamin that it most probably makes its own contribution to the overall pattern of *in vivo* response.

It is particularly instructive to compare the seasonal changes in plasma levels of 25-hydroxycholecalciferol reported by Gupta *et al.* (1974) and McLaughlin *et al.* (1974) (highest in June to September, lowest in December to April) with the seasonal variation in calcium absorption observed by Malm (1958) in prisoners, also living in a Northern climate, who were receiving a diet relatively poor in calcium (450 mg/day) but adequate in vitamin D. The highest percentage of the prisoner's 'better' balances occurred in August and September, and most of their 'worst' in January, February and March. Further careful investigation will be required to determine whether 25-hydroxycholecalciferol itself or the 24,25-hydroxy-metabolite discussed below are most likely to mediate such seasonal changes in calcium metabolism, which may be quite distinct from true vitamin deficiency.

B 1,25-DIHYDROXYCHOLECALCIFEROL

The finding of a still more polar metabolite associated with the nuclear chromatin of intestinal mucosa (Haussler *et al.*, 1968) and the demonstration that the second hydroxylation involves specific loss of tritium from the 1 position in a double-labelled tracer and occurs uniquely in the kidney (Lawson *et al.*, 1969; Fraser and Kodicek, 1970) opened a new era of excitement in the understanding of calciferol action.

The new compound was rapidly isolated, identified and synthesised (Holick *et al.* 1971a, b; Lawson *et al.*, 1971; Seemler *et al.*, 1972), proving to be the 1α-25-dihydroxy-derivative of the vitamin. Evidence from many laboratories agrees that this is by far the most potent of the cholecalciferol metabolites in inducing intestinal calcium absorption and calcium mobilisation from bone. Experiments involving the use of actinomycin D and the timing of events in relation to the metabolism of a tracer of radioactive 1,25-dihydroxycholecal-ciferol were claimed to show that it undergoes no further change before eliciting the intestinal response (Tanaka *et al.*, 1971; Frolik and DeLuca, 1971), though they have been criticised on several grounds (Kodicek, 1972).

Competitive displacement assays sufficiently sensitive to measure the minute concentrations of 1,25-dihydroxycholecalciferol which circulate in plasma have been developed (Brumbaugh *et al.*, 1974; Eisman *et al.*, 1976) and confirmatory measurements have been made by a method of extraction and bioassay, though the latter requires large blood samples (Hill *et al.*, 1974). Haussler *et al.* (1975) reported circulating levels of 32 ± 1 pg/ml in 15 normal subjects, and almost identical figures (29 ± 2 pg/ml) were obtained by Eisman *et al.* (1976). Tracer studies indicate that 1,25-dihydroxycholecalciferol has a circulating half-life of 14 h in man (Mawer *et al.*, 1976), which is consistent with the evidence of Brickman *et al.* (1976) that hypercalciuria induced by this active metabolite in normal subjects passes off with a mean half-time of 1.5 days.

As discussed in detail below, circulating concentrations of 1,25-dihydroxycholecalciferol are indeed closely correlated with physiological and pathological changes in calcium metabolism, and its role as a calcium-regulating hormone as well as a vitamin is no longer disputed.

C 24,25-DIHYDROXYCHOLECALCIFEROL

Although it is established that 1,25-dihydroxycholecalciferol plays an essential role in calcium physiology and its low concentrations in plasma can be studied by appropriate chemical as well as isotopic methods, in mass terms it forms a very small part of the total pool of cholecalciferol derivatives except in severely vitamin D-deficient animals. Under conditions of normal dietary intakes and cholecalciferol supplementation, the second most abundant metabolite found in extracellular fluid and tissues is another dihydroxy derivative which is also active in stimulating intestinal transport. This compound was originally thought to be 21,25-dihydroxycholecalciferol (Suda *et al.*, 1970) but was finally assigned the 24,25 dihydroxy-structure after more complete characterisation (Holick *et al.*, 1972).

Haddad *et al.* (1976) and Taylor, Hughes and De Silva (1976) have recently independently shown that 24,25-dihydroxycholecalciferol is equipotent with 25-hydroxycholecalciferol in displacing radioactive 25-hydroxycholecalciferol from the binding protein in rat serum and is thus included in estimates of circulating 25-hydroxycholecalciferol made by non-chromatographic assay methods. Separating the mono- and di-hydroxy metabolites by gel partition chromatography, Haddad *et al.* (1976) reported serum concentrations of 24,25-dihydroxycholecalciferol lying between 4 and 11 ng/ml in four normal adults. These levels ranged from 30 to 90 per cent of the accompanying levels of 25-hydroxycholecalciferol. Considerably lower levels were reported in normals by Taylor *et al.* (1977) and these were less than 10 per cent of the accompanying levels of 25-hydroxycholecalciferol. Similarly low normal levels have been reported in a third displacement assay developed by Graham *et al.* (1977) and the discrepancy between these figures and the high values reported by Haddad *et al.* remains to be resolved.

In the period of excitement generated by developing knowledge of the role of 1,25-dihydroxycholecalciferol, the 24,25-dihydroxy-isomer came to be regarded principally as a less-active substance formed when the renal 1-hydroxylase system was suppressed (Tanaka and DeLuca, 1974a.)

However it is now becoming clear that 24,25-dihydroxycholecalciferol has a most interesting combination of biological properties. Although at least 1000-fold less potent than 1,25-dihydroxycholecalciferol in stimulating bone resorption *in vitro* (Reynolds *et al.*, 1973), Kanis and his colleagues have recently reported that the 24,25-dihydroxy-compound enhances calcium absorption in man at doses of only 1–10 μg/day by mouth, being thus almost equipotent with 1,25 dihydroxycholecalciferol in this respect (Kanis *et al.*, 1977). In addition, evidence is referred to above that this metabolite may specifically inhibit PTH secretion (p. 391 Bordier *et al.* (1977) have claimed that 25-hydroxycholecalciferol or a further metabolite (which might be the 24,25-dihydroxy isomer) preferentially promotes bone mineralisation in clinical osteomalacia. However the latter authors provided no evidence that the small oral doses of 1,25-dihydroxycholecalciferol used for comparison were absorbed by their patients, most of whom had steatorrhoea or malabsorption due to prior gastrectomy or intestinal disease.

In their early studies of the pharmacology of 24,25-dihydroxycholecalciferol, Suda *et al.* (1970) administered large doses (6.5 nmol; 3 μg) in short-term (12 h) experiments with rats and concluded that this dihydroxy metabolite was much less active than 1,25-dihydroxycholecalciferol in stimulating intestinal absorption of calcium. However in a later paper, DeLuca and his colleagues recognised that 24,25-dihydroxycholecalciferol has remarkable intestinal activity when given at lower doses on a long-term basis (130 pmol by intraperitoneal injection, daily for 8 days; Boyle *et al.*, 1973). These authors also produced some evidence that the 24,25-compound exerts this effect only after further transformation to a still more polar metabolite, possibly the trihydroxy derivative 1,24,25-trihydroxycholecalciferol (Boyle *et al.*, 1973).

The effect of calciferol in healing the bony lesions of clinical rickets has been known for more than 50 years and its actions in increasing bone weight and mineral content were established by classical animal experiments (Mellanby, 1919a, b; Herting and Steenbock, 1955; Cramer *et al.*, 1957). However no direct action of calciferol or a metabolite in promoting bone formation at the tissue level has yet been demonstrated (Omdahl and DeLuca, 1973). The tendency of 24,25-dihydroxycholecalciferol to cause a positive calcium balance and favour bone mineralisation rather than breakdown will undoubtedly attract close attention in future studies, and if a direct anabolic response of bone to the vitamin D system does play a role in normal physiology, this metabolite certainly seems the strongest current candidate as a mediator. In view of the anabolic effects of parathyroid hormone at low doses already discussed (p. 388), it is of considerable interest that Taylor *et al.* (1977) have reported that circulating levels of 24,25-dihydroxycholecalciferol are consistently elevated in primary hyperparathyroidism.

III Distinction between Calciferol-Dependent and Calciferol-Regulated Processes

Calciferol is exceptional among vitamins in that its biological effects can be conceptually divided into strictly vitamin-*dependent* and vitamin-*regulated* processes. Both intestinal absorption of calcium and phosphate and mobilisation of these elements from bone by parathyroid hormone (the other process on which land-living vertebrates rely for correction of hypocalcaemia) are severely impaired in total vitamin D-deficiency (Harrison *et al.*, 1958; Rasmussen *et al.*, 1963; Harrison and Harrison, 1964). There is also intriguing though incomplete evidence that the mechanisms of muscular contraction include a strictly calciferol-dependent process (Curry *et al.*, 1974; Birge and Haddad, 1975; Schott and Wills, 1976).

One of the main sources of experimental difficulty in investigating these relationships is that extreme deficiency is required to demonstrate strict calciferol-dependence. For example a total of only 8 ng (20 pmol) given to a rat in divided doses over 3 days is sufficient to restore the ability of exogenous PTH to mobilise calcium from bone (Rasmussen *et al.*, 1963). Justly or unjustly, many experiments with animals thought to be vitamin D-deficient have been criticised on the ground that they ought rather to have been described as vitamin-depleted.

Another difficulty is that when calcium concentration in the intestinal lumen is high, uptake occurs principally by a passive (though saturable) process known as facilitated diffusion, whereas active transport predominates under conditions of scarcity (Wasserman and Taylor, 1969). Both processes are modulated by calciferol, but only the latter appears to be strictly calciferol-dependent and investigators have not always distinguished adequately between them. It seems clear that some animals (e.g. the rat) can be kept normocalcaemic by a sufficiently high calcium diet, even though completely vitamin D-deficient and unresponsive to PTH (Rasmussen *et al.*, 1963). This effect is presumably due to intestinal calcium uptake by the diffusional process.

Identification of strictly calciferol-dependent processes is clearly an important approach to elucidating its mechanism of action and it is noteworthy that the active intestinal absorption of calcium, renal tubular reabsorption of the ion and calcium mobilisation from bone all involve transport against a concentration gradient. Neither intestinal nor bony calcium transport are important in the physiology of fish and although vitamin D is abundant in the livers of marine teleosts, living in a virtually calcium-saturated environment, it appears to play no role in their homeostasis (Urist, 1976). However fish venturing into fresh water depend for calcium on concentration by a pump in their gill membranes while, in the sea, renal tubular transport of calcium is essential to keep the concentration of this element in the *milieu interieur* down to the physiological range. It would be of considerable interest to know whether these pumps, too, have a calciferol-dependent mechanism, since this would suggest that active calcium transport systems may represent a common locus of action of the vitamin.

The best current explanation for calciferol-dependence of the osteolytic processes stimulated by parathyroid hormone is that it is probably a consequence of the profound disturbances of intracellular and intramitochondrial calcium content which occur in the absence of vitamin D. The biochemistry of this interaction has been well reviewed by Rasmussen and his colleagues (most recently by Rasmussen and Bordier, 1974) and will not be further discussed here, since it is only marginally relevant to the normal functional interplay of PTH and the hormonal metabolite (or metabolites) of vitamin D.

The question whether the effects of calciferol or its metabolites on the kidneys contain a regulatory component or illustrate only calciferol-dependence has been more difficult to determine. It has long been known that both the calcium-retaining and the phosphaturic responses of the renal tubules to parathyroid hormone are dimished, though not abolished, in severe vitamin D deficiency (Gran, 1960; Harrison and Harrison, 1941, 1964; Arnaud *et al.*, 1966; Ney *et al.*, 1965). Furthermore, the restoration of calciferol to severely deficient rats or dogs diminishes urinary calcium excretion in the face of rising plasma calcium (Nicolaysen and Eeg-Larsen, 1956; Gran, 1960). Rasmussen and his colleagues have proposed a mechanism for these findings based on disturbance of the calcium content of tubule cells and mitochondria in the deficient state, analogous to the mechanism of calciferol-dependent bony responses already referred to (Rasmussen and Bordier, 1974).

It is virtually impossible to disentangle, convincingly, the chronic effects on bone, kidney and intestine of calciferol deprivation or pharmacological excess, even by the use of parathyroidectomised subjects. Chronic experiments have therefore contributed little to understanding the mechanisms of normal calcium and phosphate regulation.

The best evidence for a hormonal role of calciferol metabolites acting on the kidney has been provided by relatively acute administration. In a number of early studies of this type, calciferol itself appeared to enhance renal phosphate reabsorption, often to such an extent that a maximum rate of tubular reabsorption (TM_{PO_4}) could no longer be demonstrated during phosphate loading. However the doses required were entirely pharmacological and the onset of their effects was delayed for many hours (Klein and Gow, 1953; Crawford *et al.*, 1955; Ney *et al.*, 1965; Gekle *et al.*, 1969).

Puschett *et al.* (1972a) were the first to show a convincing effect of 25-hydroxycholecalciferol infused to thyro-parathyroidectomised dogs in near-physiological amounts (0.6–2.4 μg over a period of two hours). A stable and easily measurable phosphaturia produced in these animals by volume expansion and a sustaining infusion (physiological saline and calcium gluconate, with added inulin) was significantly reduced within about 30 min of starting to administer the metabolite, and phosphaturia caused by relatively large infusions of PTH was also reduced. Calciferol itself was active in these experiments, but 100 to 400-fold higher doses were required and the effect tended to be slower in onset. A similar study in which 1,25-dihydroxycholecalciferol was given as a single intravenous injection (0.6 μg) caused equally consistent anti-phosphaturia, though if anything of slightly smaller magnitude; pilot experiments with still smaller doses (25 ng) showed no effect (Puschett *et al.*, 1972b).

Similar results were obtained by Popovtzer *et al.* (1974), who infused the two metabolites at 20–100 ng/100 gm/h to intact rats and PTX rats infused with PTH. There was no significant difference between the responses to the mono- and dihydroxylated derivatives and these doses may in fact have been higher than necessary, because no significant difference was seen between responses of the two kidneys when a metabolite was infused into one renal artery. In contrast to the results of Puschett *et al.* (1972b) in dogs, the calciferol metabolites caused no antiphosphaturia in the absence of parathyroid hormone, even when the PTX rats were given infusions of calcium and phosphate. Puschett *et al.* (1975) confirmed the PTH-dependence of responses to small doses of 25-hydroxycholecalciferol in rats (25 ng/100 gm/h) and speculated that the doses of 0.3–1.2 μg/h used in dogs may have been supraphysiologic.

The foregoing descriptions of acute renal responses to the calciferol metabolites have emphasised their effects in stimulating phosphate re-absorption. However parallel increases in reabsorption of calcium and sodium were reported in all the studies cited, and changes in the rates of transport of all three ions appear to have been roughly simultaneous.

Investigations of the biochemical changes involved in these renal effects of the calciferol metabolites are so far quite incomplete. However some involvement of cyclic nucleotides is suggested by more pharmacological experiments involving combined infusion of 25-hydroxycholecalciferol and dibutyryl cyclic AMP (Puschett *et al.*, 1974) or addition of the metabolite to supraphysiologic infusions of parathyroid hormone (Popovtzer and Robinette, 1975).

It is a pity that the vital question whether these rapid renal responses to two of the calciferol metabolites are involved in normal calcium and phosphate regulation at present rests on the judgement of the reader whether the blood levels produced are likely to have been in the physiological range. Infusion of only 25 ng/100 gm/h of 25-hydroxycholecalciferol to rats is in fact an impressively low dose by comparison with normal blood levels in this species (e.g. the figure of 1–2 μg/100 ml reported by Clark and Potts (1977) in their control studies preparatory to calciferol deprivation).

Blood levels of 25-hydroxycholecalciferol do not vary with the calcium or phosphate intake, but we should recall that the renal physiology of the 24,25-dihydroxy metabolite (discussed above in the light of its interestingly anabolic character) has yet to be reported. It is much to be hoped that, in some future study, direct measurements to compare pre- and post-infusion blood levels with those seen in calcium and phosphate deprivation will put the hormonal significance of renal responses to this or another calciferol metabolite beyond question.

IV Functional Interactions

The extreme vitamin D-deficiency required for the study of calciferol-dependent processes is seen only as the result of experimental manipulation or in studies of the pathology of rickets. For the understanding of functional interaction and control mechanisms it is the calciferol-regulated processes which are important. Their study requires data obtained under near-normal *in vivo* conditions, since only these are capable of distinguishing what *does* occur from the many biochemical changes which *in vitro* evidence shows *could* occur.

A INFLUENCE OF PARATHYROID HORMONE ON CALCIFEROL METABOLISM

In spite of earlier controversy, it is now generally accepted that in conditions of normal dietary intakes and calciferol supplementation the fraction of dietary calcium absorbed by the intestine is principally controlled by the circulating level of parathyroid hormone (Parsons, 1976a; for earlier references, see Parsons and Potts, 1972). As is usually the case, other (possibly more primitive) control mechanisms can be demonstrated under conditions of gland ablation and may play a role in disease or under conditions of physiological stress. Although many details of the control mechanism remain to be worked out, the evidence now seems overwhelming that this sensitive regulation of calcium absorption in normal health depends on parathyroid hormone modulating the hydroxylation of calciferol.

Only in the case of the 1-hydroxylating system of the kidney tubule which generates 1,25-dihydroxycholecalciferol has the nature of the modulation so far been worked out in any detail. This metabolite is active at such low plasma levels that experiments on the regulation of its biosynthesis have been carried out almost exclusively by radioactive tracer techniques. A summary of two of the basic studies will illustrate the complications involved and the possibility of differences in interpretation.

Garabedian *et al.* (1972) injected labelled 25-hydroxycholecalciferol to thyroparathyroidectomised vitamin D-deficient rats on a low calcium diet, keeping the animals alive by regular injections of unlabelled 1,25-dihydroxy-cholecalciferol. Injection of small doses of parathyroid extract (5 or 10 i.u. every 6 h for 2 days) caused a twelve-fold increase in the proportion of tracer which was extractable from plasma and chromatographed in the position of 1,25-dihydroxycholecalciferol. At this dose level, PTE caused no change in serum levels of calcium or phosphate which might have mediated the effect.

Fraser and Kodicek (1973) used an *in vivo/in vitro* technique which avoided some possible sources of artifact in the *in vivo* procedure (such as changes in size of metabolite pools or rates of destruction), but introduced others of its own. They injected larger doses of PTE (30 i.u. every 6 h for 2 days) to 1 day-old chicks, and observed a four-fold increase in conversion of labelled 25-hydroxycholecalciferol to the 1,25-dihydroxy-metabolite by unfractionated kidney homogenates. These doses of PTE caused hypercalcaemia, but it seemed unlikely that this could explain the results because addition of calcium to the homogenates caused the opposite changes in enzyme activity. Experiments by Henry (1977) with kidney homogenates from chicks injected with large doses of bPTH for several hours before sacrifice also showed a marked stimulation of 1-hydroxylase activity. However experiments *in vivo* and *in vitro* by MacIntyre and his colleagues initially provided diametrically opposite evidence, suggesting that under some circumstances administration of parathyroid hormone can *decrease* formation of 1,25-dihydroxycholecalciferol. A later report from this group showed that addition *in vitro* of highly purified bPTH to suspensions of chick kidney tubules can either increase or decrease formation of labelled 1,24-dihydroxycholecalciferol, depending on the calcium concentration in the medium (Larkins *et al.*, 1974).

This clearly documents that in this system (as in most others) it is impossible to obtain definitive information on control function from experiments *in vitro*. Only biochemical modulations seen to occur under unquestionably physiological conditions can be interpreted with any confidence as having control significance.

There is therefore particular interest in the measurements of Haussler *et al.* (1975, 1976) already cited, showing that plasma levels of 1,25-dihydroxycholecalciferol are almost doubled in primary hyperparathyroidism and halved in hypoparathyroidism. Both sets of measurements were significantly different from those of a control group. Further data on the clinical correlation of levels of this hormonal metabolite of calciferol are eagerly awaited, as is the fuller investigation of its possible decrease with age, hinted at by Eisman *et al.* (1976). If confirmed, the latter may well prove connected with the age-related decrease in parathyroid function documented by Fujita *et al.* (1977), but measurements of biologically active circulating PTH will be needed for a full understanding of functional interaction between the hormones.

Regulation of the renal system responsible for introducing a second hydroxyl group to 25-hydroxycholecalciferol in the 24 position has been much less fully investigated. It is reported to be activated in kidney tissue from rats given 1,25-dihydroxycholecalciferol (Tanaka and DeLuca, 1974b) and suppressed in chick kidney by oestrogen (Tanaka *et al.*, 1976), both in pharmacological doses. At the present time, the evidence seems inadequate to establish the role of the 24-hydroxylase in normal calcium metabolism. However it is worth recalling the preliminary evidence already referred to that circulating levels of 24,25-dihydroxycholecalciferol are raised in hyperparathyroidism (Taylor *et al.*, 1977).

B DIRECT INFLUENCE ON CALCIFEROL METABOLISM OF THE PLASMA CONCENTRATION OF PHOSPHATE BUT NOT CALCIUM

Studying the part played by PTH-accelerated synthesis of 1,25-dihydroxycholecalciferol in mediating adaptation to dietary deficiency of calcium and phosphate, Tanaka and DeLuca (1974b) showed that rats maintained on a diet low in phosphorus produce the active metabolite whether they have been thyroparathyroidectomised or not. On the other hand, rats maintained on low-calcium diets, which also produce the 1,25- dihydroxy-compound, lose this ability within 48 h after thyroparathyroidectomy. Correspondingly, adaptation to a low-phosphate diet was still seen in rats receiving all their cholecalciferol as the 1,25-dihydroxy-metabolite but, under these circumstances, no adaptation occurred to a low-calcium diet (Ribovich and DeLuca, 1975.)

Parallel findings have been reported in the chick by Baxter and DeLuca (1976), who measured calcium absorption from a duodenal loop, and by Friedlander *et al.* (1977), measuring the intestinal content of calcium-binding protein. These two indications of absorptive activity were compared with 1-hydroxylase activity in homogenised kidney tissue, obtained after a period on calcium- or phosphate-deficient diets. Confirming the earlier work in rats, it was concluded that the stimulation of calcium absorption by a low-calcium diet was due entirely to increased synthesis of the active calciferol metabolite (inferentially a consequence of parathyroid stimulation). On the other hand low-phosphate intake stimulated the 1-hydroxylase in chicks much less than in the earlier rat studies, and its effect in enhancing absorption was at least in part a direct intestinal response in this species.

The potential clinical importance of this work on altered calciferol metabolism in phosphate deficiency has been most clearly brought out by Hughes *et al.* (1975) and Haussler *et al.* (1976), who provided the essential confirmation of these postulated control relationships by direct measurement of the circulating levels of 1,25-dihydroxycholecalciferol in both rat and man. This removed any possibility of artefact in the earlier *in vitro* estimates of hydroxylase activity. Intact rats showed a 4- to 5-fold increase in plasma concentration of the 1,25-dihydroxy-metabolite on low-phosphorus and low-calcium diets, whereas thyroparathyroidectomised animals responded only to the low phosphate.

The paper by Haussler *et al.* (1976) contains a particularly clear discussion of the complex physiological interaction of the steroid and peptide systems in mediating a selective increase in plasma phosphate in response to phosphate deprivation (low plasma P → increased plasma 1,25-dihydroxycholecalciferol → increased gut absorption of Ca and P and liberation of both ions from bone → depression of parathyroid secretion → hypercalciuria, hypophosphaturia and raised plasma P).

Haussler *et al.* (1976) also draw attention to an intriguing parallel between phosphate-depletion in rats and the human conditions of vitamin D-resistant rickets and absorptive hypercalciuria, suggesting that these maladies provide two clinical examples of phosphate depletion without concomitant hyperparathyroidism. They report significantly elevated circulating levels of 1,25-dihydroxycholecalciferol in 18 cases of idiopathic hypercalciuria and suggest a plausible and testable sequence of pathological changes to account for this disorder (Primary renal P leak → lowered plasma P → increased plasma 1,25-dihydroxycholecalciferol → increased gut absorption of Ca and P → depression of parathyroid secretion → hypercalciuria and hyperphosphaturia → stones).

Although in the above studies emphasis has been laid on the parallelism between increases in intestinal calcium and phosphate transport induced by 1,25-dihydroxycholecalciferol, there has long been evidence that these processes are separable and involve different mechanisms (Harrison and Harrison, 1961; Wasserman and Taylor, 1973). Thus there is still a likelihood of major changes in our understanding as further details of these complex homeostatic mechanisms are unravelled. The possibility of contributions from comparative endocrinology should not be overlooked, because MacIntyre and his colleagues have shown that injection of 1,25-dihydroxycholecalciferol causes striking hyperphosphataemia without hypercalcaemia in eels (MacIntyre *et al.*, 1976) and advanced the hypothesis that this active metabolite may originally have evolved to mediate phosphate homeostasis in the sea, where calcium is abundant but phosphorus is the limiting factor in survival of many organisms, occurring at a concentration of only 1 mg phosphorus per metric ton (Urist, 1976).

C INFLUENCE OF OTHER HORMONES

1 *Calcitonin.* At a target tissue level, it has long been clear that calcitonin can moderate the hypercalcaemia induced by toxic doses of cholecalciferol (Melancon and DeLuca, 1969). This is probably largely due to the prevention of acute osteolysis, and direct inhibition by calcitonin of the osteolytic effect of 25-hydroxycholecalciferol has been observed in tissue culture (Wener *et al.*, 1972). At relatively modest doses (1.25 m i.u./h by infusion to rats), calcitonin also steadily lowers cholecalciferol-induced calcium absorption from the intestine (Olson *et al.*, 1972).

The possibility that calcitonin may directly affect the pattern of metabolism of cholecalciferol is still undecided. An increased transformation of tritiated 25-hydroxycholecalciferol into the 1,25-dihydroxy-metabolite reported by Galante *et al.* (1972) after administration of large doses of calcitonin to rats might well have been due to compensatory secretion of endogenous PTH, while a depression of the 1-hydroxylase activity of isolated chick renal tubules described by Rasmussen *et al.* (1972) is open to the general criticisms already presented in discussing the doubtful physiological relevance of such *in vitro* observations.

2 *Prolactin.* Moderate doses of ovine prolactin (10 μg/kg/h infused for 18 h) have been shown to cause marked hypercalcuria and modest hypercalcaemia in rats (Mahajan *et al.*, 1974). The effect was unaltered by parathyroidectomy but the hypercalcaemia was 3–4 fold greater in animals deprived of their thyroids, indicating that it had probably been limited by endogenous secretion of calcitonin. Direct measurements of circulating 1,25-dihydroxycholecalciferol showed a two-fold rise after injections of ovine prolactin to chicks (Spanos *et al.*, 1976a), strongly suggesting that both effects were due to prolactin activation of renal 1-hydroxylase activity, an interaction previously shown to be possible *in vitro* (Spanos *et al.*, 1976b). A four-fold increase in plasma levels of 1,25-dihydroxycholecalciferol has been observed in lactating rats, using non-lactating females as a control (Pike *et al.*, 1977).

3 *Steroid Sex Hormones*. Kenney (1976) has shown that the activity of renal 1-hydroxylase is increased during the reproductive period in birds, and Tanaka *et al*. (1976) have produced evidence that this may be a direct effect of oestrogen. They observed tremendous enhancement of the 1-hydroxylase activity after injecting pharmacological doses of the steroid, although addition of testosterone was necessary before an effect could be seen in immature chicks. This effect, too, has been confirmed by direct measurements of plasma levels of 1,25-dihydroxycholecalciferol (Pike *et al*., 1977).

4 *Adrenocortical steroids*. The clinical association of the adrenal cortex with calcium metabolism has long been clear from the almost invariable occurrence of osteoporosis in Cushing's syndrome (Iannacone *et al*., 1960) and in patients treated chronically with anti-inflammatory steroids. Indeed, significant demineralisation of the skeleton can be detected within as little as a month after the start of intensive corticosteroid treatment (Reifenstein, 1958). These observations relate to the effect of grossly unphysiological steroid concentrations in the blood, and the same is true of many experiments carried out to analyse the mechanisms involved. However the effects of adrenalectomy do indicate that the adrenal cortex plays at least a supportive role in normal calcium metabolism, and exerts an important modulating influence on the balance of cellular activity in bone. This conclusion is borne out by some of the results of more moderate administration of exogenous steroids, shortly to be mentioned.

Many of the effects of exogenous glucocorticoids are the opposite of those produced by giving vitamin D or its active metabolites. Indeed the use of cortisone to treat vitamin D intoxication was first suggested by Anderson *et al*. as long ago as 1954, and many others have confirmed that it is highly effective. For instance 200 mg of cortisone daily restores a normal level of plasma calcium within 10 days or so in patients with severe calciferol poisoning, a result which is not achieved for several months by simple withholding of the vitamin (Verner *et al*., 1970).

The first point to be considered is therefore whether corticosteroids interfere with calciferol metabolism. Avioli *et al*. (1968) reported that administration of prednisone (30 mg/day) to normal human subjects shortened the plasma half-time of tritiated cholecalciferol and decreased the circulating concentration of a bioactive metabolite, subsequently identified as 25-hydroxycholecalciferol. On the other hand, 5 mg/day of cortisone or corresponding doses of more potent steroids given daily to rats (weighing 120–140 gm) appeared not to affect the pattern of metabolites in studies of Kimberg *et al*. (1971). A more recent study by Lukert, Stanbury and Mawer (1973) also indicated that rats treated with 5 mg/day of the more potent compound prednisolone had unchanged amounts of 1,25-dihydroxycholecalciferol in intestinal mucosa and slightly raised concentrations in the plasma, making it unlikely that altered calciferol metabolism could account for the markedly impaired intestinal calcium transport. However, Carré *et al.* (1974), again working with rats, found that treatment with prednisolone accelerated conversion of the active dihydroxymetabolite to a still more polar compound which was biologically inert.

Thus the existence of a cortisol effect on patterns of calciferol metabolism cannot be regarded as entirely settled, but it must be emphasised that those effects that have been reported were obtained with large doses of exogenous steroid.

Turning to the possibility of an effect on parathyroid hormone secretion, there is good evidence that this is increased in corticosteroid excess. Parathyroid hyperplasia has been reported in Cushing's syndrome (Wajchenberg *et al.*, 1965) and other indirect support for the association with hyperparathyroidism is cited by Fucik *et al.* (1975). The latter authors reported a statistically significant elevation of immunoreactive PTH in 11 patients receiving 15–80 mg of prednisone daily for 1 to 50 months. The measured concentration was virtually double that found in 19 controls, and these authors endorsed the proposal that the bone loss of corticosteroid excess may be partly caused by induced hyperparathyroidism. In view of evidence cited below that cortisol interferes especially with the anabolic response to PTH, this mechanism seems entirely reasonable.

The major disturbances of calcium and bone metabolism induced by the corticosteroids are probably accounted for by their direct actions on the skeleton and intestine. The most dramatic of these is perhaps the interference with active calcium uptake, first indicated by the remarkable ability of glucocorticoids to prevent the calcium hyperabsorption of sarcoidosis (Anderson *et al.*, 1954; Henneman *et al.*, 1956). Intestinal calcium absorption is also the only authenticated example of a calcium transport process whose activity is increased by adrenalectomy. Important experiments by Kimberg *et al.* (1961) and Kimberg *et al.* (1971), using gut sacs isolated after various treatments, showed that calcium transport was enhanced by adrenalectomy and inhibited by cortisone in doses as low as 2 mg daily per rat for 5–7 days. The inhibition persisted in rats simultaneously given 25-hydroxycholecalciferol (Kimberg *et al.*, 1971) or 1,25-dihydroxycholecalciferol (Favus *et al.*, 1973), and occurred in spite of the presence on their intestinal mucosa of higher levels of calcium binding protein than in normal controls. Thus its biochemical basis remains uncertain.

Studies of renal tubular reabsorption of calcium and magnesium under the influence of aldosterone and cortisol by Lemann *et al.* (1970) led to the conclusion that neither of these steroids has any direct effect on renal transport of the divalent cations.

Thus the remaining topics for discussion concern the effects of the glucocorticoids on bone. Experiments on adrenalectomised rats by Talmage and Kennedy (1970) and on rats given 5 mg of cortisol per kg per day by

Talmage *et al.* (1970) support the general conclusion that the adrenocortical hormones have no acute physiological effect on calcium homeostasis. However the exogenous cortisol did appear to reduce the rate of long-term bone turnover, while adrenalectomy caused a corresponding increase. The dose of 5 mg/kg/day was acknowledged to be more than that needed to maintain adrenalectomised rats, but is modest in comparison with the doses of more than 30 mg/kg often used by other investigators.

Such massive doses of cortisol do cause hypocalcaemia within a few hours in parathyroidectomised animals (Stoerk *et al.*, 1963). This acute hypocalcaemia is reversed by concurrent administration of parathyroid extract, consistent with the concept that it is negated by compensatory parathyroid hypersecretion in intact animals (Stoerk *et al.*, 1963), just as in human subjects (Fucik *et al.*, 1975).

It is important to be aware that the balance of action of the corticosteroids on bone is so dramatically dose-dependent. Although the hypocalcaemic tendency associated with pharmacological blood levels is due to inhibition of bone breakdown (which can readily be demonstrated *in vitro*: Raisz, 1965; Stern, 1969), doses in the clinical range principally inhibit bone formation and actually accelerate destruction of the skeleton, in part via stimulation of the parathyroids (Jee *et al.*, 1972).

V Possible Future Directions in Investigating the Patterns of Hydroxylation

Distinctive tendencies to elicit one more than another component of a highly complex overall response have been repeatedly referred to in the above characterisations of the individual calciferol metabolites. Their remarkably different specificities raise the fascinating possibility that the metabolites may have different biological roles and that physiological adaptations of calcium and phosphate metabolism may involve far more subtle changes than the rising and falling concentrations of PTH and 1,25-dihydroxycholecalciferol which are at present established. To take only one example, 24,25-dihydroxycholecalciferol may be relatively anabolic and 1,25-dihydroxycholecalciferol relatively catabolic in their effects on the skeleton. Such a relationship would be analogous to the contrasting biological significance of low and high-dose responses to parathyroid hormone and the relatively anabolic properties of its amino-terminal fragment (Herrmann-Erlee *et al.*, 1976; Parsons, 1976a).

It is true that each of the three metabolites mentioned can stimulate intestinal calcium absorption, mobilise calcium from bone and enhance its reabsorption by the renal tubule. But this black-and-white statement takes no account of dose and is reminiscent of the fact that vasopressin can contract the uterus and oxytocin suppress urine formation, if high enough doses are administered.

Full-colour understanding of the biological significance of changes in the pattern of cholecalciferol hydroxylation will require far more detailed knowledge of the selective potencies of the individual metabolites in relation to their circulating levels under different physiological circumstances. In the one end-organ system for which a detailed comparison of dose-relationships is available under conditions of continuous exposure, 25-hydroxy- and 1,25-dihydroxycholecalciferol show log dose-response regressions of identical form for the mobilisation of calcium from bone explants, the positions of the lines indicating that the dihydroxy metabolite is 100-fold more potent than the 25-hydroxy-metabolite in this respect (Raisz *et al.*, 1972a,b; Reynolds *et al.*, 1973). 24,25-Dihydroxycholecalciferol was 1000 times less potent than the 25-hydroxy-metabolite and can be assumed to play no part in stimulating bone breakdown *in vivo*, but if cholecalciferol metabolites *do* significantly modulate (and not merely facilitate) this response, 25-hydroxycholecalciferol is at least as strong a candidate as the 1,25-dihydroxy metabolite, since it circulates at a concentration 100 to 1000 times higher.

Careful, quantitative comparison of the other effects of the two dihydroxylated metabolites in rachitic animals will provide a basis for understanding the significance of their normal assayed concentrations. The controversial question of whether 25-hydroxycholecalciferol itself makes a distinctive contribution to the overall biological response will most probably require studies in which further renal metabolism is impossible, and comparisons of all three metabolites in well-dialysed anephric patients are likely to be uniquely valuable in this regard.

There can by now be little dispute that in designing such fundamentally important comparisons, it will be essential to avoid the peaks of high blood concentration which follow pharmacologically unsophisticated methods of drug delivery. It has been shown, for example, that bone breakdown elicited by high levels of calciferol metabolites long outlasts a brief period of exposure (Raisz *et al.*, 1972a). Thus the situation is precisely analogous to that discussed elsewhere for the peptide hormones, in that inappropriately high transient blood levels induced by high rates of entry to the bloodstream can profoundly distort the pattern of experimental or therapeutic results (Parsons, 1976b).

To illustrate this directly from the literature on calciferol, one example has already been mentioned of a fundamental change in characterisation of a metabolite which followed the moderation of a frankly unphysiological dose schedule.

The first report on biological activity of the metabolite subsequently identified as 24,25-dihydroxycholecalciferol described it as preferentially active in the mobilisation of bone mineral (Suda *et al.*, 1970). This was based on study of the mobilisation of calcium from bone of rats given single intravenous injections of 6.5 nm (2.7 μg), an experimental design previously used with 25-hydroxycholecalciferol by Blunt *et al.* (1968b). Subsequently Boyle *et al.* (1973), giving a 50-fold lower dose by intraperitoneal injection on eight successive days, recognised that it can stimulate intestinal calcium absorption without mobilising calcium from bone.

Even the régime used by Boyle *et al.* (1973) must have induced major daily concentration peaks and extreme caution is required in interpreting the results of such experiments. As an example of the difficulty one may cite the data of Tanaka *et al.* (quoted by Omdahl and DeLuca, 1973), who found that daily intravenous doses of 325 pmol of 1,25-dihydroxycholecalciferol (130 ng) raised the plasma calcium level almost to normal in vitamin D-deficient rats on a low calcium diet. Similar doses of 1,25-dihydroxycholecalciferol in oil given by stomach tube failed to maintain plasma calcium concentrations, whereas the same dose of 25-hydroxycholecalciferol given in the same way was extremely effective. The oral 25-hydroxycholecalciferol is likely to have led to sustained endogenous production of 1,25-dihydroxycholecalciferol, whereas each intravenous dose of the dihydroxy metabolite would be expected to produce a concentration peak well into the osteolytic range. The 25-hydroxycholecalciferol may also have acted preferentially on the kidney (Puschett *et al.*, 1972a, b). In any case, the two treatments probably raised plasma calcium by fundamentally different mechanisms and were therefore not comparable. Only if continuous infusions or delayed-release parenteral preparations of 1,25-dihydroxycholecalciferol had proved much more effective than by mouth would it have been possible to sustain the author's conclusion (Omdahl and DeLuca, 1973) that this hormone was more likely to prove effective parenterally than orally (a conclusion which is contrary to subsequent clinical experience; e.g. Mawer *et al.*, 1976).

VI Conclusion

After the great technical leaps of the last decade which established the existence of the potent metabolites of calciferol and provided methods for their measurement at circulating concentrations, we can look forward to intellectual excitement of another kind as the subtle interactions of the newly-recognised system and other endocrine mechanisms are worked out in many conditions of health and disease. Experiments based on the close imitation of normal physiological blood levels can be expected to further test our understanding of natural function and to lead to solid therapeutic advances.

References

Anderson, J., Dent, C. E., Harper, C. and Philpot, G. R. (1954). *Lancet* **2**, 720–724.
Arnaud, C. D., Rasmussen, H. and Anast, C. (1966). *J. Clin. Invest.* **45**, 1955–1964.

Aurbach, G. D. and Phang, J. M. (1974). *In* 'Medical Physiology' (Ed. V. B. Mountcastle) thirteenth edition, Vol. II, pp. 1655–1695. Mosby, St Louis.
Avioli, L. V., Birge, S. J. and Lee, S. W. (1968). *J. Clin. Endocr. Metab.* **28**, 1341–1346.
Baxter, L. A. and DeLuca, H. F. (1976). *J. Biol. Chem.* **251**, 3158–3161.
Birge, S. J. and Haddad, J. G. (1975). *J. Clin. Invest.* **56**, 1100–1107.
Blondin, J. and Rutherford, W. E. (1975). *Kidney International* **8**, 456.
Blunt, J. W. and DeLuca, H. F. (1969). *Biochemistry* **8**, 671–675.
Blunt, J. W., DeLuca, H. F. and Schnoes, H. K. (1968a). *Biochemistry* **7**, 3317–3322.
Blunt, J. W., Tanaka, Y. and DeLuca, H. F. (1968b). *Proc. Natl. Acad. Sci.* (*USA*) **61**, 1503–1506.
Bordier, P. J., Ryckewaert, A., Marie, P., Miravet, L., Guéris, J., Ferrière, C. and Norman, A. W. (1977). *In* 'Vitamin D', Proc. Third Workshop (Ed. A. W. Norman) pp. 897–911. De Gruyter, Berlin.
Boyle, I. T., Omdahl, J. L., Gray, R. W. and DeLuca, H. F. (1973). *J. Biol. Chem.* **248**, 4174–4180.
Brickman, A. S., Coburn, J. W., Friedman, G. R., Okamura, W. H., Massry, S. G. and Norman, A. W. (1976). *J. Clin. Invest.* **57**, 1540–1547.
Brumbaugh, P. F., Haussler, D. M., Bressler, H. and Haussler, M. R. (1974). *Science* **183**, 1089–1091.
Canterbury, J. M., Claflin, A. J., Lerman, S., Henry, H. L., Norman, A. W. and Reiss, E. (1976). Endocrine Society Programme: *Endocrinology* **29**, (Suppl.), 65.
Care, A. D., Bates, R. F. L., Swaminathan, R., Scanes, C. G., Peacock, M., Mawer, E. B., Taylor, C. M., DeLuca, H. F., Tomlinson, S. and O'Riordan, J. L. H. (1975). *In*. 'Calcium-regulating Hormones' (Ed. R. V. Talmage, Maureen Owen and J. A. Parsons) pp. 100–110. Excerpta Medica, Amsterdam.
Carré, M., Ayigbedé, O., Miravet, L. and Rasmussen, H. (1974). *Proc. Natl. Acad. Sci.* (*USA*) **71**, 2996–3000.
Chertow, B. S., Baylink, D. J., Wergedal, J. E., Su, M. H. H. and Norman, A. W. (1975). *J. Clin. Invest.* **56**, 668–678.
Clark, M. B. and Potts, J. T. Jnr. (1977). *Calcif. Tiss. Res.* **22** (Suppl), 29–34.
Copp, D. H. (1969). *Ann. Rev. Pharmacol.* **9**, 327–344.
Copp, D. H. (1970). *Ann. Rev. Physiol.* **32**, 61–86.
Copp, D. H. (1976). *In* 'Amer. Physiol. Soc. Hbk'. Section 7, Vol. VIII, pp. 431–442. Williams and Wilkins, Baltimore.
Cramer, J. W., Porrata-Doria, E. I. and Steenbock, H. (1957) *Endocrinology* **61**, 590–593.
Crawford, J. D., Gribetz, D. and Talbot, N. B. (1955). *Amer. J. Physiol.* **180**, 156–162.
Curry, O. B., Basten, J. F., Francis, M. J. O. and Smith, R. (1974). *Nature* (*London*) **249**, 83–84.
DeLuca, H. F. (1974). *In* 'Metabolism and Function of Vitamin D' (Ed. D. R. Fraser) pp. 5–26. Biochem. Soc., London, Spec. Publ. No. 3.
DeLuca, H. F. (1976). *J. Lab. Clin. Med.* **87**, 7–26.
Eisman, J. A., Hamstra, A. J., Kream, B. E. and DeLuca, H. F. (1976). *Science* **193**, 1021–1023.
Favus, M. J., Walling, W. M. and Kimberg, D. V. (1973). *J. Clin. Invest.* **52**, 1680–1685.
Fraser, D. R. and Kodicek, E. (1970). *Nature* (London) **228**, 764–766.
Fraser, D. R. and Kodicek, E. (1973). *Nature New Biology* (London) **241**, 163–166.
Friedlander, E. J., Henry, H. L. and Norman, A. W. (1977). *In* 'Vitamin D', Proc. Third Workshop (Ed. A. W. Norman) pp. 288–298. De Gruyter, Berlin.

Froeling, P. G. A. M. and Bijvoet, O. L. M. (1974). *Neth. J. Med.* **17**, 174–183.
Frolick, C. A. and DeLuca, H. F. (1971). *Arch. Biochem. Biophys.* **147**, 143–147.
Fucik, R. F., Kukreja, S., Hargis, G. K., Bowser, E. N., Henderson, W. J. and Williams, G. A. (1975). *J. Clin. Endocr. Metab.* **40**, 152–155.
Fujita, T., Ohata, M., Ota, K., Tanimoto, K., Hanano, Y., Funasako, M. and Uezu, A. (1977). Proc. 5th Parathyroid Conf. (Ed. R. V. Talmage and H. Copp). Excerpta Medica, Amsterdam. In press.
Galante, L., Colston, K. W., MacAuley, S. J. and MacIntyre, I. (1972). *Nature* (*London*) **238**, 271–273.
Garabedian, M., Holick, M. F., DeLuca, H. F. and Boyle, I. T. (1972). *Proc. Natl. Acad. Sci.* (*USA*) **69**, 1673–1676.
Gekle, D., Ströder, J. and Rostock, D. (1969). *Klinische Wochenschrift* **47**, 1177–1178.
Graham, R. F., Preece, M. A. and O'Riordan, J. L. H. (1977). *Calcif. Tiss. Res.* **22** (Suppl.), 416–421.
Gran, F. C. (1960). *Acta Physiol. Scand.* **40**, 132–139.
Gupta, M. M., Round, J. M. and Stamp, T. C. B. (1974). *Lancet* **I**, 586–588.
Haddad, J. G. and Chyu, K. J. (1971). *J. Clin. Endocrinol.* **33**, 992–995.
Haddad, J. G., Min, C., Walgate, J. and Hahn, T. (1976). *J. Clin. Endocrinol. Metab.* **43**, 712–715.
Haddad, J. G. and Rojanasathit, S. (1976). *J. Clin. Endocrinol. Metab.* **42**, 284–290.
Haddad, J. G. and Stamp, T. C. B. (1974). *Amer. J. Med.* **57**, 57–62.
Harrison, H. E. and Harrison, H. C. (1941). *J. Clin. Invest.* **20**, 47–55.
Harrison, H. E. and Harrison, H. C. (1961). *Amer. J. Physiol.* **201**, 1007–1012.
Harrison, H. E. and Harrison, H. C. (1964). *Metabolism* **13**, 952–958.
Harrison, H. C., Harrison, H. E. and Park, E. A. (1958). *Amer. J. Physiol.* **192**, 432–436.
Haussler, M. R., Baylink, D. J., Hughes, M. R., Brumbaugh, P. F., Wergedal, P. F., Shen, J. E., Nielsen, F. H., Counts, S. J., Bursac, K. M. and McCain, T. A. (1976). *Clin. Endocrinol.* **5** (Suppl.), 151s–165s.
Haussler, M. R., Bursac, K. M., Bone, H. and Pak, C. Y. C. (1975). *Clin. Res.* **23**, 322A.
Haussler, M. R., Myrtle, J. F. and Norman, A. W. (1968). *J. Biol. Chem.* **243**, 4055–4064.
Henneman, P. H., Dempsey, E. F., Carroll, E. L. and Albright, F. (1956). *J. Clin. Invest.* **35**, 1229–1242.
Henry, Helen L., (1977). *In* 'Vitamin D', Proc. Third Workshop (Ed. A. W. Norman) pp. 125–133. De Gruyter, Berlin.
Henry, H. L. and Norman, A. W. (1975). *Biochem. Biophys. Res. Commun.* **62**, 781–788.
Herrmann-Erlee, M. P. M., Heersche, J. N. M., Hekkelman, J. W., Gaillard, P. J., Tregear, G. W., Parsons, J. A. and Potts, J. T. Jnr. (1976). *Endocr. Res. Commun.* **3**, 21–35.
Herting, D. C. and Steenbock, H. (1955). *J. Nutr.* **57**, 469–482.
Hill, L. F., Taylor, C. M. and Mawer, E. B. (1974). *Clin. Sci. Mol. Med.* **47**, 14P.
Hirsch, P. F. and Munson, P. L. (1969). *Physiol. Rev.* **49**, 548–622.
Holick, M. F., Schnoes, H. K. and DeLuca, H. F. (1971a). *Proc. Natl. Acad. Sci.* (*USA*) **68**, 803–804.
Holick, M. F., Schnoes, H. K., DeLuca, H. F., Suda, T. and Cousins, R. J. (1971b). *Biochemistry* **10**, 2799–2804.

Holick, M. F., Schnoes, H. K., DeLuca, H. F., Gray, R. W., Boyle, I. T. and Suda, T. (1972). *Biochemistry* **11**, 4251–4255.
Hughes, M. R., Brumbaugh, P. F., Haussler, M. R., Wergedal, J. E. and Baylink, D. J. (1975). *Science* **190**, 578–579.
Iannaccone, A., Gabrilove, J. L., Brahms, S. A. and Soffer, L. J. (1960). *Ann. Int. Med.* **52**, 570–586.
Jee, W. S. S., Roberts, W. E., Park, H. Z., Julian, G. and Kramer, M. (1972). *In* 'Calcium, Parathyroid Hormone and the Calcitonins' (Ed. R. V. Talmage and P. L. Munson) pp. 430–438. Excerpta Medica, Amsterdam.
Kanis, J. A., Heynen, G., Russell, R. G. G., Smith, R., Walton, R. J. and Warner, G. T. (1977). *In* 'Vitamin D', Proc. Third Workshop (Ed. A. W. Norman) pp. 793–795. De Gruyter, Berlin.
Kenney, A. D. (1976). *Amer. J. Physiol.* **230**, 1609–1615.
Kimberg, D. V., Baerg, R. D., Gershon, E. and Graudusius, R. T. (1971). *J. Clin. Invest.* **50**, 1309–1321.
Kimberg, D. V., Schachter, D. and Schenker, H. (1961). *Amer. J. Physiol.* **200**, 1256–1262.
Klein, R. and Gow, R. C. (1953). *J. Clin. Endocr. Metab.* **13**, 271–282.
Kodicek, E. (1972). *Clin. Endocrinol. and Metab.* **1**, 305–323.
Kodicek, E. (1974). *Lancet*, **I**, 325–329.
Larkins, R. G., MacAuley, S. J., Rapoport, A., Martin, T. J., Tulloch, B. R., Byfield, P. G. H., Matthews, E. W. and MacIntyre, I. (1974). *Clin. Sci. Mol. Med.* **46**, 569–582.
Lawson, D. E. M., Pelc, B., Bell, P. A., Wilson, P. W. and Kodicek, E. (1971). *Biochem. J.* **121**, 673–682.
Lawson, D. E. M., Wilson, P. W. and Kodicek, E. (1969). *Biochem. J.* **115**, 269–277.
Lemann, J. Jnr., Piering, W. F. and Lennon, E. J. (1970). *Nephron* **7**, 117–130.
Llach, F., Coburn, J. W., Brickman, A. S., Kurokawa, K., Norman, A. W., Canterbury, Janet, M. and Reiss, E. (1977). *J. Clin. Endocrinol. Metab.* **44**, 1054–1060.
Lukert, B. P., Stanbury, S. W. and Mawer, E. B. (1973). *Endocrinology* **93**, 718–722.
Lumb, G. A., Mawer, E. B. and Stanbury, S. W. (1971). *Amer. J. Med.* **50**, 421–441.
Lumb, G. A. and Stanbury, S. W. (1974). *Amer. J. Med.* **56**, 833–839.
MacIntyre, I., Colston, K. W., Evans, I. M., Lopez, E., MacAuley, S. J., Peignoux-Deville, J., Spanos, E. and Szelke, M. (1976). *Clin. Endocrinol.* **5**, (Suppl.), 85s–95s.
Mahajan, K. K., Robinson, C. J. and Horrobin, D. F. (1974). *Lancet* **I**, 1237–1238.
Malm, O. J. (1958). *Scand. J. Clin. Lab. Invest.* **36**, (Suppl.), 1–280.
Mawer, E. B. (1977). *In* 'Vitamin D', Proc. Third Workshop (Ed. A. W. Norman) pp. 165–173. De Gruyter, Berlin.
Mawer, E. B., Backhouse, J., Davies, M., Hill, L. F. and Taylor, C. M. (1976). *Lancet* **I**, 1203–1206.
Mawer, E. B., Backhouse, J., Holman, C. A., Lumb, G. A. and Stanbury, S. W. (1972). *Clin. Sci.* **43**, 413–431.
Mawer, E. B., Lumb, G. A., Schaefer, K. and Stanbury, S. W. (1971). *Clin. Sci.* **40**, 39–53.
McLaughlin, Marilyn, Raggatt, P. R., Fairney, Angela, Brown, D. J., Lester, Eva and Wills, M. R. (1974). *Lancet* **I**, 536–538.
Melancon, M. J. Jnr. and DeLuca, H. F. (1969). *Endocrinology* **5**, 704–710.
Mellanby, E. (1919a). *Lancet*, **I**, 407–412.

Mellanby, E. (1919b). *J. Physiol.* (London) **52**, liii–liv.
Munson, P. L. (1976). *In* 'Amer. Physiol. Soc. Hbk.' Section 7, Vol. VII, pp. 443–464. Williams and Wilkins, Baltimore.
Ney, R. L., Au, W. Y. W., Kelly, G., Radde, I. and Bartter, F. C. (1965). *J. Clin. Invest.* **44**, 2003–2009.
Nicolaysen, R. and Eeg-Larsen, N. (1956). *In* 'Ciba Foundation. Symp. Bone Structure and Metabolism' (Ed. G. W. E. Wostenhome and C. M. O'Connor) pp. 175–186. Churchill, London.
Norman, A. W. and Henry, H. (1974). *Rec. Prog. Horm. Res.* **30**, 431–480.
Norman, A. W., Lund, J. and DeLuca, H. F. (1964). *Arch. Biochem. Biophys.* **108**, 12–21.
Oldham, E. B., Arnaud, C. D. and Jowsey, J. (1974). *In* 'Endocrinology 1973' (Ed. S. Taylor) pp. 261–268. Heinemann Medical Books, London.
Olson, E. B. and DeLuca, H. F. (1969). *Science* **165**, 405–407.
Olson, E. B., DeLuca, H. F. and Potts, J. T. Jnr. (1972). *Endocrinology* **90**, 151–157.
Omdahl, J. L. and DeLuca, H. F. (1973). *Physiol. Rev.* **53**, 327–372.
Parfitt, A. M. (1976). *Metabolism* **25**, 809–844; 909–955; 1033–1069; 1157–1188.
Parsons, J. A. (1976a). *In* 'Biochemistry and Physiology of Bone' (Ed. G. H. Bourne) Vol. IV, pp. 159–225. Academic Press, New York.
Parsons, J. A. (1976b). *In* 'Peptide Hormones' (Ed. J. A. Parsons) pp. 67–83. Macmillan, London.
Parsons, J. A. and Potts, J. T. Jnr. (1972). *Clin. Endocrinol. Metab.* **1**, 33–78.
Pike, J. W., Toverud, S., Boass, A., McCain, T. and Haussler, M. R. (1977). *In* 'Vitamin D', Proc. Third Workshop (Ed. A. W. Norman) pp. 187–189. De Gruyter, Berlin.
Ponchon, G. and DeLuca, H. F. (1969). *J. Clin. Invest.* **48**, 1273–1279.
Ponchon, G., Kennan, A. L. and DeLuca, H. F. (1969). *J. Clin. Invest.* **48**, 2023–2037.
Popovtzer, M. M. and Robinette, J. B. (1975). *Amer. J. Physiol.* **229**, 907–910.
Popovtzer, M. M., Robinette, J. B., DeLuca, H. F. and Holick, M. F. (1974). *J. Clin. Invest.* **53**, 913–921.
Puschett, J. B., Beck, W. S. and Jelonek, A. (1975). *Science.* **190**, 473–475.
Puschett, J. B., Fernandez, P. C., Boyle, I. T., Gray, R. W., Omdahl, J. L. and DeLuca, H. F. (1972b). *Proc. Soc. Exper. Biol. Med.* **141**, 379–384.
Puschett, J. B., Moranz, J. and Kurnick, W. S. (1972a). *J. Clin. Invest.* **51**, 373–385.
Puschett, J. B., Beck, W. S., Jelonek, A. and Fernandez, P. C. (1974). *J. Clin. Invest.* **53**, 756–767.
Raisz, L. G. (1965). *J. Clin. Invest.* **44**, 103–116.
Raisz, L. G., Trummel, C. L. and Simmons, H. (1972a). *Endocrinology* **90**, 744–751.
Raisz, L. G., Trummel, C. L., Holick, M. F. and DeLuca, H. F. (1972b). *Science* **175**, 768–769.
Rasmussen, H. and Bordier, Ph.J. (1974). 'The Physiological and Cellular Basis of Metabolic Bone Disease.' Williams and Wilkins, Baltimore.
Rasmussen, H., DeLuca, H. F., Arnaud, C. D., Hawker, C. and Von Stedingk, M. (1963). *J. Clin. Invest.* **42**, 1940–1946.
Rasmussen, H., Wong, M., Bikle, D. and Goodman, D. B. P. (1972). *J. Clin. Invest.* **51**, 2502–2504.
Reifenstein, E. C. Jnr. (1958). *Clin. Orthop.* **10**, 206–253.
Reynolds, J. J., Holick, M. F. and DeLuca, H. F. (1973). *Calcif. Tiss. Res.* **12**, 295–301.
Ribovich, M. L. and DeLuca, H. F. (1975). *Arch. Biochem. Biophys.* **170**, 529–535.

Schott, G. D. and Wills, M. R. (1976). *Lancet* **I**, 626–629.
Semmler, E. J., Holick, M. F., Schnoes, H. K. and DeLuca, H. F. (1972). *Tetrahedron Lett.* **40**, 4147–4150.
Smith, J. E. and Goodman, D. S. (1971). *J. Clin. Invest.* **50**, 2159–2167.
Spanos, E., Pike, J. W., Haussler, M. R., Colston, K. W., Evans, I. M. A., Goldner, A. M., McCain, T. A. and MacIntyre, I. (1976a). *Life Sciences* **19**, 1751–1756.
Spanos, E., Colston, K. W., Evans, I. M. S., Galante, L. S., MacAuley, S. J. and MacIntyre, I. (1976b). *Molec. Cell. Endocrinol.* **5**, 163–167.
Stamp, T. C. B., Haddad, J. G. and Twigg, C. A. (1977). *Lancet* **I**, 1341–1343.
Stanbury, S. W. and Lumb, G. A. (1966). *Quart. J. Med.* **35**, 1–23.
Stern, P. H. (1969). *J. Pharmacol. Exper. Ther.* **168**, 211–217.
Stoerk, H. C., Peterson, A. C. and Jelinek, V. C. (1963). *Proc. Soc. Exper. Biol. Med.* **114**, 690–695.
Suda, T., DeLuca, H. F., Schnoes, H. K., Ponchon, G., Tanaka, Y. and Holick, M. F. (1970). *Biochemistry* **9**, 2917–2922.
Talmage, R. V. (1975). *Calcif. Tiss. Res.* **17**, 103–112.
Talmage, R. V. and Kennedy, J. W. II. (1970). *Endocrinology* **86**, 1075–1079.
Talmage, R. V., Park, H. Z. and Jee, W. (1970). *Endocrinology* **86**, 1081–1084.
Tanaka, Y., Castillo, L. and DeLuca, H. F. (1976). *Proc. Natl. Acad. Sci.* (*USA*) **73**, 2701–2705.
Tanaka, Y. and DeLuca, H. F. (1974a). *Science* **183**, 1198–1200.
Tanaka, Y. and DeLuca, H. F. (1974b). *Proc. Natl. Acad. Sci* (*USA*) **71**, 1040–1044.
Tanaka, Y., DeLuca, H. F., Omdahl, J. and Holick, M. F. (1971). *Proc. Natl. Acad. Sci.* (*USA*) **68**, 1286–1288.
Taylor, C. M., DeSilva, P. and Hughes, S. E. (1977). *Calcif. Tiss. Res.* **22**, (Suppl.), 40–44.
Taylor, C. M., Hughes, S. E. and DeSilva, P. (1976). *Biochem. Biophys. Res. Comm.* **70**, 1243–1249.
Tucker, G., Gagnon, Ruth, E. and Haussler, M. R. (1973). *Arch. Biochem. Biophys.* **155**, 47–57.
Turton, C. W. G., Stanley, P., Stamp, T. C. B. and Maxwell, J. D. (1977). *Lancet*, **I**, 222–224.
Urist, M. R. (1976). *In* 'Amer. Physiol. Soc. Hbk.' Section 7, Vol. VIII, pp. 183–214. Williams and Wilkins, Baltimore.
Verner, J. V., Engel, F. L. and McPherson, H. T. (1970). *Ann. Int. Med.* **48**, 765–773.
Wajchenberg, B. L., Quintão, E. R., Liberman, B. and Cintra, A. B. U. (1965). *J. Clin. Endocrinol. Metab.* **25**, 1677–1681.
Wasserman, R. H. and Taylor, A. N. (1969). *In* 'Mineral Metabolism' (Ed. C. L. Comar and F. Bronner), Vol. III, pp. 321–403. Academic Press, New York.
Wasserman, R. H. and Taylor, A. N. (1973). *J. Nutr.* **103**, 586–599.
Wener, J. A., Gorton, S. J. and Raisz, L. G. (1972). *Endocrinology* **90**, 752–759.

Subject Index